AMERICAN COLLEGE OF
FOOT & ANKLE ORTHOPEDICS & MEDICINE

Review Text in Podiatric Orthopedics and Primary Podiatric Medicine

edited by

Annemarie A. Edwards, DPM, FACFAOM, FACFAS
Intermountain Health Care Physician Division
Department of Veterans Affairs Medical Center
Podiatric Medicine and Surgery
Assistant Residency Director
Externship Director
Salt Lake City, UT

John H. Walter, Jr., DPM, MS, FACFAOM, FACFAS
Chairman and Professor, Department of Podiatric Orthopedics and Biomechanics,
Temple University School of Podiatric Medicine, Philadelphia, PA
Faculty, Department of Surgery, Temple University School of Podiatric Medicine,
Philadelphia, PA
Podiatric Orthopedic Residency Director, Temple University School of Podiatric Medicine,
Philadelphia, PA

Larry R. Goss, DPM, FACFAOM, FACFAS, FAPWCA
Adjunct Clinical Instructor, Department of Podiatric Orthopedics and Biomechanics,
Temple University School of Podiatric Medicine, Philadelphia, PA
Director of Podiatric Surgical Residency, Tenet Roxborough Memorial Hospital,
Philadelphia, PA
Attending Staff, The WorldWalk Foundation, Bala Cynwyd, PA
Private Practice, Philadelphia Foot and Ankle, PC, Bala Cynwyd, PA

Published by
American College of Foot & Ankle Orthopedics & Medicine
5272 River Road, Suite 630
Bethesda, MD 20816
800-265-8263

ISBN 0-9764122-0-9

CONTENTS

CONTRIBUTORS

EDITORS

Annemarie A. Edwards, DPM, FACFAOM, FACFAS
Intermountain Health Care Physician Division
Department of Veterans Affairs Medical Center
Podiatric Medicine and Surgery
Assistant Residency Director
Externship Director
Salt Lake City, UT

John H. Walter, Jr., DPM, MS, FACFAOM, FACFAS
Chairman and Professor, Department of Podiatric Orthopedics and Biomechanics, Temple University
    School of Podiatric Medicine, Philadelphia, PA
Faculty, Department of Surgery, Temple University School of Podiatric Medicine, Philadelphia, PA
Podiatric Orthopedic Residency Director, Temple University School of Podiatric Medicine,
    Philadelphia, PA

Larry R. Goss, DPM, FACFAOM, FACFAS, FAPWCA
Adjunct Clinical Instructor, Department of Podiatric Orthopedics and Biomechanics, Temple
    University School of Podiatric Medicine, Philadelphia, PA
Director of Podiatric Surgical Residency, Tenet Roxborough Memorial Hospital, Philadelphia, PA
Attending Staff, The WorldWalk Foundation, Bala Cynwyd, PA
Private Practice, Philadelphia Foot and Ankle, PC, Bala Cynwyd, PA

CONTRIBUTORS

Robert L. Baron, DPM, FACPR, FACFAOM
Professor and Chairman, Department of Radiology, Scholl College of Podiatric Medicine at Finch
    University/Chicago Medical School
Private Practice, Oswego, IL

Jason Bruse, DPM, FACFAS
Submitted while Senior Podiatric Surgical Resident, Department of Veterans Affairs Medical Center, Salt Lake City, UT
Podiatric Surgery
Intermountain Health Care Physicians Division
Endocrine, Diabetes, and Podiatry Clinic, Ogden, UT

Cindy Bullock, DPM
Senior Podiatric Surgical Resident, Department of Veterans Affairs Medical Center, Salt Lake City, UT

Denise B. Freeman, DPM, MSE, ABPOPPM, FACFAOM, FACFAS
Associate Professor, College of Podiatric Medicine and Surgery, Des Moines University - Osteopathic Medical Center
Director, Podiatric Orthopedic Residency Program, College of Podiatric Medicine and Surgery, Des Moines University Osteopathic Medical Center
Coordinator, Lower Extremity Biomechanics Course, College of Podiatric Medicine and Surgery, Des Moines University - Osteopathic Medical Center
Coordinator, Clinical Biomechanics Course, College of Podiatric Medicine and Surgery, Des Moines University - Osteopathic Medical Center

Alexandra Grulke, DPM
Podiatric Surgical Resident, Temple University Hospital, Philadelphia, PA

Arthur E. Helfand, DPM, DABPOPPM, DABPPH
Professor Emeritus, Temple University School of Podiatric Medicine, Philadelphia, PA
Retired Chair, Department of Community Health, Aging, and Health Policy
Honorary Staff, Temple University Hospital
Honorary Staff, Thomas Jefferson University Hospital
Consultant, Temple University Institute on Aging
Past President, American Podiatric Medical Association
Past President, American Board of Podiatric Orthopedics
Past President, American Board of Podiatric Public Health

Erwin J. Juda, DPM, RPH, FACFAOM
Private Practice, Christiana, DE
Assistant Professor, Department of Podiatric Medicine, Temple University School of Podiatric Medicine, Philadelphia, PA

Franklin Kase, DPM, FACFAOM, FACFAS, ABPOPPM, FAAPSM
Chief of Podiatric Surgery, Glendale Memorial Hospital, Glendale, CA
Podiatric Medicine Director, Wound Care Center, Glendale Memorial Hospital, Glendale, CA
Peer Review and Insurance and Patient Relations Committee, California Podiatric Medical Association

Podiatric Consultant, Burbank High School, Burroughs High School, Glendale College, Occidental College, Los Angeles Police Department, Los Angeles Fire Department, Verdugo Hills Gymnastic Club

Medical Advisory Board, Southern California Association of Occupational Health Nurses

QME (Qualified Medical Examiner), California State Industrial Medical Council Expert Witness, Board of Podiatric Medicine, State of California AME (Agreed Medical Examiner)

President, California Podiatric Medical Association

Podiatric Consultant to the Los Angeles Olympic Committee

P.R. Krishna, MD, MS, FICS

Harvey Lemont, DPM, FASCP
Director, Foot Dermatology Clinic, Temple University School of Podiatric Medicine, Philadelphia, PA
Director, Laboratory of Podiatric Pathology, Philadelphia, PA

Todd C. Loftus, DPM, FACFAS
Submitted while Chief Podiatric Surgical Resident, Department of Veterans Affairs Medical Center, Salt Lake City, UT
Private Practice, Columbus, OH

Ralph E. Marcus, MD, FACR
Chief Rheumatology Section, Holy Name Hospital, Teaneck, NJ
Associate Professor of Medicine, The University of Medicine & Dentistry of NJ
Robert Wood Johnson Medical School, New Brunswick, NJ

Robert S. Marcus, DPM, FACFAOM
Founder and Director, Academy of Continuing Podiatric Medical Education
Board of Directors, American College of Foot & Ankle Orthopedics & Medicine
President, American Society of Podiatric Medicine

Roger W. Marcus, MD, FACR
Chief Rheumatology Section, Upper Chesapeake Hospital Center
Attending Physician, Franklin Square Hospital, Baltimore, MD

William J. Martin, DPM, ABPOPPM, FACFAS, FACFAOM
Associate Professor, Podiatric Surgery & Orthopedics, Temple University School of Podiatric Medicine, Philadelphia, PA

James McGuire, DPM, PT, CWS, CPED, DABPOPPM, FAPWCA
Chairman, Department of Podiatric Medicine, Temple University School of Podiatric Medicine, Philadelphia, PA
Assistant Professor, Department of Podiatric Orthopedics
Director, Advanced Wound Healing Center Foot and Ankle Institute
Director, Department of Physical Medicine Foot and Ankle Institute

Marianne J. Misiewicz, DPM
Submitted while Senior Podiatric Surgical Resident, Department of Veterans Affairs Medical Center, Salt Lake City, UT
Private Practice, Columbia, MO

Jeffrey C. Page, DPM, FACFAS, FACFAOM, FASPD, FAPWCA
Professor and Director, Arizona Podiatric Medicine Program, Midwestern University, Glendale, AZ
Attending Staff, Carl T. Hayden, VA Medical Center
Research Field Advisory Group, Department of Veterans Affairs, Podiatry Services
Clinical Associate Professor, Des Moines University
Clinical Faculty Appointment, Barry University
Adjunct Assistant Professor, California College of Podiatric Medicine

Howard J. Palamarchuk, DPM, FAAPSM
Assistant Professor, Department of Orthopedics and Biomechanics, Temple University School of Podiatric Medicine, Philadelphia, PA

Jeffrey M. Robbins, DPM, DABPPH, DABPOPPM, FACFAOM
Director Podiatry Services, Department of Veterans Health Affairs Central Office
Chief of Podiatry Section, Louis Stokes Cleveland VAMC
Professor of Podiatric Medicine, Ohio College of Podiatric Medicine
Director, Podgeriatric Fellowship Program, Louis Stokes Cleveland VAMC

Samuel J. Spadone, DPM, DABPOPPM, FAPWCA
Instructor, Department of Podiatric Medicine, Temple University School of Podiatric Medicine, Philadelphia, PA
Acting Chair, Department of Community Health and Aging, Temple University School of Podiatric Medicine, Philadelphia, PA
Acting Assistant Dean for Educational Affairs, Temple University School of Podiatric Medicine, Philadelphia, PA

Ronald L. Valmassy, DPM, DABPOPPM, FACFAOM
Professor and Past Chairman, Department of Biomechanics, California School of Podiatric Medicine
Staff Podiatrist, Center for Sports Medicine, Saint Francis Memorial Hospital, San Francisco, CA

Elizabeth J. Weber, DPM, DABPOPPM
Private Practice, Binghamton, NY

Robert B. Weber, DPM, JD, MBA, FACFAOM, FACFAS, DABPOPPM
Residency Director, Montgomery Hospital, Norristown, PA
Private Practice, Trappe, PA

Heather L. Whitesel, DPM
Senior Podiatric Surgical Resident, Department of Veterans Affairs Medical Center, Salt Lake City, UT

Kendrick A. Whitney, DPM, DABPOPPM, FACFAOM, FAPWCA
Assistant Professor, Department of Podiatric Orthopedics and Biomechanics, Temple University School of Podiatric Medicine, Philadelphia, PA
Coordinator, Pathomechanics Course, Temple University School of Podiatric Medicine, Philadelphia, PA
Director, Pedorthics Pre-Certification Courses, Temple University School of Podiatric Medicine, Philadelphia, PA

Joseph Witkowski, MD
Professor of Dermatology, Temple University School of Podiatric Medicine, Philadelphia, PA
Clinical Professor of Dermatology, University of Pennsylvania, Philadelphia, PA

Gregg K. Young, DPM
Chief Podiatric Section, Department of Veterans Affairs Medical Center, Salt Lake City, UT
Director of Podiatric Education, Department of Veterans Affairs Medical Center, Salt Lake City, UT
Staff Podiatrist, University Hospital, Salt Lake City, UT
Assistant Professor in Vascular Surgery, University of Utah School of Medicine
Adjunct Assistant Professor, New York College of Podiatric Medicine
Adjunct Clinical Faculty, Barry University College of Podiatric Medicine
Adjunct Clinical Faculty, Temple University College of Podiatric Medicine, Philadelphia, PA
Adjunct Clinical Associate Professor, University of Osteopathic Medicine and Health Sciences
Auxiliary Clinical Associate Professor, Dr. William M. Scholl College of Podiatric Medicine
Adjunct Faculty, Ohio College of Podiatric Medicine
Adjunct Assistant Professor, California School of Podiatric Medicine at Sammuel Merritt College

Michael Zapf, DPM, MPH, FACFAOM, FACFAS
Former Associate Professor, California College of Podiatric Medicine
Former Clinical Instructor, Los Angeles County/University of Southern California Medical Center
Licensed Clinical Microbiologist Technologist, State of California
Public Health Microbiologist, State of California
Private Practice, Agoura Hills, CA

FOREWORD

The American College of Foot & Ankle Orthopedics & Medicine (ACFAOM) has produced this reference text to serve as both a source for quick information for the podiatric physician, and as a study guide for the certification examinations of Podiatric Orthopedics and Primary Podiatric Medicine. The information presented is intended to give a good overview of the subject matter and to provide a suggested reading list for more in-depth information, as may be required for individual interest and need.

We would like to express our sincere thanks to all of the chapter authors for their willingness to participate and their expertise and enthusiasm for the project. We hope that the membership of ACFAOM, as well as the podiatric community in general, will find the text useful.

In addition to acknowledging the authors of this current edition, ACFAOM would like to acknowledge and thank the following editors and authors instrumental in the publication of the first edition: Marc A. Bernard, Steven R. Kravitz, Philip J. Gianfortune, Daniel P. Evans, Casimir F. Strugielski, Gerald A. Weber, Mary Ann Cardile, Lester J. Jones, Alan M. Warren, Guido A. La Porta, Maria M. Griffiths, Steven F. Boc, Donna Myers, D. Scott Malay, Thomas Maglietta, Gary Feldman, Arlene F. Hoffman, James L. Canterbury, Elizabeth Auger, Stephen Palmer, Dean Titemore and Stanley E. Weinstein.

Annemarie Edwards, DPM, Co-Editor
Larry R. Goss, DPM, Co-Editor
John H. Walter, Jr., DPM, Co-Editor
David Bernstein, DPM, President ACFAOM

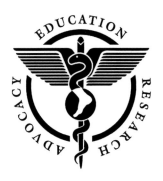

About ACFAOM

ACFAOM is The American College of Foot & Ankle Orthopedics & Medicine, the membership organization for podiatric physicians with a special interest in podiatric orthopedics and medicine. ACFAOM's mission is to support scientific study, research, and continuing education in the field of primary podiatric medicine and foot orthopedics.

ACFAOM was founded in 1949 as the American College of Foot Orthopedists (ACFAOM). The name was changed in the early 1990s to better reflect the scope and interest of the membership. Primary podiatric medicine and orthopedics has long been the backbone of podiatric practice and the forté of many podiatric physicians. Most podiatric practices today are approximately 80% medicine and orthopedics, with surgery making up the balance. Therefore, ACFAOM is the specialty college that represents the largest part of podiatric practice.

With nearly 1,000 active members, ACFAOM is the second largest specialty college affiliated with the American Podiatric Medical Association (APMA). This insures that ACFAOM members are active on behalf of the profession and that they subscribe to the highest professional standards.

ACFAOM also works closely with the American Board of Podiatric Orthopedics and Primary Podiatric Medicine (ABPOPPM), the board that administers a rigorous testing and certification program for podiatrists specializing in primary podiatric medicine and orthopedics. Fellows of the College, who may use the designation FACFAOM (Fellow of the American College of Foot & Ankle Orthopedics & Medicine) have successfully completed the certifying examination of ABPOPPM or have met other relevant and equivalent criteria. Associates of the College are Board-qualified. Thus, ACFAOM members have achieved the highest level of training and education available in the field of primary podiatric medicine and foot orthopedics. Other membership categories are available for students and residents.

ACFAOM's goals are to advance the standards of practice and the quality of services of all podiatrists who devote their professional efforts to the podiatric orthopedic and medical management of lower extremity problems and to provide opportunities for dialogue, education, advancement and improvement of all aspects of the specialty. ACFAOM promotes podiatric medicine and orthopedics to the public, to other podiatrists and to other medical professions, while advocating for the needs and interests of podiatrists in the specialty.

IMAGING/RADIOLOGY

by Robert L. Baron, Philip J. Gianfortune, Daniel P. Evans and Casimir F. Strugielski, updated for the 2004 edition by Robert L. Baron & Heather L. Whitesel

RADIATION SAFETY AND PROTECTION REVIEW

I. **Radiation exposure units**
   A. **Air:** presence of radiation in air prior to striking an object
      1. Roentgen (R) traditional unit of measurement
      2. Coulomb per kilogram (C/kg) System International (SI) or metric unit
   B. **Tissue exposure**/(absorbed dose): amount of radiation which the tissue has absorbed
      1. Radiation absorbed dose (rad) traditional unit of measurement
      2. Gray (Gy) SI unit (one Gy is equal to 100 rads)
   C. **Occupational exposure:** exposure to various types of radiation that produce the same biological effect or damage to tissue
      1. Absorbed Dose Equivalent or ADE
      2. Units
         a. Roentgen equivalent man (rem) = rads X quality factor
         b. Sievert (Sv) = Gy X quality factor; this is the SI unit

II. **Radiation exposure limits (dose limits)**
   A. **Concept:** "Non-threshold response to radiation"
      1. For any degree of exposure to radiation this exposure will result in some type of biological change or damage
   B. **Primary consideration for using diagnostic radiation**
      1. The benefit of exposure to radiation must outweigh the risk of adverse effects (tissue damage) by it
   C. **Exposure levels: NCRP report #91**
      1. Occupational
         a. Effective dose limit: 5 rems or 0.50 Sv (50 mSv)
         b. Dose limits tissues/organs

     i. Lens of the eye: 15 rems or 0.150 Sv (150 mSv)

     ii. All others: 50 rems or 0.500 Sv (500 mSv)

  c. Cumulative exposure rem X age in years: 10 mSv X age

 2. Public Exposure (Annual)

  a. Effective dose limit: 0.5 rem or 5 mSv

  b. Dose limit tissues

     i. Lens of the eye, skin, extremities: 5 rems or 50 mSv

 3. Embryo

  a. Fetal exposure total dose: 0.5 or 5 mSv

  b. Dose in one month: 0.05 rem or 0.5 mSv

 4. Maximum Permissible Dose (MPD)

  a. Traditional Formula: 5(N-18) rem (used to calculate dose limits according to age)

     i. Example: a 28 year podiatrist wishes to determine MPD 5(28 - 18) rem = 5(10) rem = 50 rems

  b. 50 rems represents the total cumulative whole body absorbed dose permitted during the course of 10 years (28 minus 18)

  c. Replacing the MPD formula is: years X 1 rem

     i. Represents cumulative absorbed dose for occupational personnel

  d. ALARA principle

     i. <u>As Low As Reasonably Achievable</u>: use of technical factors which will produce the lowest dose of radiation yet achieve a diagnostic study

      (a) A strong emphasis is placed on proper radiation safety procedures for the patient and operator

III. Effects of radiation exposure

A. Short Term Effects

 1. Results from massive amounts of whole body exposure at one specific moment in time

 2. Also known as Acute Radiation Syndrome

 3. Stages (duration of each stage is dose dependent)

  a. Initial Stage: following exposure to whole body radiation; symptoms include nausea, vomiting, and malaise

  b. Latent Stage: no symptoms or apparent remission of radiation exposure effects

  c. Manifest Illness Stage: effects are dose dependent

  d. Death or Recovery Stage: dependent on the dose received and type of medical intervention

 4. Doses for Acute Radiation Syndrome

  a. Hematopoietic death (350-1,000 rems): death usually in 10-21 days due to fever, infection, and bleeding

  b. Gastrointestinal death (1,000-10,000 rems)

     i. Death usually in 3-10 days

     ii. Symptoms include severe nausea with vomiting, diarrhea, fatigue, fever, loss of appetite, anemia, leukopenia, infection, hemorrhage in G.I., bone marrow, electrolyte imbalance

     iii. Fatal due to extensive damage to the epithelial cell lining of the GI tract

  c. Central Nervous System (CNS) Death (>10,000 rems)

     i. Death within several hours: 72 hours

     ii. Symptoms include: nervousness, confusion, loss of vision, diarrhea, burning sensation to skin

     iii. Death is attributed to cardiovascular collapse

B. Long Term Effects
   1. Exposure to small radiation amounts over longer periods of time
   2. Capable of producing: life span shortening; carcinogenesis; embryological defects: first trimester most critical; genetic mutations
   3. Local tissue responses include: loss of hair; skin reddening; skin discoloration; skin ulceration; weathered or leathery appearing skin; gonadal dysfunction; radiation induced cataractogenesis

C. Cell Sensitivity
   1. High: lymphocytes, immature red blood cells, fetal cells (all types)
   2. Moderate: epithelial cells
   3. Low: muscle, nerve (increased sensitivity in fetus and embryo)
   4. Radiosensitivity increases for cells which have a high rate of division, are immature or the least specialized
   5. Factors which determine the degree of biological or genetic damage:
      a. Amount of radiation exposure
      b. Size of area exposed
      c. Particular body area exposed
   6. LD 50/30
      a. Lethal dose that will kill 50% of the exposed population in 30 days
      b. Dose is approximately 200-300 rads or 2-3 Gy
   7. LD 50/60
      a. Lethal dose that will kill 50% of the exposed population in 60 days

IV. Radiation safety principles
   Time: the least amount of time in radiation beam reduces exposure
   Distance: the further away from radiation beam, the less exposure received
   Shielding: type and thickness of barrier material

A. Patient Protection
   1. Beam limiting devices restrict radiation beam to a specific area
      a. Cones
      b. Cylinder
      c. Aperture diaphragm
      d. Adjustable collimators
   2. Filtration (3 types)
      a. Inherent: built in by the manufacturer
      b. Added: added by the operator externally to the tube
      c. Total: represents the sum of inherent plus added filtration
   3. Total filtration is dependent on the peak or maximum kilovolts (kVp) output for a specific unit
   4. National Council of Radiation Protection recommends for total filtration:
      a. Fixed x-ray units
         i. Below 50 kVp: 0.5 mm aluminum
         ii. 50-70 kVp: 1.5 mm aluminum
         iii. Above 70 kVp: 2.5 mm aluminum
      b. Mobile x-ray units: Fluoroscopic units
         i. 2.5 mm aluminum total permanent filtration
   5. Protective attire: recommended minimum thickness
      a. Aprons (adult or child): 0.5 mm lead thickness
      b. Gloves: 0.25 mm lead thickness

6. Compensating filters: specially designed filters which provide for balanced density and contrast with one exposure of body tissues with varying thicknesses and densities
7. Exposure Factors
   a. Technique charts provide proper exposure parameters and insure consistency of films
   b. Employ lower milliamp (mA) and higher kilovolts (kVp) techniques
8. Processing
   a. Manual - adherence to time/temperature method
   b. Automatic
9. Quality assurance program
   a. Monitors the causes requiring repeat films
   b. Potential areas of concern are: processing problems, poor positioning, improper film identification, poor collimation, changes in image appearance, film artifacts
10. Film: screen selection
    a. Faster speed films paired with compatible intensifying screens reduce exposure by decreasing exposure time

B. Operator Safety

1. Shielding
   a. Barriers between operator and x-ray unit
      i. 1.5 mm lead thickness
      ii. 7 feet in height
      iii. Permanently affixed to wall or floor
2. Patient positioning
   a. Use of restraint devices and positioning aids
   b. Radiolucent sponges
   c. Cassette holders
   d. Sand bags
   e. Tape
3. Non-occupational personnel should be utilized to hold patients requiring assistance during examinations
4. Monitoring devices
   a. Film badges provide monthly reports kept minimum three years
   b. The placement is alternated on a monthly basis

SPECIALTY POSITIONS

I. Forefoot

A. Nonweightbearing

1. Causton
   a. Structures visualized: sesamoid apparatus on a longitudinal axis
   b. Film placement flat on positioning stand, align long axis of film with long axis of foot
   c. Foot placement: medial aspect of foot in contact with cassette surface
   d. Tube angle: 40° toward rear foot
   e. Central ray: prominence first metatarsal phalangeal joint
2. Holly
   a. Structure visualized: sesamoids, plantar metatarsal heads
   b. Film placement: flat on positioning stand
   c. Foot placement: posterior calcaneus in contact with cassette surface, digits toward x-ray tube, plantar flex foot to form a 75° angle with cassette

   d. Tube angle: 0°
   e. Central ray: distal aspect of the first metatarsal head
  3. Lewis
   a. Structure visualized: sesamoids, plantar metatarsal heads
   b. Film placement: flat on positioning stand
   c. Foot placement: patient prone, digits dorsiflexed on cassette
   d. Tube angle: 0°
   e. Central ray: first metatarsal prominence

B. Weightbearing
  1. Axial sesamoid
   a. Structure visualized: both sesamoids, crista first metatarsal, plantar metatarsals (2-5)
   b. Film placement: vertical, long axis of cassette parallel with positioning platform
   c. Foot placement: on 1/4 inch felt pad, dorsiflex digits against cassette front, elevate calcaneus 2 inches from platform
   d. Tube angle: 90°
   e. Central ray: plantar metatarsal heads

II. Rearfoot

A. Nonweightbearing
  1. Isherwood: Oblique Lateral
   a. Structure visualized: anterior subtalar joint
   b. Film placement: flat as in dorsoplantar foot projection
   c. Foot placement: plantar surface in contact, rotate medially 45°
   d. Tube angle: 0°
   e. Central ray: 2 cm inferior and 2 cm anterior of lateral malleolus
  2. Isherwood: Medial Oblique Axial
   a. Structure visualized: middle subtalar joint
   b. Film placement: flat as in dorsoplantar
   c. Foot placement: posterior calcaneus contact front of cassette, rotate foot and lower leg medially 30°
   d. Tube angle: 10° towards the ankle
   e. Central ray: 2 cm inferior and 2 cm anterior of medial malleolus
  3. Isherwood: Lateral Oblique Axial
   a. Structure visualized: posterior subtalar joint
   b. Film placement: flat as in dorsoplantar
   c. Foot placement: posterior calcaneus contact front of cassette, rotate foot and lower leg laterally 30°
   d. Tube angle: 10° toward the ankle
   e. Central ray: 2 cm inferior and 2 cm anterior of lateral malleolus
  4. Broden: Medial oblique
   a. Structure visualized
    i. Posterior facet: two portions
     (a) anterior portion (40° tube angle)
     (b) posterior portion (10° tube angle)
    ii. Talar: sustentaculum tali articulation (20° & 30° tube angles)
   b. Film placement: flat as in dorsoplantar projection
   c. Foot placement: posterior calcaneus on cassette front, rotate lower leg 45°, medially invert and dorsiflex the foot
   d. Tube angle: 10°, 20°, 30°, 40°

        e. Central ray: 2 cm inferior and 2 cm anterior of lateral malleolus
    5. Broden: Lateral oblique
        a. Structure visualized: posterior facet in profile
        b. Film placement: flat as in dorsoplantar projection
        c. Foot placement: posterior calcaneus in contact with cassette front, rotate lower leg 45° laterally, dorsiflex and evert the foot
        d. Tube angle: 12°, 15°, 18° (three tube angles, 3° apart)
        e. Central ray: 2 cm inferior and 2 cm anterior of medial malleolus

B. Weightbearing
    1. Harris and Beath
        a. Structures visualized: middle and posterior subtalar joint
        b. Film placement: flat as in dorsoplantar projection
        c. Foot placement: patient faces away from tube, plantar aspect on cassette, slight flexion in knees
        d. Tube angle: varies 35°-45° (measure subtalar joint to weight bearing surface on lateral weight bearing radiograph of foot)
        e. Central ray: 5 cm superiorly from prominence of posterior calcaneus

III. Clubfoot

A. Kite's Method: simulated weightbearing
    1. Dorsoplantar
        a. Structures visualized: mid foot, forefoot on dorsoplantar projection
        b. Film placement; flat as dorsoplantar projection
        c. Foot placement: supine position, knees flexed and lower leg vertical, foot flat in contact with cassette, toes held down
        d. Tube angle: direct as in a dorsoplantar projection
        e. Central ray: midtarsal region
    2. Medial-lateral
        a. Structures visualized: rear foot, midfoot, forefoot lateral perspective
        b. Film placement: flat, align long axis of cassette with long axis of foot
        c. Part placement: place child on affected side (side to be examined) lateral side of foot in contact with cassette, digits held in place, place block of wood against plantar aspect of foot to simulate weightbearing
        d. Tube angle: 0°
        e. Central ray: medial aspect midtarsal region

ADVANCED IMAGING MODALITIES

I. Magnetic Resonance Imaging

A. Basic Overview: an imaging modality capable of providing high contrast cross sectional representations of a body part without the use of ionizing radiation. MRI utilizes magnetic fields to derive information about body tissues. Mobile hydrogen ions (protons) in the body are first aligned by a stationary magnetic field, and then excited by radiofrequency pulses. As the protons relax from the pulses, they emit radiofrequency signals. The signal from a body tissue depends on the number of mobile protons, and the interactions between protons in that tissue. Spatial encoding of the signal allows cross-sectional images to be obtained in any plane. There are no known detrimental biologic effects, but MRI is avoided in the first trimester of pregnancy because of lack of data

B. Signal characteristics of body tissues: low signal=dark, high signal=white

1. Low signal on all sequences: substances with few mobile protons: air, cortical bone, tendon, fibrocartilage, ligaments. Also fast moving blood (usually)
2. Low signal on T1weighted images: most fluid, muscle
3. High signal on T1 weighted images: fat, some stages of hematoma, high protein-content fluid, slow-moving blood
4. Low signal on T2 weighted and STIR images: fat, some stages of hematoma
5. High signal on T2 weighted and STIR images: fluid: includes cysts, infection, acute fractures, chronic inflammation

C. Terminology
1. Tesla (T): measure of strength of magnetic field (most MRI units 0.3-3 T). Higher T= greater signal to noise ratio
2. TE: echo time. T2 weighting is dependent primarily on TE
3. TR: repetition time. T1 weighting is dependent primarily on TR
4. TI weighted image: TE<20, TR<600
5. T2 weighted image: TE>60, TR>2000
6. Spin Echo: a type of sequence of radiofrequency pulses which can yield either T1 weighted or T2 weighted images. Fast spin echo (FSE) is a newer technique that saves time, but results in slight blurring, which increases with echo train (ET) length. Unless a fat saturation (FS) pulse is added to an FSE sequence, fat will be high signal intensity on T2 weighted images and abnormalities can be obscured
7. Short tau inversion recovery (STIR): another type of sequence which results in a heavily T2 weighted image
8. Gradient echo (GRE, GE or FE): another type of sequence which can be either T1 or T2 weighted

D. Contrast enhancement: gadolinium contrast may be given intravenously. It accumulates in tissues based on the amount of blood flow. It may also be given intra-articularly, for MRI arthrograms

E. Indications
1. Tumors of soft tissue and bone
2. Infections of soft tissue and bone
3. Trauma of soft tissue and bone
4. Congenital anomalies including coalition
5. Avascular necrosis and osteochondrosis
6. Cartilage abnormalities
7. Arthritis
8. Screening for cause of persistent, unexplained pain (has superseded bone scan for this purpose)

F. Contraindications/Precautions
1. Cardiac pacemakers
2. First trimester of pregnancy
3. Iron and sheet metal workers (ocular foreign bodies)
4. Aneurysm clips
5. Post-op clips (for up to 4-6 weeks)
6. Cardiac valve prostheses
7. Metallic implants will create artifact
8. Claustrophobia - can use sedation or open MRI unit

II. Computed Axial Tomography (CT)

A. **Basic Overview:** cross-sectional radiographic images produced by a series of finely collimated x-ray beams, analysed by computer. Can be obtained in axial or coronal planes, and other planes can be generated from the original data set by computer

B. **Terminology**
1. Gantry: circular aperture which houses x-ray tube and detectors
2. Primary slice: original cross sections (transverse, and coronal)
3. Reformatted slice: computer produced planes other than original
4. Attenuation: the density of a tissue, measured in Hounsfield units from –2000 to +2000. Water is approximately 0. The higher the number, the denser the tissue
5. Helical CT: more recent CT scanners obtained images helically rather than as separate transverse slices. This allows for rapid, very high resolution images

C. **Contrast:** Iodinated contrast may be given intravenously, and will accumulate in tissues based on vascularity. It may also be given intra-articularly, for CT arthrograms

D. **Indications**
1. Trauma
2. Coalitions
3. Tumors of bone and soft tissue (MR better for soft tissue tumors)
4. Infection of bone and soft tissue
5. Avascular necrosis
6. Osteochondrosis dissecans (in conjunction with arthrography)
7. Arthritis

E. **Contraindications**
1. First trimester of pregnancy
2. Claustrophobia
3. Allergy to contrast agent (if employed)
4. Weight limit for gantry

III. Nuclear Medicine

A. **Basic Overview**
1. The introduction of a radionuclide isotope into the body and the analysis of its distribution and accumulation by a gamma camera
2. Bone scans have high sensitivity but low specificity

B. **Terminology**
1. Hot spot: area of increased uptake of isotope (fracture, infection)
2. Cold spot: area lacking in any isotope uptake usually due to absence of blood flow (avascular necrosis)

C. **Indications:** in most centers today, the low specificity has caused these scans to be superceded by MRI and/or CT for most patients
1. Osteomyelitis (infection)
2. Trauma
3. Inflammatory arthritis
4. Stress or occult fractures (fractures are reliably shown only >24 hours post injury)
5. Tumors
6. Non-specific pain

D. **Contraindications/Considerations**
1. Poor vascular supply
2. Immunocompromised patient
3. Renal dysfunction

E. Isotopes
   1. Technetium: uptake of Tc with any osteoblastic activity dependent upon an intact vascular supply
   2. Gallium: localizes in neoplastic and inflammatory processes, isotope binds to WBCs
   3. Indium: dependent on chemotaxis of leukocytes
   4. Ceretec (HMPOA): Tc 99 labelled WBCs; increased specificity for infection

F. Stages of a Tc-99 bone scan
   1. Phase 1: dynamic or blood flow phase (radionuclide angiogram); depends on blood flow to bone
      a. Serial images at 3 second intervals
   2. Phase 2: blood pool phase or tissue phase
      a. Represents relative vascularity to a particular area or lesion prior to skeletal uptake
      b. Scanned 1-6 minutes post injection
   3. Phase 3: delayed imaging phase (static) or bone imaging phase
      a. Represents relative osteoblastic activity
      b. Scanned 2-4 hours post injection
      c. Not accurate if patient has poor renal clearance, in which case phase 4 also performed
   4. Phase 4: delayed phase
      a. Scanned 24 hours post injection to allow for adequate tissue clearance in patients who have decreased renal activity

G. Sequencing of Nuclear Imaging (Double Trace:Technetium/Gallium Scans)
   1. To increase specificity, scans may be used in combination
   2. Technetium scan performed first due to shorter half-life
   3. Assists in differentiating cellulitis from osteomyelitis

IV. Arthrography, Tenography and Sinography

A. Basic Overview: injection of a contrast agent to visualize an area not normally seen on plain radiographs, CT or MRI

B. Contrast agents
   1. Iodinated contrast: nonionic preferred, used with plain radiographs or CT
   2. Air: a nontoxic medium, but does not provide high spatial resolution
   3. Gadolinium: used in conjunction with MRI

C. Indications
   1. Tenogram
   2. Sinogram
   3. Arthrogram: usually done in conjunction with CT or MRI

D. Contraindications
   1. Allergy to contrast agent (iodine based), unless premedication given
   2. Cellulitis

V. Venography and Angiography

A. Basic Overview: invasive tests to evaluate the vascular system of the foot and ankle via injection of a radio-opaque contrast
   1. Indications
      a. Vascular disease
      b. Trauma
      c. Arteriovenous malformation
      d. Evaluation of embolic phenomenon
      e. Tumor evaluation

2. Contrast venogram is rarely used today for the detection of DVTs; ultrasound is the standard of care as venogram is contraindicated in many possible DVT patients. D-dimer is used in conjunction with ultrasound for increased specificity in DVT workup

VI. Ultrasound

A. Diagnostic of soft tissue masses, edema, and structural abnormalities of muscle and tendon in the hands of an experienced bone radiologist

B. Also used to guide newer types of extracorporeal shock wave therapy to decrease procedural pain by guiding the shock wave therapy so it is aimed slightly off of the calcaneus

PEDIATRIC RADIOLOGY

I. **Ossification Centers:** The following ossification times are a reference only and represent an average of numerous studies. It should be noted that females tend to ossify at a faster rate than males. Skeletal maturity and development will not always occur at the same rate bilaterally

Osseous Structure	Time of Ossification
Calcaneus	Primary center: 4th fetal month Secondary Center: 5 to 8 years
Talus	Primary Center: 6th fetal month Secondary Center (if present): 8 to 9 years
Cuboid	9th fetal month
Lateral Cuneiform	6 months
Intermediate Cuneiform	12 months
Medial Cuneiform	18 months
Navicular	2.5 - 5 years
Metatarsals-1st	Primary center: 3rd fetal month Secondary center (base): 3 years
2nd-5th	Primary (diaphysis): 3rd fetal month Secondary (distal epiphysis): 3-4 years
Phalanges	Primary center (diaphysis): 3rd-4th fetal month Secondary center (proximal epiphysis): 2-4 years
Sesamoids	7-10 years

II. Osseous abnormalities

A. **Avascular Necrosis:** disorder in which lack of blood supply leads to destructive changes in involved bone (does not include traumatic OCD of talar dome)

1. Radiographic stages

a. Avascular stage: increased soft tissue density. Relative increase in density of affected bone due to hyperemic response of surrounding bone

b. Revascularization stage: mixed lucent and sclerotic changes in bone. Collapse of affected bone

c. Remodeling stage: adaptive changes to contour and density of affected bone

d. Residual deformity stage: may see return to normal density of bone with permanent adaptive changes at opposing joint surface

2. Eponyms

Eponym	Osseous Structure
Mochet-Diaz Disease	Talus
Sever's Disease	Calcaneus
Koehler's Disease	Navicular
Buschke's Disease	Cuboid
Freiberg's Disease	Metatarsal head (2-4th)
Iselen's Disease	Fifth metatarsal base (traction apophysis)
Theiman's Disease	Phalanges (questionable existence)
Renandier's Disease	Tibial sesamoid
Trevor's Disease	Fibular sesamoid

B. Rickets
1. Secondary to lack of vitamin D intake and/or metabolism
2. Calcification of the cartilage in the zone of provisional calcification diminishes while cartilage cells continue to proliferate leading to a widening of the epiphyseal plate and irregularity in the zone of provisional calcification
3. Radiographic Presentation: osteopenic changes, thinning of cortex, physeal dysplasia (widening and irregular), metaphysis flares leading to a cupped appearance, bowing of long bones

C. Scurvy (Vitamin C deficiency)
1. Cessation of the proliferation of the cartilage cells in the epiphyseal plate
2. Cartilage mineralization continues resulting in a widened and sclerotic zone of provisional calcification

D. Lead Intoxication (Plumbism)
1. Primarily obtained through inhalation or ingestion
2. Radiographic presentation: marked increase in density in metaphysis where lead is incorporated into the bone. Lead lines (thickened sclerotic metaphyseal bands) are considered a normal finding up to four years of age
3. In reference to the radiographic presence of lead lines in lead intoxication
   a. Density: represents the concentration of lead in the ingested material
   b. Width: duration of exposure or ingestion of lead
   c. Number of bands: related to the number of incidences of exposure

E. Battered child syndrome
1. Radiographic presentation: the presence of spiral and/or transverse fractures of the long bones, or metaphyseal corner fractures. Multiple fractures in various stages of repair. Marked periosteal activity in diaphysis of long bones due to "grabbing and twisting motion" of abuser

F. Developmental Variants
1. Bifid epiphysis: a vertical cleft in the epiphysis resembling a fracture
2. Cone-shaped epiphysis: a common variant which may or may not be associated with an underlying abnormality
3. Clinodactyly: congenital curly toe
4. Delta phalanx: a triangular asymmetry of a phalangeal bone resulting from premature partial closure of the epiphyseal plate
5. Polydactyly: the formation of extra or supernumerary digits. May form as a separate entity or form in association with another digit giving a syndactylized appearance. It may also appear as a cleft or bifid digit
   a. May be associated with a variety of congenital syndromes

   b. Pre-axial (15%): on medial aspect closest to the hallux
   c. Post-axial (85%): on the lateral aspect closest to the fifth toe
   d. Type A: fully developed digit
   e. Type B: rudimentary duplication
G. **Brachydactyly/brachymetatarsia:** an abnormally shortened digit or metatarsal often associated with trauma in childhood, juvenile rheumatoid arthritis, Turner's syndrome, Ollier's disease, multiple hereditary exostoses, pseudohypoparathyroidism or pseudo-pseudohypoparathyroidism, and other congenital syndromes
H. **Vestigial metatarsal:** rudimentary metatarsal, usually an incomplete polymetatarsia; often confused with an os intermetatarseum
I. **Macrodactyly:** a focal gigantism associated with neurofibromatosis

BIOMECHANICAL EVALUATION OF PEDAL RADIOGRAPHS

Proper evaluation of radiographs is based on dorsoplantar and lateral weight-bearing projections taken in the normal angle and base of gait.

   I. **Normal adult osseous relationships**

   A. **Rearfoot Analysis**

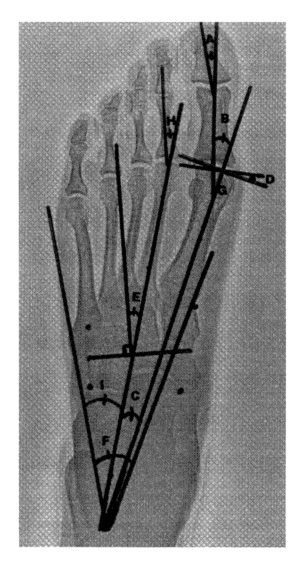

Biomechanical angles on a Plantar-dorsal view
A = Hallux Interphalangeus Angle
B = Hallux Abductus Angle
C = Metatarsus Primus Adductus Angle
D = Proximal Articular Set Angle
E = Metatarsus Adductus Angle
F = Talo-calcaneal Angle
G = Tibial Sesamoid Position (3)
H = Digital Abductus Angle (2nd)
I = Forefoot Angle

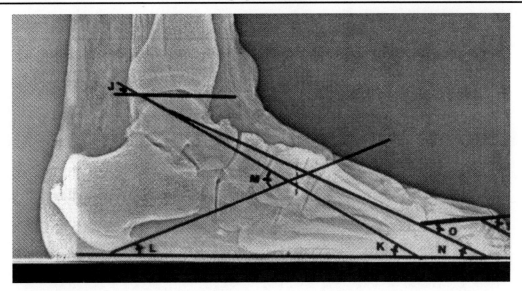

Biomechanical angles on a medial-lateral view
J = Talo-tibial Angle
K = Talar Declination Angle
L = Calcaneal Inclination Angle
M = Lateral Talo-calcaneal Angle

N = First Metatarsal Declination Angle
O = Hallux Dorsiflection Angle
P = Hallux Interphalangeus Angle

1. Longitudinal Axis of the Rearfoot
2. Longitudinal Axis of the Hindfoot
3. Greater Tarsal Axis (most often utilized): represents a line parallel to the distal lateral aspect of the body of the calcaneus
4. Lesser Tarsus Angle = Greater Tarsus Axis to Lesser Tarsus Axis
    a. Normal value: 10°-15°
    b. Increases with pronation as well as skew foot formation
5. Forefoot Adductus Angle = Greater Tarsus Axis to Metatarsus Axis
    a. Normal value: 8°-14°
    b. Defines linear relationship between forefoot and rearfoot
    c. Increases with metatarsus adductus
    d. Decreases or negative angle in severe flatfoot deformities or following trauma to the midfoot region
    e. Both axes are radiographically present at birth, making it useful in pediatric cases
6. Talocalcaneal Angle = Bisection of Talar Neck To Calcaneal Bisection
    a. Normal value: 17°-21°
    b. Increases with pronation and decreases with supination; may diminish or have negative value with clubfoot deformity
7. Talar Declination Angle
    a. Normal value: 15°-20°
    b. Compares bisection of talar neck to the weight bearing surface
    c. Increases with pronation and decreases with supination
    d. Angle may approach 90° with vertical talus formation
8. Calcaneal Inclination Angle
    a. Normal value: 18°-22°
    b. The angle formed by comparing the proximal and distal aspects of the calcaneal inferior surface with the weight bearing surface
    c. Increases with supination or pes cavus and decreases with pronation or pes planus

B. Midfoot Analysis
1. Lesser Tarsus Axis
   a. Axis formed by points consisting of the four corners
      i. Distal medial first cuneiform
      ii. Proximal medial navicular
      iii. Distal lateral cuboid
      iv. Proximal lateral cuboid
   b. Midpoint of the medial wall of the lesser tarsal bones, as well as a midpoint of the lateral wall, is measured
   c. These two midpoints are connected with a line
   d. Perpendicular line is drawn to the line connecting the midpoints. This line represents the lesser tarsus axis
2. Metatarsus Adductus Angle = Lesser Tarsus Axis to Metatarsal Axis
   a. Normal value: 10°-15°
   b. Used to assess adduction of the forefoot relative to midfoot
   c. Assists in assessment of H.A.V.
3. Total Adductory Angle = Metatarsus Adductus Angle + First IM Angle
   a. Greater than 30° should consider a proximal procedure for correction of HAV

C. Forefoot Analysis
1. Biomechanical assessment of hallux abducto valgus deformity
   a. First intermetatarsal angle
      i. Normal value: 8°- 12°
      ii. Angle formed by the bisections of the first and second metatarsals
   b. Hallux abductus angle
      i. Normal value: 0°- 15°
      ii. Angle formed by the bisections of the first metatarsal and proximal phalanx
   c. Hallux interphalangeus angle
      i. Normal value: 0°-8°
      ii. Angle formed by the bisections of the proximal and distal phalanges
   d. Proximal articular set angle
      i. Normal value: 0°-8°
      ii. Angle formed by comparing the functional articular surface of the first metatarsal head with the bisection of the first metatarsal
   e. Distal articular set angle
      i. Normal value: 0°-5°
      ii. Angle formed by comparing the effective articular surface of the base of the proximal phalanx to its longitudinal axis
   f. Metatarsus primus elevatus
      i. Elevation of the first metatarsal compared to the second metatarsal
   g. First metatarsal protrusion distance
      i. Normal value: ± 2.0 mm
      ii. Compares the relative length of the first and second metatarsals
   h. Tibial sesamoid position
      i. Graded 1-7 based on its position relative to the bisection of the first metatarsal

RADIOGRAPHIC EVALUATION OF INFECTION

I. **Terminology**
   A. **Emphysema:** radiolucent appearance of air or gas in the soft tissue
   B. **Sequestrum:** walled-off portion of sclerotic avascular bone
   C. **Cloaca:** defect or sinus in cortical bone for the discharge of pus and debris
   D. **Involucrum:** the walling off or arrest of infection with new bone formation
   E. **Marjolin's Ulcer:** malignant degeneration of chronic sinus tract or ulcer base to squamous cell carcinoma
   F. **Sclerosing Osteitis of Garre:** an attenuated form of osteomyelitis characterized by marked sclerotic changes in the involved bones

II. **Routes of Contamination**
   A. **Hematogenous**
   B. **Direct Inoculation**
   C. **Contiguous Spread of Infectious Process**

III. **Hematogenous Osteomyelitis**
   A. **Most commonly affects young or debilitated elderly patients**
   B. **Location dependent on vascular pattern**
      1. Infantile Pattern: Vascular supply penetrates epiphysis leading to epiphyseal and joint involvement
      2. Childhood Pattern: Vessels unable to penetrate open physeal plate resulting in infection affecting the metaphyseal region
      3. Adult Pattern: Re-establishment of vascular supply to epiphysis as plate closes leading to epiphyseal and joint involvement

IV. **Direct Inoculation:** Direct implantation of infective organism by puncture wound, open wound, or open fracture
   A. **Radiographic Presentation:** soft tissues show deep tissue plane involvement and early periosteal reaction; cortical destruction precedes medullary involvement

V. **Contiguous Spread of Infection**
   A. **Spread of infectious process to bone from a surrounding source**, i.e.: ulceration or cellulitis. Most common route of infection in the foot
   B. **Radiographic presentation:** soft tissue changes precede osseous findings. As infectious process deepens, periosteal involvement is followed by changes in the cortex. Medullary involvement is then seen following cortical destruction

VI. **Radiographic Presentation of Infectious Processes**
   A. **Plain film analysis**
      1. Radiographic findings lags clinical presentation by 7-10 days
      2. Soft tissue changes
         a. Deep soft-tissue swelling adjacent to the area of bony involvement
         b. Obliteration of fascial planes
         c. Emphysema associated with gas producing organisms
      3. Osseous changes

　　　a.　Periosteal reaction
　　　b.　Loss of cortical integrity
　　　c.　Focal osteopenia
　　　d.　"Moth-eaten" lucencies in the medullary canal
　　　e.　Both CT and MRI may assist in delineating the extent of medullary involvement

VII. Nuclear Imaging

A. Technetium scan

1. Used to differentiate cellulitis from osteomyelitis, but significant false-positive and false-negative rate, especially in children and diabetic patients

Technetium Scan	Phase 1	Phase 2	Phase 3
Cellulitis	increased	increased	normal
Acute Osteomyelitis	increased	increased	increased
Chronic Osteomyelitis	normal	normal	increased

B. Gallium scan

1. Gallium tagged to WBCs and indicator of body's response to an inflammatory process
2. Cellulitis and osteomyelitis will result in an increased uptake in areas of inflammation

C. Computed Tomography

1. Assists in delineating medullary involvement of infection and in identifying plantar compartment abscess formation
2. Can result in overestimating the level of cellulitis, as it is difficult to differentiate cellulitis from edema
3. Best modality for assessment of endosteal and periosteal involvement

D. Magnetic Resonance Imaging

1. Highest sensitivity and specificity of any imaging technique
2. T-1 weighted image: decrease in signal intensity in medullary canal with presence of osteomyelitis
3. T-2 weighted image: increase in signal intensity in medullary canal with presence of osteomyelitis

MRI IN MUSCULOSKELETAL INJURY OF THE FOOT AND ANKLE

I. Achilles Tendon (axial & sagittal are best planes)

A. Complete tear (T2 and clinical); take in plantarflexion to approximate if reattachment is feasible

B. Degeneration of tendon (T1 or proton density weighted sequences and on IR sequences)

C. Pathologic changes are usually 2-6cm proximal to calcaneus

II. Os Trigonum (axial CT or MRI)

A. CT for ossicle or fracture

B. MRI for cystic changes on both sides of a synchondrosis from chronic disruption. Good for visualization of adjacent structures such as FHL

C. Clinical via diagnostic injection of lidocaine or mix of corticosteroid and lidocaine

III. Accessory Soleus

A. Radiographs (obliteration/changes in Kager's triangle)

   B. **CT or MRI** (signal characteristics of mm)
   C. **Clinical** (soft tissue mass; pain after exercise; possible Ischemia within mm. Or compartment like syndrome)

IV. **Tendon Injury Classification**
   A. **Grade I tendon injury:** thickened tendon with splitting of fibers (possible linear signal vs. normal heterogeneous signal)
   B. **Grade II tendon injury:** focal thinning
   C. **Grade III tendon injury:** complete disruption
   D. **Tendinosis:** loss of normal striation and discoloration. MRI findings: thickening of tendon with or without internal signal and high T2 peri-tendon
   E. **Paratendinitis:** increase signal on T2 peri-tendon. Otherwise normal thickness and signal intensity

V. **PTT**
   A. **Most common injured flexor tendon**
   B. **Largest flexor tendon** (1.5-2 times the diameter of the other flexors)
   C. **Tears seen most often behind the medial malleolus**, at the navicular, or 2-3 cm proximal to the navicular
   D. **CT or MRI;** MRI more sensitive and specific as well as shows internal structural changes
   E. **The Magic Angle:** artifact when the tendon passes at 55 degrees to the magnetic field that produces what looks like an increased signal within the tendon on T1 and proton density weighted images. This increase in signal is noted in structures with normally low signal with highly ordered collagen fibrils (i.e., tendons). This can be avoided by imaging the foot in various degrees of flexion and thus changing areas of the "magic angle"
   F. **Also look for osteophytes, thickening flexor retinaculum, degeneration or loss of spring ligament associated with PTT pathology**

VI. **FHL**
   A. **Tears seen in ballerinas and in sports involving "toeing off" from hallux**
   B. **Os trigonum can impinge FHL**
   C. **High signal on T2 MRI peri-tendon in FHL tendon sheath can be a normal finding**

VII. **Tarsal Tunnel Syndrome**
   A. **50% idiopathic**
   B. **50% mechanical**
      1. Ganglion cysts (lobulated discrete structure with uniformly high signal on T2)
      2. Nerve sheath tumors (variable signal but along anatomic distribution of n.)
      3. Varicosities (high signal T2 and IR signal)
      4. Tenosynovitis (high signal on T2 surrounding tendons)
      5. Abductor hallucis hypertrophy (esp. if symptomatic during exercise)
      6. Hindfoot valgus
      7. Post-traumatic fibrosis (scar tissue = low signal on T1 and T2)

VIII. **MCL (Deltoid)**
   A. **MRI**
   B. **CT**
   C. **Posterior tibiotalar and tibiocalcaneal ligaments most easily visualized**

    D. **Posteriotibial uniformly thick with heterogeneous signal on MRI**

    E. **Tibiocalcaneal variable thickness with low signal intensity usually**

    F. **High T2**; 60-67% of posterior tibiotalar ligaments are avulsion with avulsion fx/osseous fragment common

IX. Accessory Navicular

    A. **4-21% of population**

    B. **Female >male**

    C. **Associated with PTT injury**

    D. **3 Types**

        1. True sesamoid within PTT (os tibiale externum; usually asymptomatic)

        2. Ossification along medial aspect of navicular via cartilaginous synchondrosis; most common (sypmtomatic due to assoc. with PT tears or synchondrosis alone)

        3. Fusion of type II; prominent medial process of navicular (gorilloid or cornuate navicular)

    E. **MRI advantageous as it allows assessment of PTT**

    F. **Radionuclide Bone Scan shows increased activity at site of synchondrosis**

X. LCL

    A. **Inversion injury accounting for approximately 90% of all ankle sprains**

    B. **ATF** (most commonly injured)

    C. **CF** (next most commonly injured)

    D. **PTF** (rarely injured)

    E. **Plain radiographs, stress radiographs, arthrograms, surgical exploration**

    F. **Talar tilt** (lines drawn parallel to talar dome and tibial plafond)

    G. **Normal talar tilt is 0-13 degrees**

    H. **Talar tilt >10 degrees with instability and >5 degrees difference with contralateral side**

    I. **Anterior translation of talus >6mm or difference of >3mm difference with contralateral side=instability**

    J. **Calcaneal-fibular ligament extrinsic to capsule and attached to peroneal tendon sheath**; thus can be evaled with arthrography of ankle. (i.e., extravasation of contrast into peroneal tendon sheath = torn CF ligament. However, only if acute as chronic scar tissue may give a false positive)

    K. **ATF and CF typically low signal**; PTF intermediate signal normally

    L. **Magnetic resonance arthrography highly sensitive and specific.** Use clinical suspicion to deem whether warranted or not

XI. Peroneal Tendon Injuries

    A. **Ruptures and tenosynovitis not as common, but associated with chronic LCL tears**

    B. **MRI most helpful**

    C. **Isolated tomography rare unless local anesthetic desired in tendon sheath for diagnostic purposes**

    D. **Peroneus longus most commonly injured with acute tear; however isolated peroneus brevis tears possible also.** Inspect most medial aspect of brevis tendon alongside fibula if tendon tear not immediately visible in surgery

    E. **Acute tear usually approximately at calcaneal-cuboid joint just distal to os peroneum**

    F. **Avulsion of base of 5th obviously almost always involve peroneus brevis**

    G. **Chronic tears usually longitudinal splits within tendon and at level of lateral malleolus or distal**

H. **Increased mechanical stress associated with chronic tears**
1. Osseous spurring on fibula
2. Tears of LCL and superior retinaculum
3. Abnormal accessory mm (peroneus quartus or distally lying/hypertrophied peroneus brevis mm belly)
4. Peroneal tendon subluxation
5. Hypertrophied peroneal tubercle
6. Flat or convex tip of lateral malleolus
7. Flattening or retromalleolar groove
8. Small avulsion fx fragment from post-lateral malleolus (avulsion of superior peroneal retinaculum)

XII. **Peroneal Tendon Splits**

A. **Tendon appears thickened or attenuated with areas of abnormal signal extending through its substance**
B. **C-shape of peroneus brevis tendon can alter morphology and partly cover peroneus longus tendon**
C. **Increased T2 signal in tendon sheath and surrounding soft tissues**
D. **May be no signal changes in tendon however, and only have an irregular contous with clefts**

XIII. **Anterolateral Impingement Syndrome**

A. **Entrapment of abnormal soft tissue in the anterolateral ankle gutter**
B. **Trauma etiology most likely; an accessory fascicle of the anterolateral tibiofibular ligament also associated with this syndrome though**
C. **MRI useful for evaluation of patient's with confusing clinical presentation or those in which conservative therapy has failed**
D. **Anterolateral gutter best seen on axial images usually**
E. **Anterolateral gutter defined by the ATF ligament anteriorly, the lateral malleolus laterally, and the talus medially**
F. **The anterolateral gutter normally has a fat signal on MRI as fibrofatty tissue is usually located there.** Fluid signal filling the gutter and encompassing a distinct soft tissue mass separate from the ATF ligament aids correct diagnosis

XIV. **Sinus Tarsi Syndrome**

A. **MRI helpful again due to fat in sinus tarsi and contrast**
B. **Sagittal T1 and IR sequences helpful**
C. **T1 weighted images normally high signal; IR sequences normally dark**
D. **T2 in sagittal or coronal planes also helpful**
E. **Sinus tarsi syndrome evaluated as three main MRI patterns:** (1) T1 and T2=low signal; fibrosis, (2) T1=low signal with T2=high signal; synovitis or inflammation, and (3) T1=lobulated low signal intensities and T2=high signal; synovial cysts
F. **Associated findings of LCL and PTT tears**
G. **Acute or subacute ankle injury may give false positive; correlate with clinical findings**

XV. **Plantar Fasciitis**

A. **Clinical findings obviously a mainstay;** however, can also evaluate with radiographs, 3-phase bone scan, and MRI

B. **MRI may be helpful with atypical presentation**
C. **Enthesophyte with poorly defined margins may suggest a seronegative arthritis**
D. **Linear calcification within fascia may be associated with CPPD**
E. **Normal plantar fascia is a thin linear low signal tissue on all MRI sequences and measures approximately 3mm in thickness**
F. **Plantar fasciitis usually presents >5mm in thickness with increased T2 signal**
G. **IR or fat-suppressed sequences may show increase in adjacent bone marrow of calcaneus**
H. **Increase in T2 noted in plantar fascia and surrounding soft tissue**

XVI. Calcaneus Fractures

A. **Sander's CT Classification** (in detail in Trauma chapter) and radiographs are the primary evaluation tools
B. **CT advantageous for STJ evaluation, evaluation of flexor and peroneal tendons, and evaluation of comminution**
C. **Spiral CT scanning allows for 2 dimentional and 3 dimentional reformations**
D. **If patient is splinted or casted can place patient's foot flat on table and perform 2mm acquisitions from rearfoot proximally to calcaneocuboid joint.** At this point thin 1mm two dimentional reformations can be done in the sagittal and axial planes. If axial plane imaging is only possible then perform a coronal reconstruction. 3-D reconstruction may be necessary for complex fragment spatial orientation
E. **Coronal plane best for evaluation of posterior facet of STJ.** Middle facet, flexor tendons, and peroneal tendons also best visualized in this plane. Axial reconstruction for evaluation of calcaneocuboid joint. Sagittal reconstruction for Bohler's angle depression

XVII. Stress Fractures

A. **Evaluate with bone scan, CT, or MRI if subtle radiographic changes to further explore.** Also helpful if radiographs not demonstrative but clinical symptoms suspicious
B. **Bone scanning allows assessment of other bone structures, but has low specificity**
C. **CT good for midfoot tarsal fractures.** Sagittally oriented fractures common and seen on coronal imaging. Trabecular thickening, increased marrow attenuation, and later thickening of cortex and periosteal thickening
D. **MRI primarily shows marrow edema.** T1=low signal and T2 and IR=high signal. T1 and IR recommended for evaluation. Low specificity a drawback of MRI however

XVIII. Osteochondritis Dissecans

A. **Most commonly in talus in foot and ankle**
B. **CT and MRI with and without contrast used for evaluation**
C. **Coronal plane best in CT and MRI**
D. **MRI better for cartilage and fluid visualization.** Fragment may below signal indicating sclerosis or have a marrow signal

XIX. Growth Plate Injuries

A. **Multiplanar capabilities of MRI helpful in locating a bone bar**
B. **Bone bar appears black on brighter physeal background**

XX. Tarsal Coalitions

A. **Calcaneonavicular and talocalcaneal coalitions most common**

B. **Fibrous, cartilaginous, or bony coalitions** (or a mix thereof)

C. **CT and MRI best tools**

D. **CT best in coronal plane for STJ coalitions and axial for calcaneonavicular coalitions**

E. **Fibrous or cartilaginous coalitions may give the sustentaculum tali a medial plantar slope.** Middle facet landmarks changed sometimes. Cystic changes in areas of coalitions may also be noted

XXI. **Lisfranc Injuries**

A. **MRI for joint alignment and Lisfranc ligament visualization**

B. **Lisfranc ligament noted as hypointense band on oblique axial imaging**

DIAGNOSIS OF BONE TUMORS

I. **Evaluation:** The key factors to assess when evaluating a bone tumor are:

A. **Patient's age and sex**

B. **Location**
    1. Which bone(s) is/are involved?
    2. Region of bone involved (epiphysis, diaphysis, metaphysis)

C. **Pattern of destruction**
    1. Permeative: no visible margin or border, tumor blends imperceptibly with surrounding bone
        a. Primary malignancies, metastasis, acute osteomyelitis
    2. Moth-eaten: only sporadic margin noted with some blending into surrounding bone
        a. Multiple myeloma, eosinophilic granuloma
    3. Geographic: border or demarcation of lesion visible
        a. Benign tumors, cysts, chronic osteomyelitis

D. **Type of Matrix**
    1. Osseous: fluffy amorphous mineralization
    2. Cartilaginous: punctate calcifications or rings of calcifications
    3. Fibrous or fibro-osseous: ground glass appearance

E. **Periosteal reaction**
    1. Single layer
    2. Multiple lamellation (onion skin)
    3. Codman's Triangle (suggests a very aggressive lesion)
    4. Perpendicular periosteal reaction
    5. Sunburst periosteal reaction
    6. Velvet periosteal reaction

C. **Signs and Symptoms**
    1. Blood work
    2. Physical findings
    3. Response to medication/treatment

II. Common areas of occurrence for bone tumors

EPIPHYSIS	METAPHYSIS	DIAPHYSIS
Giant Cell Tumor	Osteogenic Sarcoma	Ewing's Sarcoma
Chondroblastoma	Osteoblastoma	Chondrosarcoma
	Osteoid Osteoma	Myeloma
	Chondrormyxoid Fibroma	Metastasis
	Non-ossifying Fibroma	
	Chondrosarcoma	
	Fibrosarcoma	
	Enchondroma	

III. Aggressive vs. Nonaggressive

Aggressive	Nonaggressive
lesion is permeative or moth-eaten	lesion is geographic, distinct borders
lesion is merging with surrounding bone	lesion is distinct from surrounding bone
fast aggressive growth	slow non-aggressive growth
lesion may be large (> 6 cm)	periosteal buttressing
mulitlaminar periosteal reaction	well defined unilaminar periosteal
sun burst reaction	reaction
Codman's triangle	
onion skin	
spiculated	

IV. Metastases: rare below the knee, except from lung, breast and renal cell carcinoma

Type of lesion	Site in Males most common to least common	Site in Females most common to least common
Lytic	Lung	Breast
	Kidney	Lung
	Bladder	Kidney
	Colon	Uterus-Cervix
Blastic	Prostate	Breast
	Breast	GI tract
Mixed	Lung	Breast
		Uterus-Cervix

V. Bone Tumors

A. Osseous Lesions

1. Osteoid Osteoma
    a. Sex: male 2: female 2
    b. Age: second to third decade
    c. Location: 50% in tibia, also in talus, calcaneus, phalanges
    d. Appearance: lucent nidus < 1 cm with sclerotic rim; periosteal reaction; hot Tc bone scan; extensive bone sclerosis
    e. Clinical: dull pain, worse at night, relieved with aspirin

2. Osteoblastoma
    a. Sex male>female
    b. Age: second to third decade
    c. Location: 30%-40% in spine, also in femur, tibia, and small bones of feet
    d. Appearance: lucent nidus > 1 cm with sclerotic rim; expansile; less sclerotic than osteoid osteoma
    e. Clinical: pain similar to osteoid osteoma
3. Osteosarcoma
    a. Sex: male 1.5: female 1.0
    b. Age: peak age 10 to 25 years old
    c. Location: usually metaphyseal, 40% femur, 16% tibia
    d. Appearance: periostitis, onion skin, sunburst, Codman's triangle metaphyseal medullary lesion
    e. Clinical: 50% elevated alkaline phosphatase; 20% 5 year survival; pain, swelling
4. Parosteal Sarcoma (3% to 4% of all osteosarcomas)
    a. Age: most over 20 years of age
    b. Location: lower 2/3's femoral metaphysis, proximal tibia, and humerus
    c. Appearance: lobulated mass of amorphous ossification, sessile base, rarely has aggressive periostitis
    b. Clinical: mass with dull aching pain; 80-90% 5 yr survival rate
5. Periosteal Sarcoma (rare)
    a. Age: 10 to 25 years old
    b. Location: diaphyseal, arises from bone surface
    c. Appearance: soft tissue mass with bony spicules and calcifications
    d. Clinical: pain and swelling; prognosis worse than parosteal but better than osteosarcoma

B. Cartilaginous Lesions
1. Enchondroma
    a. Sex: male = female
    b. Age: 10 to 50 years
    c. Location: 50% small tubular bones hands and feet, humerus, femur, flat bones
    d. Appearance: geographic lucent lesions, may be expansible, may have "ground glass" punctate calcifications
    e. Clinical: painless unless pathologic fracture
        i. Ollier's Disease: multiple enchondromatosis
        ii. Mafucci's Syndrome: multiple enchondromas with hemangiomas
2. Chondroblastoma
    a. Sex: male 2: female 1
    b. Age: 2nd and 3rd decade (75% teenagers)
    c. Location: epiphyseal, 50% around knee, also distal femur and tibia
    d. Appearance: geographic, lytic with sclerotic margins; 50% have internal calcifications
    e. Clinical: usually painful with joint effusion
3. Chondromyxoid Fibroma (very uncommon)
    a. Sex: male>female
    b. Age: 4 to 79 years old
    c. Location: 76% in lower extremity, tibia common, also in femur, fibula, tarsus
    d. Appearance: ovoid, loculated lucent area, sclerotic rim, geographic cortical expansion, rarely calcified

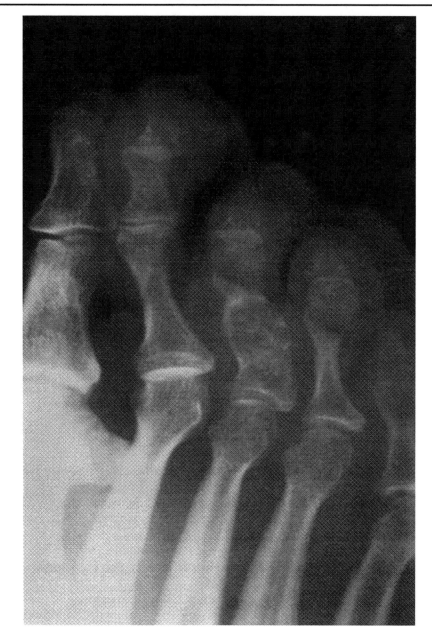

Enchondroma proximal phalanx 3rd digit

      e. Clinical: vague pain
4. Osteochondroma (most common in the foot; 10-15% of foot bone tumors)
      a. Age: 1st, 2nd, 3rd decade
      b. Location: metaphysis of long bones
      c. Appearance: arises at epiphysis and grows toward diaphysis, cartilage, capped bony excrescence, pedunculated, sessile or calcific in shape, subungual has fibro cartilage cap, all others have hyaline cartilage. Matrix is stippled, expansile, and lytic in appearance. Nonpainful unless it grows prominent and causes soft tissue trauma
      d. Clinical: mechanical pain only (nerve or vessel impingement)
5. Chondrosarcoma
      a. Age: mean of 40

   b. Location: centrally or peripherally in pelvis, femur, tibia, and humerus

   c. Appearance: malignant degeneration of osteochondroma, enchondroma, or periosteal chondroma; lucent, geographic, with punctate calcifications

   d. Clinical: pain of months or years duration

  6. Bizarre parosteal osteochondromatous proliferation (rare, benign)

   a. Age: 3rd and 4th decade of life

   b. Location: 72% occur in hands and feet, metaphyseal

   c. Appearance: appears as disorganized osteochondroma without continuity from underlying osseous medulla

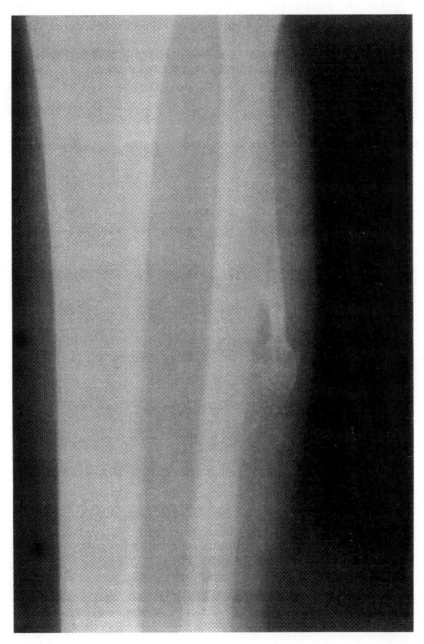

Osteochondroma fibula

C. Fibrous Lesions
1. Non-ossifying fibroma (fibro-cortical defect)
   a. Incidence: 30%-40% children have one, natural regression in most instances
   b. Location: NOF-eccentric in medullary space; FCD-arises in cortex (histologically identical)
   c. Appearance: geographic with sclerotic rim, usually in lower extremity
   d. Clinical: asymptomatic unless pathologic fracture; **Do not biopsy**
2. Ossifying fibroma (aka intracortical fibrous dysplasia, osteofibrous dysplasia)
   a. Age: seen in early childhood, progresses for 5: 10 yrs then stabilizes
   b. Location: tibia and fibula
   c. Appearance: bubble-like ground glass appearance
   d. Clinical: painless, tibial bowing, 25% have pathologic fracture
3. Fibrous dysplasia
   a. Appearance: 75% monostotic, 25% polyostotic, unilateral involvement in lower extremity, geographic intramedullary lesion with ground glass appearance, may be expansible, may have painful skeletal deformities
   b. Clinical: Albright's Syndrome: a polyostotic fibrous dysplasia, cafe au lait spots, endocrine dysfunction
4. Fibrosarcoma (uncommon malignant fibrous lesion)
   a. Age: 3rd to 6th decade of life
   b. Location: metaphyseal long bone, especially distal femur
   c. Appearance: lytic lesion in metaphysis of long bone, no bone reaction, no calcified or ossified matrix present, excessive bony destruction
   d. Clinical: very painful
5. Malignant Fibrous Histiocytoma
   a. Age: median age 41
   b. Location: may arise secondary to other lesion
   c. Appearance: ends of long bone lytic with no matrix characteristics, high grade aggressive tumor
   d. Clinical: poor prognosis

D. Cysts and Cyst-like Lesions
1. Aneurysmal bone cyst
   a. Sex: female > male
   b. Age: 10 to 20 years old
   c. Location: 50% predilection for long bones, also spine and small tubular bones
   d. Appearance: lytic expansible loculated lesion, composed of blood filled cavities (soap bubbles)
   e. Clinical: painful, previous trauma may play a role in location
2. Unicameral Bone Cyst
   a. Sex: male > female
   b. Age: 2 to 49 years
   c. Location: 90% arise in proximal humerus or femur, metaphysis or diaphysis, calcaneus and flat bones
   d. Appearance: no cortical thinning, sclerotic rim, non-expansible, may have fallen fragment sign
   e. Clinical: asymptomatic unless pathologic fracture
3. Epidermoid cyst
   a. Age: 2nd, 3rd, 4th decade
   b. Location: skull or terminal phalanges

   c. Appearance: geographic lucency
   d. Clinical: uncommon lesion of squamous epithelium-keratin and cholesterol crystals, associated with history of digital trauma
  4. Interosseous Lipoma (rare benign lesion within the marrow)
   a. Location: metaphysis of tubular bones, any skeletal site is possible
   b. Appearance: loculated lucent geographic lesion with cortical expansion, may have calcific focus
   c. Clinical: asymptomatic unless pathologic fracture
  5. Interosseous ganglion
   a. Sex: male > female

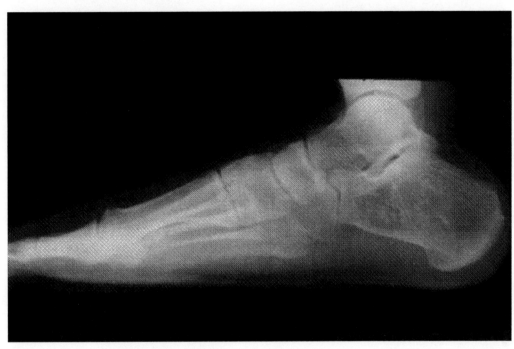

Unicameral bone cyst calcaneus

   b. Age: 14 to 73 years, average age is 40
   c. Location: subchondral lesion, ends of long bones, distal tibia most common
   d. Appearance: geographic circular lucency with thin sclerotic rim, no mineralization
   e. Clinical: may have pain or be asymptomatic

E. Miscellaneous Lesions
  1. Ewings' Sarcoma
   a. Sex: male 3 > female 2
   b. Age: peak 10 to 20 years
   c. Location: 60% to 67% in lower extremity or pelvis, femur most common
   d. Appearance: permeative destructive lesion, onion skin periostitis, Codman's triangle
   e. Clinical: pain and swelling, low grade fever; 5 year survival poor if located in axial skeleton
  2. Lymphoma
   a. Sex: male 2 > female 1
   b. Age: mean age 29 to 44
   c. Location: 75% in tubular bones, most common femur and humerus - diaphyseal or metaphyseal

      d.   Appearance: small destructive foci, elliptical in shape, endosteal scalloping

      e.   Clinical: 90% have localized pain, pathologic fractures

  3. Multiple myeloma

      a.   Sex: male 2>female 1

      b.   Age: 45 to 80 years old

      c.   Location: flat bones most common, may involve long bones

      d.   Appearance: punched out geographic lesions, may be destructive or expansible

      e.   Clinical: pain 6 months to 7 years duration, weakness, weight loss, poor prognosis

  4. Giant cell tumor

      a.   Sex: male = female

      b.   Age: 20 to 40 years

      c.   Location: 50%-60% around the knee, distal femur, proximal tibia - metaphyseal or epiphyseal

      d.   Appearance: lytic lesion geographic or permeative, may be expansible, locally aggressive. No matrix calcification, can be mistaken for an enchondroma

      e.   Clinical: painful mass with possible pathologic fracture

  5. Pigmented Villonodular bursitis

      a.   Cartilage destruction

      b.   No bone formation

RADIOLOGY OF JOINT DISEASES

I. Non-inflammatory Disorders

  A. Osteoarthritis (Degenerative Joint Disease): most common skeletal joint abnormality

    1. Primary osteoarthritis: degeneration of a joint in absence of precipitating factor

    2. Secondary osteoarthritis: degenerative changes precipitated by insult or injury

      a.   Age: likelihood increases with advancing years (>50-60 years) males < 45, females > 45

      b.   Sex: primary degenerative joint disease largely affects females, secondary degenerative joint disease - males

      c.   Location: larger weightbearing joints (ankle infrequent unless secondary type)

         i. Midtarsus (first M-C joint) and MPJ (hallux limitus/rigidus)

      d.   Appearance: osteophyte formation, eburnation, subchondral cysts joint mice (intra-articular osseous fragment), joint collapse, deformity and malalignment

      e.   Clinical: limited range of motion, crepitus, palpable enlargement of joint

  B. Inflammatory Disorders

    1. Sero-Negative arthritis

      a.   Psoriatic arthritis: 3%-7% of patients with psoriasis will develop PA

         i. Age: around 40 years of age, increasing incidence in children of juvenile form

         ii. Sex: males 2-3:1 females

         iii. Location: distal interphalangeal joints most consistent, IPJ of hallux, calcaneus

         iv. Appearance

            (a) acro-osteolysis (distal tuft resorption)

            (b) periostitis

            (c) ivory phalanx (distal phalanx of hallux)

            (d) interphalangeal joint involvement of hallux

            (e) abnormal widening of joint spaces

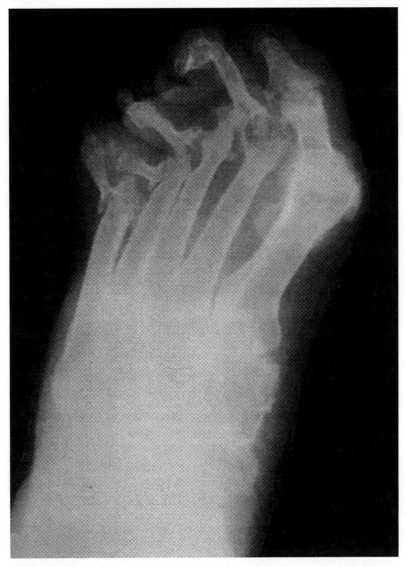

Psoriatic arthritis

        (f) normal mineraliation (in contrast to RA)
        (g) pencil-in-cup deformity of MPJs
     v. Clinical: cocktail sausage enlargement of the digits; equal involvement of hands and feet
        (a) possible neuropathic component
        (b) asymmetrical involvement
        (c) joint changes may precede skin changes
  b. Reiter's Disease: endemic (venereal) and epidemic (post-dysenteric)
     i. Age: 20-40 years of age - young adult males most typical
     ii. Sex: males (endemic) - females and children (epidemic)
     iii. Location: sacroiliac joint, calcaneus and pedal digits (MPJ, PIPJ, and IPJ of hallux)
     iv. Appearance: similar to PA but without hand involvement, often exuberant infra-calcaneal spur formation
     v. Clinical: feet affected 90%, oligoarticular and asymmetrical, urethritis, conjunc-

tivitis and poly arthritis (triad), balanitis and keratoderma blennorhagicum

  c. Ankylosing spondylitis

     i. Age: 15-35 years of age (late 20s to early 30s most common)

     ii. Sex: males (90%)

     iii. Location: sacroiliac joints, spine, and calcaneus

     iv. Appearance: bilateral sacroilitis with changes in SI joint leading to fusion, bamboo-spine with syndesmophytosis, pedal changes nondescript and similar to PA and Reiter's disease, whiskering effect (entheses) at tendinous insertions of calcaneus

     v. Clinical: oligoarticular and asymmetrical, positive HLA B - 27 antigen

  d. Gastroenteropathies (ulcerative colitis and Crohn's Disease)

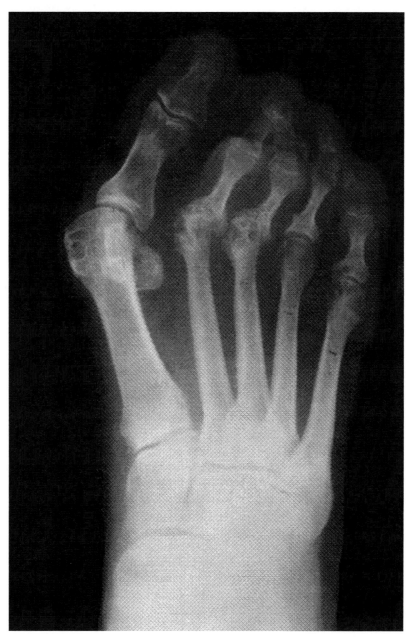

Rheumatoid arthritis

       i. Age: tendency to affect young adults

      ii. Sex: males and females

     iii. Location: sacroiliac joints

     iv. Appearance: soft tissue edema, peri-articular osteopenia, joint space narrowing and erosions (less severe than RA), periostitis and sclerosis, spondylitis similar to ankylosing spondylitis

      v. Clinical: migratory type of arthritis which usually follows onset of colitis or enteritis, symmetric affect on peripheral joints, erytherna nodosum

2. Sero-Positive arthritides

   a. Rheumatoid arthritis

      i. Age: 40 years of age

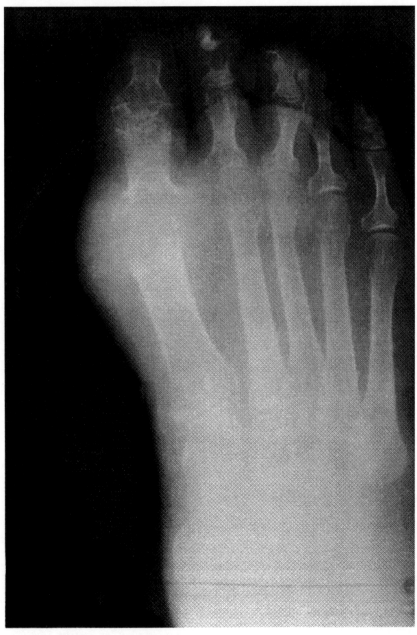

Gout first metatarsal phalangeal joint

        ii. Sex: below 40, females 3; males 1, 40 and over, females = males

        iii. Location: carpal and metacarpal joints, metatarsophalangeal joints, midfoot (T-N joint), and calcaneus

        iv. Appearance: peri-articular soft tissue edema, joint space widening, juxta-articular osteopenia initially, erosive changes (medial plantar aspect of metaheads), uniform joint space narrowing, calcaneal erosions (retro-calcaneal and inferior bursa), ankylosis, main-en-lorgnette, swan-neck, and boutonniere deformities of the hand

        v. Clinical: HAV most common pedal deformity, fibular deviation of digits 1-4, flexion deformity of DIPJs and PIPJs, extension deformity of MPJs

3. Crystalline-Induced arthritides

    a. Gouty arthritis: hyperuricemia due to over production of uric acid or diminished renal excretion, primary: unknown etiology or genetic enzyme defect, secondary: known disorder or medication (thiazide diuretic)

        i. Age: incidence increases after age 40

        ii. Sex: males 90% and females 10% (increases following menopause)

        iii. Location: first MPJ and other small peripheral joints

        iv. Appearance: extra-articular involvement a hallmark, joint effusion and edema, tophi formation (sodium urate deposits), C-shaped erosions with overhanging ridge of bone (Martel's sign), calcification of tophi ankylosis

        v. Clinical: monarticular in early stages, acute attack lasts 3-7 days, can have hyperuricemia without gout symptoms, permanent osseous changes after several acute episodes

    b. Pseudogout (CPPD disease): calcium pyrophosphate dihydrate

        i. Age: 50-60 years of age (middle-aged to elderly)

        ii. Sex: both male and female

        iii. Location: knee most common, hip, ankle, T-N, C-C, T-C, and metatarsophalangeal joints of foot

        iv. Appearance: presence of calcification of articular cartilage and peri-articular tissue

        v. Clinical: positive birefringence of crystals under polarized microscopy, clinically similar to gout although attacks less painful, acute attacks can last one day up to 2 weeks, association with diabetes, hypertension, and atherosclerosis

4. Miscellaneous arthritides

    a. Neurotrophic joint disease: joint destruction secondary to loss of proprioception and deep sensation (Charcot joint)

        i. Age: 5th to 7th decade but can occur at anytime

        ii. Sex: males and females both affected

        iii. Hypertrophic Form

          (a) Stages

            (i) destructive

            (ii) coalescent

            (iii) remodelling

          (b) Location: ankle, subtalar, and midtarsal joints

          (c) Appearance: joint distention, increased density of bone and soft tissue, osseous debris, dislocation, disorganization, destruction

          (d) Clinical: most common secondary to diabetes

        iv. Atrophic form (Diabetic osteolysis)

          (a) Location: primarily non-weightbearing joints, MPJs

           (b) Appearance: resorption of articular end resembling "licked candy stick"

           (c) Clinical: encountered primarily in the forefoot

  b. Diffuse idiopathic skeletal hyperostosis: characterized by ligamentous ossification and calcification

     i. Age: middle aged and elderly (>50 years of age)

     ii. Sex: males > females

     iii. Location: spine, peripheral joints, calcaneus

     iv. Appearance: whiskering of tendinous attachment to bone (enthuses)

     v. Clinical: 20% have concurrent diabetes, HLA B-8 antigen (40%)

  c. Pulmonary hypertrophic osteoarthropathy

     i. Age: 40-60 years of age

     ii. Sex: males primarily

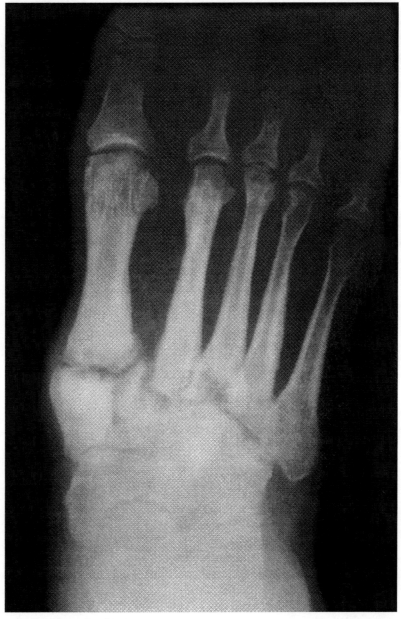

Neurotrophic joint disease

         iii. Location: tibia, fibula, radius, ulna, metacarpals, metatarsals, and phalanges

         iv. Appearance: digital clubbing, symmetrical arthritis and periostitis (triad) periostitis in metaphysis and diaphysis of long bones

         v. Clinical: usually a sequelae to a major thoracic disorder (bronchogenic carcinoma), bilateral and symmetrical involvement

    d. Inflammatory erosive osteoarthritis: interphalangeal arthritis characterized by acute inflammatory attacks and eventual ankylosis

         i. Age: 4th to 6th decades

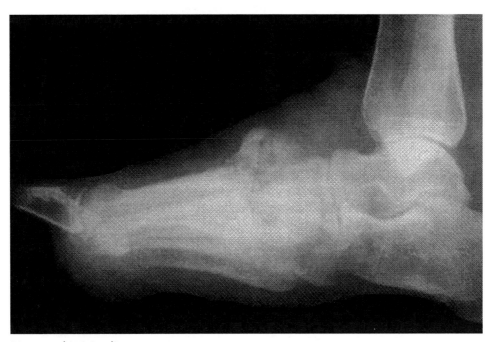

Neurotrophic joint disease

         ii. Sex: female

         iii. Location: IPJ of hands, MCP and CMC joints, symmetrical involvement

         iv. Appearance: "gull-wing" appearance of IPJs

         v. Clinical: course can run months to years, resolves or progresses to resemble RA

   5. Collagen vascular disorders

    a. Scleroderma

         i. Age: third to fifth decades

         ii. Sex: females > males

         iii. Location: fingers, wrist, ankles, and feet

         iv. Appearance: diffuse osteoporosis, soft tissue atrophy, tuftal resorption, soft tissue calcification in subcutaneous tissue

         v. Clinical: Raynaud's phenomenon, soft tissue thickening and swelling, pain and stiffness in extremities

         vi. Associated syndrome

               C: calcinosis

               R: Raynaud's phenomenon

               E: esophageal abnormality

               S: sclerodactyly

               T: telangiectasia

  b. Systemic Lupus erythematosus
    i. Age: females during child bearing years, rare over age 45
    ii. Sex: females > males
    iii. Race: blacks > whites
    iv. Location: small joints of hand, knee, wrist, and shoulder
    v. Appearance: joint space narrowing, deforming non-erosive arthropathy of hands and feet, soft tissue calcification, osteonecrosis
    vi. Clinical: malaise, weakness, fever and weight loss, skin rash, symmetrical polyarthritis, spontaneous tendon rupture
  c. Polyarteritis Nodosa
    i. Age: 20-50 years of age
    ii. Sex: men > females
    iii. Location: lower extremities
    iv. Appearance: plain film changes unusual, soft tissue swelling periostitis of tibia and fibula
    v. Clinical: variable features dependent upon extent of disease; renal involvement 75%-80%, peripheral vascular involvement leading to gangrene

OSTEOPOROSIS

 I. **Definition:** a condition of decreased mass per unit volume of normally mineralized bone. Factors to consider include age, race, gender, and body size. It is the most common skeletal disorder encountered. Normal bone is comprised of cortical bone (80%) and trabecular bone (20%)

 II. **Incidence:** of the disorders which cause a diminished bone mass, involutional bone loss is the most common cause of osteoporosis. Primary and secondary for-ins of osteoporosis

 III. **Clinicopathology:** Age related (involutional) bone loss begins in the 35-40 year old age group. Females lose up to 35% of their cortical bone and 50% of the trabecular bone (males about 2/3rds of these amounts) in their lifetime. A woman who experiences menopause at the average age of 51 will likely lose up to 50% of her total skeletal mass by the age of 75

 IV. **Risk Factors/Etiologies**

  A. **Race and family history:** African Americans have greater bone mass and less incidence of osteoporosis than Caucasians and Asians
  B. **Age and Sex:** peak bone mass at age 35
  C. **Nutrition:** the need for calcium increases with age
   1. Malabsorption of Vitamin D
  D. **Endocrine Factors**
   1. Hypogonadism
   2. Hyperthyroidism
   3. Hyperparathyroidism: effects of parathyroid hormone
   4. Hyperadrenalism
  E. **Weightbearing activity and stature:** sedentary lifestyle of the elderly and lack of mechanical stress on the body predisposes them to osteoporosis
  F. **Nulliparity**
  G. **Amenorrhea**

H. Excessive ETOH Intake and Cigarette Smoking
1. Toxic to bone forming cells
2. Interferes with intestinal Ca absorption

V. Diagnosis

A. Plain radiographs: of little screening value. Loss of up to 35% of density before evident on x-ray
1. Radiogrammetry
   a. Jhamaria's Calcaneal Index: Evaluation of the compressive and tensile trabecular pattern of the calcaneus as viewed on a lateral projection (Grade 0 - severely osteoporotic, Grade 5 - normal)
   b. Singh's Index: Based on evaluation of trabecular of the femoral head
   c. Rule of Thirds, Halves: Based on the cortical thickness of the middiaphysis of second metatarsal on an AP projection (both cortices two-thirds total width and trabecular bone one-third.) Cortical bone loss = 1% year. After age of forty subtract 10% of the cortical thickness for every decade of life. After forty both cortices equal 50% of thickness and trabecular bone constitutes remaining 50%. This is only a general guideline adapted from the metacarpal index, subject to weightbearing influences on the second metatarsal

B. Quantitative CT: measures bone density at the wrist and spine - can also measure trabecular density - less precise than absorptiometry

C. Absorptiometry (Single and Dual Photon)
1. Single and Dual: measured at the wrist
2. Dual: spine and hip

D. Dual energy x-ray absorptiometry: can measure bone density at all sites in the body

VI. Types of Involutional Osteoporosis

A. Type I Post-Menopausal: 55-75 years of age
1. Increased osteoblastic activity
2. Increased resorption
3. Bone loss: trabecular (intracapsular fracture)
4. Lab values: normal except urine Ca+ increased and PTH function decreased

B. Type 2 Senile or age-related: >70 years of age females, >80 years of age males
1. Decreased osteoblastic activity
2. Decreased formation
3. Bone loss: cortical and trabecular (extracapsular fracture)
4. Lab values: normal except increased PTH function

C. Primary Osteoporosis: no underlying disorder responsible

D. Secondary Osteoporosis: bone loss secondary to underlying disorder such as:
1. Steroid therapy
2. Myeloma
3. Metastases
4. Gastric surgery
5. Anticonvulsant therapy
6. Heparin therapy
7. Hyperparathyroidism
8. Diabetes
9. Alcoholism
10. Hypogonadism
11. Anorexia

COMPLEX REGIONAL PAIN SYNDROME TYPE I AND II
(FORMERLY RSD AND CAUSALGIA)

I.   **Definition:** Complex regional pain syndrome represents a diversely challenging clinical entity. A disorder affecting the sympathetic nervous system, its main characteristic is pain usually disproportionate to the incident or injury responsible for inciting it. The key to success in treating complex regional pain syndrome seems to rest on the early recognition of the signs and symptoms associated with it. In this way, a diagnosis can be made and a treatment regimen instituted. Left untreated, complex regional pain syndrome progresses through three stages, each stage more resistant to treatment than the previous one.

  A. **Alternate Terminology**
    1. Reflex sympathetic dystrophy
    2. Algodystrophy
    3. Causalgia major
    4. Causalgia minor
    5. Neurodystrophy
    6. Post-traumatic dystrophy
    7. Shoulder hand syndrome
    8. Sudeck's atrophy

II. **Proposed Etiology of Complex Regional Pain Syndrome** (exact pathophysiology unknown)

  A. **Trauma:** often minor, is a leading precipitating factor of CRPS I
    1. Accidental
      a. Sprain
      b. Fracture
      c. Burn
    2. Surgical
      a. Extremity (neuroma removal has high incidence in Podiatric surgery)
      b. Tight cast
      c. Nerve damage
  B. **Metabolic Disorders**
    1. Ischemic heart disease and myocardial infarction
    2. Cerebral/spinal cord lesions
    3. Infection
    4. Vascular disease
    5. Musculoskeletal disorders
  C. **Idiopathic**

III. **Clinical Signs and Symptoms of Complex Regional Pain Syndrome**

  A. **Pain:** burning or aching in nature; localized to site of injury initially but spreads to involve entire extremity
  B. **Hyperesthesia**
  C. **Edema:** pitting or non-pitting (at some time during course of disease; possibly prior to seeking medical advice)
  D. **Decreased motor function**
  E. **Tremor**
  F. **Vasomotor irregularity**
    1. Raynaud's phenomenon

2. Vasoconstriction
3. Vasodilation
4. Hyperhidrosis

G. **Radiographic changes**
1. Spotty osteoporosis
2. Generalized osteoporosis
3. Joint abnormalities

IV. **Diagnosis of Complex Regional Pain Syndrome:** There is no one test that confirms the diagnosis. Diagnosis is dependent on clinical presentation early in the course of the disease. Many times the clinical presentation is confusing as pt may present in any stage. Not every pt follows the typical scenario, and children and adolescents usually present and are treated differently. The following modalities or findings may assist in establishing the diagnosis:

A. **History of injury or infection**
B. **Persistent burning or aching pain exaggerated for the type of complaint**
C. **Hyperesthesia and hyperirritability at certain trigger points** (if undiagnosed may even progress to multi-limb or hemi-body involvement)
D. **Plain film radiography**—spotty loss of bone density
E. **Three phase Tc99 bone scan:** uptake of involved extremity in early phases and uptake demonstrating periarticular involvement in later phases. Decreased uptake may be observed in the early stage of Complex Regional Pain Syndrome due possibly to vasoconstriction
F. **Type I (RSD) vs. Type II (causalgia) have had the following diagnostic criteria:**
1. Type I (b, c, and d=dx)
   a. An initiating event of trauma/immobilization
   b. Continuing hyperalgesic pain (unproportional to initiating event)
   c. Edema at one time during dz course, variances of integumental vascularity, or abnormal sudomotor activity in area of pain
   d. Absence of differential diagnoses (poststroke pain syndrome, peripheral neuropathy, postherpetic neuralgia, myofascial pain, radiculopathy, infectious arthritis, Raynaud's, Buerger's dz, traumatic vasospasm, etc.)
2. Type II (a, b, and c=dx)
   a. Continual pain status post nerve injury; not limited to nn. distribution, however
   b. Edema at one time during dz course, variances of integumental vascularity, or sudomotor activity in area of pain
   c. Absence of differential diagnoses as listed above

V. **Stages of Complex Regional Pain Syndrome**

A. **Stage I - Acute Hyperemic Phase** (Average duration 1-3 months): most responsive to treatment
1. Onset of severe burning pain localized to the site of injury
2. Hyperesthesia
3. Localized edema
4. Muscle spasm
5. Stiffness and limited mobility
6. Vasospasm: initially skin is warm, red, and dry then becomes cyanotic, cold, and sweaty
7. Hyperhidrosis
8. Hair and nail growth may actually improve in this stage
9. Can be reversed with sympathetic blockade

10. John Buckholz, DPM in Fundamentals of Foot Surgery, further divides the first stage into two distinct and separate phases. Phase IA is the initial response of the affected area with vasoconstriction and hypothermia which lasts for approximately 2-6 weeks. In Phase IB, the opposite and traditional presentation becomes apparent in the form of vasodilation, hyperthermia, erythema, and hyperhidrosis. According to Buckholz, this phase lasts anywhere from 2 to 6 months

11. Normal Radiographs; bone scan may be abnormal

B. Stage 2-Dystrophic Ischemic Phase (Average duration 3-6 months)
1. Spreading edema-becomes brawny
2. Pain more severe and diffuse
3. Skin moist, cyanotic, and cold

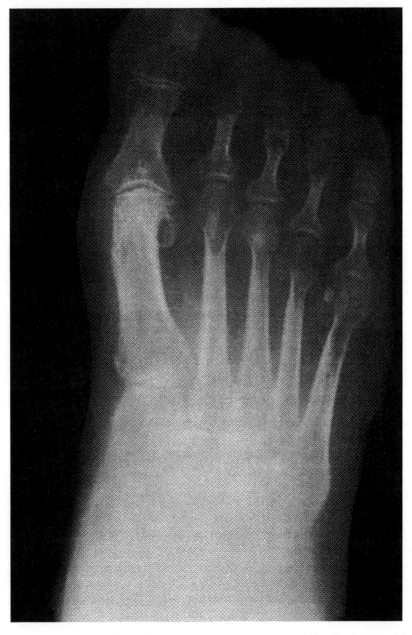

Reflex sympathetic dystrophy

4. Nails become brittle and ridged
5. Hair becomes scant
6. Muscle wasting and atrophy becomes prominent
7. Subchondral osteopenia; bone scan may be abnormal
8. Sympathetic block may be effective although larger or prolonged series may be necessary

C. **Stage 3-Atrophic Phase** (6-12 months; usually becomes irreversible)
1. Pain continues and can become intractable and involve entire extremity
2. Marked trophic changes
3. Skin becomes smooth, shiny, and tight
4. Muscle atrophy
5. Generalized osteoporosis/bone demineralization (Sudeck's atrophy notable on radiographs)
6. Flexor contractures and weakness of interphalangeal joints
7. Pain exacerbated by cold
8. Aggressive treatment necessary: sympathetic blockade, counseling, physical therapy

IV. CRPS in Children and Adolescents

1. Etiology of major trauma is less likely
2. Female>Male
3. First described in adolescents in the 1970s
4. Clinical symptomatology more severe at initial presentation than adult CRPS (children without autonomic symptomatology usually have multiple sites of pain)
5. Cold extremity more common than a warm extremity in adolescents
6. Hyperhidrosis is less common in adolescent CRPS
7. Trophic changes less common in adolescent CRPS
8. Adolescent CRPS is more effectively treated with conservative therapy vs. pharmacologic
9. Conservative therapy should include aggressive physical therapy (5-6 hours per day), contrast bath therapy, TENS, etc.
10. TENS therapy more helpful in children than in adults
11. Aggressive PT (may need narcotic meds to complete PT) more helpful in children than sympathetic blockade. Blockade should be reserved for recalcitrant cases

V. Treatment of CRPS in Adults

1. No single treatment effective in all cases; multidisciplinary approach recommended
2. Mild cases respond to physical therapy/modalities
3. Moderate cases usually need an anticonvulsant/antidepressant analgesic therapy added for the patient to tolerate physical therapy
4. B-blockers, alpha-blockers, alpha-antagonists, and calcium channel blockers used for treatment
5. Severe cases or cases with sympathetic dysfunction necessitate regional anesthetic blockade to tolerate physical therapy. These patients have shown response to spinal analgesia
6. Clinical trials with ketamine-midazolam anesthesia showing promising results. Others in trial include guanethidine (IV regional), bupivicaine (lumbar sympathetic blockade), pamidronate (po), phenoxybenzamine (po), and methylprednisone with lidocaine (parenteral)
7. Morphine pump implantation or spinal stimulator used

8. Preemptive analgesia via epidural catheter at a minumum of 12 hours prior to surgical procedures and 3 days postoperatively reported by Cramer et.al in JFAS Vol. 39 (6). Highly recommended
9. Sympathectomy showed promise initially, but long term results show return of symptomatology to the area in a multitude of studies
10. TENS unit therapy helpful in early phases, but may actually exacerbate symptomatology in later stages
11. Motor cortex stimulation in the brain for severe hemi-body CRPS pts. reported

RADIOLOGY OF DIABETES MELLITUS

I. **The radiographic evaluation of diabetes mellitus generally assesses the following three areas:**

   A. **Vascular Changes**
      1. Vascular pathology is accelerated in the diabetic population
      2. Manifested radiographically as vascular calcification
      3. Presence of Mockenberg's medial calcinosis at the digital level increases suspicion of diabetes mellitus

   B. **Neurotrophic Arthropathies** (Charcot joint disease)
      1. Atrophic arthropathy
         a. Affects non weight bearing joints
         b. Pedal involvement: usually at metatarsal phalangeal joint level
         c. Radiographic appearance
            i. Loss of normal osseous architecture with a tapering of the long bones (licked-candy stick)
            ii. No fragmentation or profound periosteal activity is noted
         d. Diabetic osteolysis (diabetic osteopathy)
            i. See osteolysis followed by reformatting of osseous components
            ii. May represent a viral infection of bone
      2. Hypertrophic neuroarthropathy
         a. Affects weight bearing joints
         b. Pedal involvement: MPJ, Lis Franc, and rearfoot joint levels
         c. Stages
            i. Destructive
               (a) marked increase in soft tissue contour and density due to inflammatory process
               (b) destruction and fragmentation of bone
               (c) fragmentation occurs at a joint level with osseous components maintaining a portion of the cartilaginous surface
               (d) sharding of bone
               (e) fine particulate debris
               (f) loss of normal anatomical alignment
            ii. Coalescent
               (a) decrease in soft tissue inflammation
               (b) fragments begin to unite
               (c) resorption of the fine particulate debris
            iii. Remodeling

(a) no evidence of soft tissue inflammation
(b) fusion of osseous components is completed
(c) may have loss of normal osseous configuration or alignment

C. **Infection evaluation**
1. Plain film analysis
    a. Baseline films critical for early assessment
    b. Inflammatory response may not occur due to vascular status
    c. Early periosteal reaction and cortical and medullary destruction
    d. Sclerosis of bone may represent attenuated infectious process
    e. Charcot joint disease may be differential diagnosis
2. Nuclear imaging
    a. Bone scans of limited value
    b. Will be "hot" in both osteomyelitis and Charcot
    c. Isotope labeled WBC's somewhat increases specificity for osteomyelitis (i.e., Ga 67, In 111, Tc 99 HMPAO, or Ceretec), but Charcot joint can be positive with these agents also
3. Computed Tomography
    a. less sensitive than MRI; used when MRI contraindicated or not available
4. MRI
    a. Utilized to assess extent of marrow involvement
    b. TI weighted image will show decrease in signal intensity
    c. T2 weighted image will show increase in signal intensity
5. Bone biopsy: in suspected cases of osteomyelitis a bone biopsy may be needed to confirm diagnosis

THYROID AND PARATHYROID DISEASES

I. **Hyperthyroidism (Graves' Disease)**

A. **Findings**
1. Increased osteoblastic and osteoclastic activity with a net loss of bone
2. Stimulates bone growth in the young and bone loss in adults
3. New bone formation is seen along metatarsals, metacarpals, and phalanges of the hands and feet
4. Periostitis along shafts of tubular bones
5. Cone shaped epiphyses
6. Asymmetrical shortening of metacarpals
7. Will cause thyroid acropachy in 1% of patients
8. Insidious swelling of hands and feet
9. Clubbing of fingers
10. Exophthalmus

II. **Hypothyroidism**

A. **Two syndromes**
1. Congenital - thyroid deficiency leads to cretinism
2. Acquired - juvenile myxedema
B. **Radiographically identical**
1. Retardation of maturity and growth of skeleton

2. Delayed appearance and fusion of ossification centers
3. Ossific centers start at diffuse areas which eventually coalesce
4. Bands of increased density at ends of long bones
5. Slipped capital epiphysis femur results in coxa vara
6. Vertebral flattening, kyphosis
7. Brachycephalic
8. Bone changes may regress in adult cretins

III. Hyperparathyroidism

A. **Primary:** usually due to solitary adenoma of a parathyroid gland 3rd to 5th decade
   1. Causes generalized osteitis fibrosa cystica
   2. Increased osteoclastic activity
   3. Subperiosteal bone resorption
   4. Localized destruction cause intramedullary or intra cortical translucencies called brown tumors or osteoclastomas filled with fibrous connective tissue or brown mucoid material
   5. Cortical definition lost causing "lace-like appearance of bone"
   6. Sites commonly affected in lower extremity
   7. Sesamoids
       a. Tufts of terminal phalanges
       b. Femur, tibia, calcaneal borders
B. **Secondary:** secondary to chronic renal failure, vitamin D deficiency, rickets
   1. Skeletal changes similar to primary with addition of arterial and soft tissue calcifications and osteosclerosis
C. **Tertiary:** escape of PT gland from regulatory effects of serum calcium
   1. Skeletal changes similar to primary and secondary

IV. Pseudohypoparathyroidism

A. **Findings**
   1. Sex-linked dominant, shows in 2nd decade
   2. Decreased serum calcium
   3. Normal parathyroid hormone level
   4. Skeletal changes
       a. Dwarfism
       b. Moonface
       c. Brachydactyly
       d. Cone-shaped epiphysis
       e. Ectopic calcifications/ossifications

V. **Pseudo-pseudohypoparathyroidism (Albrights' hereditary osteodystrophy):** Incomplete genetic manifestation of pseudohypoparathyroidism with the same skeletal changes but normal serum calcium

SKELETAL CHANGES ASSOCIATED WITH RENAL DISEASE

I. Renal Glomerular Failure

A. **Renal osteodystrophy**
   1. Osteosclerosis

2. Thick trabecular pattern "chalky bone"
3. "Rugger jersey" or sclerotic lines upper and lower border of vertebrae
4. Osteoporosis
5. Osteomalacia: generalized demineralization with Loosers' lines
6. Osteitis fibrosa cystica (rare)
7. Subchondral trabecular resorption
8. Fibrosis
9. New bone formation
10. Metastatic calcifications - arterial, ocular, periarticular, cutaneous-avascular necrosis

B. Dialysis bone disease
1. 30% have distinct articular and peri-articular erosions of the hands and feet
2. 50% have associated adjacent soft tissue calcifications of the IPJ
3. Progressive bone loss leads to fractures from minor trauma
4. Increased incidence of osteomyelitis and septic joints
5. Bone diseases become more complex with prolonged dialysis

II. Renal Tubular Failure

A. Syndromes produce renal tubular acidosis
1. Wilson's disease
2. Vitamin D resistant rickets

B. Radiographic changes
1. Similar to those of rickets and osteomalacia
2. Widening of growth plates
3. Metaphyseal changes
4. Bowing of long bones
5. Dwarfism

PAGET'S DISEASE (OSTEITIS DEFORMANS)

I. Identifying information

A. Disease of unknown etiology (possibly slow viral infection)
B. Mono or polyostotic (more common) forms
C. Males 2:1 females
D. Age: mid-life (> 40)
E. Lab values: elevated serum alkaline phosphatase levels (>20 X), marked increase in isotope uptake in Technetium bone scan
F. Stages
1. Destructive phase (osteoclastic activity)
   a. Subchondral destruction of bone extending into the metaphysis
   b. Blade of grass pattern of destruction in the diaphysis
2. Combined phase (osteoclastic and osteoblastic activity)
   a. Most common stage encountered
   b. Widened appearance of bone with thickening of cortices and trabecular pattern
3. Sclerotic phase (osteoblastic activity)
   a. Angular deformity
   b. Long medullary space
4. Malignant Degeneration
   a. Reported in 6% of cases
   b. Osteosarcoma (50%)

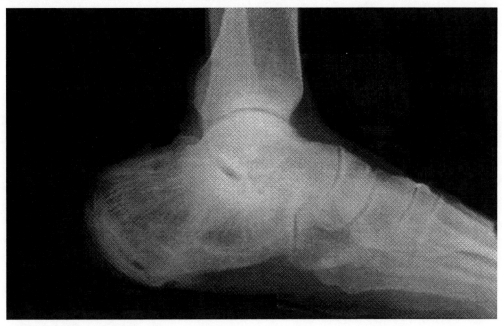

Paget's (combined stage)

        c. Fibrosarcoma (25%)
        d. Chondrosarcoma (rare)

II. Radiographic appearance

A. Findings

1. Stage dependent
2. Calcaneus most commonly affected pedal bone
3. Initial bone resorption osteoporosis circumscripta
4. Marked increase in bone density with coarsened trabecular patterns
5. Hair on end or cotton wool appearance of flat bones
6. Angular deformities of long bones including lateral curvature of femur and anterior bowing of tibia (saber shin deformity)
7. Increase in size of bone a common finding in later stages leading to change in shoe, hat size
8. Pathological fractures
9. May see marked bone destruction, periosteal activity, soft-tissue masses with malignant degeneration

BONE HEALING AND FRACTURE REPAIR

I. Stages of Fracture Repair

A. Inflammatory Stage

1. Immediate (up to 10% of cycle)

B. Reparative Stage

1. 2-8 weeks (up to 40% of cycle)

C. Remodelling Stage

1. 6 weeks-2 years (up to 70% of cycle)

II. Delayed Union: Adequate interval of time from injury to union without radiographic or clinical evidence of union for location and type of fracture, usually up to six months. Clinical union precedes radiographic union by as much as 2 to 4 weeks

  A. Causes of Delayed Union
1. Soft tissue interposition
2. Excessive soft tissue destruction
3. Disruption of vascular supply
4. Inadequate immobilization
5. Distraction of fragments
6. Inadequate internal fixation

III. Non-Union: All reparative processes of healing bone have ceased with union highly improbable. Failure of a fracture or osteotomy to heal within 6 to 8 months

  A. Causes of Non-Union
1. Excessive motion
2. Infection
3. Gap or defect wider then 5.0 mm
4. Lack of vascular supply
5. Tension at bony ends (bone heals with compression and fails in tension)
6. Compound fracture or severe comminution
7. Insecure fixation
8. Immobilized for insufficient time
9. Ill-advised open reduction
10. Distraction by screws or plate

  B. Location: metaphyseal most difficult to treat
1. Cancellous bone: repairs rapidly
   a. Rich vascular supply
   b. Lack of callus

  C. Types of Bony Callus Encountered in Non-Union
1. Hypervascular: characterized by varying amounts of hypertrophic callus formation. Rich blood supply fully capable of biologic reaction
   a. Elephant's foot
      i. Hypertrophic and rich in callus
      ii. Insecure fixation or premature weightbearing
   b. Horse's hoof
      i. Mildly hypertrophic and poor in callus
      ii. Moderately unstable fixation with plate/screws
      iii. Minimal callus, insufficient for union
   c. Oligotrophic
      i. Not hypertrophic and callus absent
      ii. Major displacement or distraction of fragments
2. Avascular: lack of vascular callus formation and necrotic or atrophic bony ends. Usually requires stable fixation and bone graft
   a. Torsion wedge: avascular intermediate fragment (butterfly)
   b. Comminuted
      i. More then one avascular intermediate fragment
      ii. No callus
   c. Defect

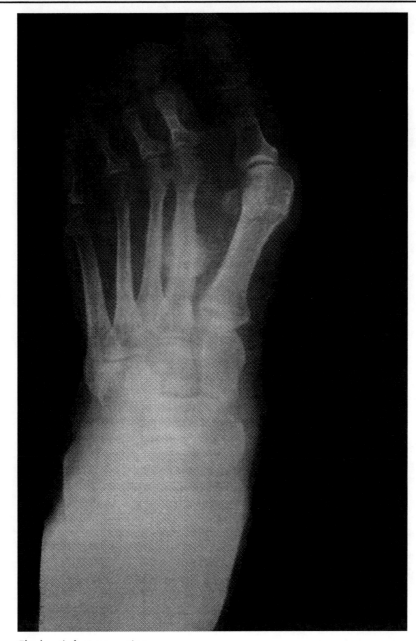

Elephant's foot non-union

        i. Loss of diaphyseal fragment
       ii. Ends viable but union impossible
      iii. Fracture ends atrophy
      iv. Compound fractures, sequestration in osteomyelitis, and resection of tumors
   d. Atrophic
        i. Intermediate fragments missing
       ii. Scar w/o osteogenic potential develops
      iii. Ends atrophic and osteoporotic

D. Treatment: two primary objectives
  1. Healing of non-union
  2. Restoration of function

E. **Radiographic Findings of Non-Union:** The radiographic criterion of non-union consists of serial radiographs once a month over three consecutive months without evidence of bony activity or repair at the fracture or osteotomy site
  1. Sclerosis at fracture ends (capped with vascular supply unable to advance)
  2. Failure to show any progressive change in a 3 month interval
  3. Progressive bowing in sequential x-rays (long bones)
  4. Increased atrophy above and below fracture site
  5. Excessive callus with lucent interval (false callus)
  6. Absence of remodelling
F. **Bone Scan** (Tc99)
  1. Hot in a true non-union where osteogenic potential remains
  2. A cold spot or photon deficient area indicates lack of vascularity and may be seen in the early development of a non-union
  3. Decreased uptake centrally and increased uptake (hot spot) at ends consistent with a pseudoarthrosis

IV. **Synovial Pseudoarthrosis:** variant or terminal form of non-union with formation of dense scar tissue and false joint with serum loculated in cicatricial mass. Can occur subsequent to either hypervascular or avascular non-union. Less then 5% occurrence rate. Congenital form is associated with neurofibromatosis. The acquired form is characterized by pain, instability and bowing. Radiographically, sclerotic margins resulting in capping of medullary canal with lucent gap between fragments

FRACTURE CLASSIFICATION SYSTEMS

I. **5th Metatarsal Base Fractures**
  A. **Stewart Classification**
    1. Type I: Jone's fracture, transverse fracture at the diaphyseal metaphyseal junction
    2. Type II: Intra-articular avulsion fracture
    3. Type III: Extra-articular avulsion fracture
    4. Type IV: Intra-articular comminuted fracture
    5. Type V: Extra-articular avulsion fracture of the apophysis

II. **Lisfranc Dislocations**
  A. **Hardcastle Classification**
    1. Type A: Homolateral or homomedial, where all the metatarsals dislocate in the same direction
    2. Type B: Partial incongruity, where less than all the metatarsals dislocate in a medial or lateral direction
    3. Type C: Divergent, medial dislocation of the first metatarsal and partial or total lateral dislocation of the lesser metatarsals

III. **Classification of Navicular Fractures**
  A. **Watson-Jones**
    1. Type I: Avulsion fracture of the tuberosity by the posterior tibial tendon
    2. Type II: Dorsal lip fracture
    3. Type III: Fracture of the body of the navicular

BIBLIOGRAPHY

Adler A, Carlton R. Principles of Radiographic Imaging: An Art and Science. Chapter 3 Basic Radiation Protection. Delmar Publishers, Albany, 1992.

Allen, G. et al; "Epidemiology of complex regional pain syndrome: a retrospective chart review of 134 patients"; Pain 80 (1999): 539-544.

Anderson, D. et al; "Complex Regional Pain Syndrome of the Lower Extremity: A Retrospective Study 33 Patients"; JFAS 38 (6); 1999. 381-387.

Aronoff, G. et al , "American Academy of Disability Evaluating Physicians (AADEP) Position Paper: Complex Regional Pain Syndrome I (RSD): "Impairment and Disability Issues"; American Academy of Pain Medicine 3 (3); 2002.

Ballinger PW. Merril's Atlas of Radiographic Positions and Procedures, 9th edition. Chapter 2 Radiation Protection. C.V. Mosby, St. Louis, 1995.

Bandyk, D. etal; "Surgical Sympathectomy for Reflex Sympathetic Dystrophy Syndromes"; J of Vascular Surgery 35 (2); 269-277.

Bareither D. Lower Extremity Anatomy Course Handout. Scholl College of Podiatric Medicine. Basic Biomedical Sciences, 1996-97.

Baron RL, Strugielski CF. X-Ray Positioning. Part 1: Weightbearing Projections. Podiatric Staff, February 1989.

Baron RL, Strugielski CF. X-Ray Positioning. Part 2: Non Weightbearing and Partial Weightbearing Projections. Podiatry Today, March, 1989.

Baron RL, Strugielski CF, Knight B. X-Ray Positioning. Part 3: Specialty Radiographs. Podiatry Today, September 1989.

Bennett, D. et al; "Spinal Cord Stimulation for Complex Regional Pain Syndrome I (RSD): a Retrospective Multicenter Experience from 1995 to 1998 of 101 Patients"; Neuromodulation 2 (3), 1999; 202-210.

Berquist TH. Radiology of the Foot and Ankle. Raven Press, New York, 1989.

Birklein, F. et al; "Neurological Findings in Complex Regional Pain Syndromes-Analysis of 145 Cases"; Acta Neurol. Scand 2000: 101: 262-269.

Bontrager KL, Anthony BT. Textbook of Radiographic Positioning and Related Anatomy. Multi-Media Publishing, Inc., Denver, 1988.

Broden B. Roentgen examination of the subtalar joint in fractures of the calcaneus. Acta Radiol 31:85, 1949.

Brower, Anne C.; Arthritis in Black and White; WB Saunders Company; Philadelphia, 1997.

Bushong S. Radiologic Science for Technologist. Chapters 26, 28, 29, 30, 32. C.V. Mosby Co., St. Louis, 1988.

Carlson, L. et al; "Treatment of Reflex Sympathetic Dystrophy Using the Stress-Loading Program"; Journal of Hand Therapy; July-September 1988; 149-154.

Causton J. Projection of the sesamoid bones in the region of the first metatarsophalangeal joint. Radiology 9:39, 1943.

Cramer et al; "Preemptive Analgesia in Elective Surgery in Patients with Complex Regional Pain Syndrome: A Case Report"; JFAS 39 (6): 387-391; 2000.

Crim, Julia R. and Sanders, Richard K.; Osteochondral Injuries; Seminars in Ultrasound, CT, and MRI; Vol 22 (4): 352-370; August 2001.

Crim, Julia; Talus Fractures; E-Medicine Journal; 27 June 2001; Vol 2 (6).

Clinics in Podiatric Medicine and Surgery. Vol. 5, No. 4 October 1988. Radiation Safety pp 759-766.

Current Trends in Foot and Ankle Imaging, OKU; American Academy of Orthopedic Surgeons: 315-332

Das, A. et al; "Syringomyelia and Complex Regional Pain Syndrome as Complications of Multiple Sclerosis"; Arch Neurol. Vol 56; Aug 1999: 1021-1024.

Dixon, Larry, M.D. Benign and Malignant Lesions of Bone: A Study Guide. Department of Radiology. University of Chicago, 1996-97.

Dunn, D. et al; "Chronic Regional Pain Syndrome as Complications, Type I: Part II"; AORN 72 (Oct. 20000: 643-653.

Edeiken J, Dalinka M, Karasick D. Edeikens' Roentgen Diagnosis of Diseases of Bone, Vols. 1-2. Williams and Wilkins, Baltimore, 1990.

Forrester DM, et al. Radiology of Joint Disease. Aspen, Rockville, MD, 1988.

Gerber L et al. Psoriatic Arthritis. Gruber & Stratton; Orlando, 1985.

Greenfield GB. Radiology of Bone Diseases. Lippincott, Philadelphia, 1988.

Greenfield GB, Arrington JA. Imaging of Bone Tumors. J.B. Lippincott, Philadelphia, 1995.

Greenspan A. Orthopedic Radiology: A Practical Approach. J.B. Lippincott, Philadelphia, 1988.

Grech et al. Diagnosis of Metabolic Bone Disease. W.B. Saunders, Philadelphia, 1985.

Harbut, R. et al; "Successful Treatment of a Nine-Year Case of Complex Regional Pain Syndrome Type I (Reflex Sympathetic Dystrophy) with Intravenous Ketamine-Infusion Therapy in a Warfarin-Anticoagulated Adult Female Patient"; Pain Medicine; Vol 3 (2); 2002: 147-155.

Harris RI, Beath T. Etiology of peroneal spastic flatfoot. J Bone Joint Surg (Br) 30:624, 1948.

Hogan, C. et al; "Treatment of Complex Regional Pain Syndrome of the Lower Extremity"; J Am Acad Orthop Surg 2002; Vol 10 (4): 281-289.

Holly EW. Radiography of the tarsal sesamoid bones. Medical Radiography and Photography 31:73, 1955.

Isherwood I. A radiological approach to the subtalar joint. J Bone Joint Surg (Br) 43:566, 1961.

Janig, W. et al; "Complex Regional Pain Syndrome is a Disease of the Central Nervous System"; Clin Auton. Res (2002); Vol 12: 150-164.

Keifer, R. et al; "Ketamine-Midazolam Anesthesia for Intractable Complex Regional Pain Syndrome-Type I (CRPS-1); Poster Presentation Dept. of Neurology Drexel Univ.; Philadelphia.

Kirkpatrick, Douglas P. et. al.; The Snowboarders Foot and Ankle; www.highcountryhealth.com/articles/sbfoot.htm.; 2001.

Kissel, et al. Bizarre Parosteal Osteochondromatous Proliferation: An Unusual Bone Tumor. JAPMA 85:6, 301-305, 1995.

Kite HJ. Principles involved in the treatment of congenital clubfoot. J Bone Joint Surg 21:595, 1939.

Kite HJ. The Clubfoot. Grune and Stratton, NY 1964. Isherwood I. A radiological approach to the subtalar joint. J Bone Joint Surg (Br) 43:566, 1961.

Lewis RW. Non-routine views in roentgen examinations of the extremities. Surg Gynecol Obstet 69:38, 1938.

Meisel A. et al. Atlas of Osteoarthritis. Lea & Febiger, New York, 1984.

Merrill's Reference of Roentgenographic Positions and Standard Radiographic Procedures. Volume #1, Ninth Edition, C.V. Mosby, St. Louis, 1995.

Mirra JM. Bone Tumors. Lea & Febiger, Philadelphia, 1989.

MRI of the Foot and Ankle; Current Problems in Diagnostic Radiology; Lucas, Philip et. al.; Vol 26 (5) Sept-Oct. 1997: 209-268.

Netherlands Committee on Bone Tumors: Radiographical Atlas of Bone Tumors, Vol 1 and 2. Williams and Wilkins, Baltimore, 1966.

National Council on Radiation Protection (NCRP) Report #91. Recommendations on limits for exposure to ionizing radiation. Bethesda, MD, 1987 NCRP Publication.

National Council on Radiation Protection (NCRP) Report #54. Medical radiation exposure of pregnant and potentially pregnant women. Bethesda, MD, 1977 NCRP Publication.

Nordin BEC. Metabolic Bone and Stone Disease. Churchill Livingstone, New York, 1984.

Pearlman et al; Traumatic Classifications of the Foot and Ankle. J Foot Surg 28:6, 55 1581,1989.

Primer on Rheumatic Diseases. Arthritis Foundation. 1188 Arthritis Foundation, Atlanta.

Reflex Sympathetic Dystrophy Syndrome. Reflex Sympathetic Dystrophy Syndrome Association of America. P.O. Box 821. Haddonfield, New Jersey 08033, 1995.

Resnick and Niwayama. Diagnosis of Bone and Joint Disorders. Second Edition. Saunders, Philadelphia, 1988.

Resnick, Donald; Bone and Joint Imaging; WB Saunders Company, Philadelphia, 1996.

Rheumatologic Disorders: Diagnosis and Management. Syntex Pharmaceutical Company, 1983.

Schmidt, C. et al; "Severe Complex Regional Pain Syndrome Type II After Radial Artery Harvesting"; Ann Thorac. Surg 2002; Vol 74: 1250-1.

Seidelmann & Shook, Drs.; Feb; A Foot and Ankle Seminar: MRI & Surgery; Cleveland, Feb. 4-5, 2000.

Son, B.C. et al; "Motor Cortex Stimulation in a Patient with Intractable Complex Regional Pain Syndrome Type II with Hemibody Involvement"; J Neurosurg. Vol 98: 175-179: 2003.

Sprawls P. Physical Principles of Medical Imaging. Chapters 32 and 33. Aspen, Rockville, MD, 1987.

Statkiewicz - Sherer, Visconti, Ritenour. Radiation Protection in Medical Radiography. Chapters 3, 4, 6, 7, 8, 9. C.V. Mosby, St. Louis, 1993.

Strugielski CF, Knight B, Baron RL. Radiographic Artifacts. What they are, their cause and correction. Podiatry Today, June 1990.

Wasmer, G. et al; "Vascular Abnormalities in Reflex Sympathetic Dystrophy (CRPS 1): Mechanisms and Diagnostic Value"; Brain (2001): Vol 124: 587-599.

Whitney AK. Radiographic Charting Technic. Philadelphia, 1996.

Weisman SD. Radiology of the Foot. Second Edition. Williams and Wilkins, Baltimore, 1989.

Weiss L, Docks G, Freedland J. Lauge-Hasen classification: A Clockwork Injury. J Foot Surg 22:3, 192-197, 1993.

CHAPTER 1
IMAGING/RADIOLOGY

1.   Short Tau Inversion Recover (STIR) in magnetic resonance imaging results in an image more heavily
       weighted in which of the following sequences?

       A.   T1
       B.   T2
       C.   Neither, it is equally weighted

2.   Patients can have an MRI if they have vessel clips implanted during surgery such as greater saphenous vein
       harvest for CABG surgery?

       A.   True
       B.   False

3.   When can stress fractures be reliably shown via nuclear medicine studies?

       A.   Immediately
       B.   > 6 hours after injury
       C.   > 24 hours after injury

4.   Which of the following test/tests are the standard of care in DVT workup?

       A.   Contrast venogram
       B.   Ultrasound
       C.   D-dimer
       D.   B and C
       E.   None of the above

5.   Technetium scanning to differentiate between cellulites and Osteomyelitis has a significant false-positive
       and false-negative rate in which of the following patient populations?

       A.   Post-menopausal women and male patients
       B.   Rheumatoid arthritis patients
       C.   Children and diabetic patients
       D.   Equal in all populations

6.   The "Magic Angle" refers to which of the following?

       A.   The angulation needed between the tube angle and the central ray in radiographs
       B.   The false artifact in an MRI when a tendon passes 55 degrees to the magnetic field
       C.   Another name for Bohler's angle

7.   Which differential diagnosis is least likely to be considered with giant cell tumor due to calcifications often
       seen with this diagnosis?

       A.   Enchondroma
       B.   Pigmented villonodular synovitis/bursitis
       C.   Periosteal sarcoma
       D.   Epidermoid cyst

8.   Which podiatric surgery has a higher incidence of complex regional pain syndrome (CRPS)?

        A.   Digital arthroplasty
        B.   Distal metatarsal osteotomy
        C.   Neuroma removal

9.   Which one variable is most often noted in both adult and adolescent complex regional pain syndrome (CRPS) at initial presentation?

        A.   Edema
        B.   Hyperhidrosis
        C.   Warm extremity
        D.   Trophic changes

10.   Sanders CT classification is used for evaluation of which type of fractures?

        A.   Talar fractures
        B.   Epiphyseal plate fractures
        C.   Calcaneal fractures
        D.   Ankle fractures

LABORATORY MEDICINE

Michael A. Zapf

LABORATORY TESTS

I. **Purpose**

   A. **Diagnosis**

   B. **Screening for disease to detect presence in a population of asymptomatic individuals**

   C. **Monitoring effects of therapy**

II. **Normal Values**

   A. **Normal values presented for tests discussed in this chapter are from a wide range of sources.** They include the widest ranges reported in the reference texts listed at the end of this chapter and those from various reference laboratories used by the author of this chapter. They are of limited value and not meant to apply to any particular patient, laboratory, or testing method or to establish or rule out any particular disease state. Clinicians are advised to consult the normal ranges from their own reference laboratory. When performing laboratory testing in the office, be aware of the limitations of the normal ranges printed on package inserts or reference texts. Factors such as individual laboratory techniques, population variations, sampling errors, and distance from the laboratory can cause a test result to vary from the reference ranges

   B. **Sensitivity:** True positives or that proportion of patients who have a disease that test positive

   C. **Specificity:** True negatives or that proportion of patients who do not have the disease who test negative

   D. **SI Units:** (Système International d'United) International method by which all laboratory tests can be reported; most laboratories use conventional reference ranges that can be converted, if desired, into the international units

III. **General precautions for taking the sample**

   A. **Fasting:** Preferred for 8-12 hours prior to test for glucose, phosphorus, cholesterol, triglycerides, potassium, and BUN

   B. **Collection:** One puncture for all tubes

   C. **Tourniquet:** When in place for longer than 1-2 minutes, electrolytes, lactate, and pH are affected

D. Exposure of blood to bright light degrades bilirubin

E. Refrigeration: Creatinine deteriorates at room temperature

F. IM Injections: When injected within 8 hours creatine kinase and lactic dehydrogenase can be increased

G. Serum: Liquid part of clotted blood required for enzymes and electrophoresis

H. Plasma: Liquid part of anticoagulated blood adequate for all but enzymes and electrophoresis

I. Medications: May affect results

IV. Chemistry evaluations

A. Acid phosphatase: (male 0. 13-0.63 U/ml; female 0.01-0.56 U/ml; prostatic 0-0.5 U/dl). Elevated in bone disease such as Paget's disease and prostatic disease

B. Albumin (adult 3.5-5.0 g/dl)
1. Usually measured by protein electrophoresis
2. Makes up to 65% of total protein
3. Levels are elevated in dehydration states and diabetic ketoacidosis
4. Levels are decreased with protein loss from kidney damage, hemorrhage, and burns

C. Albumin/globulin (A/G) ratio (adult 1.0-2.5)
1. Indirect measurement of globulin levels can be calculated by subtracting the albumin level from the total protein level
2. Low A/G ratios seen in liver disease, malnutrition, diarrhea, and other disorders
3. Increased ratios are uncommon
4. Some believe it should no longer be ordered since electrophoresis is widely available

D. Alkaline phosphatase (AP) (adult: 13-100 IU/L; infants and children up to age 12 years: 350 IU/L) AP levels are elevated with bone metabolism, pregnancy, liver disease, and taking drugs such as allopurinol, colchicine, Indocin, penicillins, and oral antidiabetes medications

E. Alanine aminotransferase (ALT/SGPT) (adult 1-21 U/L) ALT levels are elevated up to 50 times normal in liver disease and to a lesser extent in bone disease

F. Aspartate aminotransferase (AST/SGOT) (adult 7-27 U/L)
1. Low specificity
2. AST levels are elevated in liver, skeletal muscle, kidneys, and cardiac and pancreas disorders
3. Levels are also elevated after MI but normal in angina pectoris
4. AST levels peak 24-36 hours after injury and fall to normal in 6 days
5. May be 20-100 times normal in acute viral hepatitis
6. Many drugs can cause the levels to be increased

G. Bilirubin (total: 0.1-1.2 mg/dl; conjugated/direct: <0.3 mg/dl; unconjugated/indirect: 0.1-1.0 mg/dl)
1. Jaundice is seen when levels of bilirubin rise above 2 mg/dl
2. Bilirubin is formed from breakdown of hemoglobin to bilirubin (direct) or is converted to bile (indirect) in the liver
3. Levels become elevated if there is excess hemolysis, poor liver function, or obstruction
4. Laboratories can easily measure total and direct; indirect can be calculated

H. Calcium (adult: 8.5-10.5 mg/dl; newborn 7.4-14.0 mg/dl; infant: 5.0-6.0 mg/dl; child 9-11.5 mg/dl)
1. Calcium levels are elevated in bone disease and hyperparathyroid conditions
2. Phosphorus levels usually fall as calcium levels rise

I. Carbon dioxide (adult normals in venous whole blood: 2-26 mM/L; in plasma or serum: 24-30 mM/L); elevated in metabolic alkalosis and decreased in metabolic alkalosis conditions such as diabetic ketoacidosis and renal failure

J. Chloride (adult: 100-106 mEq/L; newborn: 94-112 mEq/L; infant 95-110 mEq/L; child: 98-108 mEq/L); chloride levels are increased in acidotic states, decreased in alkalosis and generally follow potassium levels unless patients are taking potassium-sparing diuretics

K. Cholesterol (total) (adult: 120-220 mg/dl; infant: 70-175 mg/dl; child: 120-240 mg/dl)
   1. Cholesterol tests measure the tendency to form atherosclerosis
   2. Recent food and alcohol intake and many drugs affect results
   3. Cholesterol is found in all tissues and in circulation as both protective HDL and risk increasing LDL
   4. Hyperlipidemia can be caused by liver disease, renal failure, hypothyroidism, diabetes mellitus, obesity, alcohol use, and medications

L. Creatinine (adult male: 0.6-1.5 mg/dl; adult female: 0.2-0.9 mg/dl; infant to 6 years 0.3-0.6 mg/dl; older child: 0.4-1.2 mg/dl); levels are elevated in renal disease (very specific) and levels generally follows BUN levels

M. Creatine kinase (CK) (adult male: 17-148 U/L; adult female: 10-79 U/L)
   1. Infrequently ordered screening test but is a sensitive indicator of cardiac muscle damage
   2. Elevated in necrosis or atrophy of cardiac or skeletal muscle
   3. CK-MB isoenzyme used to evaluate for MI
   4. CK-BB isoenzyme is increased in malignant hyperthemia

N. Serum gamma-Glutamyl Transpeptidase (GGT, GGTP) (adult: 11-63 U/L); GGT is a sensitive indicator that is elevated in alcoholism and other conditions affecting the liver

O. Glucose (adult serum or plasma: 70-110 mg/dl; adult whole blood: 60-100 mg/dl; newborn: 30-80 mg/dl; child:- 60-100 mg/dl)
   1. Elevated in diabetes and Cushing disease and for those on steroid treatment
   2. Elevations above 500 mg/dl with low CO_2 associated with ketoacidosis
   3. World Health Organization defines any fasting measurement > 140 mg/ dL on more than one occasion or any test >200 mg/dl as evidence of diabetes; consider confirming with glycosylated hemoglobin

P. Lactate dehydrogenase (LD) (adult 45-240 U/L)
   1. Elevated LD with other tests being normal may indicate a hemolyzed specimen
   2. Extreme LD elevations are seen in myocardial infarction and certain types of anemia
   3. Measurement of isoenzymes can increase diagnostic specificity
   4. Lesser elevations point to hepatitis or damage to muscle or organs

Q. Magnesium (Mg) (adult 1.5-2.1 mEq/L; newborn: 1.4-2.9 mEq/L; child: 1.6-2.6 mEq/L)
   1. Levels are increased with increased dietary intake (antacids or cathartics), decreased renal function, or gastrointestinal absorption
   2. Levels are decreased in ketoacidosis, alcoholism, and several other disease states especially gastrointestinal or renal disturbances

R. Phosphorus (adult serum: 3.0-4.5 mg/dl; pediatric: 4.0-7.0 mg/dl)
   1. Most found in bone
   2. Always order with and compare to calcium levels
   3. Levels are elevated in kidney disease, hypoparathyroidism, hyperthyroidism, severe muscle injury, bone healing, and others
   4. Levels are decreased in hyperparathyroidism, renal disorders, chronic use of aluminum hydroxide antacids, diabetic acidosis, osteomalacia and others. In Vitamin D deficient states (osteomalacia) the PTH is elevated thus lowering Phosphorus levels

S. Potassium (K) (adult: 3.5-5.0 mEq/L, infant: 3.6-5.8 mEq/L; child 3.5-5.5 mEq/L)
   1. Needed for normal nerve and muscle impulse and influenced by acid-base disturbances
   2. High or low levels are cardiotoxic and can contraindicate elective surgery
   3. Many causes for both elevated and decreased levels; common cause of decreased

level is diuretic therapy with inadequate potassium and chloride supplementation

T. Protein (total) (adult total protein: 6.0-8.6 g/dl; adult albumin: 3.5-5.6 g/dl; adult globulin: 2.3-3.5 g/dl; newborn total: 4.6-7.4 g/dl; infant: 6.0-6.7 g/dl; child 5.9-8.1 g/dl)
1. Increased in hypergammaglobulinemias (best diagnosed with protein electrophoresis) or hypovolemic states
2. Decreased in nutritional deficiencies, decreased protein synthesis (liver disease), increased loss, increased catabolism (e.g., fever, inflammation) and dilution with fluids or water intoxication

U. Protein electrophoresis (PE)
1. Test separates total protein into five parts: albumin and the four globulin fractions, alpha-1, alpha-2, beta, and gamma
2. Can evaluate serum protein abnormalities
3. Normal ranges exist for each fraction of the PE at various age ranges

V. Sodium (Na) (adult serum: 135-145 mEq/L; infant: 134-150 mEq/L; child: 135-145 mEq/L)
1. Regulates acid-base equilibrium
2. Protects against fluid loss
3. Needed for normal muscle function
4. Increase is uncommon and usually due to dehydration
5. Decrease is caused by many conditions including overhydration, diuretic use, hepatic failure, and diabetic acidosis

W. Triglycerides (adult 30-175 mg/dl)
1. Synthesized from carbohydrates and stored in adipose tissue
2. Provide energy to skeletal and cardiac muscle
3. Found in very-low-density lipoproteins
4. Provide a good estimate of lipoproteins
5. Elevated by high carbohydrate diet, emotional stress, estrogen use, and oral contraceptives

X. Urea nitrogen (BUN) (adult 8-45 mg/dl; infant: 5-15 mg/dl; child: 10-36 mg/dl)
1. The end product of protein metabolism which occurs mostly in the liver
2. If the kidneys cannot excrete urea, it accumulates in blood
3. Increase is called azotemia, and high levels correlate with renal disease
4. Always compare BUN levels with serum creatinine

Y. Uric acid (adult men: 4.0-8.5 mg/dl; adult women: 2.3-7.3 mg/dl; pediatric: 2.2-5.8 mg/dl)
1. An end product of purine metabolism
2. Is cleared from the blood by the kidneys
3. Levels are increased with excessive production, such as lymphoproliferative conditions, or decreased kidney function
4. Thiazide diuretics, stress, fasting, and foods high in purines cause levels to be elevated

Z. Osmolality-serum: (282 - 295 mOsm/kg water; a serum osmolality of 285 mOsm correlates with a urine specific gravity of 1.010
1. Tests ability to maintain fluid balance status
2. In severe dehydration the value increases due to increase in BUN, glucose and sodium concentration
3. Levels increased (hyperosmolality) in renal disease, CHF, DM, Azotemia, hypernatremia and others
4. Levels decreased (hypoosmolality) in hyponatremia, low salt diet, excess water intake
5. Dehydration causes both serum and urine osmolality to increase

V. Immunologic and rheumatologic tests for antibody-dependent immunologic disorders

    A. Total lymphocyte count (adult: 1,000-3,000 cells/mm^3, childhood: 3,000-4,000 cells/mm^3)

        1. A measure of the total number of lymphocytes in the body

        2. Gives a good estimate of cellular immune system

        3. Elevated in myeloproliferative disorders and decreased in immunocompromised states

        4. When abnormal counts are found, the subpopulation responsible should be investigated

    B. Measuring lymphocyte subpopulations

        1. Lymphocyte subpopulations such as T-cells, T-helper cells, suppressor-T cells, and B-cells can be measured as both the percentage of all lymphocytes and as an absolute number of cells/mm^3

        2. HIV Infection causes a selective decrease in T-helper cells with a concomitant increase in the T-suppressor cell to T-helper cell ratio

        3. With autoimmune diseases there is often an increase in the number of T-helper cells

    C. Quantitation of immunoglobulins (Qigs)

        1. Quantitative measurement can be made of the three major immunoglobulins: IgG, IgM and IgA, each has its own age-specific reference range

        2. These tests can measure the general state of immune function but are not very specific

        3. Elevated levels of IgG correlate with chronic infection, chronic inflammation, autoimmune disease, and neoplasm

        4. IgE measurement measures allergic responses

    D. Autoantibodies

        1. Detection and quantitation of autoantibodies are ordered when an autoimmune etiology is suspected

        2. Most results are reported in titers; presence of a titer increases suspicion of the presence of an underlying disease

        3. Many autoimmune diseases are silent for long periods of time after autoantibodies are encountered

        4. Some examples are as follows:

Test	Reference range	Possible Disorder
ANA	≤1:40	Multiple systemic Rheumatologic disorders (95% specific for SLE)
Islet cell	None	Type I diabetes
Rheumatoid factor	<1:20	Rheumatoid arthritis
Sm antigen	None	Positive in 30% SLE

    E. Complement Activation

        1. Many antibody-mediated immunologic disorders, such as rheumatologic diseases and gram-negative infections, are associated with a production of complement-fixating antibodies

        2. Specific sites on the antibody molecules bind and activate the complement cascade, resulting in damage to the target cell, which results in an increased activation and decreased level of complement

        3. Complement can be measured as total complement or, preferably, by the amount of the components, which is called split products (e.g., C3, C4, C4d); each has its own reference range, and its absence is often associated with specific disease states (e.g., SLE) or a propensity to develop pyogenic infections

        4. C3 (adult normal: 70-150 mg/dl) is increased in subacute inflammation and decreased in immune-complex disease, especially SLE

        5. C4 (adult normal: 10-30 mg/dl) is decreased in SLE

VI. Acute inflammatory reactants: These tests measure acute and chronic inflammatory, neoplastic, and infectious states; unexplained mild and transient increases are common; occasionally an extreme elevation is noted in the absence of disease; not infrequently the tests are normal in patients with active disease. APR refers to protein acute phase reactants that increase in any inflammatory situation

   A. Erythrocyte sedimentation rate (ESR) / Sed rate algorithm for Westergren upper limit of normal for adult males: (age)/2 reported in mm/hr; for adult females: (age + 10)/2, reported in mm/hr, newborns: 0-2 mm/hr; child: 3-13 mm/hr
      1. Measures the distance that red blood cells (RBCs) fall in plasma over a period of time
      2. Wintrobe method is better for mild elevations and Westergren method is better for higher levels
      3. Reference ranges are age and sex dependent for both methods
      4. In patients with cancer, an ESR > 100 mm/hr might indicate metastasis
   B. C-reactive protein (CRP) (adult normal: < 8 mg/L)
      1. A plasma protein that can rise as much as 30 fold after a tissue injury from a previously almost undetectable level
      2. Quite useful in following the progress of rheumatic diseases
      3. Levels rise and fall faster than the ESR thus more sensitive
      4. Rises caused by surgery should fall by the third day
      5. Persistent elevation should alert a clinician to the possibility of a postoperative complication

VII. Pregnancy testing: Human chorionic gonadotropin (HCG) is produced by the placenta during pregnancy and can be measured in serum as soon as 10 days after conception

   A. Urine analysis HCG
      1. Latex agglutination test easily performed in the office
      2. Urine HCG can detect pregnancy as early as the fourth day after missed menstruation and is 95% reliable by the tenth to the fourteenth day
      3. A first morning voided urine is needed for the test
   B. Serum immunoassay of HCG (Normal in males and non-pregnant females is 0.1 IU/L but has been reported as high as 5-10 IU/L)
      1. The immunoassay test for HCG becomes positive as early as ten days after conception
      2. More than 95% reliable by fourteenth day and starts to drop in the third month

VIII. Urinalysis: is divided into three parts: visual, chemical and microscopic. The chemical usually consists of a combination of tests usually performed with dried reagents on a "dipstick." The microscopic is performed on a sediment formed from a centrifuged portion of the urine looking for crystals and formed elements, such as white and red blood cells. The specimen of choice is first morning, mid-stream clean catch urine. Positive chemistry tests should be confirmed by more specific or exacting tests. Formed elements are reported as the number per high power field (hpf) when a test tube of urine is concentrated by centrifugation and the "plug" is examined with a microscope. The concentration (osmolality) of the urine can affect the appearance of the formed elements

   A. Visual - Color: Urine color can indicate the presence of metabolites such as bilirubin (yellow) or hemoglobin (red) or the presence of colored chemicals that "stain" the urine; not all laboratories report color
   B. Chemical
      1. Specific gravity (adult normal: 1.002-1.030)

    a.   Specific gravity is usually measured by a urinometer or a refractometer and is a measure of the concentrating ability of the kidneys and the hydration state of the patient

    b.   Chemistry tests on urine - usually done with "dipstick"

2.   Osmolality – (average is about 500 - 800 mOsm)

    a.   Better measure of urine concentration than specific gravity

    b.   In AM should be about 3X serum level

    c.   Increased in dehydration and low on diruretics or inability of kidneys to concentrate urine

3.   pH: Provides an indication of add-base balance of the body and is useful in the characterization of urine crystals

4.   Protein: Levels are elevated in kidney disease or when there is excess protein load as can occur with inflammatory and myeloproliferative disorders

5.   Glucose: Measurable glucose in the urine is present when the patient's glycemia exceeds approximately 180 mg/dl or if there is damage to kidney (less likely); the lack of ability of the dipstick to measure galactose makes it unsuitable in some pediatric situations

6.   Ketones: Present in urine during starvation and diabetes mellitus (ketoacidosis)

7.   Blood: Blood in the urine can result from lysed RBCs; also measures myoglobin present after muscle injury or from RBCs that have lysed in the circulation

8.   Bilirubin: The test measures conjugated bilirubin that may be elevated after liver damage

9.   Urobilinogen: Urobilinogen elevation in the urine correlates with any cause of elevated serum bilirubin; test is of little clinical value

10. Nitrite: A test for bacteria in the urine that converts the naturally occurring nitrates to nitrite

11. Leukocyte esterase - Test measures an enzyme found in white blood cells (WBCs); its absence might indicate an absence of an infection, but a negative test should not substitute for the microscopic analysis of WBCs in the urine

C. Microscopic - Formed elements: the "microscopic" part of the urinalysis

1.   RBCs (adult normal: < 3/hpf): Increased numbers found in urinary system diseases (including infection) as well as appendicitis and intestinal disorders

2.   WBCs (adult normal: < 5/hpf): Pyuria, or the presence of white blood cells in the urine, indicates inflammation or infection of the urinary tract; acute infections can produce more than 50 WBCs/hpf

3.   Bacteria: Bacteria seen in the urine may indicate an infection but is not considered a reliable test; presence of WBCs is more reliable

4.   Epithelial cells can be distinguished by their shape

5.   Squamous cells are usually found in the distal urethra, but they are also found in the vagina and the vulva; in a female's specimen, they indicate that the specimen might not be a clean catch, which lessens its value as an accurate specimen

6.   Transitional epithelial cells line much of the urinary tract, and their presence in numbers greater than a few cells should be investigated

7.   Renal tubular cells are found in increased numbers when infection or damage has occurred to the renal tubules

8.   Casts are formed when various proteins that have precipitated in the renal tubules break loose and flow in urine

    a.   Hyaline casts, formed from protein, occur normally in small numbers with slight increases after exercise; large numbers may non-specifically indicate renal damage

    b.   Red blood cell casts, even when reported as hemoglobin casts or blood casts, indicate renal disease or, less likely, endocarditis

      c.   White blood cell casts carry the same significance as white blood cells

      d.   Tubular epithelial cell casts may indicate tubule pathology

      e.   Granular casts are described as fine or coarse; they can be transiently present in small numbers after exercise in normal individuals; and large numbers or persistently preset suggest renal disease

      f.   Waxy casts are thought to be formed from the breakdown of granular casts

      g.   Fatty casts indicate renal damage or the possibility of damage to the body's fat or bone marrow storage areas

9.   Crystals: A variety of crystals form in the urine, some only in acid and some only in basic urine; urine standing at room temperature enhances the development of crystals; however, the presence of crystals does not necessarily indicate disease

      a.   Calcium oxalate crystals are relatively common but possibly indicate hypercalciuria or hyperparathyroidism

      b.   Uric acid crystals are frequently found in acid urine; high amounts might indicate increased purine metabolism

      c.   Amorphous crystals are commonly encountered; they are defined as urates, in acid urine and phosphates if the urine is alkaline; these are of minimal significance

      d.   Calcium phosphate crystals are found in alkaline urine; they are of minimal significance

      e.   Cystine crystals may indicate the presence of metabolic disorders

      f.   Leucine or tyrosine crystals may indicate the presence of amino acid metabolism or other disorders

      g.   Sulfonamide crystals are found during treatment with some sulfur-containing drugs

10. Mucous threads are commonly found in normal individuals and are seen in increased numbers with inflammatory conditions of the urinary tract

11. Trichomonas vaginalis is a protozoan parasite whose presence confirms infection

IX. Complete blood count (CBC) and coagulation abnormalities

A. **The complete blood count** (CBC, or sometimes, hemogram) is performed on whole, anticoagulated blood; CBC measurements include the numbers of WBCs, the WBC differential, the RBC count, hemoglobin (Hgb), hematocrit (Hct), RBC indices, and an estimation of the number of platelets

    1.   White blood count (adult normal: 4,500-11,000/µl, at 1-4 years: 1,500-8,500/µl)

      a.   Infections usually cause an increase in the WBC count to 17,000 or more

      b.   Other causes of an increase include trauma, including recent surgery, and some medications

      c.   Severe increases might indicate leukemia

      a.   Important information is found by determining the percentage of the types of WBCs (the differential)

      e.   Low levels might be hereditary, or secondary to immunosuppressive medications

      f.   Total WBC = 4,500 – 10.000/µl

    2.   WBC differential

      a.   Neutrophils (also called PMNs or polymorphonuclear cells, "segs" or segmented neutrophils) (adult normal: 56%; at 12 months: 28%; at 4 years: 39%) (1,800 – 7,500/µl

         i.   The neutrophil count is increased in infection, inflammation, tissue damage, recent surgery, diabetic ketoacidosis, and from many medications

        ii. An increase in immature forms, called bands, is referred to as a shift to the left

   iii. The presence of band cells or myelocytes, both of which are immature forms of granulocytes, are thought to indicate an overtaxed bone marrow that cannot produce enough mature forms to answer a challenge

   iv. Less than normal neutrophil levels place the patient at an increased risk of infection

 b. Lymphocytes (adult normal: 34%; at 12 months: 61%; at 4 years: 50%)

   i. Transient lymphocyte increases are often seen in viral diseases

   ii. Leukemias cause persistent elevations of the lymphocyte count

   iii. Special reactive or atypical lymphocytes are seen in viral hepatitis, infectious mononucleosis, and other disorders

   iv. Total lymphocyte count is 1,500 – 4,000/μl

 c. Monocytes (normals: <5% after 12 months): Increases in monocyte numbers can often be associated with malignancies and rheumatologic disorders (200-900/ml)

 d. Eosinophils (normals: <4% after 12 months): Increases are seen in allergic reactions and parasitic infection or infestations (0-700/μl)

 e. Basophils (normals: <1%): Increases, without concomitant increases in PMNs, are usually results of myeloproliferative disorder (0-150/μl)

3. RBCs: RBCs develop from nucleated normoblasts that extrude their nuclei and develop into reticulocytes, which are released into the circulation from marrow sites and quickly develop into typical erythrocytes. Erythrocytes live and function for about 120 days, transporting oxygen and carbon dioxide on their hemoglobin molecules; at the end of their life span, they are engulfed by phagocytes. Erythrocytes are broken down into iron that is recirculated, amino acid-rich globin, and a part that is ultimately excreted as urobilinogen in urine and feces

 a. RBC count (adult normals males: 4.6-6.2 million/μl; adult females: 4.2-5.4 million/μl; newborn: 4.0-6.3 million/μl; 12 months: 3.6-5.0 million/μl)

   i. By definition anemia is a low RBC count; causes of anemia include diet, medications, systemic disease, and blood loss

   ii. Polycythemia, or too many RBCs, is characteristic of a physiologic response to low levels of oxygen or certain kidney tumors

 b. Mean corpuscular volume (MCV) (adult normal: 82-98 μm^3; 12 months: 87-100 μm^3)

   i. MCV forms the basis for anemia classification

   ii. Microcytic anemias, such as iron deficiency or chronic disease, have low MCVs

   iii. Macrocytic anemias, such as those of alcoholic liver disease, have high MCVs

   iv. Normocytic anemias are further divided into two categories:

    1) Those with high reticulocyte counts indicate increased RBC production secondary to hemolysis or blood loss, and

    2) Those with low reticulocyte counts indicate decreased RBC production such as found with bone marrow suppression

 c. RBC shape and size (normally 0.2-μm thick and 6.7-7.8-μm in diameter)

   i. Anisocytosis refers to a collection of varying size RBCs, a condition of some anemias

   ii. Acanthocytosis, or spur cells, have spike-like projections on the surface of the cell and are seen in some enzyme-deficiency conditions and after splenectomy

   iii. Other conditions to be aware of include the presence of large red blood cells (macrocytes), small cells (microcytes), inclusion bodies (e.g., Heinz, Howell-Jolly), and shapes like poikilocytosis and schistocytes

   iv. Sickle cells have unusual hemoglobin molecules that present as sickle cell disease or thalassemia

     d. Mean corpuscular hemoglobin concentration (MCHC) (adult normal: 32%-36%; 12 months: 27%-33%): A calculated value describing the hemoglobin concentration in the average RBC

     e. Mean corpuscular hemoglobin (MCH) (adult normal 27-31 pg; 12 months: 22-32 pg): A calculated value that is increased in macrocytic anemias and decreased in microcytic anemias

     f. Hemoglobin (Hgb) (adult normal male: 13.5-18 g/dl; female: 12-16 g/dl; newborn: 14-20 g/dl; 12 months: 11.2-14 g/dl; 3 years: 11.2-12.5 g/dl): Low values are indicative of anemia

     g. Reticulocyte count (adult normal 0.5%-1.5%; 25,000-75,000 cells/µl)
       i. Reticulocytes are immature RBCs
       ii. The reticulocyte count is useful for dividing normocytic anemias into those of decreased or increased production

     h. Platelets/thrombocytes (adult normal 150,000-400,000/µl; newborns: 150,000-250,000/µl): Hemorrhagic conditions are evident with low platelet levels

B. Coagulation tests: A routine evaluation of coagulation can be accomplished with a platelet count, bleeding time, prothrombin time, an activated partial thromboplastin time or the platelet function analysis; more specific tests are available if any of these is found to be abnormal or if there is a family history of clotting abnormalities

  1. Bleeding time (BT) (adult normal 1.5-9.5 minutes):
     a. Time to clot from a standardized skin puncture
     b. BT > normal usually indicates a problem with platelet numbers or function
     c. Poorly standardized and subject to technique errors
     d. Repeated and pediatric tests unpleasant

  2. Platelet Function Analysis (PFA) - automated test to replace BT

  3. Activated partial thromboplastin time (APTT/PIT) (adult normal 25-38 seconds)
     a. PTT measurements evaluate the intrinsic and common clotting pathways
     b. Prolonged values indicate increased risk of bleeding
     c. The PTT is used to monitor heparin therapy

  4. Prothrombin test (PT) (adult normals < 2 seconds from control): A prolonged PT identifies defects of the vitamin K-dependent path of the extrinsic and common pathways

X. Synovial fluid: Aspirated under strict sterile technique, synovial fluid is normally clear and pale yellow. In normal synovial fluid a mucin clot is compact, there are fewer than 200 WBCs/mm³, and the differential shows less than 25% polymorphonuclear cells. Normal synovial fluid will string out 4-6 cm from the end of a needle from which it is slowly expressed. Glucose concentration should be within 20 mg/dl of the serum glucose value. The pH is 7.2-7.6, and crystals are absent

A. RBCs in the joint can indicate either bleeding during taking the sample or the presence of blood in the joint

B. WBCs in the joint above normal levels indicate inflammation or infection

C. Mucin in the joint will clot with the addition of 2% acetic acid; a poor clot usually correlates with a high WBC concentration, suggesting an infection or inflammation

D. Crystals of uric acid (gout), CPPD (pseudogout), cholesterol, corticosteroid, or lithium heparin are often identified using polarized light microscopy

E. Glucose conversion to lactate can be a valuable early indication of joint infection; infectious arthritis can result in joint glucose levels <50% of the serum levels; and other inflammatory conditions cause a lesser decrease

Y. Arterial blood gases

Arterial blood gases (ABG) are used to evaluate the respiratory and acid-base systems; as a rule, the sum of the PO_2 and PCO_2 should be less than 140 mm Hg

   A. pH (adult normal: 7.35-7.45): The pH is regulated by physiologic buffers (bicarbonate, Hgb, protein, and phosphate) and the excretion of metabolic acid products by the lungs (CO_2) and kidneys (ammonium ions)

   B. PO_2 (adult normal: 75-105 mm Hg): Hypoxemia or low levels of PO_2 indicate low respiratory levels, low cardiac output, abnormal hemoglobins, or increased O_2 consumption

   C. PCO_2 (adult normal: 33-44 mm Hg): High rates of ventilation such as might occur with hyperventilation result in decreased PCO_2 levels. High levels indicate poor lung function

   D. HCO_3 (adult normal: 22-26 mEq/L): Bicarbonate concentration is usually calculated from measured values of pH and PCO_2 using the Henderson-Hasselbalch equation; levels are increased in acidotic conditions, and the converse is also true

   E. BE (base excess): (adult normals: -2-+2 mEq/L): Negative values of base excess indicate a decrease is available buffer; a condition found in increased acid production

   F. O_2 saturation (adult normal > 95%): A calculated value indicating the relative amount of O_2 being carried by the Hgb compared to the total amount of Hgb in the blood; venous blood is 65%-75% saturated

ORGAN SYSTEM ANALYSIS

   I. Cardiovascular disease: Creatine kinase (CK) and lactate dehydrogenase (LD) are called the cardiac enzymes because they are such invaluable markers of myocardial injury

   A. CK is an enzyme found in high concentrations in cardiac muscle. CK is the first enzyme elevated when the myocardium is damaged; and the CK-MB form of the enzyme (called an isoenzyme) is exclusively found in heart muscle and is more specific than a general CK measurement

   B. LD is present in high concentration in virtually all muscle; exercise and strenuous physical activity, as well as cardiac damage and pulmonary disease, elevate LD levels; and an isoenzyme, LD-1, is more specific for cardiac muscle

   C. Aspartate aminotransferase (AST/SGOT) levels increase in response to cardiac damage

   D. Arterial blood gasses assess the adequacy of ventilation and perfusion and evaluate metabolic acidosis

   E. Troponin is a complex of proteins in cardiac muscle that elevates after cardiac injury in 4-8 hours to a level above 1.2 ng/dl. (The normal value or troponin is <o.06 ng/ml.) The complex is made up of non-specific troponin B and cardiac specific I and C, either of which can be used as a marker. Together they are sometimes given the name troponin "T". While CPK-MB levels return to normal after 2 days, the tropnonin level remains increased for up to 10 days permitting late diagnosis of a cardiac event

   II. Central nervous system (CNS) and peripheral nervous system: Refer to the reference texts for discussions of cerebrospinal fluid analysis

   III. Endocrine

   A. Thyroid function: Hypothalamus → TRH → pituitary → TSH → thyroid → ↑ inactive T4 → ↑ active T3 → ↓ TRH and ↓ TSH

1. Hypothyroidism – cold intolerance, weight gain, dry skin, fatigue, myxedema
   a. See ↑ TSH and ↓ Free T4 (↓ negative feedback of T4 on TSH)
2. Hyperthyroidism – weight loss, fatigue, heat intolerance, nervousness, palpitations, Graves disease and goiter
   a. Hashimoto's thyroiditis or secondary to pituitary or hypothalamic disease
   b. See ↓ TSH and ↑ T4 and ↑ T3
   c. TSH – single most important thyroid test. Rule of Thumb: For screening purposes a normal TSH indicates a normal thyroid. Danesse (1996) advises that a sTSH obtained every five years in all adults is cost effective. It will detect early thyroid disease and minimize the risks associated with its sequelae such as lipid disorders, altered mental status and dysrhythmia
   d. If the TSH level is clearly elevated (suggesting hypothyroidism), confirmation with a total or a free- T_4 test is appropriate
   e. If the TSH level is undetectable (suggesting hyperthyroidism), confirmation with a total or free-T_4 test would be helpful
   f. If the TSH level is subnormal but borderline (also suggesting hyperthyroidism), a total or free-T_4 test may be helpful. Ultimately, a TRH stimulation study may be required to further define thyroid function

B. **Parathyroid:** The parathyroid controls serum calcium and, indirectly, serum phosphorus; these two tests provide a good window into parathyroid function. Parathyroid hormone, itself, can be measured by a variety of techniques, each with its own normal range. Elevated levels of PTH indicate hyperparathyroidism; patients with hyperparathyroidism demonstrate hypercalcemia and hypophosphatemia. In Vitamin D deficient states there is a decrease in serum calcium with a corresponding increase in PTH. Elevated PTH will attempt to raise Calcium levels and lower phosphate levels

C. **Diabetes:** During a fasting state the plasma concentration of glucose is maintained by the breakdown of glycogen (glycogenolysis) and the conversion of protein to glucose (gluconeogenesis). Insulin and glycogen are intimately involved in these processes. Other hormones, including growth hormone, glucocorticoids, thyroid hormones, and epinephrine also have effects on blood sugar levels. Random and fasting glucose tests form the basis for diabetes diagnosis. Diabetic control during the previous three months is monitored by measuring glycosylated hemoglobin. Measuring glycosylated blood proteins, such as fructosamine, is a measure of blood sugar control over the prior three weeks
   1. Glucose measurements – The American Diabetes Association Expert Committee in committee states that diabetes can be detected by any of three positive tests. To confirm the diagnosis, there must be a second positive test on a *different* day
      a. A fasting blood glucose of 126 mg/dL or greater on two or more tests on different days
      b. A random glucose level of 200 mg/dL or greater when symptoms are present but must be confirmed on another day with a positive fasting plasma glucose or a positive oral GTT
      c. A 2-hour oral glucose tolerance test (GGT) of 200 mg/dL at the 2-hour mark repeated on two different days. The Committee urges that this test be phased out as too unreliable
   2. Glycohemoglobin (Glycerated hemoglobin, glycosylated hemoglobin, Ghb, and Hemoglobin A1c HbA1c)
      a. Test gives a sense of the level of glucose control of the diabetic patient in the previous 3 months
      b. Glucose binds permanently and irreversibly to RBC hemoglobin

      c. Reference ranges vary depending on the method used; generally, a 1% rise in Ghb levels translates into a 35 mg/dl increase in serum glucose

      d. In terms of control, 7% is considered good control (equal to a daily average of 150 mg/dl), 10% is fair (240 mg/dl), and 12% is poor (300 mg/dl)

      e. A level of 5.5% corresponds to an average blood glucose of 100 mg/dl

      f. Test has low sensitivity and high specificity

      g. Normal values do not rule out impaired glucose intolerance

      h. The test can be ordered any time of day without regard for food intake

      i. The diagnosis of diabetes is not made on the basis of this test alone

    2. Insulin tolerance levels: See prior for a discussion of the insulin tolerance test and how it is used with glucose tolerance testing to diagnose diabetes; diabetes-in-situ is the condition where there is a normal glucose tolerance test and an abnormal insulin tolerance test

    3. Insulin levels are measurable with an Immunoassay. Levels elevated in islet cell tumors and in NIDDM. Elevated insulin levels correlate with ASO

IV. Gastrointestinal disease: Gastric disorders are not well monitored by the routine blood chemistry tests; consider the measurement of gastrin, pepsinogen, and insulin to evaluate this system

V. Liver. Hepatic damage can result in 4 scenarios: ↓ hepatocyte synthesis, direct hepatic injury, obstructive biliary injury and improper bilirubin clearance

A. Decreased ability for proteins synthesis

    1. Albumin, fibrinogen and serum protein decreased

    2. Decreased binding proteins for copper and iron

    3. Prolonged prothrombin time

    4. Rule of Thumb: albumin levels of < 1.0 g/dl and Prolonged Prothrombin times with INR of > 1.5 are seen in patients with severe, chronic and end-stage liver disease

B. Direct injury to hepatocytes (60% of liver cells)

    1. Enzymes from hepatocytes released: AST/SGOT, ALT/SGPT and LDH all elevated

    2. Rule of Thumb: AST and ALT > 10X normal = severe liver damage

    3. Hepatitis or drug damage/toxicity

C. Obstruction of biliary tree

    1. Alk Phos, GGT and 5-NT all elevated

    2. Rule of Thumb: Alk Phos 10X normal in absence of bone disease = obstruction

    3. Albumin, total protein, AST and ALT all near normal

D. Improper biliary clearance

    1. Breakdown product of hemoglobin cleared by liver

    2. "Conjugated - direct" form elevated in liver damage or biliary obstruction

    3. Note: "unconjugated-indirect" form from blood hemolysis

    Note: y-Glutamyl transferase (GGT) levels are elevated in liver disease; the level increases rapidly after alcohol consumption and is a good marker for both acute and chronic alcoholism; GGT levels are also increased in pancreatitis, kidney disease, diabetes mellitus, and prostate cancer

VI. Musculoskeletal and joint disease

A. CK is elevated in many diseases of muscle, including polymyositis and muscular dystrophies, but is normal in most joint diseases and atrophic muscle states; along with LDH and AST/SGOT, CK is elevated in malignant hypothermia

B. Rheumatoid arthritis (RA)

1. Tests for rheumatoid arthritis (RA) include the presence of rheumatoid factor (RF) in the serum and poor mucin clotting of synovial fluid
2. A significant titer for RF is > 1:80
3. SLE, Sjogren's, and other connective diseases can also have elevated RFs
4. ESR and C-reactive protein are usually elevated in RA
5. RF tests are usually negative in psoriatic arthritis

C. Gout

1. Shows the presence of urate crystals in polarized light microscopy
2. Although serum uric add levels are usually elevated, up to a third of gout patients have uric acid levels within the normal range
3. Recent aspirin use may artificially lower the uric acid value
4. There is a modest increase in the WBC count and ESR during an attack

D. Septic arthritis has characteristic findings in synovial fluid analysis; a gram's stain can be useful for bacterial diagnosis and acid-fast stain for mycobacteria

E. Polymyalgia rheumatica has a marked increase in ESR, a mild anemia, and sometime a decrease in albumin; serum enzymes, such as AP and AST/SGOT, are increased in some patients

F. Osteoarthritis: Results of routine chemistry tests are uniformly negative and not helpful

VII. Nutritional Status

A. Hemoglobin – decreases in anemia <14 g/dL for men and <12 g/dL for women

B. Hematocrit – decreases in anemia < 37% for men and < 36% for women

C. Albumin (normal 3.5-5.0 g/dL)

1. Levels <3.5 g/dL (<2.8 g/dL severe) nutritional deficiency
2. Correlates with long term wasting and not short term dietary change
3. Prealbumin (normal 15-40 mg/dL) (AKA thyroxine-binding prealbumin or transthyrettin [TTHY])
   a. Replacing albumin in some centers
   b. <5 mg/dL is severe nutritional deficiency

D. Total Protein Serum (normal 6.0 – 8.0 g/dL) - Levels <6.0 mg/dL result in low osmotic pressure so that fluids and nutrition do not flow into cells

E. Total lymphocyte count (normal 1,500 – 3,000 cells) Rule out chemotherapy, infection and autoimmune diseases as cause of low value. <800 cells is severe decrease

F. Transferrin (normal 180-260 mg/dL)

1. Iron deficiency causes transferrin levels to rise even with proper nutrition
2. This test valuable with iron levels normal
3. < 100 mg/dL severe; 100-150 mg/dL moderate and 150-170mg/dL mild nutritional deficiency

G. Nitrogen balance studies - Measure urine nitrogen compared to 24 hour protein intake

VIII. Renal status: Kidney function is normal when the glomerular filtration rate (GFR) and tubular function are normal; a decrease in kidney function results in an increase in nitrogenous end products (uremia), hyperkalemia, and acidosis; tubular damage results in acidosis, hypokalemia, hypophosphatemia, and hypouricemia

A. Blood urea nitrogen (BUN normal = 10-20 mg/dl): High urea levels are indicative of poor kidney function; urea clearance from the kidney can be used to measure GFR, and BUN should be run with and compared to serum creatinine

    B. Serum creatinine: Creatinine levels rise with poor kidney function; it is a more sensitive and specific test of renal function than BUN

    C. Urine creatinine levels

        1. Levels are very stable and vary only when its excretion via the kidney is compromised

        2. Creatinine clearance has become a popular way to measure GFR

        3. GRF is synonomous with Creatinine Clearance Rate

        4. A traditional test involves collecting a 24-hour urine sample although it can be done with as little as a 2-hour sample; an easier method to estimate GFR can be determined by a calculation involving serum creatinine levels

        5. Normal creatinine levels < 1.0 mg/dl

        6. Creatinine of 2 mg/dl = 50% ↓ GFR and creatinine of 4 mg/dl = 75% ↓ GFR

    D. Urinalysis is important in assessing kidney function

IX. Pancreas: With any acute injury to the pancreas, serum amylase rises within 6 hours. Serum pancreatic isoamylase (isoenzymes of amylase) can identify the specific amylase of the pancreas (as opposed to that of the salivary glands). Amylase levels fall before that of lipase. Both lipase and amylase levels should be ordered in suspected pancreatitis. Normal ranges for both tests depend on the assay method used

    A. Amylase: A useful marker for pancreas activity but it is also found in salivary glands; isoenzymes can separate pancreatic from salivary amylase

    B. Lipase: The only organ of the body containing lipase is the pancreas; thus, it is a more or less specific test for pancreatitis when the test is available

X. Respiratory disease: Arterial blood gasses and pH measurements assess the adequacy of ventilation and perfusion and evaluate metabolic acidosis

XI. Prostate disease

    A. Measurement made of PSA – prostate specific antigen. Normally slowly increases with age

    B. Normals: Age 40-49<2.5 ng/ml, 50-59< 3.5ng/ml, 60-69<4.5ng/ml, 70-79<6.5ng/ml

    C. More than 5-8% increase in 1 year is abnormal

    D. Elevations seen in inflammation and CA

    E. Rectal examination before the test does not influence the result

    F. Not specific - only 30 of 100 men with elevation of PSA have cancer

    G. Nearly 75% of men with results from 3-10 ng/ml have BPH (benign prostatic hyperplasia)

BIBLIOGRAPHY

Cowan, DF, Olano, JP. A Practical Guide to Clinical Laboratory Testing, 1st edition. Blackwell Science, Inc. 1997.

Danese MD, Powe NR, Sawin CT, et al. Screening for mild thyroid failure at the periodic health examination: a decision and cost effectiveness analysis. JAMA 1996;276:285-92.

Deska, K, Pagana, TJ, et al. Mosby's Manual of Diagnostic and Laboratory Tests, 2nd edition. Mosby Year Book 2002.

Henry, JB, editor. Clinical Diagnosis and Management by Laboratory Methods, W B Saunders Co, 2001.

Helfand M, Redfern CC, Sox HC. Screening for thyroid disease. Ann Intern Med 1998;129:141-3.

Howanitz JH, Howanitz PJ, eds. Laboratory Medicine: Test Selection and Interpretation. Churchill Livingston, New York, 1991.

McPhearson, RA Editor, Tietz Clinical Guide to Laboratory Tests, W B Saunders Co, 2002.

Pribor HP, Hurlbut TA. The Laboratory Consultant. Lea & Febiger, Philadelphia, 1992.

Speicher CH. The Right Test, A Physician's Guide to Laboratory Medicine, 2nd ed. W.B. Saunders Co., Philadelphia, 1990.

Tietz NW, Finley PR, Pruden EL. Clinical Guide to Laboratory Tests, 2nd ed. W.B. Saunders Co., Philadelphia, 1990.

Tilkian SM, Conover MB, Tilkian AG. Clinical Implications of Laboratory Tests. C.V. Mosby Co., St. Louis, 1987.

Wallach MD. Interpretation of Diagnostic Tests, 5th ed. Little Brown and Co., Boston, 1992.

CHAPTER 2
LABORATORY MEDICINE

1.   Which of the following is not typically included in a CBC?

    A.   Differential leukocyte count
    B.   Total erythrocyte count
    C.   Reticulocyte count
    D.   Total leukocyte count
    E.   Hemoglobin levels

2.   Which of the following are true regarding the fasting blood glucose test?

    A.   Elevated levels can be confirmed with a glycosylated hemoglobin test
    B.   Values are decreased in patients receiving steroid therapy
    C.   Ketoacidosis can result from mild increases in blood glucose levels
    D.   Diabetes can be diagnosed with a single test with results over 140 mg/dl

3.   Which of the following are associated with glucose intolerance (elevated glucose levels in a glucose tolerance test)?

    1.   Cushing's disease
    2.   Gestational diabetes mellitus
    3.   Non-insulin-dependent diabetes mellitus
    4.   Chronic pancreatitis

        A.   Only 1 and 3 are correct
        B.   Only 2 and 4 are correct
        C.   Only 1, 2, and 3 are correct
        D.   Only 4 is correct
        E.   All are correct

4.   A young type 1 diabetes patient presents to your office for a nail procedure and starts to "feel funny". The first step in testing a patient who has suspected diabetic ketoacidosis is:

    A.   Serum glucose levels
    B.   Plasma glucose levels
    C.   Hemoglobin A1C
    D.   Urine strip for glucose and ketones
    E.   Arterial blood gas (ABG)

5.   Which test(s) are helpful in trying to determine if a joint inflammation is caused by a bacterial infection:

    1.   Glucose concentration in joint fluid
    2.   Gram stain of the joint fluid
    3.   CBC
    4.   Serum glucose levels
    5.   WBC levels in the joint fluid

A.   Only 1 and 2 are correct
B.   Only 1, 2 and 3 are correct
C.   Only 1, 2, 3 and 4 are correct
D.   Only 2 and 5 are correct
E.   All are correct

6.   According to the American Diabetes Association a diagnosis of diabetes can be made when:

1.   Repeated random plasma glucose >200mg/dl on two tests on different days
2.   A single fasting glucose test >126mg/dl
3.   2 repeated fasting glucose tests on different days >126mg/dl
4.   A single 2 hour GTT >300mg/dl
5.   Repeated 2 hour GTT on different days >200mg/dl
6.   A single "elevated" HgbA1C test

A.   Only 1 and 3 are correct
B.   Only 1 and 5 are correct
C.   Only 3 and 5 are correct
D.   Only 3, 5 and 6 are correct
E.   All are correct

7.   A patient with bone pain might have a diagnosis of osteomalacia. What test findings are true in this condition?

1.   Hypocalcemia
2.   Hypercalcemia
3.   Elevated parathyroid levels (PTH)
4.   Decreased parathyroid levels (PTH)
5.   Elevated phosphorus serum levels
6.   Decreased phosphorus serum levels

A.   Only 1 is correct
B.   Only 2 is correct
C.   Only 1, 3 and 5 are correct
D.   Only 2, 4 and 6 are correct
E.   Only 1, 3 and 6 are correct

8.   Regarding test for Musculoskeletal and joint disease the following is true:

A.   CK (Creatine Kinase) is usually elevated in joint diseases
B.   A rheumatoid factor >1:80 is diagnostic of rheumatoid arthritis
C.   Urate crystals seen in dark field microscopy is positive for gout
D.   ESR and CRP and elevated in rheumatoid arthritis
E.   Abnormal mucin clots are frequently seen in osteoarthritis

9.   In the assessment of nutritional status for wound healing, you would order a nutritional consult if you found which of the following:

A.   Hemoglobin of 16 g/dl
B.   Hematocrit of 41%
C.   Prealbumin level of 5 mg/dl
D.   Albumin level of 4 g/dl
E.   Total lymphocyte count of 3,500/ul

10.   In the consideration of prescribing an antibiotic that is cleared by the kidney, which of the following tests
       would tend to make you decrease the dose of the medication?

       A.   Serum albumin of 7 g/dl
       B.   Fasting serum glucose of 225 mg/dl
       C.   High urine specific gravity and osmolality
       D.   Serum BUN (blood urea nitrogen) of 14 mg/dl
       E.   Serum creatinine of 3 mg/dl

Chapter 3

PHARMACOLOGY

Erwin J. Juda

I. Conventional Analgesics

- **A. Epicritic** (Superficial Pain)
  1. Noxious stimulation of superficial somatic structures elicits sharp lancinating type of pain
  2. Generally well localized beginning and ending abruptly
  3. Not effectively relieved by conventional analgesics, the use of adjuvant analgesics alone or as an adjunct may prove beneficial (e.g., neuropathic pain)
- **B. Protopathic** (Deep Pain)
  1. Noxious stimulation of visceral structures presenting a dull aching type of pain
  2. Generally poorly defined with insidious onset and slow recession
  3. Very effectively relieved by conventional analgesics

II. Narcotic Agonist Analgesics (Opioids)

- **A. Opioid Analgesics**
  1. Morphine Sulfate
     - a. 10 to 30 mg po every 4 hours (Immediate Release)
     - b. 10 mg IM every 4 hours
     - c. MS Contin and Oramorph-SR: 15-60 mg po q8-12 h (Sustained Release)
     - d. Kadian: 20-100 mg po q12-24 h (Sustained Release)
  2. Levorphanol Tartrate (Levo-Dromoran)
     - a. 2 mg po or subcutaneously every 6 to 8 hours
  3. Hydromorphone (Dilaudid)
     - a. 2 to 4 mg po every 4 to 6 hours
  4. Methadone (Dolophine)
     - a. 2.5 to 10 mg po, SC or IM every 3 to 4 hours
  5. Meperidine (Demerol)
     - a. 50 to 150 mg po, SC or IM every 3 to 4 hours
  6. Codeine
     - a. 15 to 60 mg po, SC, IV or IM every 4 to 6 hours
  7. Oxycodone (Roxicodone, OxyContin)
     - a. 5 mg po every 6 hours (Immediate Release)
     - b. 10 to 40 mg po q8-12 hours (Sustained Release)
  8. Propoxyphene HCL (Darvon)
     - a. 65 mg po every 4 hours

   9. Propoxyphene Napsylate (Darvon-N)
      a. 100 mg po every 4 hours
   10. Oxymorphone (Numorphan)
      a. 0.5 mg IV or 1-1.5 mg IM every 4 to 6 hours
B. Actions
   1. Analgesia
      a. Exert their major effect by interacting with opioid receptors in the CNS
      b. The three primary opioid receptors are indicated as follows:
         i. MU Receptor - Supraspinal analgesia, respiratory depression, euphoria and physical dependence
         ii. Kappa Receptor - Spinal analgesia, sedation and pupillary constriction
         iii. Sigma Receptor - Dysphasia, hallucinations and psychomimetic effects
   2. Suppression of Cough Reflex
      a. Direct suppression of the cough center in the medulla
   3. Sedation
   4. Euphoria
   5. Preanesthetic Medication
C. Primary Adverse Effects
   1. Respiratory Depression
      a. Direct inhibition of respiratory center in brainstem
      b. Opioids are contraindicated in those with decreased respiratory reserve (e.g., emphysema) or excessive respiratory secretions (e.g., COPD)
   2. Nausea and Vomiting
      a. Direct stimulation of the chemoreceptor trigger zone
   3. Excessive Sedation or Drowsiness
   4. Physical or Psychological Dependence
   5. Hypotension
      a. Inhibits vasomotor center in brainstem causing peripheral vasodilation
   6. Constipation
      a. Decreased gastrointestinal motility
   7. Miosis
      a. Stimulation of Edinger-Westphal nucleus of oculomotor nerve causes characteristic pinpoint pupils
      b. Diagnostically important since most other causes of coma or respiratory depression produce dilation of the pupil
   8. Urinary Retention
      a. Decreased contractility of ureters and bladder
      b. Opioids should be used cautiously in patients with prostatic hypertrophy or urethral stricture
D. Drug Interactions
   1. MAO Inhibitors
      a. Seizures, coma, apnea and possible death particularly with Meperidine (Demerol)
      b. Mechanism - Unknown
   2. Tricyclic Antidepressants
      a. Seizures, hypotension, coma and possible death
      b. Mechanism - Unknown
   3. Antipsychotics
      a. Excessive hypotension and sedation especially with Phenothiazine group
      b. Mechanism - Pharmacologic synergism

    4. CNS Depressants

       a. Potentiates respiratory depression and sedation

E. Combination Products

    1. Oxycodone - Aspirin (Percodan)

    2. Oxycodone - Acetaminophen (Percocet, Roxicet, Tylox)

    3. Hydrocodone - Acetaminophen (Vicodin, Lortab, Anexsia, Zydone)

    4. Hydrocodone - Ibuprofen (Vicoprofen)

    5. Dihydrocodeine - Aspirin (Synalgos-DC)

    6. Codeine - Aspirin - Butalbital (Fiorinal w/Codeine)

    7. Codeine - Aspirin (Empirin w/Codeine)

    8. Codeine - Acetaminophen (Tylenol w/Codeine)

    9. Propoxyphene HCL - Aspirin (Darvon Compound-65)

    10. Propoxyphene Napsylate - Acetaminophen (Darvocet-N)

III. Narcotic Mixed Agonist - Antagonist Analgesics

A. Narcotics that stimulate one receptor but block at another receptor are classified as mixed agonist - Antagonist Analgesics (listed in descending order of antagonistic activity)

    1. Buprenorphine (Buprenex)

       a. 0.3 mg IM or slow IV every 6 hours in patients over age 13. Not recommended for children

       b. Strongest antagonist of this group equipotent with Naloxone

    2. Butorphanol (Stadol, Stadol-NS)

       a. 1 mg IV or 2 mg IM every 3 to 4 hours

       b. 1 mg Intranasally (1 spray in only one nostril). May repeat in 60-90 minutes. The initial 2 dose sequence can be repeated in 3 to 4 hours

    3. Nalbuphine (Nubain)

       a. 10 mg IV, SC or IM every 3 to 6 hours

    4. Dezocine (Dalgan)

       a. 5 to 20 mg IM every 3 to 6 hours

    5. Pentazocine (Talwin, Talwin-NX)

       a. 50 to 100 mg po every 3 to 4 hours

       b. Weakest antagonist of this group

       c. All members of this group can precipitate withdrawal symptoms

IV. Narcotic Antagonists

    A. Naloxone (Narcan)

       1. Rapidly reverses the coma and respiratory depression of opioid overdose

       2. 0.4 to 2 mg IV can cause reversal as quickly as within 30 seconds. Dose is repeated at 2 to 3 minute intervals up to total of 10 mg

       3. Produces no pharmacologic effects in normal individuals

    B. Naltrexone (Revia)

       1. Used for opiate-dependence maintenance programs and alcoholism due to longer duration of action

       2. Single oral dose of 50 mg can block the effect of injected heroin up to 48 hours

    C. Nalmefene (Revex)

       1. Supplied in two dosage strengths

         a. 100 mcg for post-operative narcotic reversal

         b. 1 mg for management of heroin overdose in addicts

V. Central Analgesics

    A. Tramadol (Ultram)

        1. Atypical centrally acting synthetic analgesic approved for moderate to moderately severe pain

        2. Exerts a dual mechanism of action

            a. Binds to MU - opioid receptor

            b. Inhibits reuptake of Norepinephrine and Serotonin

        3. Analgesia comparable to acetaminophen/Codeine and Aspirin/Codeine combinations

        4. Most common adverse effects include dizziness, vertigo, nausea, constipation and headache

        5. May enhance seizure risk in patients taking anticonvulsants and neuroleptics

        6. Drug interactions with MAO inhibitors and CNS depressants

        7. Not an NSAID - has no anti-inflammatory activity

        8. Seizure risk is increased with doses above the recommended range, in patients taking opioids, MAO inhibitors and neuroleptics as well as those with history of seizures or recognized risk such as head trauma, alcohol and drug withdrawal and CNS infections

        9. Contraindicated in patients with history of anaphylactoid reactions to Codeine and other opioids

        10. Do not use in opioid-dependent patients and not recommended in those with history of drug dependence or abuse

            Dosage:

            a. Initiate with 25 mg/day in AM and titrate in 25 mg increments as separate doses every 3 days for total of 100 mg/day (25 mg qid) for chronic pain patients who do not need immediate pain relief

            b. After titration completed, 50-100 mg po q4-6 hours can be given not to exceed 400 mg/day (300 mg/day if over age 75)

    B. Tramadol/Acetaminophen (Ultracet)

        1. Combination product consisting of 37.5 mg Tramadol with 325 mg Acetaminophen

        2. Indicated for management of acute pain for 5 days or less

        3. Dosage: 2 tablets po q4-6 hours prn pain not to exceed 8 tablets per day

VI. Salicylates

    A. Salicylic Acid Derivatives

        1. Aspirin (Acetylsalicylic Acid, ASA)

            a. 325 to 650 mg po every 4 hours

            b. Rheumatic disorders may require 3.2 to 6 g/day

        2. Salsalate (Disalcid)

            a. Usual adult dose is 3,000 mg/day in divided doses

        3. Sodium Salicylate

            a. 325 to 650 mg po every 4 hours

        4. Choline Salicylate (Arthropan)

            a. 870 mg po every 3 to 4 hours

        5. Magnesium Salicylate (Magan)

            a. 650 mg po every 4 hours

        6. Choline Magnesium Trisalicylate (Trilisate)

        7. Diflunisal (Dolobid)

            a. Not a true salicylate since not hydrolyzed to form salicylic acid as the others but is labeled as a derivative

            b. 500 mg po every 8 to 12 hours

8. Sodium Thiosalicylate (Rexolate)
   a. Injectable Salicylate for IM use
   b. Acute gout dosage: 100 mg IM q 3-4 hours x 2 days, then 100 mg/day until asymptomatic

B. Actions
1. Analgesic
2. Antipyretic
3. Anti-inflammatory - Irreversible inhibition of enzyme prostaglandin H Synthase (Cyclooxygenase) to block the conversion of arachidonic acid to prostaglandins

C. Primary Adverse Effects
1. Gastrointestinal Effects
   a. Most common adverse effect especially in higher doses up to 70% of patients
   b. May contraindicate Salicylates in active peptic ulcer disease
2. Hypersensitivity
   a. Incidence is highest in patients with asthma, nasal polyps and recurrent rhinitis
   b. Hypersensitivity is most common with aspirin of the group and could include urticaria, bronchospasm and anaphylaxis
3. Reye's Syndrome
   a. Use of Salicylates especially aspirin in children or teenagers with influenza (flu) or chickenpox should be avoided
   b. Acute life-threatening condition characterized by vomiting and lethargy leading to delirium and coma
4. Salicylism
   a. Tinnitus, hearing loss or vertigo are signs of toxicity seen at high dosage levels
5. Hyperuricemia
   a. Serum uric acid levels are elevated at usual analgesic doses of Salicylates (<2 g/day) due to decreased uric acid excretion that could precipitate an acute gout attack
   b. Salicylates at higher anti-inflammatory dosage levels can decrease serum uric acid

D. Drug Interactions
1. Anticoagulants
   a. Increased bleeding and hypoprothrombinemia effects of Warfarin
   b. Mechanism - Protein binding displacement
2. Insulin
   a. Hypoglycemia
   b. Mechanism - Increased circulating concentration of Insulin
3. Sulfonylureas
   a. Hypoglycemia
   b. Mechanism - Protein binding displacement

VII. Acetaminophen (Tylenol)

A. Analgesic and antipyretic effects only
B. No anti-inflammatory activity
C. Alternative for aspirin to treat mild to moderate pain in those patients intolerant to aspirin, have a history for peptic ulcer or hemophilia, are taking anticoagulants or uricosuric drugs or at risk for Reye's syndrome
D. Excessive or overdosage associated with hepatotoxicity
E. Usual adult dosage - 325 to 650 mg po every 4 to 6 hours

ADJUVANT ANALGESICS

I.   **Tricyclic Antidepressants** (TCAs)

A. **Amitriptyline** (Elavil)
B. **Imipramine** (Tofranil)
C. **Nortriptyline** (Pamelor)
D. **Desipramine** (Norpramin)
   1. Tricyclic Antidepressant Group:
       a. Mechanism of Analgesia - may be related to inhibition of Norepinephrine and/or serotonin reuptake
       b. TCAs have proarrhythmic effects involving an increased risk for Torsade De Pointes
       c. Baseline EKG should be done and repeated after achieving therapeutic dose
       d. Avoid use in CHF especially if ejection fraction is 35% or less, ischemic heart disease, bundle branch block, benign prostatic hypertrophy and narrow angle glaucoma
       e. Initial dose for Amitriptyline:
              25 mg po hs if under age 65
              10 mg po hs if over age 65
       f. Therapeutic window for Amitriptyline is 10-100 mg/day
       g. Titration - increase by 10-25 mg at weekly intervals - Titrate to analgesia or side effects
       h. Therapeutic onset - 5 days to more than 4 weeks

II. **Anticonvulsants** - Considered second-line therapy for most neuropathies

A. **Gabapentin** (Neurontin)
   1. Mechanism of analgesia - unknown, structurally related to Gamma-Aminobutyric Acid (GABA) but does not interact with GABA receptors
   2. Inhibits N-type calcium channels
   3. Explored for its usefulness in pain from shingles
   4. Has attractive pharmacokinetic properties in that it does not bind to plasma protein, is not metabolized by the liver and is eliminated unchanged by renal excretion
   5. Initial dose - 300 mg po qd
   6. Titration - rapidly increase to 300-400 mg po tid-qid
   7. Therapeutic onset - several days to 2 weeks

B. **Carbamazepine** (Tegretol)
   1. Mechanism of analgesia - inhibits sodium channel activity
   2. Best agent for lancinating sharp pain
   3. FDA approved to treat trigeminal neuralgia
   4. Carries a black box warning for blood dyscrasias including agranulocytosis and aplastic anemia
   5. Hepatotoxicity is also a significant risk
   6. Baseline CBC w/diff, reticulocyte count, serum iron and monitored weekly x4 then every 3-6 months thereafter
   7. Baseline SMA-12 and hepatic function tests monitored periodically
   8. Initial dose - 100 mg po bid
   9. Titration - titrate dose upward every 7 days with range at 800-1200 mg daily in 3 or 4 divided doses

C. **Sodium Channel Blockers**
   1. Mexiletine (Mexitil)

        a. Mechanism of analgesia - sodium channel blocking activity decreases spontaneous firing of peripheral nerve fibers

        b. Contraindicated in liver failure, ventricular conduction defects and 2nd or 3rd degree heart block

        c. Initial dose - 150 mg po bid-qid

        d. Titration - 150 mg qd x 3 days, then bid x 3 days, then increase to maximum of 10 mg/kg/day

  2. Lidocaine Patch 5% (Lidoderm)

        a. Mechanism of analgesia - blocks neuronal sodium channels

        b. 10 cm x 14 cm patch contains 700 mg Lidocaine

        c. Systemic absorption is minimal and directly related to skin surface covered and duration of patch application

        d. At least 95% (665 mg) of the Lidocaine remains in a used patch with absorption being $3 \pm 2\%$ of the dose

        e. FDA approved to treat post-herpetic neuralgia

        f. Dosage - apply up to 3 patches over most painful area only once for up to 12 hours within a 24 hr period

  3. Lidocaine Cream 3% (LidaMantle)

        a. Mechanism of analgesia - blocks neuronal sodium channels

        b. Lidocaine 3% in an acid mantle base

        c. Skin acidifier base is formulated to provide an acid pH of 5.5 acting as an efficient vehicle for transporting Lidocaine into skin

        d. Dosage - apply to affected area bid - tid

  4. Lidocaine 2.5%/Prilocaine 2.5% (Emla, Emla anesthetic)

        a. Mechanism of analgesia - blocks neuronal sodium channels

        b. Eutectic mixture of Lidocaine 2.5% and 2.5% of Prilocaine

        c. Emla - Cream formulation available in 5 g with Tegaderm dressings and 30 g tube

        d. Emla anesthetic - disc formulation with 1 g Emla emulsion with surface contact of 10 square centimeters

D. Selective Serotonin Reuptake Inhibitors (SSRIs)

  1. Paroxetine (Paxil)

  2. Citalopram (Celexa)

        a. Mechanism of analgesia - inhibits reuptake of serotonin

        b. Generally less effective here than tricyclic antidepressants

        c. Trial may be warranted in patients unable to tolerate TCAs

        d. Paroxetine - reduced pain but less effective than Amitriptyline or Imipramine

        e. Citalopram - more effective than placebo in one study for decreasing diabetic neuro-pathic pain

        f. Paroxetine dose - 40 mg po qd

        g. Citalopram dose - 20-40 mg po qd

  3. Venlafaxine (Effexor, Effexor-XR)

        a. Mechanism of analgesia - inhibition of Norepinephrine and/or serotonin reuptake

        b. Structurally novel antidepressant chemically unrelated to TCAs

        c. Gaining interest because it combines the reuptake inhibition of Norepinephrine and serotonin without the anticholinergic effects as a theoretic advantage over TCAs

        d. Disadvantage - adverse reactions include elevated blood pressure and/or hypertension, irritability and insomnia

        e. Dosage - 75 mg/day up to 225 mg/day

  4. Clonidine (Catapres - TTS)

       a.   Mechanism of analgesia - inhibition of sympathetic activity

       b.   Alpha-2 receptor agonist

       c.   C-fiber type pain may have an element of sympathetic mediation which can be overcome with Clonidine

       d.   A clinical trial of Clonidine (Catapres-TTS-3) applied topically for one week can help to disclose likelihood of success

       e.   Patch application rotated to different sites in areas of hyperalgesia to decrease risk of dermatologic reactions

       f.   Initial dose - 0.1-0.3 mg Patch q 7 days

       g.   Titration - titrate to analgesia or side effects such as dizziness, dry mouth and orthostatic hypotension

E. NMDA Receptor Antagonists

   1.   Dextromethorphan

       a.   Mechanism of analgesia - blockade of N-Methyl-D-Aspartate receptors

       b.   D-Isomer of Levorphanol which is a low affinity antagonist to the Glutamate receptor subtype NMDA

       c.   Activation of NMDA receptor by Glutamate and Aspartate is believed to play a role in "wind-up" or second pain

       d.   Can block NMDA receptors in the spinal cord but also in the brain which can reverse learned inhibitions and induce transient psychosis

       e.   Dose needed to produce sufficient analgesia remains undefined with dosage range at 30-150 mg tid

   2.   Baclofen (Lioresal)

       a.   Mechanism of analgesia - pre & post-synaptic blockade of GABA receptors

       b.   Muscle relaxant used for intermittent neuropathic pain and considered a first-line agent for trigeminal neuralgia

       c.   Initial dose - 5-10 mg po tid

       d.   Titration - increase by 10 mg every other day until analgesia or side effects

       e.   Therapeutic onset - several days

   3.   Topical Capsaicin (Capsin)

       a.   Mechanism of analgesia - depletion of neuropeptide substance - P and C-fiber desensitization

       b.   Recommended for focal or localized areas of neuropathic pain

       c.   Larger areas of treatment not feasible due to increased irritation exposure and cost

       d.   Dosage - 0.025-0.075% strength applied tid-qid

       e.   Best if used on qid basis to maintain neuropeptide depletion

       f.   Therapeutic onset - 4-6 weeks

III. Miscellaneous Agents:

A. Calcium Channel Blockers

   1.   Nifedipine (Procardia)

   2.   Ziconotide

B. Calcitonin - Salmon (Miacalcin)

   1.   One spray (200 IU) per day administered intranasally, alternating nostrils daily

C. Alpha-Lipoic Acid

   1.   OTC Nutritional supplement also known as Thioctic Acid

   2.   Antioxidant used to help eradicate free radicals

   3.   Believed to be beneficial in improving Insulin sensitivity

4. The recommended dose is 200 mg per day although studies have ranged up to 1,800 mg per day in divided doses for diabetic neuropathy

ANTI-ANXIETY DRUGS

I. **Benzodiazepines**
   A. **Anxiolytic**
      1. Oxazepam (Serax)
         a. 10 to 30 mg po 3 or 4 times daily
         b. Good choice in elderly patients or those with liver disease since inactivated by Glucuronidation
      2. Lorazepam (Ativan)
         a. 2 to 6 mg/day in divided doses
      3. Alprazolam (Xanax)
         a. 0.25 to 0.5 mg po tid
         b. Drug of choice for panic disorders and agoraphobia
      4. Chlordiazepoxide (Librium)
         a. 5 to 10 mg po 3 or 4 times daily
         b. Also used for acute alcohol withdrawal
      5. Diazepam (Valium)
         a. 2 to 10 mg po 3 or 4 times daily
         b. Given by IV infusion for seizures - Drug of choice for status epilepticus, drug or toxin induced seizures
         c. Good skeletal muscle relaxant to treat spontaneous muscle spasms
      6. Clorazepate Dipotassium (Tranxene)
         a. 15 to 60 mg/day in divided doses
   B. **Actions**
      1. Facilitates Gamma-Aminobutyric Acid (GABA) inhibition of neuronal activity in the limbic and cortical areas of CNS
      2. Generalized Anxiety Disorders
      3. Situational Anxiety (e.g., Podiatric Surgical Procedures)
      4. Panic Disorders and Agoraphobia
         a. Drug of Choice - Alprazolam (Xanax)
      5. Seizures
         a. Drug of Choice - Diazepam (Valium) for status epilepticus
      6. Muscle Relaxation
         a. Increases presynaptic inhibition in the spinal cord
         b. Diazepam (Valium) useful for muscle strain and for spasticity seen in multiple sclerosis and cerebral palsy
   C. **Primary Adverse Effects**
      1. Drowsiness and Confusion
      2. Physical and Psychological Dependence

II. **Miscellaneous Anxiolytics**
   A. **Buspirone** (Buspar)
      1. Second generation Nonbenzodiazepine anxiolytic exerts effect as a serotonin receptor partial agonist

2. Lacks anticonvulsant and muscle relaxant properties
3. Drug of choice for chronic anxiety
4. Relieves anxiety without the sedation, hypnotic or CNS depressant effects seen with Benzodiazepines
5. Usual Dose - 5 mg po 3 times daily

B. Hydroxyzine (Atarax, Vistaril)
1. Antihistamine with anti-emetic activity
2. Useful for patients with a history of drug abuse due to low tendency for being habit forming
3. 50 to 100 mg po prior to procedure and up to 3 or 4 times daily for anxiety

C. Meprobamate (Equanil, Miltown)
1. Less effective than Benzodiazepine group
2. Strong sedative properties
3. 400 mg po 3 or 4 times daily

D. Chloral Hydrate
1. Often used in children, elderly and institutionalized patients
2. Metabolized to Trichlorethanol with rapid onset and short duration of action
3. Contraindicated in renal or hepatic impairment, cardiac disease and gastritis
4. Adult Dose - 500 mg-1 gram po 30 minutes prior to surgery
5. Child Dose - 50 mg/kg/day up to 1 gram on single dose

ANTIBIOTICS

I. Penicillins

A. General
1. Bactericidal inhibitors of cell wall synthesis
2. Major cause of resistance due to production of B-Lactamases (Penicillinases)
3. Renal clearance can be slowed by co-administration of Probenecid

B. Natural Penicillins
1. Penicillin G (Pfizerpen, Wycillin)
   a. Only parenteral formulations are currently in use, the oral formulations are no longer available
   b. 600,000 to 1.2 million units/day IM Procaine Penicillin G
   c. 1.2 million units/day IM Benzathine Penicillin G
2. Penicillin V (Pen-Vee K, Veetids)
   a. Acid stable
   b. 250-500 mg po qid
3. Spectrum of Activity
   a. Streptococci
   b. Non-Penicillinase producing Staphylococci
   c. Non-Penicillinase producing Gonococci
   d. Anaerobes except Bacteroides

C. Penicillinase-Resistant (Semisynthetic) Penicillins
1. Nafcillin (Unipen)
   a. 500 mg IM every 4 to 6 hours; 3 to 6 g IV/day
   b. 250-500 mg po every 4 to 6 hours
2. Oxacillin
   a. 500 mg po every 4 to 6 hours

        b.   250 mg - 1 g IV every 4 to 6 hours
3. Dicloxacillin (Dynapen, Pathocil)
        a.   125-250 mg po every 6 hours
4. Cloxacillin (Cloxapen)
        a.   250-500 mg po every 6 hours
5. Spectrum of Activity
        a.   All Staphylococci except Methicillin-resistant Staph (MRSA)
        b.   Streptococci

D. Aminopenicillins
1. Ampicillin (Totacillin, Principen)
        a.   250-500 mg po tid-qid
        b.   15-20 mg/kg/day IV up to total 4 gm daily slow infusion
2. Amoxicillin (Amoxil, Trimox, Wymox)
        a.   250-500 mg po tid
        b.   Oral agent of choice for enterococcus if susceptible
3. Bacampicillin (Spectrobid)
        a.   400 mg po every 12 hours
4. Spectrum of Activity for class of agents above:
        a.   Streptococci
        b.   Slight increased activity against Enterococci
        c.   Not active against most Staphylococci
        d.   Gram-negative organisms such as E-coli, Proteus Mirabilis, Shigella and Salmonella

E. Extended-Spectrum Penicillins
1. Ticarcillin (Ticar)
        a.   3 g IV every 3, 4 or 6 hours
2. Piperacillin (Pipracil)
        a.   3 g IV every 6 hours
3. Carbenicillin (Geocillin)
        a.   382-764 mg po qid
4. Spectrum of Activity for class of agents above:
        a.   Increased gram-negative coverage including most Enterobacter and some Pseudomonas Aeruginosa
        b.   Streptococci
        c.   Not active against most Staphylococci

F. Penicillin/B-Lactamase Inhibitor Combinations
1. Ampicillin - Sulbactam (Unasyn)
        a.   3 g IV or IM every 6 hours
2. Amoxicillin - Clavulanate (Augmentin)
        a.   250-500 mg po every 8 hours preferably with glass of water or 875 mg po bid with a full glass of water
        b.   Since both strengths contain the same amount of Clavulanic Acid, two 250 mg tablets are not equivalent to one 500 mg tablet
        c.   Drug of choice for bite wounds
3. Ticarcillin - Clavulanate (Timentin)
        a.   3.1 g IV every 6 hours
4. Piperacillin - Tazobactam (Zosyn)
        a.   3.375 g IV every 6 hours or 4.5 g IV every 8 hours
        b.   Piperacillin has best anti-pseudomonal activity of group
5. Spectrum of Activity

       a. All Staphylococci except Methicillin-resistant Staph (MRSA)

       b. Anaerobes including Bacteroides

       c. Gram-negative coverage - E-Coli, proteus mirabilis, most enterobacter and some pseudomonas aeruginosa

  6. Drugs of choice in diabetic foot infections

       a. The combination of Clindamycin (Cleocin) and Ciprofloxacin (Cipro) is also an excellent alternative especially in PCN-allergic patients. Clindamycin with a Quinolone (Ciprofloxacin) is effective for diabetic foot infections and polymicrobial osteomyelitis

G. Primary Adverse Effects

  1. Hypersensitivity Reactions

       a. Most important adverse reaction of Penicillins seen in 5-10% of patients

       b. Maculopapular rash occurs most commonly with Ampicillin and incidence increased with co-administration of Allopurinol

  2. Diarrhea

  3. Nephritis

  4. Neurotoxicity

  5. Platelet Dysfunction

H. Drug Interactions

  1. Parenteral Penicillins - Aminoglycosides

       a. Effect - Inactivation of certain Aminoglycosides

       b. Mechanism - Unknown, do not mix parenteral Aminoglycosides and Penicillins in same solution

  2. Penicillins (Ampicillin) - Allopurinol

       a. Effect - Markedly increased rate of Ampicillin-induced skin rash

       b. Mechanism - Possible Allopurinol potentiation of Ampicillin rashes

II. Cephalosporins

A. General

  1. Bactericidal inhibitors of cell wall synthesis

  2. Are relatively resistant to Penicillinases but are sensitive to Cephalosporinases

  3. Probenecid can also slow their excretion

B. First Generation - Parenteral

  1. Cefazolin (Ancef, Kefzol)

       a. 500 mg - 1 g IV or IM every 6 to 8 hours

       b. Drug of choice for surgical prophylaxis

  2. Cephapirin (Cefadyl)

       a. 500 mg - 1 g IV or IM every 4 to 6 hours

  3. Cephradine (Velosef)

       a. 1 g IV qid

C. First Generation - Oral

  1. Cephalexin (Keflex, Keftab)

       a. 250-500 mg po tid-qid

       b. Drug of choice for Methicillin-sensitive Staph Aureus (MSSA), streptococci, E-coli and proteus

  2. Cefadroxil (Duricef)

       a. 500 mg-1 g po qd-bid

  3. Cephradine (Velosef)

   a. 250-500 mg po tid-qid
  4. Spectrum of Activity for first generation Cephalosporins:
   a. All Staphylococci except Methicillin-resistant Staph
   b. Streptococci except Enterococci
   c. Anaerobes except Bacteroides Fragilis
   d. Gram-negative - Proteus Mirabilis, E-coli and Klebsiella Pneumoniae (<u>Acronym Peck</u>)

D. Second Generation - Parenteral
  1. Cefuroxime (Zinacef)
   a. 750 mg - 1.5 g IV or IM every 8 hours
  2. Cefonicid (Monocid)
   a. 1 g IV or IM once daily
  3. Cefoxitin (Mefoxin)
   a. 1-2 g IV or IM every 6 to 8 hours
  4. Cefotetan (Cefotan)
   a. 1-2 g IV or IM every 12 hours
  5. Cefmetazole (Zefazone)
   a. 2 g IV every 6 to 12 hours

E. Second Generation - Oral
  1. Cefaclor (Ceclor)
   a. 250-500 mg po tid
  2. Cefuroxime (Ceftin)
   a. 125-250 mg po bid
  3. Cefprozil (Cefzil)
   a. 250-500 mg po every 12 hours
  4. Loracarbef (Lorabid)
   a. 400 mg po every 12 hours
  5. Spectrum of Activity for second generation Cephalosporins:
   a. Staphylococci but slightly less active than first generation
   b. Streptococci - Same coverage as first generation
   c. Gram-negative - Haemophilus Influenzae, Enterobacter, and Neisseria in addition to gram negatives covered by first generation (<u>Acronym Henpeck</u>)
   d. Same Anaerobic coverage as first generation

F. Third Generation - Parenteral
  1. Cefotaxime (Claforan)
   a. 1-2 g IV or IM every 8 hours
  2. Ceftizoxime (Cefizox)
   a. 1-2 g IV or IM every 8 to 12 hours
  3. Cefoperazone (Cefobid)
   a. 1-2 g IV or IM every 12 hours
  4. Ceftriaxone (Rocephin)
   a. 1-2 g IV or IM once or twice daily
  5. Ceftazidime (Fortaz, Tazidime, Tazicef, Ceptaz)
   a. 1-2 g IV or IM every 8 to 12 hours

G. Third Generation - Oral
  1. Cefixime (Suprax)
   a. 200 mg po every 12 hours or 400 mg po once daily
  2. Ceftibuten (Cedax)
   a. 400 mg po qd

3. Cefpodoxime Proxetil (Vantin)
   a. 400 mg po q 12 hours
4. Cefdinir (Omnicef)
   a. 300 mg po q 12 hours or 600 mg po qd
   b. Excellent activity against Staph Aureus including PCN-resistant Staph Aureus while maintaining good gram-negative coverages
   c. Causes "red-colored" stools due to forming GI complexes with iron
5. Cefditoren Pivoxil (Spectracef)
   a. A prodrug hydrolyzed to Cefditoren
   b. Contraindicated in patients allergic to milk proteins since it contains sodium casein-ate as an inactive ingredient. Lactose intolerance differs from this since lactose is milk sugar rather than protein
   c. Contraindicated in patients with carnitine deficiency since Pivoxil salt is cleaved to Pivolate and excreted by kidneys depleting carnitine along with it
   d. 200 mg po q 12 hours
6. Spectrum of Activity for third generation Cephalosporins
   a. Inferior to first generation in regard to activity against Gram-positive Cocci
   b. Streptococci - Same as first and second generation
   c. Similar Anaerobic coverage with Bacteroides coverages varying with each agent
   d. Enhanced activity against gram-negative organisms as above second generation including Serratia Marcescens

H. Fourth Generation - Parenteral
1. Cefepime Hcl (Maxipime)
   a. High level of activity against both gram-positive and gram-negative organisms
   b. Considered to have increased activity against Pseudomonas Aeruginosa than Ceftazidime (Fortaz)
   c. 1-2 g IV or IM every 12 hours

I. Primary Adverse Effects
1. Hypersensitivity Reactions
   a. Cephalosporins should be used with caution in patients allergic to Penicillin with approximately 10% cross-reactive sensitivity
   b. Cephalosporins should not be given to any patient with a history of anaphylaxis to Penicillin
   c. Allergic responses to Cephalosporins alone are low at about 1-2%
2. Disulfiram-like Reaction
   a. Certain Cephalosporins such as Cefamandole and Cefoperazone can block alcohol oxidation allowing increased levels of Acetaldehyde
3. Bleeding
   a. Bleeding can occur with Cefamandole or Cefoperazone due to anti-vitamin K effects
   b. Administration of vitamin K can reverse the problem

J. Drug Interactions
1. Parenteral Cephalosporins - Aminoglycosides
   a. Effect - Increased nephrotoxicity
   b. Mechanism - Suspected competition for renal elimination
2. Cephalosporins - Oral anticoagulants
   a. Effect - Augmented Warfarin effects
   b. Mechanism - Anti-platelet effects of certain parenteral Cephalosporins such as Cefamandole and Cefoperazone

III. Penem and Monobactam Group

  A. Ertapenem (Invanz)
1. Penem class antibiotic reserved for severe limb or life-threatening infection
2. Activity against gram-positives, gram-negatives except pseudomonas and anaerobes
3. 1 g IV or IM qd

  B. Imipenem - Cilastatin (Primaxin)
1. Carbapenem group antibiotic with broadest spectrum of activity than any available antibiotic
2. Used for severe limb or life-threatening infections in diabetic patients including gas formers such as necrotizing fasciitis
3. Associated with high incidence of causing seizures
4. Cross-reactivity is possible in those with demonstrated history of Penicillin allergy
5. 500 mg IV every 6 to 8 hours as slow IV infusion

  C. Aztreonam (Azactam)
1. Member of Monobactam group
2. Only active against gram-negative Aerobes
3. No activity against gram-positive nor Anaerobic organisms
4. Can be used in place of Aminoglycosides for severe gram-negative infection
5. 1 g IV every 8 hours

IV. Macrolide Antibiotics

  A. Macrolide Antibiotics
1. Erythromycin (E-Mycin, Ery-Tab, ERYC, EES)
  a. 250-500 mg po qid
  b. 500 mg IV every 6 hours
2. Troleandomycin (TAO)
  a. 250-500 mg po qid
3. Azithromycin (Zithromax)
  a. 500 mg po on first dose followed by 250 mg po once daily on days 2 through 5
4. Clarithromycin (Biaxin, Biaxin-XL)
  a. 250-500 mg po every 12 hours
5. Dirithromycin (Dynabac)
  a. Enteric-coated tablet formulation
  b. 500 mg po qd

  B. Primary Adverse Effects
1. Epigastric Distress
  a. Most common adverse effect
2. Cholestatic Jaundice
  a. Occurs especially with Estolate salt form of Erythromycin
  b. Patients with hepatic dysfunction should not be treated with Erythromycin since it accumulates in the liver
3. Ototoxicity
  a. Transient deafness can occur especially at high dosages of Erythromycin

  C. Drug Interactions
1. Erythromycin, Clarithromycin - Theophylline
  a. Effect - Increased Theophylline toxicity
  b. Mechanism - Decreased Theophylline renal clearance
2. Erythromycin - Oral anticoagulants

       a. Effect - Increased anticoagulant activity with hemorrhage

       b. Mechanism - Unknown, possible reduced clearance of Warfarin

  3. Erythromycin - Digoxin

       a. Effect - Increased Digoxin toxicity in about 10% of patients

       b. Mechanism - Digoxin is metabolized by GI bacteria in about 10% of patients

V. Aminoglycosides

Bacteriostatic inhibitors of protein synthesis

Administered parenterally since not absorbed orally very well

A. Aminoglycosides

1. Streptomycin
   a. 1-2 g/day IM only in divided doses
2. Gentamicin (Garamycin)
   a. Preferable dose is 3-5 mg/kg IV or IM <u>once daily</u>
   b. 3 mg/kg/day in 3 equal doses every 8 hours IV or IM has been the previous standard
3. Kanamycin (Kantrex)
   a. Total daily dose of 1.5 g IV or IM in 2 or 3 equal doses
4. Tobramycin (Nebcin)
   a. 3 mg/kg/day in 3 equal doses every 8 hours IV or IM
5. Amikacin (Amikin)
   a. 15 mg/kg/day IV or IM in 2 or 3 equal doses
6. Netilmicin (Netromycin)
   a. 1.5-2 mg/kg IV or IM every 12 hours

B. Primary Adverse Effects

1. Ototoxicity
   a. Irreversible deafness directly related to high peak plasma levels
2. Nephrotoxicity
   a. Mild renal impairment to severe acute tubular necrosis
3. Neuromuscular paralysis
   a. Seen mostly after large intraperitoneal or intrapleural doses

C. Drug Interactions

1. Aminoglycosides - Parenteral Cephalosporins
   a. Effect - Increased nephrotoxicity
   b. Mechanism - Suspected competition for renal elimination
2. Aminoglycosides - Parenteral Penicillins
   a. Effect - Inactivation of certain aminoglycosides
   b. Mechanism - Unknown, do not mix parenteral Aminoglycosides and Penicillins in same solution
3. Aminoglycosides - Loop diuretics
   a. Effect - Increased 8th cranial nerve damage with possible irreversible hearing loss
   b. Mechanism - Synergistic auditory toxicity

D. Aminoglycoside Monitoring

1. BUN and serum creatinine every 3rd day until stable, then weekly
2. Baseline audiogram and repeated on periodic basis
3. Peak level - drawn 20-30 minutes after administration of dose. Relates to dosage amount. If peak is too high then lower dosage and if too low then increase dose
4. Trough level - drawn immediately prior to next dose. Relates to time interval. If trough is elevated then need to spread out dosing time interval

VI. Glycopeptide Antibiotics

A. Vancomycin (Vancocin)

1. Bactericidal against all gram-positive organisms including Methicillin-resistant Staph Aureus (MRSA)
2. No activity against gram-negative nor Anaerobic organisms
3. Oral form of drug used to treat antibiotic-induced Pseudomembranous colitis produced by Clostridium Difficile
4. Nephrotoxicity is less frequent than with earlier preparations but may still occur
5. Ototoxicity has been implicated associated with high serum levels
6. Most significant adverse effect is "Red Man" or "Red Neck" syndrome associated with histamine release and can be related to the speed of administration so therefore infuse slowly over 60 minutes
7. Oral dose for C. Difficile is 125 mg qid
8. 1 g slow IV infusion over 45-60 minutes every 12 hours

VII. Anti-Anaerobes

A. Clindamycin (Cleocin)

1. Primarily used in treatment of Anaerobic infections such as Bacteroides Fragilis
2. Most serious adverse effect is Pseudomembranous colitis as result of superinfection with Clostridium Difficile
3. Diarrhea as primary manifestation seen in up to 20% of individuals
4. 300 mg po every 8 to 12 hours
5. 600-900 mg IV every 12 hours

B. Metronidazole (Flagyl)

1. Extensive use in treatment of Anaerobes including Bacteroides and Clostridia infections
2. Most common adverse effects involve the GI tract such as nausea, vomiting, cramps and epigastric distress
3. Most notable drug interaction is with alcohol resulting in a Disulfiram-like reaction due to accumulation of Acetaldehyde
4. Drug of choice for C. Difficile induced Pseudomembranous colitis - 500 mg po q 6 hours
5. 500 mg slow IV infusion over 60 minutes q 6 hours

VIII. Quinolones

A. General

1. Inhibits bacterial DNA gyrases resulting in a bactericidal effect
2. Bactericidal with good coverage against most common gram-negative bacteria
3. Variable coverage for Staph when used alone
4. Contraindicated in pregnancy and children due to cartilage toxicity

B. Quinolones

1. Ciprofloxacin (Cipro)
   a. Second generation Fluoroquinolone
   b. 400 mg slow IV infusion over 60 minutes q 12 hours
   c. 500-750 mg po q 12 hours
2. Levofloxacin (Levaquin)
   a. Third generation Quinolone
   b. 500 mg po or slow IV infusion over 60 minutes qd
   c. 750 mg po qd for complicated skin and skin structure infection
3. Gatifloxacin (Tequin)

        a. Fourth generation Quinolone

        b. 400 mg po or slow IV infusion over 60 minutes qd

    4. Moxifloxacin (Avelox)

        a. Fourth generation Quinolone

        b. 400 mg po or slow IV infusion over 60 minutes qd

        c. The fourth generation Quinolones has activity against gram-negatives, gram-positives and anaerobes useful as intermediary agents in polymicrobial involvement such as diabetic foot infections

C. Primary Adverse Effects

    1. EKG changes

        a. May have potential to prolong the QT interval especially with the newer generational agents (e.g., Gatifloxacin)

        b. Should not be used in patients with known prolongation of the QT interval, patients with uncorrected hypokalemia, and those taking antiarrhythmic agents

        c. Must be used with caution in patients taking other medications that are known to prolong the QT interval (e.g., tricyclic antidepressants)

    2. Photosensitivity reactions

        a. Avoid excessive exposure to sunlight or artificial ultraviolet light sources (e.g., tanning beds)

    3. CNS disturbances

        a. Headache, dizziness and lightheadedness are most prominent

    4. Nephrotoxicity

        a. Crystalluria has been reported in high doses

    5. Tendon ruptures

        a. Achilles and other tendon ruptures requiring surgical repair or resulting in prolonged disability have been reported with Ciprofloxacin and other Quinolones

D. Drug Interactions

    1. Gatifloxacin (Quinolones) - Antiarrhythmic agents/TCAs

        a. Effect - Life threatening cardiac arrhythmia including Torsade De Pointes

        b. Mechanism - Unknown, suspected prolongation of QT interval

    2. Quinolones - Multivalent cations (Antacids - Ca, Al, Mg)

        a. Effect - Antacids decrease effects of Quinolones

        b. Mechanism - Chelation binding decreases GI absorption

    3. Quinolones - Theophylline

        a. Effect - Increased Theophylline toxicity

        b. Mechanism - Inhibition of hepatic metabolism of Theophylline

    4. Quinolones - Sucralfate (Carafate)

        a. Effect - Decreased effects of Quinolones

        b. Mechanism - Chelation binding decreases GI absorption due to aluminum salt contained in Sucralfate

IX. Broad-Spectrum Antimicrobials

A. Tetracyclines

    1. Tetracycline (Panmycin, Sumycin)

        a. 250-500 mg po bid-qid

    2. Demeclocycline (Declomycin)

        a. 150 mg po qid or 300 mg po bid

    3. Doxycycline (Vibramycin, Vibratab)

        a. Drug of choice for Lyme Borrelia

          b. Alternate agent of choice in PCN-Allergic patients for bite wounds and syphilis

          c. 100 mg po qd-bid

    4. Minocycline (Minocin, Vectrin)

          a. Oral alternative to Vancomycin for Methicillin-resistant Staph Aureus (MRSA)

          b. 100 mg po bid

    5. Oxytetracycline

          a. 250 mg po bid-qid

B. Primary Adverse Effects

    1. Gastric Distress

          a. Epigastric distress is common from gastric mucosal irritation but can be minimized with food except no dairy products

    2. Bone and Dentition Effects

          a. Deposition in bone and primary dentition occurs during calcification in growing children

          b. Causes brownish-yellow discoloration and hypoplasia of teeth

          c. Avoid use during pregnancy or in children younger than 8 years

    3. Hepatotoxicity

    4. Photosensitivity

          a. Severe sunburn reactions can occur when exposed to sunlight or ultraviolet rays

          b. Seen most frequently with Doxycycline and Demeclocycline

    5. Superinfections

          a. Broad-spectrum activity could result in overgrowth of Candida or resistant Staphylo-cocci

C. Drug Interactions

    1. Tetracyclines - Multivalent Cations (Dairy products and antacids - Ca, Al, Mg)

          a. Effect - Decreased effects of Tetracyclines

          b. Mechanism - Chelation binding decreases GI absorption

    2. Tetracyclines - Digoxin

          a. Effect - Increased Digoxin toxicity in about 10% of patients

          b. Mechanism - Tetracycline is metabolized by GI bacteria in about 10% of patients

X. Streptogramins

A. Quinupristin/Dalfopristin (Synercid)

    1. Both agents are bacteriostatic alone but are <u>synergistic</u> when used in the 30:70 combination and become bactericidal

    2. Inhibits protein synthesis by irreversibly binding to the 70 S ribosome

    3. Reserve use to treat gram-positive infections unresponsive to other antibiotics including Vancomycin (e.g., VRE-Vancomycin resistant enterococcus)

    4. 7.5 mg/kg IV q 12 hours for complicated skin structure infections caused by staph Aureus (<u>MSSA</u>) or strept pyogenes

    5. 7.5 mg/kg IV q 8 hours for limb or life-threatening infections with Vancomycin resistant enterococcus faecium (VREF)

XI. Oxazolidinones

A. Linezolid (Zyvox)

    1. Bacteriostatic activity against PCN-resistant Strept Pneumoniae, MRSA and Vancomycin-resistant enterococcus (VRE)

    2. Inhibits early step in protein synthesis that is involved in binding MRNA during start of translation

3. Oral dosing is equivalent to IV dosing
4. 600 mg IV or po q 12 h for MRSA or VRE
5. 400 mg po q 12 h for uncomplicated skin structure infection

XII. Anti-Mycotic Drugs

A. **Griseofulvin** (Fulvicin U/F, Fulvicin P/G, Gris-Peg, Grisactin)
    1. Disrupts the mitotic spindle and inhibits fungal mitosis
    2. Fungistatic against only dermatophytes
    3. Possible cross sensitivity in Penicillin allergic patients since derived from Penicillium
    4. Absorption is enhanced when taken with a meal with high fat content
    5. Available in microsize and ultramicrosize formulations
    6. Ultramicrosize increases GI absorption approximately 1.5 times that of the microsize but no evidence that the lower dosage confers any significant clinical differences
    7. Contraindicated in patients with acute intermittent porphyria due to hepatotoxicity
    8. Tinea Pedis - 750 mg-1 g po microsize or 660-750 mg po ultramicrosize per day in divided doses for 4 to 8 weeks
    9. Tinea Unguium - 750 mg-1 g po microsize or 660-750 mg po ultramicrosize per day in divided doses minimal 6 months up to 12-18 months

B. **Ketoconazole** (Nizoral) (Azole Group)
    1. Can be either fungistatic or fungicidal depending on dose
    2. Effective against broad range of systemic mycoses including Candida and Dermatophytes resistant to Griseofulvin
    3. Major drawback is association with hepatic toxicity including fatalities
    4. Blocks adrenal steroid synthesis with possible gynecomastia
    5. 200-400 mg po daily

C. **Fluconazone** (Diflucan) (Azole Group)
    1. Fungistatic against systemic mycoses and agent of choice for cryptococcal meningitis due to cerebrospinal fluid penetration
    2. Available for oral and IV administration
    3. Agent of choice for disseminated fungal infections in immunocompromised patients
    4. 100-400 mg po daily

D. **Itraconazole** (Sporanox) (Azole Group)
    1. Fungistatic against broad range of systemic mycoses
    2. Most notable adverse effect is a black box warning to avoid use of Itraconazole in patients with cardiac dysfunction such as CHF or a history of CHF
    3. Potent inhibitor of the cytochrome P450-3A4 isoenzyme system which elevates plasma levels of drugs metabolized by this pathway
    4. Contraindications:
        a. CHF or a history of CHF
        b. Coadministration with Quinidine, Triazolam (Halcion), oral Midazolam (Versed), Dofetilide (Tikosyn) or Pimozide (Orap)
        c. HMG-CoA reductase inhibitors - "Statin Drugs" such as Lovastatin (Mevacor), Atorvastatin (Lipitor), etc.
        d. Pregnancy and in women contemplating pregnancy
    5. Elevation of liver enzymes greater than twice the normal range occurs in about 4% of patients
    6. Gastrointestinal effects are also seen in about 4% of patients
    7. Hepatic enzyme levels should be obtained prior to treatment as baseline and monitored approximately monthly during therapy

8. Dosage: (best taken after a full meal)
9. Tinea Pedis - 100 mg po qd x 28 consecutive days or 200 mg po bid x 7 consecutive days
10. Onychomycosis - 200 mg po bid for one week on and three weeks off for 3 monthly cycles as pulse therapy

E. **Terbinafine** (Lamisil) (Allylamine Group)
1. Fungicidal against dermatophytes
2. Most notable adverse effect is a black box warning for rare cases of liver failure leading to death or hepatic transplantation in patients with and without pre-existing liver disease
3. Not recommended for patients with chronic or active liver disease
4. Inhibits CYP2D6-mediated metabolism which may have clinical relevance for drugs metabolized by this enzyme such as beta blockers, tricyclic antidepressants, selective serotonin reuptake inhibitors and monoamine oxidase inhibitors
5. Adverse effects include headache, GI effects, rash, neutropenia, visual and taste disturbances
6. Hepatic function monitoring should be done as baseline and repeated by week 6 (mid-cycle) and at end of therapy
7. Can be taken without regard to food or meals
8. Onychomycosis Dosing: 250 mg po qd for 12 consecutive weeks

F. **Drug Interactions for Azole Group and Griseofulvin**
1. Itraconazole - Quinidine, Triazolam, Midazolam, Dofetilide, Pimozide
   a. Effect - Serious cardiac events such as arrhythmia, cardiac arrest or sudden death
   b. Mechanism - Inhibition of cytochrome P450-3A4 isoenzyme
2. Itraconazole - HMG - CoA reductase inhibitors ("Statins")
3. Ketoconazole
   a. Effect - Increased levels of statin drugs with Rhabdomyolysis
   b. Mechanism - CYP3A4 hepatic enzyme metabolism
4. Ketoconazole - H2 Antagonists, proton pump inhibitors, antacids
   Itraconazole
   a. Effect - Inactivation of Imidazoles
   b. Mechanism - Imidazoles require acidic Ph. alteration of Ph by H2 antagonists, protein pump inhibitors and antacids
5. Ketoconazole - Itraconazole, Phenytoin (Dilantin)
   a. Effect - Decreased effect of Imidazoles
   b. Mechanism - Increased metabolism by Hydantoin induction of hepatic enzymes
6. Griseofulvin - Oral Anticoagulants
   a. Effect - Decreased effect of Warfarin
   b. Mechanism - Unknown
7. Griseofulvin - Oral Contraceptives
   a. Effect - Unintended pregnancy
   b. Mechanism - Griseofulvin-induced increase in hepatic metabolism

ANTI-DIABETIC AGENTS

I. **ADA Optimal Control of Diabetes Mellitus**

A. **Fasting blood glucose between 80 and 120 mg%**
B. **Bedtime glucose between 100 to 140 mg%**
C. **Glycosylated hemoglobin less than 7%**

II. Insulin Preparations

A. Rapid-Acting (3-4 hours)

1. Insulin Lispro (Humalog)
   a. Human Insulin analog developed by recombinant DNA technology available by prescription only
   b. Differs structurally by switching 2 amino acids proline and lysine, hence the name Lispro
   c. Indicated for patients with type I and type II diabetes mellitus
   d. Peak serum levels occur earlier, are higher, and of shorter duration than regular human Insulin allowing administration closer to meals
   e. May be administered within 15 minutes before or immediately after a meal
   f. Hyperglycemic events are less frequent and provides better control of post-prandial glucose excursions
2. Insulin Aspart (Novolog)
   a. Recombinant Insulin analogue produced by replacement of proline by aspartic acid, thus the name Aspart
   b. Indicated for control of hyperglycemia in adult patients
   c. Absorption is 2 to 3 times faster than regular Insulin due to a low association to hexamers in the mixture
   d. Should be administered immediately before a meal about 5 to 10 minutes before eating
   e. More effective than regular Insulin in controlling post-prandial hyperglycemia in type I patients

B. Short-Acting (6-12 hours)

1. Regular Insulin (Crystalline Zinc Insulin - CZI)
   a. Zinc complex solution of Bovine, Porcine or human Insulin
   b. Given subcutaneously and can be given IV in emergencies
2. Semilente Insulin
   a. Very fine zinc precipitate Insulin suspension

C. Intermediate-Acting (12-24 hours)

1. Isophane (NPH) Insulin
   a. NPH - Neutral Protamine Hagedorn - CZI Insulin with positive charged peptide protamine at neutral Ph
   b. Zinc complexes with protamine
   c. Larger particle size than regular
2. Lente Insulin
   a. Larger precipitate size than Semilente allows for slower onset and longer duration of action

D. Long-Acting (24-36 hours)

1. Protamine - Zinc Insulin
   a. Larger particle size than NPH Insulin
2. Ultralente Insulin
   a. Larger particle size then Lente Insulin
   b. Extended Insulin Zinc suspension which is poorly soluble, therefore delayed onset and prolonged duration of action
3. Insulin Glargine (Lantus)
   a. Differs structurally by switching 2 amino acids glycine and arginine, hence the name Glargine
   b. Indicated for type I & II in adults and type I DM in children

      c. Long acting "peakless" Insulin characterized by slow absorption and a flat plasma Insulin profile with no peak

      d. This compound is less soluble than native human Insulin at physiological PH and precipitates in skin after subcutaneous injection resulting in delayed absorption

      e. Administered once daily at bedtime

E. Primary Adverse Effects

    1. Hypoglycemia

      a. Can occur from Insulin overdose, exercise or inadequate caloric intake

    2. Immune Disorders

      a. Production of anti-Insulin antibodies

    3. Hypersensitivity Reactions

      a. Local urticaria and erythema

    4. Lipodystrophy

      a. Alternating injection sites can minimize subcutaneous fat dystrophy

F. Drug Interactions

    1. Insulin - Alcohol

      a. Effect - Hypoglycemia

      b. Mechanism - Inhibition of gluconeogenesis

    2. Insulin - Beta Blockers

      a. Effect - Prolonged hypoglycemia with masking of hypoglycemia symptoms (tachycardia)

      b. Mechanism - Beta-blockers blunt sympathetic mediated responses to hypoglycemia

    3. Insulin - MAO Inhibitors

      a. Effect - Hypoglycemia

      b. Mechanism - Inhibition of gluconeogenesis

    4. Insulin - Salicylates

      a. Effect - Hypoglycemia

      b. Mechanism - Increased circulating concentration of Insulin

III. Type II Diabetes Mellitus - Characterized by 3 fundamental defects

A. Decreased peripheral glucose utilization

B. Increased hepatic glucose production

C. Insufficient Insulin secretion

IV. Oral Sulfonylureas - Cause an increase in the amount of Insulin secreted in response to a carbohydrate challenge

A. Short-Acting Agents (6-10 hours)

    1. Tolbutamide (Orinase)

      a. Rapidly absorbed first generation compound

B. Intermediate-Acting Agents (12-24 hours)

    1. Acetohexamide (Dymelor)

      a. Has uricosuric properties thus may be beneficial in diabetics with gout

    2. Tolazamide (Tolinase)

      a. Slowly absorbed

      b. Has a mild diuretic effect

    3. Glipizide (Glucotrol, Glucotrol-XR)

      a. Rapidly absorbed but can be delayed with food in single or divided doses

    4. Glyburide (Diabeta, Micronase, Glynase Prestab)

      a. Also exerts a mild diuretic effect

        b.   Second generation compounds such as Glipizide and Glyburide are up to 200 times more potent than first generation agents

        c.   1.25-20 mg in single or divided doses

        d.   Glynase Prestab is micronized form dosed at 0.75-12 mg

    5.   Glimepiride (Amaryl)

        a.   Once daily dosing with duration of action of approximately 24 hours-1-4 mg po qd

C. Long-Acting Agents (>24 hours)

    1.   Chlorpropamide (Diabinese)

        a.   Causes adverse effects more frequently than other sulfonylureas

        b.   Most likely of group to cause Disulfiram-like reaction when alcohol is consumed

D. Drug Interactions

    1.   Sulfonylurea - Alcohol

        a.   Effect - Hypoglycemia and Disulfiram-like reactions

        b.   Mechanism - Decreased elimination and altered metabolism involving Aldehyde Dehydrogenase

    2.   Sulfonylurea - Anticoagulants

        a.   Effect - Hypoglycemia

        b.   Mechanism - Inhibits hepatic metabolism of sulfonylurea

    3.   Sulfonylurea - MAO Inhibitors

        a.   Effect - Hypoglycemia

        b.   Mechanism - Unknown

    4.   Sulfonylurea - NSAIDS or salicylates

        a.   Effect - Hypoglycemia

        b.   Mechanism - Protein binding displacement

    5.   Sulfonylurea - Thiazide Diuretics

        a.   Effect - Hyperglycemia

        b.   Mechanism - Thiazide diuretics decrease Insulin secretion

V. Meglitinides

A. Repaglinide (Prandin)

    1.   Oral hypoglycemic for type II NIDDM

    2.   A "sulfonylurea-like" agent stimulating endogenous Insulin release

    3.   Differs from sulfonylureas in chemical structure and receptor binding site in pancreatic beta cells

    4.   Potassium channel blockade depolarizes beta cell to open calcium channels allowing Insulin secretion

    5.   Most beneficial in post-prandial control hence the name Prandin

    6.   0.5-4 mg po taken 15-30 minutes before each meal

    7.   Advantages:

        a.   Post-prandial control without greatly affecting FBS

        b.   Insulin release is <u>glucose dependent</u>

        c.   More rapid onset and shorter duration than sulfonylureas

        d.   Dose individualization from meal to meal

    8.   Disadvantages:

        a.   Hypoglycemia although less than sulfonylureas

B. Nateglinide (Starlix)

    1.   An amino acid derivative of D-Phenylalanine with pharmacologic actions similar to Repaglinide

    2.   Indicated as monotherapy or in combination with Metformin for type II DM

3. Considered to have a more rapid onset and shorter duration of action than Repaglinide
4. 120 mg po tid taken 1 to 30 minutes before a meal
5. Patients with near goal glycosylated hemoglobin may begin therapy with 60 mg dose

VI. Biguanides

A. Metformin (Glucophage)
1. Oral hypoglycemic for type II NIDDM
2. Differs from sulfonylureas in mechanism of action by increasing peripheral metabolic responses to endogenous Insulin
3. Increases peripheral glucose utilization and decreases hepatic glucose production
4. Can be effective alone or in combination with sulfonylureas with synergistic action since the two drugs improve glucose levels by different but complementary mechanisms
5. Most serious adverse effect is lactic acidosis
6. Contraindicated in patients with renal disease or impairment with serum creatinine levels >1.5 in men and >1.4 in women
7. 500 mg po bid is usual starting dose progressing to 850-1,000 mg po bid with AM and PM meals
8. Contraindicated in hepatic disease
9. D/C therapy 48 hrs. prior and after iodinated contrast dye studies

B. Glyburide/Metformin (Glucovance)
1. Combines the two most widely prescribed oral antidiabetic agents in a single pill
2. Available in three dosing strengths: 1.25 mg/250 mg, 2.5 mg/500 mg and 5 mg/500 mg

VII. Alpha-Glucosidase Inhibitors

A. Acarbose (Precose)
1. Ideal choice for post-prandial control
2. In contrast to sulfonylureas, Acarbose does not enhance Insulin secretion
3. Anti-hyperglycemic action results from a competitive reversible inhibition of pancreatic alpha-amylase and intestinal alpha-glucosidase hydrolase enzymes
4. Pancreatic alpha-amylase hydrolyzes complex starches to oligosaccharides in the small intestine
5. Alpha-glucosidase hydrolyzes oligosaccharides, trisaccharides and disaccharides to glucose in the small intestine
6. Indicated as monotherapy as an adjunct to diet in treating type II NIDDM
7. May also be used with a sulfonylurea to enhance glycemic control
8. Contraindicated in diabetic ketoacidosis, cirrhosis, inflammatory bowel disease, colonic ulceration and chronic intestinal digestive disorders
9. Due to its mechanism of action, Acarbose alone should not cause hypoglycemia
10. Most common adverse reactions are GI related such as abdominal pain, diarrhea and flatulence
11. Initial dose is 25 mg (half of a 50 mg tablet) given orally 3 times daily at the start of each main meal
12. Maximum recommended dose is 100 mg po tid
13. Hypoglycemia in combination therapy requires glucose - no fruit juice or complex starches

B. Miglitol (Glyset)
1. Same mechanism of action, indications and contraindications as Acarbose (Precose)
2. 25 mg po tid at the start (with the first bite) of each main meal

VIII.   **Thiazolidinediones**

    A.   **Rosiglitazone Maleate** (Avandia)

       1.   Increases peripheral glucose utilization

       2.   Decreases hepatic glucose production

       3.   Increases Insulin sensitivity through modulation at the Insulin receptor site

       4.   Approved for monotherapy or in combination with Metformin (Glucophage)

       5.   There is an increased incidence of heart failure associated with the use of Avandia in combination with Insulin

       6.   Edema in the lower extremities is an adverse drug effect in addition to the CHF potential noted above with podiatric implication

       7.   4-8 mg po qd or in divided doses twice daily

       8.   Liver enzyme testing is recommended as initial baseline, every two months for the first year and periodically thereafter

       9.   Use may result in resumption of ovulation in premenopausal anovulatory patients with potential for pregnancy

    B.   **Pioglitazone HCL** (Actos)

       1.   Actions similar to above agent

       2.   Approved for monotherapy in type 2 diabetes or in combination with a Sulfonylurea, Metformin or Insulin

       3.   15-45 mg po qd as monotherapy

       4.   15-30 mg po qd in combination therapy

       5.   Liver enzyme testing is recommended as initial baseline, every two months for the first year and periodically thereafter

       6.   Use may result in resumption of ovulation in premenopausal anovulatory patients with potential for pregnancy

ANTI-HYPERTENSIVES

    I.   **Diuretics**

    A.   **Thiazide-Related Diuretics**

       1.   Chlorothiazide (Diuril)

       2.   Hydrochlorothiazide (Hydrodiuril, Esidrix)

       3.   Chlorthalidone (Hygroton)

       4.   Metolazone (Zaroxolyn)

       5.   Indapamide (Lozol)

          a.   Inhibit active reabsorption of NaCl in the ascending loop of Henle and distal convoluted tubule

          b.   Adverse effects include electrolyte disturbances such as hypokalemia and hyponatremia

          c.   Can cause hyperglycemia by decreasing Insulin secretion

          d.   Can elevate serum uric acid levels and exacerbate gout

          e.   Interacts with Lithium by decreasing Lithium renal clearance and can interact with oral hypoglycemics by elevating glucose levels

    B.   **Loop Diuretics**

       1.   Furosemide (Lasix)

       2.   Bumetanide (Bumex)

       3.   Ethacrynic Acid (Edecrin)

4. Torsemide (Demadex)
   a. Inhibit active reabsorption of NaCl in the ascending limb of the loop of Henle
   b. Known as high ceiling diuretics due to high capacity for NaCl and water excretion
   c. Most notable adverse effect is for dose related ototoxicity
   d. Hypokalemia and electrolyte imbalances are other adverse effects
   e. Interact with aminoglycosides to increase ototoxicity and with Phenytoin to cause a decreased effect of the diuretic action

C. **Potassium-Sparing Diuretics**
   1. Spironolactone (Aldactone)
   2. Triamterene (Dyrenium)
   3. Amiloride (Midamor)
      a. Inhibit sodium reabsorption and potassium secretion in the distal tubule
      b. Not potent diuretics when used alone - most often are combined with other agents
      c. Contraindicated in renal insufficiency
      d. Interact with ACE inhibitors and potassium supplements which could lead to hyper-kalemia

II. Sympatholytic Agents - Central Acting

A. **Methyldopa** (Aldomet)
   1. Activates presynaptic inhibitory and postsynaptic alpha-receptors in the CNS to reduce sympathetic outflow
   2. Used to treat mild to moderate hypertension often combined when a diuretic alone is not successful
   3. Sexual dysfunction can occur which tends to reduce compliance
   4. Adverse effects include drowsiness, dry mouth and GI upset

B. **Clonidine** (Catapres)
   1. Stimulates postsynaptic alpha-2 receptors in the CNS to reduce total peripheral resistance
   2. Useful in treating all degrees of hypertension
   3. Common adverse effects include drowsiness, dry mouth and constipation
   4. Also available as transdermal patch under name Catapres-TTS discussed under adjuvant analgesics for sympathetic mediated pain for possible podiatric application in reflex sympathetic dystrophy (RSD)

C. **Guanabenz Acetate** (Wytensin)
   1. Activates central alpha-receptors to inhibit sympathetic outflow
   2. Mostly for mild to moderate hypertension
   3. Most common adverse effects are sedation and dry mouth

III. Sympatholytic Agents - Peripheral Acting

A. **Beta Blockers**
   1. Propranolol (Inderal)
   2. Nadolol (Corgard)
   3. Metoprolol (Lopressor, Toprol-XL)
   4. Atenolol (Tenormin)
   5. Timolol (Blocadren)
   6. Acebutolol (Sectral)
   7. Pindolol (Visken)
      a. Exerts effects at both beta-1 and beta-2 receptors
      b. Blockade of beta-1 receptors reduces heart rate and contractility

      c. Blockade of beta-2 receptors increases airway resistance

      d. Easiest way to remember beta receptors is that beta-1 = cardiac (one heart) and beta-2 = pulmonary or bronchial (two lungs)

      e. Used to treat mild to moderate hypertension

      f. Adverse effects include bronchoconstriction, which can be serious and even lethal in asthma, arrhythmias, sexual impairment, and decreased glucose, which could lead to pronounced hypoglycemia

   8. Drug interactions as noted below:

      a. Beta Blocker - Epinephrine

         i. Effect - Initial hypertensive episode followed by bradycardia

         ii. Mechanism - Beta blockade allows alpha-receptor stimulation increasing BP, which stimulates baroreceptors causing bradycardia

      b. Beta Blocker - Verapamil

         i. Effect - Effects of both drugs are increased

         ii. Mechanism - Pharmacologic synergism

      c. Beta Blocker - Insulin

         i. Effect - Prolonged hypoglycemia with masking of hypoglycemia symptoms (tachycardia)

      d. Beta Blocker - NSAIDS

         i. Effect - Impaired antihypertensive effect of beta blockers

         ii. Mechanism - NSAIDS inhibit renal prostaglandin synthesis allowing unopposed vasopressor activity

      e. Beta Blocker - Theophylline

         i. Effect - Antagonistic activity increasing airway resistance

         ii. Mechanism - Pharmacologic antagonism

      f. Beta Blocker - H2 Antagonists

         i. Effect - Increased effects of beta blockers

         ii. Mechanism - H2 antagonists can inhibit first pass hepatic metabolism of beta-blockers

B. Alpha-1 Adrenergic Blockers

   1. Prazosin (Minipres)

   2. Terazosin (Hytrin)

   3. Doxazosin (Cardura)

   4. Tamsulosin (Flomax)

      a. Are selective alpha-1 receptor antagonists

      b. Used to treat hypertension especially in presence of CHF

      c. Often combined with a diuretic and beta blocker

      d. Adverse effects include orthostatic hypotension

C. Mixed Alpha and Beta Blockade

   1. Labetalol (Normodyne, Trandate)

      a. Alpha and beta-receptor antagonist

      b. Available as oral and IV formulations

      c. Used to treat hypertensive emergencies and the hypertension of pheochromocytoma

   2. Carvedilol (Coreg)

IV. ACE Inhibitors

A. Captopril (Capoten)

B. Enalapril (Vasotec)

   C. Lisinopril (Zestril, Prinivil)

   D. Benazepril (Lotensin)

   E. Ramipril (Altace)

   F. Quinapril (Accupril)

      1. Action exerted by blocking the enzymatic conversion of angiotensin I to angiotensin II which is a potent vasoconstrictor

      2. Lower peripheral vascular resistance along with decreased sodium and water retention

      3. Useful in the treatment of hypertension and CHF

      4. Major advantage over other antihypertensives is for minimal electrolyte disturbances and fewer adverse effects

   G. Drug Interactions:

      1. ACE Inhibitor - Indomethacin

         a. Effect - Decreased hypotensive effect of ACE Inhibitor

         b. Mechanism - Interference with plasma renin activity and vasopressor response

      2. ACE Inhibitor - Potassium Supplements

         a. Effect - Hyperkalemia

         b. Mechanism - Unknown

      3. ACE Inhibitor - Capsaicin (Zostrix)

         a. Effect - Exacerbates coughing associated with ACE Inhibitors

         b. Mechanism - Unknown

V. Angiotensin II Receptor Antagonists

   A. Losartan (Cozaar)

   B. Valsartan (Diovan)

   C. Irbesartan (Avapro)

   D. Candesartan (Atacand)

   E. Telmisartan (Micardis)

   F. Eprosartan (Teveten)

      1. Angiotensin II receptor antagonists block the vasoconstrictor and Aldosterone-secreting effects of angiotensin II by selectively blocking the binding of angiotensin II to the angiotensin I receptor

      2. These agents do not inhibit the angiotensin converting enzyme (ACE)

      3. Additionally, this group of agents does not cause the non-productive cough associated with ACE inhibitors

VI. Calcium Channel Blockers

   A. Verapamil (Calan, Isoptin, Covera-HS)

   B. Nifedipine (Procardia, Adalat)

   C. Diltiazem (Cardizem)

   D. Amlodipine (Norvasc)

   E. Nicardipine (Cardene)

   F. Isradipine (DynaCirc)

   G. Felodipine (Plendil)

      1. Inhibit entry of calcium into cardiac and smooth muscle to reduce peripheral vascular resistance

      2. All calcium channel blockers are vasodilators

      3. Useful to treat hypertension in patients with diabetes, asthma, angina and peripheral vascular disease

4. These agents have an intrinsic natriuretic effect and do not usually require the addition of a diuretic
5. Most notable adverse effect is a negative inotropic effect which can contraindicate use in depressed cardiac function (e.g., CHF)
6. Drug Interactions:
    a. Calcium Blocker - Calcium Salts
        i.   Effect - Clinical effects of calcium blockers are reversed
        ii. Mechanism - Pharmacologic antagonism
    b. Calcium Blocker - Quinidine
        i.   Effect - Hypotension, arrhythmia
        ii. Mechanism - Decreased elimination of Quinidine
    c. Calcium Blocker - H2 antagonists
        i.   Effect - Hypotension
        ii. Mechanism - Inhibition of hepatic metabolism of calcium channel blockers

ANTI-RHEUMATIC DRUGS

I. **Acute Gouty Arthritis**
    A. **Colchicine**
        1. Exact mechanism of action in gout is unclear but Colchicine does inhibit leukocyte migration, cellular mitosis and phagocytosis
        2. Also reduces lactic acid production which in turn decreases uric acid deposition
        3. The anti-inflammatory activity of Colchicine is somewhat specific for gout and rarely effective in other arthritides, which has labeled the drug as a "Diagnostic Indicator"
        4. Primarily used for acute attacks of gout with relief of pain and inflammation within 12-24 hours if given early enough
        5. Most significant adverse effect seen in nearly 80% of patients are gastrointestinal such as nausea, vomiting, abdominal cramps and, in particular, diarrhea
        6. Chronic use can lead to myopathy, hepatic toxicity and agranulocytosis
        7. Contraindicated in patients with serious GI, hepatic dysfunction, blood dyscrasias and cardiac dysfunction
        8. Initial dose is 1-1.2 mg po followed by 0.5-1.2 mg every 1 to 2 hours until pain relieved or nausea, vomiting or diarrhea occurs
        9. Surgical prophylaxis for gout patients - 0.5 or 0.6 mg po tid for 3 days prior and 3 days after surgery
    B. **Indomethacin** (Indocin)
        1. Drug of choice for acute non-infectious arthritis
        2. Generally preferred to the more disease-specific Colchicine because of the high incidence for severe diarrhea
        3. Adverse effects include headache and also gastrointestinal but to lesser extent than Colchicine
        4. Acute gout dose is 50 mg po tid until pain tolerable and then reduced. Tenderness and warmth usually subside in 24 to 36 hours and edema in 3 to 5 days
    C. **Other NSAID Alternatives**
        1. Naproxen and Sulindac are increasingly being used as substitutes for Colchicine in acute attacks
        2. Naproxen (Naprosyn) - 750 mg po followed by 250 mg po tid until attack subsides

3. Sulindac (Clinoril) - 200 mg po bid x 7 days

II. Chronic Gouty Arthritis

A. Allopurinol (Zyloprim)

1. Xanthine Oxidase inhibitor preventing the conversion of Xanthine to uric acid
2. Definitive diagnosis of gout is established on identification of the classic negatively birefringent crystals of Monosodium Urate
3. Although gout is associated with hyperuricemia, elevated levels of uric acid are seen in a variety of disorders
4. Hyperuricemia can be primary as seen in gout or secondary to acute and chronic leukemia, multiple myeloma, psoriasis, renal disease, starvation diets and the use of diuretics
5. Traditionally regarded as the agent of choice in "overproducers" as opposed to "undersecretors" as determined by 24-hour urine specific for urate clearance
6. Allopurinol lowers both serum and urinary levels by inhibiting the formation of uric acid
7. The use of Allopurinol to inhibit urate formation avoids the hazard of increased renal excretion imposed by uricosuric agents
8. Salicylates can be given concurrently with Allopurinol without compromising its action
9. Most serious adverse effect is hypersensitivity with rash, which could progress to Stevens-Johnson Syndrome, vasculitis and even death. Discontinue at first sign of any rash
10. Other adverse effects include renal impairment and hepatic toxicity
11. Interacts with Ampicillin to increase rate of Ampicillin-induced skin rash
12. Half life of Allopurinol is short at 2 hours but is metabolized to Oxypurinol which has a longer half life and still inhibits Xanthine Oxidase allowing once daily dosage
13. Dosage Range - 200-300 mg po daily

B. Probenecid

1. Uricosuric agent reducing urate levels by preventing renal tubular reabsorption of uric acid
2. Inhibits excretion of other drugs such as Penicillin, Cephalosporins, NSAIDS and Methotrexate
3. In contrast to Allopurinol, salicylates antagonize the effect of uricosuric agents
4. Uricosuric agents can precipitate a gout attack whereby Colchicine or Indomethacin may be required during therapy
5. Usual Dose - 500 mg po bid

C. Sulfinpyrazone (Anturane)

1. Uricosuric agent inhibiting the reabsorption of uric acid similar to Probenecid
2. Dose - 100-200 mg po bid

III. Symptom-Modifying Anti-Rheumatic Drugs (SMARDs)

A. Salicylates

1. Discussed Under Analgesic Section

B. NSAIDS

2. Discussed Under Separate Heading

C. Corticosteroids

1. Discussed Under Separate Heading

IV. Disease-Modifying Anti-Rheumatic Drugs (DMARDs)

A. Antimalarials
1. Hydroxychloroquine (Plaquenil)
2. Chloroquine (Aralen)
    a. Exact anti-inflammatory mechanism is unknown but known to have immunosuppressant activity

B. Gold Compounds
1. Aurothioglucose (Solganal)
2. Gold Sodium Thiomalate (Aurolate)
    a. Both are IM injectables containing 50% Gold
    b. Weekly Injections - First dose 10 mg, second week 25 mg, third and subsequent weekly injections at 25-50 mg until 1 g given
    c. If no improvement after total cumulative dose of 1 g, then necessity of Gold therapy should be re-evaluated
3. Auranofin (Ridaura)
    a. Oral formulation containing 29% Gold
    b. Used in more advanced stages of RA
    c. Associated with serious gastrointestinal effects, dermatitis and mucosal membrane lesions
    d. 3 mg po bid or 6 mg po qd

C. Chelating Agents
1. Penicillamine (Cuprimine, Depen)
    a. Metabolite of Penicillin used as chelating agent, which can chelate with gold, iron salts and antacids and should not be given concurrently
    b. Possesses immunosuppressant activity
    c. Adverse effects are extremely serious including blood dyscrasias, renal impairment, optic neuritis, drug fever and autoimmune disorders

D. Immunosuppressants
1. Azathioprine (Imuran)
2. Cyclophosphamide (Cytoxan)
3. Cyclosporin A (Sandimmune)

E. Methotrexate (Rheumatex)
1. Folate Antagonist
2. Inhibits DNA synthesis in mononuclear cells and suppresses interleukin-2 production & IL-1 activity
3. Most commonly used "anchor drug" in combination therapy
4. Considered to be the new gold standard as the most effective DMARD
5. Generally well tolerated and inexpensive
6. Potential toxic effects include bone marrow suppression, pulmonary fibrosis, interstitial pneumonitis, hepatotoxicity and increased susceptibility to infection
7. Baseline testing should include CBC, creatinine, albumin, liver function tests, hepatitis B and C serology & chest X-ray
8. CBC and liver function tests to be repeated at 4-8 week intervals
9. Interacts with NSAIDS to increase MTX toxicity
10. Dosage: 7.5-15 mg/week po or sc (range 5-20 mg/week)

F. Leflunomide (Arava)
1. Pyrimidine antagonist
2. Immunomodulatory agent with anti-inflammatory activity
3. Prodrug metabolized to an acute metabolite
4. Teratogenic and is classified in pregnancy category X

5. Contraindicated in pregnant women and pregnancy must be avoided both during treatment <u>and</u> after treatment prior to the completion of the drug elimination procedure

6. Undergoes extensive enterobiliary reabsorption with the active metabolite still detectable up to 2 years after the drug is discontinued

7. Accelerated drug elimination procedure - Cholestyramine (Questran) 8 gm tid x 11 days

8. Can elevate liver enzymes and liver function tests should be performed initially at monthly intervals

9. Risk of hepatic toxicity is increased by concurrent use of Methotrexate

10. Adverse effects include diarrhea, nausea, headache, respiratory infection, rash and alopecia

11. Interacts with Rifampin which increases its action

12. Dosage: Loading dose of 100 mg qd x 3 d then 20 mg qd

G. Etanercept (Enbrel)

1. TNFR blocker

2. Binds specifically to tumor necrosis factor (TNF) and blocks its interaction with cell surface receptors

3. Indicated as subcutaneous injection to reduce signs and symptoms of moderately to severely active RA in those who have had an inadequate response to one or more DMARDs

4. Can be used in combination with Methotrexate in those who do not respond to MTX alone

5. Also indicated for polyarticular juvenile rheumatoid arthritis

6. Contraindicated in patients with sepsis and should be discontinued if patient develops a serious infection

7. Vaccination with live vaccines should not be administered concurrently

8. Adverse effects include injection site reaction, upper respiratory infection, rhinitis, dizziness, pharyngitis and cough

9. Specific drug interaction studies have not been conducted

10. Dosage: 25 mg injected SC twice a week

H. Infliximab (Remicade)

1. Monoclonal antibody that binds specifically to tumor necrosis factor alpha

2. Currently indicated to treat moderately to severely active Crohn's disease with recent approval for RA

3. May cause hypersensitivity reactions (urticaria, dyspnea, hypotension) and should be discontinued if reactions are severe

4. Adverse reactions include infusion related reactions, upper respiratory infections, autoimmune antibodies, headache, nausea & fatigue

5. Dosage: 5-10 mg/kg IV infusion given sporadically once a month or every 2 months in a two hour outpatient procedure in combination with Methotrexate

I. Anakinra (Kineret)

1. Interleukin-1 (IL-1) receptor antagonist

J. Protein A Immunoabsorption (Prosorba Therapy)

1. FDA approved procedure for severe RA in those patients who failed on multiple DMARDs including Methotrexate

2. Blood is drawn from one arm and passed through a cell separator machine to separate plasma

3. The plasma is passed through a prosorba column to remove antibodies

4. The treated plasma and blood cells are then recombined and returned to the patient through a vein in the other arm

5. Is administered in 12 weekly procedures each lasting 2 to 2-1/2 hours in length
6. Treatment is expensive (approximately $1,500 per treatment or a total of $18,000 for the 12 week course)

V. Miscellaneous Agents

A. Nutraceuticals

1. Glucosamine
   a. "Chondroprotective" nutritional supplement
   b. Amino sugar precursor to Glycosaminoglycans (GAGs)
   c. GAGs form hydrophilic macromolecules called Aggrecan containing large amounts of chondroitin sulfate
   d. Commercially produced from the chitin of shellfish (crab, lobster or shrimp shells)
   e. Oral route most common but can be administered IV, IM and intra-articular
   f. Dosage: 1500 mg/day
2. Chondroitin Sulfate
   a. Most abundant Glycosaminoglycan in cartilage
   b. Structurally similar to Heparin and is generally contraindicated in patients on anticoagulant therapy
   c. Dosage: 1200 mg/day (400 mg po tid)

B. Antibiotics

1. Minocycline (Minocin)
   a. Direct suppressive effects on B and T cell function
   b. Suppresses release of metalloproteinases
   c. May cause a lupus-like condition in some patients on long term use characterized by joint pain, lethargy, fever, Raynaud's phenomenon and a butterfly rash

C. Hyaluronic Acid Substitutes

1. Hylan G-F 20 (Synvisc)
2. Hyaluronan (Hyalgan)
   a. Hyaluronic acid substitutes
   b. Intra-articular viscosupplementation with high molecular weight fractions of sodium Hyaluronate or cross linked polymers of Hylans is aimed at improving the elasticity & viscosity of synovial fluid
   c. Indicated for treatment of pain in OA of the knee joint only in patients who failed to respond to conservative nonpharmacologic therapy and simple analgesics
   d. Following intra-articular administration, both agents move slowly into synovium, permeate articular cartilage to slowly move through joint tissues and eventually pass through the lymph system into systemic circulation
   e. Complete hepatic metabolism yields CO_2 and H_2O in about 7 days or less
   f. Contraindicated in avian allergies to avian proteins, feathers or egg products since extracted from chicken/rooster combs
   g. Contraindicated with quaternary ammonium disinfectants for skin preparation which cause precipitation of drug
   h. Do not administer concomitantly with other intra-articular injectables nor in presence of joint effusion
   i. Adverse reactions include injection site pain, knee pain & swelling, rash, ankle edema, hemorrhoid problems and phlebitis with varicosities
   j. Advise patients to avoid strenuous or prolonged (1 hour or more) weight bearing activities for up to 48 hours after treatment

    k. Dosage:

Hylan G-F20 (Synvisc) - 2 ml (16 mg) once weekly for total cycle of 3 injections using 18-22 g needle

Hyaluronan (Hyalgan) - 2 ml (20 mg) once weekly for total cycle of 5 injections using 20 g needle

CORTICOSTEROIDS

I. **General**

  A. **Glucocorticoids are the principal steroids used by podiatrists to treat a wide range of inflammatory disorders**

  B. **Major physiological glucocorticoid produced by adrenal cortex is Hydrocortisone (Cortisol)**

  C. **Normal daily production is about 20-30 mg Hydrocortisone**

  D. **Mechanism of action influenced by metabolic effects on protein, lipid and carbohydrate metabolism and anti-inflammatory effects**

  E. **Protein catabolic effects leads to skeletal muscle weakness and wasting. Destruction of skeletal protein matrix results in osteoporosis**

  F. **Carbohydrate metabolism effects involve accelerated glucose production and decreased peripheral utilization elevating plasma glucose levels**

  G. **Steroids affect lipid metabolism by decreasing rate of glucose uptake by adipose tissue**

  H. **Anti-inflammatory effect due to ability to inhibit enzyme phospholipase A2 responsible for releasing arachidonic acid as the precursor for prostaglandins and leukotrienes**

  I. **Primary classification of glucocorticoids is based on plasma and physiologic half-life in ability to suppress Adrenocorticotropic Hormone (ACTH)**

II. **Classification**

  A. **Short-Acting** (8-12 hrs.)
1. Hydrocortisone
2. Cortisone

  B. **Intermediate-Acting** (18-36 hrs.)
1. Prednisone
2. Prednisolone
3. Methylprednisolone
4. Triamcinolone
5. Paramethasone

  C. **Long-Acting** (36-54 hrs.)
1. Dexamethasone
2. Betamethasone

III. **Injectable Glucocorticoids** - The agents listed below represent a select group of commonly used injectable steroids in podiatry. Generally, the phosphate and succinate salts are considered short acting with actions lasting several days up to a week or two. Acetate, Diacetate, Tebutate, Acetonide and Hexacetonide salts are all considered long-acting with effects lasting from weeks to even months. The number of steroid injections to a specific anatomic area is well documented in the literature not to exceed 3 or 4 times per year. "Steroid Flare" is a common post injection problem due to a crystal-induced synovitis seen most commonly with the repository acetate type suspensions.   Starts shortly after injection and rarely continues beyond 48-72 hours.   Usually treated symptomatically with local ice application and analgesics

- **A. Short-Acting Injectables**
    1. Hydrocortisone Sodium Succinate (Solu-Cortef)
        a.   100-500 mg IV or IM
    2. Methylprednisolone Sodium Succinate (Solu-Medrol)
        a.   10-40 gm IV or IM
    3. Dexamethasone Phosphate (Decadron, Hexadrol, Dalalone)
        a.   4 mg/ml concentration
        b.   0.8-1 mg for small joints
    4. Betamethasone Phosphate (Celestone Phosphate)
        a.   0.5-1 mg for small joints
- **B. Long-Acting Injectables**
    1. Triamcinolone Acetonide (Kenalog)
        a.   2.5-5 mg for small joints
    2. Methylprednisolone Acetate (Depo-Medrol)
        a.   4-10 mg in small joints
    3. Dexamethasone Acetate (Decadron-LA, Dalalone-DP, TDX-LA)
        a.   4-16 mg
    4. Betamethasone Acetate/Phosphate (Celestone Soluspan)
        a.   0.5-1 cc in most foot disorders

IV. Topical Corticosteroids

- **A. Following topical absorption, corticosteroids enter systemic circulation and are metabolized the same as systemically administered steroids**
- **B. Primary effects due to anti-inflammatory activity for most causes of cutaneous inflammation including mechanical, thermal, chemical, microbial and hypersensitivity reactions**
- **C. Topical Formulation Selection:**
    1. Ointments are occlusive and generally preferred for dry scaly lesions
    2. Creams are more drying than ointments in a vanishing base and are usually best suited for weeping or oozing lesions and intertriginal areas
    3. Gels, lotions, solutions and aerosol vehicles are most useful on hairy areas
        a.   Generally ointments and gels are considered more potent than cream or lotion products
        b.   Urea can help to enhance penetration of steroids by hydrating skin
        c.   Application of steroids under plastic or saran wrap for occlusion dramatically increase skin penetration but could lead to maceration and increased systemic effects
        d.   Some of the more common and newer topical agents are noted below
        e.   Dosage for topical steroids usually is to apply sparingly 2-4 times daily to affected areas
- **D. Super High Potency**
    1. Clobetasol Propionate (Temovate 0.05%)
    2. Betamethasone Dipropionate (Diprolene 0.05%)
    3. Halobetasol Propionate (Ultravate 0.05%)
- **E. High Potency**
    1. Amcinonide (Cyclocort 0.1%)
    2. Halcinonide (Halog 0.1%)
    3. Fluocinonide (Lidex 0.05%)

      4.   Desoximetasone (Topicort 0.25%)
      5.   Diflorasone Diacetate (Psorcon-E, Florone 0.05%)

  F. Mid-Range Potency
      1.   Fluticasone Propionate (Cutivate 0.005%)
      2.   Flurandrenolide (Cordran 0.05%)
      3.   Triamcinolone Acetonide (Kenalog 0.1%, Aristocort 0.1%)
      4.   Fluocinolone Acetonide (Synalar 0.025%)
      5.   Betamethasone (Valerate 0.1%)
      6.   Mometasone (Elocon 0.1%)

  G. Mild Potency
      1.   Alclometasone Dipropionate (Aclovate 0.05%)
      2.   Desonide (Tridesilon 0.05%)
      3.   Dexamethasone (Decadron 0.1%)
      4.   Hydrocortisone (Hytone 0.5%, 1%, 2.5%)

V. Steroid-Related Complications

  A. Musculoskeletal System
      1.   Osteoporosis and risk for spontaneous pathologic fractures are most significant reasons to limit long-term use
      2.   Affects all bones especially vertebrae, ribs and long bones
      3.   Steroid myopathy is most prominent in lower extremities
      4.   Implicated in avascular necrosis of bone
      5.   Growth failure in children with irreversible height loss

  B. Endocrine System
      1.   Weight gain and obesity
      2.   Redistribution of subcutaneous fat rounding facial contour in the classic "Moonface" and dorsocervical fat pad accumulation causing the typical "Buffalo Hump"
      3.   Glucose intolerance with progression to corticosteroid-induced diabetes
      4.   Steroids may increase the requirement for Insulin or oral hypoglycemic agents in diabetes

  C. Cardiovascular System
      1.   Hypertension as result of weight gain along with sodium and water retention

  D. Gastrointestinal System
      1.   Development of peptic ulceration or exacerbation of pre-existing ulcer disease

  E. Dermatologic System
      1.   Subcutaneous fat atrophy
      2.   Striae, purpura and local burning or sensitivity from topical use
      3.   Delayed wound healing

  F. Immune System
      1.   Suppression of cellular and immunologic defense mechanisms

  G. Ocular Effects
      1.   Development of posterior subcapsular cataracts and increase in intraocular pressure

  H. Psychological Effects
      1.   Range from euphoria, irritability, paranoia to even steroid-induced psychoses

NSAIDS

I. General - Primary mechanism of action involves inhibition of cyclooxygenase (COX) activity and prostaglandin synthesis. Have analgesic and antipyretic effects. Metabolism is mostly dependent on hepatic biotransformation. COX-1 is important for platelet aggregation, regulation of blood flow in the kidney and stomach, and regulation of gastric acid secretion. COX-2 is induced during pain and inflammatory stimuli.

II. Propionic Acid Derivatives
    A. Ibuprofen (Motrin, Advil, Nuprin)
        1. 300-800 mg po tid-qid
    B. Fenoprofen Calcium (Nalfon)
        1. 300-600 mg po tid-qid
    C. Ketoprofen (Orudis, Oruvail, Orudis-KT, Actron)
        1. 25-50 mg po tid-qid
        2. Oruvail is sustained-release dosed at 75 mg po bid
    D. Naproxen (Naprosyn, EC-Naprosyn, Aleve, Naprelan)
        1. 250-500 mg po bid
        2. EC-Naprosyn is enteric-coated sustained-release dosed at 375-500 mg po bid
        3. Naprelan is extended release tablet dosed at two tablets of either 375 mg or 500 mg po qd
    E. Naproxen Sodium (Anaprox, Anaprox-DS)
        1. 275-550 mg po bid
        2. Primarily promoted for analgesia since sodium salt allows for quicker absorption
    F. Flurbiprofen (Ansaid)
        1. 50-100 mg po bid-tid
    G. Oxaprozin (Daypro)
        1. 1200 mg (600 mg x2) po qd

III. Acetic Acid Derivatives
    A. Indomethacin (Indocin, Indocin-SR)
        1. 25-50 mg po bid-tid
        2. Indocin-SR is sustained release formulation dosed at 75 mg po bid
        3. Drug of choice for acute non-infectious arthritis (e.g., Gout)
        4. Headache is common adverse effect believed to be due to serotonin release not effectively relieved by aspirin nor Acetaminophen. Diphenhydramine (Benadryl) has antihistaminic and antiserotonin activity which may be of benefit
        5. Not an innocuous drug with serious GI disturbances and renal effects
    B. Sulindac (Clinoril)
        1. 150-200 mg po bid
        2. NSAID of choice in renal impairment due to "Renal Sparing" effect
        3. Has mild Aldose Reductase inhibition activity which may be useful in diabetics with neuropathy
    C. Tolmetin (Tolectin, Tolectin-DS)
        1. 200-600 mg po tid
    D. Etodolac (Lodine, Lodine-XL)
        1. COX-2 "Preferential" Inhibitor
        2. 200-400 mg po bid-tid
        3. Lodine-XL available in 400 mg & 600 mg dosage forms
    E. Diclofenac Sodium (Voltaren, Voltaren-XR)
        1. "Delayed Release" enteric-coated formulation
        2. 50-75 mg po bid
        3. Voltaren-XR is extended release tablet dosed at 100 mg po qd or bid

F. Diclofenac Potassium (Cataflam)
   1. "Immediate Release" conventional tablet promoted for analgesia since conventional tablet dissolves faster
   2. 50 mg po tid

G. Diclofenac Sodium/Misoprostol (Arthrotec)
   1. Arthrotec-50 po bid-tid
   2. Arthrotec-75 po bid
   3. Direct ulcerogenic effects minimized with addition of Misoprostol but diarrhea can pose a problem in a significant number of patients

H. Ketorolac Tromethamine (Toradol)
   1. Indicated only for short term management of moderately severe pain requiring analgesia at the opioid level for up to 5 days
   2. Only NSAID available in injectable format
   3. 30 mg IV or 60 mg IM under age 65
   4. 15 mg IV or 30 mg IM over age 65
   5. 10 mg po every 4 to 6 hours

IV. Oxicams

A. Piroxicam (Feldene)
   1. 10 mg po bid or 20 mg po qd

B. Meloxicam (Mobic)
   1. COX-2 "Preferential" Inhibitor
   2. 7.5 mg po qd; may be increased to maximum dosage of 15 mg po qd

V. Fenamates

A. Meclofenamate Sodium (Meclomen)
   1. 50-100 mg po tid-qid
   2. Diarrhea is common and can be serious enough to limit therapy with either of the Fenamates

B. Mefenamic Acid (Ponstel)
   1. Indicated only for analgesia for therapy less than a week
   2. 250 mg po every 6 hours

VI. Naphthylalkanones

A. Nabumetone (Relafen)
   1. 1,000 mg po qd or 500-750 mg po bid
   2. Promoted for lower GI effects due to non-acidic entity
   3. COX-2 "Preferential" Inhibitor

VII. Benzene Sulfonamides

A. Celecoxib (Celebrex)
   1. Selective COX-2 inhibitor that may also be referred to as a COX-1 sparing agent
   2. GI effects markedly reduced but not necessarily eliminated
   3. Cannot use in patients allergic to ASA, NSAIDS and Sulfonamides since molecular structure similar to sulfonamides
   4. Indicated for OA, RA, intestinal polyps to reduce number of polyps in those with familial adenomatous polyposis, and acute pain

5. Dose:
    100 mg po bid or 200 mg qd for OA
    100-200 mg po bid for RA
    400 mg po bid for intestinal polyps
    600 mg/day on 1st day, then 400 mg/day thereafter for acute pain

B. Valdecoxib (Bextra)
1. Selective COX-2 inhibitor
2. Indicated for RA, OA and primary dysmenorrhea. Contraindicated in patients allergic to ASA, NSAIDS and sulfonamides
3. Available in 10 mg & 20 mg tablets
4. Dose:
    10 mg po qd for OA & RA
    20 mg po bid prn for primary dysmenorrhea

VIII. Methylsulfonyls

A. Rofecoxib (Vioxx)
1. Highly selective COX-2 inhibitor that may also be referred to as a COX-1 sparing agent
2. GI effects are markedly reduced but not necessarily eliminated
3. Currently indicated for osteoarthritis, acute pain and primary dysmenorrhea
4. Available in both tablet and liquid suspension forms
5. 12.5-25 mg po qd for osteoarthritis
6. 50 mg po qd for acute pain not to exceed 5 days

IX. COX Inhibitor Classification

A. COX-1 Specific Inhibitors
Aspirin

B. COX Non-specific Inhibitors
Bulk of most commonly used NSAIDS such as Ibuprofen, Indomethacin, Naproxen

C. COX-2 Preferential Inhibitors
Etodolac (Lodine)
Nabumetone (Relafen)
Meloxicam (Mobic)

D. COX-2 Specific Inhibitors
Celecoxib (Celebrex)
Rofecoxib (Vioxx)
Valdecoxib (Bextra)

X. Primary Adverse Effects

A. Gastrointestinal
1. Nausea, vomiting, diarrhea and GI ulceration

B. CNS
1. Most frequent is frontal headache especially with Indomethacin in 25-50% of patients
2. Dizziness, lightheadedness and mental confusion can also occur

C. Acute Pancreatitis
1. Has occurred most notably with Sulindac

D. Hematologic Effects
1. Neutropenia and thrombocytopenia especially with Indomethacin

E. Hypersensitivity Reactions

1. Include urticaria, pruritis and acute asthmatic attacks
2. Cross-sensitivity in aspirin-allergic patients

XI. Drug Interactions
A. NSAIDS - Oral Anticoagulants
1. Increased bleeding and hypoprothrombinemic effects of Warfarin
2. Mechanism - Protein binding displacement combined with antiplatelet effects
B. NSAIDS - Beta Blockers
1. Impaired antihypertensive effect of beta-blockers
2. Mechanism - NSAIDS inhibit renal prostaglandin synthesis allowing unopposed vasopressor activity
C. NSAIDS - Lithium
1. Increased Lithium toxicity
2. Mechanism - Decreased Lithium renal clearance
D. NSAIDS (Indomethacin) - ACE Inhibitors
1. Decreased hypotensive effect of ACE inhibitors
2. Mechanism - Interference with plasma renin activity and vasopressor response
E. NSAIDS - Methotrexate
1. Increased Methotrexate toxicity
2. Mechanism - Decreased renal clearance of Methotrexate

SKELETAL MUSCLE RELAXANTS

I. Central Acting
A. Carisoprodol (Soma)
1. 350 mg po tid or qid
B. Chlorphenesin Carbamate (Maolate)
1. 400 mg po qid
C. Chlorzoxazone (Paraflex, Parafon Forte DSC)
1. 250-500 mg po tid-qid
D. Cyclobenzaprine (Flexeril)
1. 10 mg po tid
E. Metaxalone (Skelaxin)
1. 800 mg (400 mg x2) po tid-qid
F. Methocarbamol (Robaxin)
1. 1-1.5 g po tid-qid
G. Orphenadrine Citrate (Norflex)
1. 100 mg po bid
H. Diazepam (Valium)
1. 2-10 mg po tid-qid
I. Baclofen (Lioresal)
1. 40-80 mg po daily in divided doses
J. Tizanidine (Zanaflex)
1. 4-8 mg po, which can be repeated at 6 to 8 hour intervals not to exceed 36 mg/day

II. Direct Acting
A. Dantrolene Sodium (Dantrium)

1. 25-100 mg po 2 to 4 times daily
2. Associated with high risk potential for hepatotoxicity
3. IV Dantrolene is used to treat malignant hyperthermia
4. All skeletal muscle relaxants have potential to cause CNS effects such as drowsiness or lightheadedness and GI effects

PEDIATRIC DOSING GUIDELINES

I.   **Young's Rule**

$$\frac{Age}{Age + 12} \times Adult\ Dose = Child\ Dose$$

II. **Clark's Rule**

$$\frac{Weight\ (in\ pounds) \times Adult\ Dose}{150} = Child\ Dose$$

III. **Cowling's Rule**

$$\frac{Age\ At\ Next\ Birthday\ (in\ years) \times Adult\ Dose}{24} = Child\ Dose$$

IV. **Fried's Rule For Infants**

$$\frac{Age\ (in\ months) \times Adult\ Dose}{150} = Infant\ Dose$$

V.   **Grain Rule for Acetaminophen/Aspirin Dosing**

One Grain (approximately 65 mg) for each year of age

e.g., 5 year old child may take one standard adult 5 gr (325 mg) tablet

BIBLIOGRAPHY AND SUGGESTED READING

Burnham, Teri Hines - Senior Managing Editor. Drug Facts and Comparisons, 56th Edition, pp. 2205. Facts and Comparisons, Wolters Kluwer Company, St. Louis, 2002.

Cunha, Burke A. - Editor. The Medical Clinics of North America. Antibiotic Therapy - Part I, pp. 1530. W.B. Saunders Company, Philadelphia, November 2000.

Cunha, Burke A. - Editor. The Medical Clinics of North America. Antibiotic Therapy - Part II, pp. 192. W.B. Saunders Company, Philadelphia, January 2001.

Joseph, Warren S. Handbook of Lower Extremity Infections, pp. 236. Churchill Livingstone, New York, 1990.

Pfeifer, Michael A. - Editor-In-Chief. Resource Guide 2002, pp. 136. Diabetes Forecast, January 2002.

Dunkin, Mary Anne. Drug Guide 2002, pp. 32-52. Arthritis Today, January/February 2002.

Juda, Erwin J. Corticosteroids: Their Use and Abuse. Advances in Podiatric Medicine and Surgery, Volume 2. Kominsky, Stephen J. - Editor In Chief. Mosby - Yearbook, St. Louis, 1996.

Barenholtz, Hedva A., and Bellamy, C., Duane. Atypical Analgesics and Pain, pp. 54-69. U.S. Pharmacist, June 1995.

Stoklosa, Mitchell J. Pharmaceutical Calculations, 6th Edition, pp. 93-95, Lea S. Febiger, Philadelphia, 1974.

Roth, Richard D. Glucocorticoids: Use in the Management of Rheumatic Disorders. Musculoskeletal Disorders of the Lower Extremities, pp. 437-448. Edited by Oloff, Lawrence M. W.B. Saunders Company, Philadelphia, 1994.

Kaschak, Thomas J. Pharmacologic Management of Inflammatory Joint Disease. Musculoskeletal Disorders of the Lower Extremities, pp. 397-436. Edited by Oloff, Lawrence M.   W.B. Saunders, Philadelphia, 1994.

Christ, Daryl. High Yield Pharmacology, pp. 122. Lippincott Williams & Wilkins, Philadelphia, 1999.

Rosenfeld, Gary C. and Loose-Mitchell, David S. Pharmacology, 3rd Edition, pp. 445. Lippincott Williams & Wilkins, Philadelphia, 1998.

Ament, Paul W., Bertolino, John G. and Liszewski, James L.   Clinically Significant Drug Interactions, pp. 1745-1753. American Family Physician, March 15, 2000.

Paauw, Douglas S. Commonly Overlooked Drug Interactions. pp. 93-97. Emergency Medicine, March 2001.

CHAPTER 3
PHARMACOLOGY

1.   Acute withdrawal symptoms can be precipitated in opioid-dependent patients when given:

      A.   Methadone (Dolophine)
      B.   Tramadol (Ultram)
      C.   Pentazocine (Talwin)
      D.   Meperidine (Demerol)
      E.   Levorphanol (Levo-Dromoran)

2.   Blockade of Beta-2 receptors will result in:

      A.   Bronchoconstriction
      B.   Increased cardiac contractility
      C.   Tachycardia
      D.   Decreased airway resistance
      E.   None of the above

3.   Anti-pseudomonal activity is associated with all of the following except:

      A.   Ciprofloxacin (Cipro)
      B.   Cefuroxime (Maxipime)
      C.   Cefepime (Zinacef)
      D.   Piperacillin (Pipracel)
      E.   Ceftazidime (Fortaz)

4.   Which of the following drugs have the potential for proarrhythmic effects associated with prolongation of the QT interval?

      A.   Gatifloxacin (Tequin)
      B.   Amitriptyline (Elavil)
      C.   Azithromycin (Zithromax)
      D.   A and B
      E.   B and C

5.   Hepatic toxicity can occur with all of the following except:

      A.   Carbamazepine (Tegretol)
      B.   Gabapentin (Neurontin)
      C.   Methotrexate (Rheumatrex)
      D.   Leflunomide (Arava)
      E.   Terbinafine (Lamisil)

6.   The use of Itraconazole (Sporanox) is contraindicated with what group of drugs?

      A.   HMG CoA reductase inhibitors
      B.   Proton pump inhibitors
      C.   ACE inhibitors
      D.   Xanthine Oxidase inhibitors
      E.   Alpha-Glucosidase inhibitors

7.   Which of the following is primarily used to regulate bedtime glucose control?

        A.   Insulin Lispro (Humalog)
        B.   Nateglinide (Starlix)
        C.   Insulin Glargine (Lantus)
        D.   Glimepiride (Amaryl)
        E.   Insulin Aspart (Novolog)

8.   Mr. Jones is on Warfarin (Coumadin) for atrial fibrillation and has been given a prescription for Griseofulvin to treat onychomycosis. The anticoagulant effect of his Warfarin would be:

        A.   Increased
        B.   Neutralized
        C.   Decreased
        D.   Unaltered

9.   Which of the following agents would be most appropriate to treat a polymicrobial diabetic foot infection in a Penicillin-allergic patient?

        A.   Ticarcillin – Clavulanate
        B.   Clindamycin – Ciprofloxacin
        C.   Vancomycin – Levofloxacin
        D.   A and B
        E.   B and C

10.   The NSAID considered to have a "renal-sparing" effect is:

        A.   Indomethacin (Indocin)
        B.   Ketoprofen (Orudis)
        C.   Piroxicam (Feldene)
        D.   Sulindac (Clinoril)
        E.   Etodolac (Lodine)

NEUROLOGY

*by Gerald A. Weber and Mary Ann Cardile,
updated for 2004 edition by Sam Spadone*

INTRODUCTION

Neurological disorders affecting the lower extremity continue to represent a significant, as well as diverse, number of conditions. The pathogenesis of these entities poses a distinct challenge to the podiatric clinician in terms of timely diagnosis, prognosis, and treatment, including pertinent consultation. This chapter is intended to provide a concise reference to the clinician for a methodical approach toward the various neuro-muscular disorders affecting the lower extremity.

I. **Neurological systems affecting the lower extremity**

A. **Central nervous system** (CNS)
1. Principally entails the brain and spinal cord
2. Functionally comprised of five divisions:
    a. The cerebral hemispheres and cortex consists of the frontal, parietal, temporal, and occipital lobes. These variously process sensory inputs, initiate complex volitional movements, and allow integration of sensory feedback and motor function
    b. The cerebellum together with the basal ganglia (caudate nucleus, putamen, globus pallidus) affects movement, muscle tone, and coordination
    c. The diencephalon (thalamus, hypothalamus, epithalamus, and subthlamus) serves as a relay station for transmitting sensory, motor, and homeostatic information. The thalamus is considered the gateway to conscious perception of sensation
    d. The brainstem (medulla, pons, and midbrain) functions to control the head and neck, as well as to process sensory information carried by the cranial and spinal nerves. Also involved with maintenance of vital functions
    e. The spinal cord's major function is to connect the peripheral and autonomic systems with the brain by receiving their afferent information and sending out efferent information. Reflex activity is initiated by spinal neurons and these also play a significant role in modulating volitional movements

B. **Peripheral nervous system** (PNS)
1. Consists of cranial and spinal nerves and their associated ganglia (posterior and anterior roots), which form nerve plexuses (e.g., lumbosacral) and subsequently branch into progressively smaller peripheral nerve branches

    2. Sensory peripheral nerve fibers are responsible for skin and joint enervation, while the motor fibers are engaged in supplying enervation to the musculature

C. Automatic Nervous System (ANS)

    1. Comprises the sympathetic and parasympathetic systems. Fibers of both are represented in the peripheral nervous systems (note that there is no parasympathetic enervation in the free lower extremity)

    2. Primary function is the enervation of involuntary structures (i.e., sympathetic enervation to the blood vessels of the lower extremities)

II. Clinical assessment of a suspected neurological deficit affecting the lower extremity

A. Eliciting an appropriate history

    1. Chief complaint

      a. Symptoms should reflect a neurogenic origin, though these may often be of a vague and non-specific nature

      b. Generalized complaints (may range from paresthesia, to numbness, tingling, electric-like shocks, unsteadiness during gait, sharp stabbing pains, burning, coldness and/or itching) may represent a sensory and/or autonomic dysfunction

      c. Weakness, stiffness, instability, spasticity, cramping, and fatigue often depict the presence of an underlying deficit of the motor system

    2. Location

      a. The distribution of symptoms will invariably characterize the level of the responsible lesion(s)

      b. Spasm and/or tightness, causing a flexion positioning of the fingers, wrist, elbow, knee, and/or ankle indicates an underlying disorder of contralateral cortical origin

      c. A unilateral flaccid foot drop reflects a peroneal palsy

      d. A "pins and needles" sensation in a stocking distribution of both feet and ankles is consistent with a sensory polyneuropathy

    3. Onset

      a. Refers to the relative acuteness, chronicity, or insidious nature of the chief concern

      b. An acute process may often reflect a traumatic or vascular insult

      c. A gradual and insidious development of signs and symptoms often reflects an underlying metabolic, structural, functional, or hereditary process. Acute onset of toxic or metabolic processes manifests with disturbances of higher cortical functions

    4. Course of the affliction typically belies the nature of the underlying pathologic process

      a. Toxic, infectious, metabolic, and neoplastic etiologies invariably proceed in a progressive pattern

      b. Vascular (ischemic) causes will characteristically induce a static deficit

    5. Duration

      a. Regardless of the etiology, the duration of the condition will correlate directly with the virulence of the underlying disorder

    6. Past medical history

      a. Correlations to neuropathology may often be traced to underlying conditions such as diabetes mellitus, thyroid disorders, collagen vascular diseases, pernicious anemia, and infections such as syphilis, etc.

    7. The age of the patient will help determine the probability of various differential diagnoses

      a. Using myopathic weakness as an example, involvement of the legs of a child is more likely related to Duchenne's or Becker's muscular dystrophy. However, after the third or fourth decade of life, such findings are more apt to be associated with polymyositis. Progressive paraparesis is more likely the result of an underlying spinal dysraphism in a child; multiple sclerosis should be suspected for the same presentation in an adult

8. Additional factors in the patient's history to be considered include:
   a. Gender
   b. Socioeconomic factors
   c. Occupation
   d. Past surgical history
   e. Family history
   f. Exacerbating factors
   g. Alleviating factors
   h Prior treatment and response

B. The sensory evaluation
   1. Observation
      a. Findings indicative of underlying sensory impairment include dystrophic skin and nails, ulcerations, dermal lesions (e.g., tufting of hair, port-wine stains, soft tissue masses, sinus tracts that may be seen in the lumbosacral region of patients with underlying spinal dysraphisms), and Charcot joint deformities
   2. Combined discriminatory sensation
      a. An impairment of these parameters (including stereognosis, graphesthesia, and two-point tactile discrimination) reflects a deficit of higher cortical sensory function (i.e., CNS deficit of the parietal lobe of the brain). However, these findings can be present in dense peripheral neuropathies; testing touch localization and double simultaneous extinction may help identify the level of involvement. Touch localization is assessed by having the patient, with eyes closed, identify where they are touched. Inability to do so suggests a cortical lesion. Double simultaneous extinction is assessed by having the patient, again with eyes closed, identify two points touched simultaneously (e.g., left hallux and right fifth toe). Inability to identify both parts touched implicates a cortical lesion
         i. <u>Stereognosis</u> - Simple objects, such as a key or coin, are placed into the palm of a patient's hand with his or her eyes closed; an inability to discern the object is consistent with a parietal lobe lesion (but see above). The same test may be performed by pressing objects into the plantar surface of the foot
         ii. <u>Graphesthesia</u> - A letter or number is traced onto the extended palm of a patient with his or her eyes closed; inability to discern the figure in the presence of grossly normal sensation indicates cortical pathology. Care must be taken to insure that the figures traced onto the skin appear the same from both the examiner's and the patient's perspectives
         iii. <u>Two-point discrimination</u> - Assesses cortical sensory integration as well as peripheral nerve function. When a deficit is noted diffusely over extremities as well as the truncal region, the underlying pathology is likely of a cortical nature. Two identical stimuli (these should be of small diameter but not sharp) are applied, alternating from a single one to both being applied simultaneously, first at a distance of several inches apart, then progressively closer together. Upon the soles of the feet, a patient should normally perceive two points of stimulation until the stimuli are only millimeters apart (norms have been established for different areas of the foot); on the trunk the normal two-point discrimination distance threshold is three to four inches

3. Light touch
   a. Assesses the integrity of the anterior spinothalamic tracts and the posterior columns
   b. The stroking of the skin with a cotton ball, small brush, or nylon filament should be perceived within the distribution of all peripheral nerves and dermatomes

4. Vibratory (pallesthesia) sensation
   a. A function of the posterior columns
   b. Assessed with a tuning fork (128 cycles/sec.) over bony prominences. More quantitative measures (e.g., the biothesiometer) are available
   c. The tuning fork is applied distally, and then moved proximally as the perception dissipates
   d. Depending on the observed pattern of sensory deficits, loss of vibratory sensation may indicate a mononeuropathy simplex, mononeuropathy multiplex, polyneuropathy, or radiculopathy

5. Proprioception (another posterior column mediated function)
   a. With patient's eyes closed, joint position sense at the first and fifth MPJ's is assessed by moving the respective digits slightly into dorsiflexion and plantarflexion in a random fashion and having the patient identify which position the joint is in. Inability to identify joint position is consistent with posterior column impairment or peripheral neuropathy. When moving the digits, they should be grasped by the proximal phalanges medially and laterally, not dorsally and plantarly

6. Pain and temperature
   a. A function of lateral spinothalamic tract integrity
   b. Application of a sharp pin alternating irregularly with a blunt object to skin within the distribution of peripheral nerves, as well as dermatome distributions with the patient's eyes closed. Inability to perceive the difference is indicative of a deficit
   c. Temperature sensation may be assessed using an ice cube or a metal object at room temperature. Failure to perceive either as cold is abnormal

7. Deep tendon reflexes
   a. To be described under the motor examination. However, realize that a deficit of the posterior (sensory) spinal root ganglia will produce a diminution of the reflex due to a compromised receptor reflex arc. These may also be affected by intraspinal pathology

8. Lower extremity dermatome distributions
   a. Dermatomes reflect the sensory enervation of the skin by various posterior spinal roots
   b. The L_4 distribution supplies the medial (dorsal and plantar) aspect of the hallux, foot, and lower leg, crossing the patella to innervate the lateral thigh
   c. The L_5 distribution supplies the central dorsal and plantar regions of the foot. More proximally it innervates the anterior lateral aspect of the leg
   d. The S_1 distribution is the dorsal and plantar aspects of the foot including the fifth digit, continuing proximally to encompass the posterolateral aspect of the leg and thigh
   e. The S_2 distribution provides enervation to the plantar and posteromedial aspect of the heel, as well as the posteromedial aspects of the leg and thigh

C. **The motor examination**
   Both CNS (upper motor) and PNS (lower motor) deficits may be assessed through employment of the same clinical tests
   1. Observation - The patient should be surveyed for the presence of instability, spasticity, drop foot, and ataxia. The patient should be inspected for any abnormal movements, e.g.,

tremors, fasciculations, and exaggerated or atypical associated movements

a. Fasciculations are visible twitching of muscle fibers without motion at the joint crossed. Fasciculations indicate peripheral denervation of metabolic, immunologic, or compression neuropathies

b. Resting tremor (typically of fingers) may manifest with a pin rolling motion and is suggestive of basal ganglia disease

c. Intention tremor (conspicuous only upon engaging in an action such as past pointing), particularly seen in the fingers is indicative of cerebellar dysfunction

d. Athetosis consists of slow, writhing movements of the face and joints of the extremities, including alternating repetitive movements of the smaller joints of the fingers and toes, alternating between flexion and extension in an involuntary and irregular fashion, which occurs at rest or during purposeful movements. Athetosis is indicative of basal ganglia and/or extrapyramidal dysfunction

e. Chorea manifests with involuntary rapid, jerky, purposeless, and repetitive movements of the head and extremities with grimacing of the face. Chorea may occur at rest or while engaging in movement and is indicative of basal ganglia and/or extrapyramidal tract disease

f. Dystonia is the persistent posturing (or attitude) of one or more joints of an extremity in an athetoid movement. Dystonia often manifests as overextension or inversion of the foot. This phenomenon may progressively evolve to engage multiple proximal joints as well as the trunk and neck (known in the latter case as torticollis). Dystonia is indicative of basal ganglia and extrapyramidal disorders

g. Tics are habitual and persistent movements (or mannerisms) that the patient cannot voluntarily suppress. These actions range from repetitive sniffing, clearing of the throat, protrusion of the chin, and blinking, to a complex of movements. Tics do not imply any particular pathologic process and may be seen in psychiatric as well as neurological disease

h. Asterixis consists of arrhythmic lapses of sustained posture and is typically evoked by having the patient maintain outstretched arms while the hands are dorsiflexed and the fingers extended. In this case, asterixis manifests in nonrhythmic flexion movements of the fingers or hands. Asterixis is usually due to hepatic or other metabolic and toxic encephalopathies, though it may be caused by hypercapnia and anticonvulsants such as phenytoin

i. Myoclonus is the involuntary and sudden (unpredictable) shock-like contractions of muscle groups and is irregular in rhythm and amplitude. With few exceptions, these movements are asynchronous and asymmetrical

   i. Rapid and faster than chorea

   ii. May be related to a seizure disorder (e.g., atypical petit mal and akinetic) particularly when focal to one extremity. Observation should additionally include detection of contractures and muscle atrophy, as well as for mental alertness and comprehension

2. Muscle tone should be evaluated with respect to individual muscle (i.e., tibialis anterior, peroneus brevis, tibialis posterior) in contrast to muscle groups. The assessment occurs with palpation of the tendonous insertion of each respective muscle with the tendon in a state of maximum stretch. Muscle tone should be classified as follows:

a. Hypotonia (decreased tone) is most often indicative of a peripheral (lower motor) neuropathy or myopathy, although an initial state (3-6 months) of hypotonia may follow acute CNS processes and precede a subsequent CNS (upper motor) induced state of spasticity

b. Normal tone

c. <u>Hypertonia</u> (increased tone) is invariably the result of a CNS (upper motor neuron) lesion or major mental disorder

d. <u>Clonus</u> is a manifestation of hypertonicity which, when present, is evoked by applying multiple repetitive end-range of motion stretches to the affected muscle/tendon. Clonus appears in either an unsustained or sustained state following repetitive stretching of the tendon. In the former, a rapid, rhythmic jerking alternating state of muscle contraction and relaxation ensues; in the latter the affected enters a fixed "clasp-knife" type of spasm for several seconds before relaxing which is known as spasticity. Spasticity implies an upper motor neuron lesion. Clonus that persists while a sustained stretch is applied reflects pyramidal tract impairment

3. Muscle power, as with muscle tone, should be assessed relative to individual muscles in contrast to groups of muscles

a. Muscle power is universally assessed on a 5-point scale (Polio Foundation Classification):

0/5 - no muscle activity

1/5 - muscle fasciculation only

2/5 - muscle activity, although unable to overcome gravity

3/5 - muscle activity able to overcome gravity, but no additional resistance

4/5 - muscle able to overcome some resistance applied by the examiner

5/5 - muscle able to overcome substantial applied resistance

b. Resistance should not be applied until the muscle demonstrates a 3/5 capacity

c. Because the muscles of the lower extremity are so large and powerful. Daniels and Worthingham employed a scale of 4⁻/5 (reflecting movement against minimal resistance), 4/5 (reflecting movement against moderate resistance), and 4⁺/5 (indicating movement against considerable but less than full resistance). This is important when considering a tendon transfer, thus only a + 4/5 can be utilized

d. Because the muscles of the lower extremity are so powerful, considerable weakness may be present before it is apparent on clinical testing. For this reason, dynometric evaluations or assessment in which the patient is asked to overcome the force of their body weight may be necessary to detect sub clinical weakness

4. Muscle mass

a. Muscle girth should be inspected to assess relative degrees of atrophy and hypertrophy

b. Atrophy (decreased size) may be indicative of decreased enervation due to a peripheral (lower motor) lesion, disuse atrophy as seen in contractures that may have been induced secondary to a spastic condition but also in painful musculoskeletal conditions, or finally, muscle mass will diminish in myopathy. Regardless of the origin, atrophy is invariably a finding occurring after changes in tone or power

c. Hypertrophy may occur due to perpetual spasm (i.e., spasticity, tetany, or myotonic dystrophy) or the result of pseudohypertrophy (i.e., the calf of patients with Becker's and Duchenne's muscular dystrophy) in which muscle tissue is replaced with lipofibrous deposition

5. Superficial reflexes

a. There are a number superficial reflexes, the most important of which is the extensor-plantar or Babinski's sign. The remaining superficial reflexes are rarely assessed in podiatric practice and are best interpreted only if present on the asymptomatic side. Unlike the deep tendon reflexes, apart from the extensor-plantar response, both upper and lower motor neuron lesions diminish the superficial reflexes. An up going or positive Babinski's sign indicates an underlying upper motor lesion affecting the pyramidal tract

   i. The Babinski sign is elicited by stroking the lateral aspect of the sole of the foot from proximal to distal, then over the metatarsal heads, producing an extension and/or fanning of the digits. Other confirmatory reflexes producing the same effect: include Chaddock's sign, Oppenheim's sign, and Gordon's sign but these are not as reliably elicited as the extensor-plantar response

   ii. Bing is elicited by applying a noxious agent (pin) to the dorsal hallux. This maneuver should normally induce a flexor withdrawal response; patients with pyramidal tract lesions may extend the hallux towards the noxious stimulus

6. Deep tendon reflexes

   a. The main muscle stretch reflexes and their associated spinal segments are the: patellar tendon reflex (L_2-$\underline{L_4}$), the tendoachilles reflex (L_5-$\underline{S_1}$), the biceps reflex (C_5-C_6), the brachioradialis reflex (C_6-C_7), and the triceps reflex (C_7-C_8)

   b. Reflexes are assessed by tapping lightly on the mildly stretched tendon of the associated muscle

   c. The reflex assesses the pathway between the sensory afferent nerves, the synaptic relay within the spinal cord, and the descending motor nerves

   d. <u>Three classification systems are commonly employed 0-4 and 0-5</u>

0/4 - no response	0/4 - no response	0/5 - no response
1/4 - hyporeflexic	1/4 - hyporeflexic	1/5 - hypotonia
2/4 - normal	2/4 – normal	2/5 - normal
3/4 - hyperreflexic	3/4 – brisk	3/5 - exaggerated response
4/4 - clonus	4/4 – hyperactive	4/5 – unsustained clonus
		5/5 – sustained clonus

   e. Hyporeflexia may denote sensory pathway impairment, lower motor neuron compromise, intraspinal disease, or primary myopathy. Cerebellar impairment may decrease reflexes secondary to generalized hypotonia and often produces prolonged undamped oscillations known as pendular reflexes

   f. Hyperreflexia invariably denotes an upper motor neuron disorder

7. Cerebellar function:

   a. Dysmetria is the inability to accurately modulate the amplitude of motion and can be demonstrated by having the patient (with eyes open) reach out to touch the examiner's finger. The patient with dysmetria will have difficulty making contact with the target in one smooth motion. Similarly, the patient may be asked, with eyes closed, to touch the tip of the index finger to the tip of their nose. Again, dysmetria will manifest as the inability to do so in one smooth motion. Past pointing is a form of dysmetria that involves consistent errors in the same direction and is a sensitive index of cerebellar impairment. Intention tremor is a form of limb ataxia manifesting with unintentional horizontal oscillations that disrupt the smooth motion of a limb to its intended target and can be the earliest finding in cerebellar disease

   b. Dysdiadochokinesia is the inability to successfully perform rapid alternating movements (e.g., supinating and pronating the wrist or slapping of the hands on one's thighs when sitting). This is a later and more specific index of cerebellar dysfunction

   c. Nystagmus may manifest as horizontal, vertical, or rotatory motion of the eyes when following an object. Again, nystagmus is a later and more specific confirmatory indication of cerebellar disease

   d. Romberg's (sign) test

      i. With a patient standing erect in the narrowest base of support consistent with maintaining balance with the eyes open, the patient is then asked to close his or her eyes. A positive Romberg's sign is loss of balance. It is important when performing this test that the examiner position him or herself so that the patient will not fall if the test is positive *and to assure the patient of this fact* (anxiety over the possibility of falling not uncommonly leads to false positive tests)

    ii. Romberg's sign cannot be assessed in patients who are unable to maintain their balance with their eyes open

    iii. Ataxia (to be discussed under gait evaluation)

D. Assessing autonomic function

Several clinical tests may aid in the diagnosis of autonomic nervous system dysfunction

1. Blood pressure response to standing
   a. Patients with orthostatic hypotension (a manifestation of autonomic impairment) will experience a fall in blood pressure of 30/15 when assessed in the standing position as compared to that assessed while lying prone for 10-15 minutes. In compensation, the pulse rate should increase from 11-29 beats per minute until the blood pressure equalizes. This test is also positive in hypovolemia and the use of certain medications; these conditions must be excluded before attributing positive results to autonomic neuropathy

2. Valsalva maneuver
   a. A patient exhales into a manometer or against a closed glottis for 10-15 seconds, creating a markedly increased intrathoracic pressure. Normally blood pressure should fall at this point with accompanying reflex tachycardia. Failure of heart rate to increase during the positive intrathoracic: pressure phase of the Valsalva maneuver indicates sympathetic dysfunction. Failure of subsequent heart rate to slow during blood pressure rising indicates parasympathetic impairment

3. Galvanic skin (sweat) resistance test (sudomotor function)
   a. A string galvanometer indicates the resistance of skin to the passage of a weak galvanic current. An increase in sweating lowers resistance, while a state of anhidrosis causes increased resistance
   b. Other tests of autonomic function include lacrimal function, the cold pressor test, pupillary reaction, and the quantitative sudomotor axon reflex test

E. Gait analysis

1. Spastic hemiplegia
   a. This gait disturbance induced by lesions of the pyramidal tract in the contralateral hemisphere
   b. The arm of the affected side is weak and stiff (to varying degrees) while being maintained in a position of abduction at the shoulder, flexion at the elbow, with varying degrees of flexion of the wrist and fingers during ambulation
   c. The affected lower extremity is maintained with varying degrees of stiffness with the hip adducted and flexed, the knee flexed, with plantarflexion and inversion of the foot and ankle, as well as flexion of the digits
   d. The affected limb will initially swing outward at the hip to avoid scraping the foot on the floor, then inward toward the trunk, producing a circumductory motion

2. Spastic paraplegia (diplegia)
   a. This gait pattern results either from lesions at the level of the brain or spinal cord that affect the pyramidal tracts
   b. Both legs are involved in a bilateral and symmetrical fashion (diplegia differs only from the standpoint of concurrent fine motor impairment of both hands)
   c. The legs are typically found in either an extended or slightly flexed position at the

hips and knees with adduction of the hips

    d. The patient ambulates with a short stride as the trunk moves from side to side in an attempt to compensate for the slow and stiff movements of the legs

    e. Depending upon the severity of the underlying lesion and/or duration prior to treatment, the patient may present with a crossing of their legs in a scissor-type gait

    f. A broad base of support with excessive pronation and contractures of the Achilles and peroneal tendons is common

3. Festinating gait

    a. This gait is associated with Parkinson's disease and other disorders of the basal ganglia

    b. During ambulation, the trunk is bent forward and the patient's arms are maintained in a slightly flexed position anterior to the trunk and devoid of any arm swing

    c. The legs are stiff and bent flexed at the knees and hips

    d. Ambulation takes the form of short, rigid steps and the patient's feet barely clear the ground in a shuffling fashion

    e. Once forward or backward motion is initiated, the upper portion of the body advances ahead of the lower portion, appearing to pursue or overtake their center of gravity

    f. These patients invariably have difficulty with gait initiation, often requiring a push to get them started

    g. After the initial period of short rigid steps, the pattern becomes progressively more rapid, thus placing the patient at risk of falling

4. *Marche à Petits Pas*

    a. This gait pattern is similar to festination except that patients with this gait do not progress to more rapid steps upon forward locomotion

    b. There is often loss of normal associated movements with the possible appearance of intermittent bizarre features such as dancing or hopping movements

    c. Patients with this condition may experience generalized weakness and predisposition to fatigue

    d. Etiologies are the same as those of the festinating pattern. Diffuse cerebral disturbances, most notably those of arteriosclerotic origin, also give rise to this gait pattern

5. Choreoathetotic gait

    a. Conditions such as Sydenham's chorea, Huntington's chorea, and athetosis and other related conditions affecting the basal ganglia and extrapyramidal system are the most common etiologies of this gait pattern

    b. Involuntary movements and abnormal posturing of the face, neck, and hands characterize this gait. In advanced stages, the large proximal joints of the extremities joints are involved as well as the trunk

    c. There is often jerking of the head with grimacing of the face and protrusion of the tongue. Squirming, twisting motions of the trunk and limbs are also seen

    d. While one arm may be thrust in the air, the other may remain behind the body, with the wrist and fingers engaging in alternating motions of pronation, supination, flexion, and extension, respectively

    e. During ambulation the legs advance in a slow and awkward manner as the feet are maintained in an equinus (sometimes dorsiflexed) or equinovarus attitude and the patient maintains a ground contact on the metatarsophalangeal region

    f. Variations include: more purposeless movements and hypotonia in Sydenham's chorea, a grotesque or waltz-like gait in Huntington's chorea, and more distal joint involvement (writhing movements) in athetosis

6. Dystonic (musculorum deformans) - Vaulting gait
    a. Although the etiology is unknown, some believe it may be due to neurotransmitter dysfunction
    b. The initial presentation is typically that of a limp caused by inversion and/or plantarflexion of the foot
    c. At times, distortion of the pelvis may produce the same gait pattern
    d. In the initial stages of the disease, patients ambulate on the lateral aspect of their feet. As the condition progresses, the patient develops other postural abnormalities which may include elevation of one shoulder or one hip, as well as twisted postures of the trunk
    e. As the condition progresses, the evolution of progressive muscle spasms causes patients to walk with their knees flexed. This is followed by a progressive lumbar lordosis and flexion at the hip
    f. The advanced and late stages will reveal the presence of torsion persisting to the extent of torticollis and/or tortipelvis, with lordosis and scoliosis, ultimately impeding ambulation
7. Apraxia
    a. This condition results from frontal lobe cortical defects causing loss of integration between the cortex and basal ganglia
    b. The trunk is maintained in slight flexion with the feet farther apart than usual
    c. The patient advances with slow, shuffling, hesitant steps, although no resting tremor or pill-rolling characteristic of Parkinson's disease is present
    d. The hallmark of the gait, in addition to the short shuffling pattern, is the inability to engage in purposeful movements (e.g., kicking a ball)
8. Senile apraxia
    a. The etiology of this condition is believed to be the same as that found in the apraxic presentation. However, there is not any overt cerebral disease
    b. There is an inherent loss in the vestibulotruncal righting reflex, predisposing the patient to fall when even a slight misstep causes the patient's center of gravity to shift with an inability to adapt
9. Cerebellar ataxia
    a. This gait results from cerebellar disease of any etiology
    b. The mildest form of involvement manifests as the inability to engage in tandem gait without losing balance
    c. Other characteristics with more overt and/or progressive involvement include a swaying and staggering gait as well as titubation of the head
10. Spastic ataxia
    a. This condition is invariably the result of cortical impairment involving the pyramidal tract superimposed on cerebellar pathology
    b. Gait will invariably be either a combination of hemiplegia or paraplegia (diplegia), with accompanying cerebellar ataxia of the affected limbs
11. Sensory ataxia
    a. Sensory ataxia is the result of posterior column dysfunction or disease of the posterior spinal roots. Occasionally, sensory ataxia results from bilateral parietal lobe disease
    b. Patients present with a broad base of gait. The legs are flung abruptly forward and outward with an audible stomping on ground contact
    c. Patients characteristically watch the ground and their feet during gait
12. Steppage gait

    a. Steppage gait results from advanced peripheral (lower motor) impairment that produces denervation of dorsiflexory extrinsic muscles of the foot eventuating in foot drop

    b. Patients with this condition are unable to dorsiflex and evert their feet. In compensation, they flex their knees and hips in order to allow their feet to clear the ground during swing phase. Ambulation is accomplished with a conspicuous foot-slap on ground contact

IV. Disorders of the brain

A. Cerebrovascular accidents

Cerebrovascular accidents (CVA's) occur when the oxygen supply to the brain is suddenly impeded, leading to anoxia and neuron death, with resultant deficits in speech, cognitive, motor, and sensory function. This may be due to trauma, neoplasms, atheroschlerotic thrombosis, embolism, hemorrhage, ruptured aneurysm, and other etiologies. Hypertension, smoking, diabetes mellitus, and hyperlipidemia are common predisposing conditions.

Clinical presentations vary according to which arterial supply is affected:
1. The middle cerebral artery is very commonly affected. Clinically one observes contralateral hemiplegia and deficits of the upper extremity (less so of the legs and feet)
2. CVA's of the anterior cerebral artery characteristically result in hemiplegia, motor deficits, and sensory deficits of contralateral lower extremity
3. The basilar artery is the least commonly affect by cerebrovascular accidents of the three major arterial systems in the brain. Disease of this artery leads to impaired balance and coordination
4. Lacunar infarcts occur when a small watershed vessel becomes occluded. The deficits produced by these lesions can be very dense and localized. In addition, they can be modality specific
5. Cerebrovascular accidents can be occlusive (the majority of cases) or hemorrhagic

Diagnosis:
1. History - Usually the history is positive for a predisposing medical condition. Episodes are usually not convulsive in nature but may be of abrupt or insidious onset. CVA's are frequently preceded by transient ischemic attacks (TIA's), described as dizziness, diplopia, blurred vision, impaired speech, or other neurological deficits. Such prodromes usually last several minutes or hours
2. Physical examination:

A comprehensive and methodical approach based on the body region and affected system(s) is paramount for prompt assessment and treatment. An outline of characteristic clinical findings in the lower extremity is presented here

    a. Sensory deficits in:
      i. proprioception - e.g., unstable gait
      ii. touch - e.g., no stereognosis, two-point discrimination, etc.

    b. Motor deficits:
      i. Flaccid paralysis (e.g., foot drop) may last from days to weeks; if the paralysis persists, prognosis diminishes. If paralysis lasts over three months, the impairment may be permanent. Return of tone and function is customarily observed in the proximal muscle groups first

    c. Cognitive impairment:

Loss of speech, short-term memory, and learning ability may be appreciable. When these deficits are severe, the prognosis is poor

   d. Gait abnormalities:

      i. Hip adductor spasticity, with potential scissor gait and/or flexion contracture of the hip. When severe, patient is unable to ambulate

      ii. Diminished knee flexion, leading to knee contractures and/or circumducted gait, with compensatory hip lifting

      iii. Depending on which muscle groups are affected, various foot deformities may develop. Spasticity of the tibialis anterior results in a varus foot type. Equinus foot deformity arises from spasticity of the gastrocnemius and soleus muscles. Equinovarus may be due to the above muscles being affected in addition to the tibialis posterior, flexor digitorum longus, and flexor hallucis longus. Claw toes may be the presenting digital deformities. Dependent upon the severity of the deformities, ambulation may or may not be possible

  3. Radiographic and laboratory findings - MRI of the brain has demonstrated ischemic areas within hours following a stroke. CT scanning visualizes infarcted regions (and resultant cavitation) within a few days. CT with contrast is a sensitive test for subdural hematomas. These exams have largely replaced arteriography (which is the definitive diagnostic procedure) due to its slight risk of complications, namely that of infarct extension. Laboratory testing is basically noncontributory and nonspecific in noninfectious and vascular etiologies of CVA's. EMG demonstrates the degree and distribution of muscle function loss. For example, drop foot may be due to excessive ankle plantarflexory activity or diminished dorsiflexory power. Treatment:

   a. Discourage bed rest

   b. Early mobilization via active and passive range of motion exercises

   c. Night splint and footboard to avoid equinus

   d. Trapeze for upper extremity mobility

   e. Standing balance exercises

   f. Ankle-foot orthoses (AFO)

   g. Knee-ankle-foot orthoses (KAFO)

   h. Quad cane

   i. Functional electrical stimulation (e.g., transcutaneous stimulation of the peroneal nerve during gait)

   j. Surgery may be required to release contractures (e.g., tendoachilles lengthening, digital fusions, tendon transfers such as the SPLATT procedure)

B. Neoplasms:

Clinical findings are similar to those seen in CVA's and depend upon the area of the brain involved. The evolution of signs and symptoms may be insidious in nature. Treatment entails addressing deficits as well as immediate oncologic evaluation and treatment

C. Infectious processes:

  1. These most commonly take the form of bacterial meningitis, subdural empyema, brain or epidural abscess, or intracranial thrombophlebitis

  2. Hematogenous spread, contiguous extension, cerebral surgery, shunting, and lumbar punctures often seed infection

  3. Diagnosis is made via blood cultures, radiographs, and CT scans of skull and chest, and lumbar puncture. Pleocytosis in the CSF is diagnostic of infection. Abnormally high spinal pressure, increased CSF protein levels, and positive CSF cultures are supportive findings. Treatment:

   a. Intravenous bactericidal antibiotics

   b. Osmotic diuretics (e.g., mannitol and urea) to reduce cerebral edema

      c. Anticonvulsants if seizures occur

      d. Adequate but not excessive parenteral fluids

D. Seizure disorders:

1. Seizures are paroxysmal cerebral neuron discharges
2. Seizures may be due to hyponatremia, hypocalcemia, hypoglycemia, ethanol withdrawal, drug use or withdrawal, toxins, CVA, head trauma, and neoplasms of the brain, etc.
3. Seizures in the frontal lobes cause abnormal motor findings that begin in distal extremities
4. Chronic and recurrent seizures comprise epilepsy (now referred to as "seizure disorder"). These seizures may be either partial (e.g., Jacksonian) or generalized (e.g., grand mal and petit mal)
5. Diagnosis is made by history, laboratory findings, and electroencephalography (EEG). Management of seizures:
   a. Assess cardiorespiratory function, administer oxygen and insert an airway if possible
   b. Start i.v. infusion of normal saline with vitamin B complex and give a bolus of 50 cc 50% glucose
   c. Infuse diazepam at 2 mg/minute, up to 20 mg total. Also infuse phenytoin at 50 mg/minute to a maximum of 18 mg/kg. If the seizure persists, consider a drip of either (but not both) of the above. If the seizure still persists, consider neuromuscular blockade or general anesthesia with halothane
   d. Antiepileptic therapy
      i. Phenytoin (Dilantin) is gold standard
      ii. Also used: carbamazepine (Tegretol), Valproate, clonazepam, gabapentin, and barbituates
      iii. Stress the importance of adequate sleep since deprivation may precipitate seizures

E. Parkinson's disease

1. This leading neurological disorder in elderly is due to loss of pigmented neurons in the substantia nigra of the basal ganglia, resulting in dopamine depletion
2. Clinically one observes initially a "pill- rolling" tremor of the thumb and index finger. Muscle stiffness and rigidity manifests with slowness of movement, limited range of motion, decreased agility, and expressionless facies
3. Gait reveals a loss of postural reflexes with bowed head, bent trunk, flexed knees, and loss of arm swing. A small-stepped festinating or shuffling gait pattern is characteristic
4. Autonomic dysfunction may manifest with hyperhidrosis, hypotension, and incontinence of bowel and bladder
5. Memory loss and cognitive defects may be associated findings
6. Parkinsonism may be primary or secondary; the latter group being due to metabolic, neoplastic, toxic, infectious, traumatic, degenerative, or other etiologies. Treatment:
   a. In the initial stages of disease, anticholinergics (e.g., benztropine mesylate or Cogentin); antihistamines (e.g., amantadine, diphenydramine); or tricyclic antidepressants (e.g., amitryptyline [Elavil] or imipramine [Tofranil]) may be helpful
   b. In the later phases of the illness medications that increase striatal dopamine levels or act as dopaminergic agonists are required. These include levodopa/carbidopa (Sinemet), bromocriptine, and monoamine oxidase inhibitors such as L-deprenyl
   c. Management also includes reassurance; patient and family education; psychotherapy (if needed), and physical therapy for maintaining mobility, range of motion, tone, and strength. Gait training may be helpful

F. Demyelinating diseases:

1. Examples are multiple sclerosis (MS), Friedreich's ataxia, and amyotrophic lateral sclerosis (ALS)
2. Clinical signs of MS include diplopia, blindness (especially central scotoma), nystagmus, dysesthesia, ataxia, spastic paresis, and urinary disturbance. This disorder occurs predominantly in young adults and an immunologic or viral cause is suspected. Acute attacks are treated with steroids. Baclofen, along with physical therapy, is used to address spasticity
3. ALS results in progressive generalized muscle atrophy, fasciculations, and weakness, with possible hyperreflexia and spasticity. Upper and lower motor neuron findings are seen. Men are affected twice as often as women, particularly during the fourth through seventh decades of life. Diagnosis may be made by muscle biopsy (shows group fiber atrophy), EMG (reveals denervation and fasciculations) and elevated CPK levels. Treatment is palliative physiotherapy. The outcome, at present, is uniformly fatal
4. Friedreich's ataxia is characterized by a cavus foot deformity, ataxia, kyphoscholiosis, arreflexia, and impaired proprioception and vibratory perception. It is observed by puberty and due to an autosomal recessive condition

G. **Cerebellar disorders** - Cerebellar disorders are comprised of two categories:
1. Midline syndrome is due to chronic alcoholism or lesions of the spinocerebellum. This syndrome causes ataxia, instability, nystagmus, and tremors
2. Lateral syndromes are due to lesions of the pontocerebellum. Contralateral hypotonia, tremor, and tilting in direction of lesion during ambulation are seen

H. **Cerebral palsy**
1. By definition, cerebral palsy is motor dysfunction evident by age two due to nonprogressive, static brain pathology
2. The incidence is 1 per 1000 live births
3. The most frequent comorbid finding is birth weight below 2500 g (2.5 kg.)
4. Etiologies may be prenatal (e.g., fetal deprivation syndrome, infections, malformations, microcephaly), perinatal (e.g., birth trauma, hypoxia, acute metabolic disturbance), or postnatal (e.g., head trauma, toxins, intraventricular hemorrhage)
5. The classification of CP is based on etiology, body distribution, and physiologic (motor) types
6. Physiologic types include:
   a. Spastic
   b. Athetotic
   c. Ataxic
   d. Atonic
   e. Tremor
   f. Rigidity
   g. Mixed

CLINICAL PRESENTATIONS

I. **Spastic**

   A. **Hemi-, di-, mono-, tri-, or quadriplegic forms are seen**

II. **Dyskinetic**

   A. **Hypotonic, choreoathetotic, and dystonic forms are seen**

III. Ataxic

IV. Mixed

   A. Areas involved
1. Monoplegia involves one limb
2. Paraplegia involves both lower limbs
3. Hemiplegia is the unilateral involvement of both the upper and lower extremities
4. Triplegia - three limbs
5. Quadriplegia - all four limbs (also known as tetraplegia)

   B. Positional deformity
1. Shoulder - adducted, flexed, and internally rotated
2. Flexion of elbow, hand, wrist
3. Thumb is adducted
4. Hip is adducted, flexed, and internally rotated with the knee flexed
5. Ankle in equinus

   C. Physiologic (motor) types

Spastic: initially manifests with acute flaccid paralysis, hypertonia and hyperreflexia appear later

1. Spastic hemiplegia is most common (less so is dyskinetic, and spastic tri- and quadriplegia)
2. Initially this presents with flaccid paralysis on one side, hypertonia and hyperrflexia develop later
3. The difference between spastic paraplegia and diplegia is that in later subtype, fine motor involvement of hands is noted
4. Only in the spastic form of CP is there an incidence of musculoskeletal deformities disproportionate to that seen in the general population. Athetosis presents with poor coordination, along with involuntary, coarse, rhythmic, continuous writhing movement, especially of hands and feet. Tremor consists of involuntary, purposeless, rhythmic oscillatory movements. Ataxia - presents with imbalance, incoordination, and a wide base of gait
   a. The diagnosis of CP rests on the presence of chronic motor dysfunction; delay in reaching developmental landmarks and the development of protective reflexes; the persistence of primitive reflexes (asymmetrical tonic neck reflex, Moro reflex, foot placement reaction); positive extenuating factors (e.g., low birth weight, etc.); equinus, low varus and/or equinovarus foot deformity, and scissor gait
   b. Associated findings in CP: include mental retardation, learning disability, impaired speech, epilepsy, and visual problems
   c. Physical therapy is a mainstay of the management of CP. Passive stretching of the gastrocsoleal muscles is commonly necessary
   d. Orthotics and braces (e.g., AFO's) are employed
   e. Inhibitory casting to maintain the knee 5° - 15° flexion is used
   f. Antispasmotic medications (Dantrolene, diazepam, Baclofen, etc.)
   g. Cerebellar stimulation
   h. Gait analysis may be helpful in designing intervention strategies and assessing their effectiveness
   i. Tendon lengthenings and transfers (e.g., VAL, Velpius, SPLATT) are employed and are more successful for spastic rather than athetoid type
   j. Appropriate osteotomies, and arthrodeses are used to address rigid deformities

k. Adductor myotomy of hip with neurectomy of anterior branch of obturator nerve may be performed

V. Spinal cord diseases

A. Spinal muscular atrophies affect the lower motor neurons, are clinically apparent by childhood, display clinical heterogeneity and are classified by age of onset and neuroanatomic locus of the responsible lesion
  1. Infantile form (Werdnig-Hoffman disease)
      a. Is a common cause of "floppy infant syndrome"
      b. Is discernable in neonatal period
      c. Causes symmetric weakness in all extremities, the trunk, and the respiratory system
      d. Reduced DTR's, sucking, crying
      e. Etiology is autosomal recessive
      f. Life expectancy is only a few years
  2. Childhood form (Kugelberg-Welander syndrome)
      a. Is characterized by later onset, slower progression, and improved prognosis
      b. Autosomal dominant and recessive forms exist
      c. Ventilatory function is spared
  3. Secondary form may be due to lead toxicity, hexosaminidase deficiency, or plasma cell dyscrasias
  4. Post-polio syndrome
      a. Is characterized by slowly progressive weakness appearing years after the initial polio episode
      b. Initially affects previously compromised muscles but later previously uncompromised muscles may be involved
  5. Localized forms
      a. Examples: Facioscapulohumeral
      b. Scapuloperoneal
      c. These are slowly progressive, with no sensory nor UMN involvement

B. Transverse myelitis
  1. Etiologies may be viral (herpes zoster or simplex, polio, rabies, syphilis, HTLV 1 or 2); fungal; parasitic; pyogenic (e.g., staphyloccal, streptococcal, or pneumococcal); tuberculous; or degenerative (ALS, MS; etc.)
  2. Signs and symptoms include pain, bladder and bowel incontinence, flaccid paralysis, sensory loss, fever, diminished DTR's, and positive Babinski reflexes
  3. Diagnosis may be made on the basis of elevated protein and or immunoglobulins in the CSF, CT or MRI scan of spine; myelography; somatosensory evoked potentials; etc.

C. Traumatic/Structural myelopathies
  1. Etiologies may entail: DJD; lordosis or scoliosis; transverse transection; vertebral fractures; stenosis or spondylolisthesis (i.e., anterior slippage of a superior vertebrae [usually L5 or L4] with resultant sensory and motor impairments with reduced DTR's)
  2. Radiation may cause sensorimotor disorders. These may be reversible if they arise soon after exposure to radiation. Deficits arising as a late effect of radiation exposure are usually permanent
  3. Electrical injuries may directly impact neural function (deficits appear immediately after the insult) or through consequent vascular occlusion (later onset of deficits)
  4. Symptoms include loss of volitional movement, sensory loss distal to the level of injury, and bladder and bowel incontinence

5. Diagnosis may be made on the basis of radiographs, MRI or CT scans, myelography, and somatosensory evoked potentials. If somatosensory evoked potentials cannot be demonstrated, this indicates complete spinal block, conversely, the return of somatosensory evoked potentials indicates improvement

D. Spinal neoplasms

1. Spinal neoplasms may be intra medullary (e.g., gliomas, ganglioneuroma, ependymomas, meduloblastomas, and astrocytomas) or extramedulary. Extramedullary lesions are further subdivided into intradural and extradural lesions
2. Examples of intradural extramedullary lesions include meninglomas; neurofibromas; arachnoid, teratomatous, epidermoid/dermoid cysts, and syringomyelia
3. Examples of extradural lesions include chordomas, hematomas, and metastatic lesions
4. Clinical features based on site and size of the neoplasm and consequently on which spinal tracts are compromised
5. Diagnosis via: X-rays (may show degenerative changes of vertebrae, foramen enlargement, calcifications); MRI or CT scan; myelogram (discerns subtypes); lumbar puncture; etc.

E. Spinal dysraphisms

1. Spinal dysraphisms are congenital defects most commonly arising in the lumbosacral segment
2. These are due to incomplete development or closure of dorsal midline of the neural tube during fetal development
3. Classification is based on whether the lesions are clinically overt or occult
4. Neurologic deficits in these conditions may be due to traction or compression of the nerve fibers
   a. Overt lesions with open defects:
      i. Myelomeningocele presents as a protruding mass of spinal cord elements
      ii. Meningocele present as a protruding mass containing dermal and fibrous tissue but no spinal cord elements
      iii. Syringomyelia is due to cavitary lesions of the cord and may be associated with characteristic fractures or dislocations. Syringomyelia is characterized by dissociated sensory loss in which pain and temperature sensation are impaired with preservation of light touch and proprioception. Neurologic deficits are usually noted in a cape-like pattern. Note that this lesion is far more common in the cervical and thoracic regions of the cord than in the lumbosacral segment
   b. Occult lesions with dosed defects may present without apparent neurologic sequelae. Examples include:
      i. Diasternatomyelia, which is due to traction
      ii. Spinal dermal sinus
      iii. Intraspinal neoplasms
      iv. Tense filum terminale
   c. Signs and symptoms of spinal dysraphisms:
      i. These initially present in the foot as cavus, planus, metatarsus adductus, equinus, in-toe, or out-toe deformities with abnormal gait
      ii. Dermal markers (e.g., tufts of hair) may be seen on the lower back
      iii. Urinary incontinence may be present
      iv. Numbness, paresthesias, and reduced pinprick sensation are common
      v. Up going Babinski reflexes may be seen

VI. Disorders of the autonomic nervous system

A. Orthostatic hypotension is idiopathic with reduced plasma norepinephrine that fails to rise adequately when patient goes from prone to the upright position resulting in a fall in blood pressure

B. Shy-Drager syndrome manifests with orthostatic hypotension despite normal plasma norepinephrine responses

C. Primary autonomic failure (<u>familial</u> dysautonomia, Riley-Day syndrome)
1. Affects those of Eastern European descent
2. Is associated with severe delay in reaching developmental milestones
3. Prior to age three, patients may exhibit episodic vomiting, hyperhidrosis, and excessive irritability
4. After age three, tachycardia, hypertension, thermal instability, and self-mutilation may appear

D. Reflex sympathetic dystrophy (RSD):
1. Is synonymous with causalgia, Sudeck's atrophy, and post-traumatic osteoporosis
2. Now known as "Corplex Regional Pain Syndrome." There are 2 types
3. Usually manifests as burning pain in varying levels of severity, usually out of proportion to the injury sustained
4. Etiology is unknown but has been theorized to be due to an incomplete nerve lesion arising after trauma resulting in exaggerated autonomic responsiveness
5. Associated findings include edema, pallor, and coolness of involved area
   a. Stages of RSD
       i. Stage one (occurring within days to weeks)
          (a) Pain typically burning in nature
          (b) Focal edema
          (c) Hyperesthesia in the affected region
          (d) Cyanosis, coolness of skin and hyperhidrosis with subsequent alternating periods of warm, dry skin and hypohidrosis
          (e) Muscle spasms
          (f) No overt radiographic findings
          (g) In mild cases, the condition may be self-limiting at this point with complete resolution
       ii. Stage two (occurs after approximately three months and lasting to approximately six months) is characterized by:
          (a) Progressive diffuse edema evolving from a soft to brawny state
          (b) A decrease in pain and hypesthesia as compared to that noted in stage one
          (c) Toenails become brittle and sometimes grooved
          (d) Decreased hair growth
          (e) Mechanical and thermal alloydnia (Hendler test with an alcohol swab)
          (f) Radiographs begin to reveal spotty osteoporosis with subsequent diffuse regional osteoporosis at the end of this period
       iii. Stage three (after six months) is characterized by:
          (a) Severe dystrophic, brittle and grooved nails, sometimes with onycholysis
          (b) Severe trophic changes of the skin and hair with the former taking on a glassy, cyanotic appearance
          (c) Atrophy of subcutaneous fat
          (d) Muscle atrophy
          (e) Decreased joint range of motion
          (f) Contractures
          (g) Marked and diffuse bone atrophy

VII. Peripheral Neuropathies

  A. Peripheral neuropathies are a heterogeneous family of conditions affecting the peripheral nervous system (PNS). These may be purely sensory, motor, or mixed in character

  B. Types of peripheral neuropathy:

  1. Radiculopathies are diseases of the spinal roots (anterior and/or posterior)
     a. Forms (Etiologies) include:
        i. Traumatic (e.g., herniated disc, status- post vertebral fracture, etc.)
        ii. Neoplastic (e.g., neurofibroma)
        iii. Infectious (e.g., poliomyelitis, in which the anterior horn cells are exclusively affected; *syphilis,* which affects the posterior horn cells exclusively; and *herpes zoster*, that typically affects the dorsal ganglia but which can involve the motor fibers as well)
        iv. Secondary to underlying structural deformity (e.g., scoliosis, spina bifida, osteoarthritis, spinal dysraphisms)
        v. Rheumatologic (e.g., anklylosing spondylitis)
        vi. Inflammatory (e.g., chronic inflammatory polyradiculopathy [CIP])
        vii. Degenerative (e.g., anterior lateral sclerosis, Kugelberg-Welander disease, Werdnig-Hoffman disease)
        viii. Metabolic (e.g., diabetes mellitus, most specifically the mononeuropathy multi-plex form of diabetes mellitus will often present with intercurrent and/or exclu-sive radicular involvement)
     b. Symptoms:
        i. These may be quite vague in nature, particularly in the initial stages, and include perceptions of heaviness, fullness, tightness, or fatigue
        ii. Paresthesias, cramping, burning, numbness, and/or lancinating pains may often ensue
        iii. Symptoms may either be confined to focal distal regions of the foot or leg (e.g., arch, calf) or follow specific dermatome and/or myotome distributions (e.g., L_4, L_5, S_1, etc.)
        iv. Pain and other symptoms may be radiating in nature. For instance, there may be pain down buttocks and back of thigh (often described as sciatic pain) or along the anterior thigh
     c. Clinical findings:
        i. Will either be sensory, motor, or mixed in nature, depending upon the spinal roots involved (e.g., anterior, posterior, or both, usually in the form of compromise of the mixed spinal nerve)
        ii. Clinical findings (e.g., diminished sensation, decreased muscle tone or power, or diminished reflexes) will follow specific radicular distribution patterns: Note that diminution of reflexes may be due to compromise of either the anterior or posterior root
     d. Testing is useful not only to confirm the diagnosis but also to estimate the prognosis for recovery and document the extent of recovery after therapeutic interventions
        i. Nerve conduction studies typically reveal decreased amplitudes within affected nerve distributions
        ii. Electromyographic (EMG) studies typically reveal acute and/or chronic denerva-tion of muscles within the afflicted myotome(s)
        iii. MRI typically reveals the nature and anatomic locus of the responsible lesion(s)

e. Treatment is invariably dependent on the underlying etiology
  i. Physical therapy is often employed
  ii. Neurosurgical or orthopedic consultation may be indicated
  iii. Foot and/or ankle-foot orthoses may help manage the sequellae of radiculopathies without impacting the underlying pathology

2. Mononeuropathy Multiplex is the impairment of multiple (two or more) noncontiguous peripheral nerves attributed to a common underlying etiology
  a. Forms (etiologies) include:
    i. Metabolic (e.g., diabetes)
    ii. Granulomatous (e.g., sarcoidosis)
    iii. Inflammatory (autoimmune/connective tissue, e.g., polyarteritis nodosa, rheumatoid arthritis, and systemic lupus erythematosus)
    iv. Infectious (e.g., leprosy, herpes zoster)
    v. Neoplastic (e.g., neurofibromatosis, direct metastasis from bone and lymph tissue)
    vi. Vascular (e.g., ischemic neuropathy with peripheral vascular disease)
  b. Symptoms
    i. May be sensory and/or motor in nature when present within the distribution of the affected nerves
  c. Clinical findings
    i. Sensory deficits including proprioception, pallesthesia, light touch, and sharp/dull sensation will present within the distribution of the affected nerves
    ii. Motor involvement will manifest decreased muscle tone of muscles within the distribution of affected peripheral nerves at the earliest stage, then followed by progressive muscle weakness
    iii. Deep tendon reflexes
      Patellar - will only be affected if the peroneal/femoral nerve(s) and/or associated spinal roots are involved
      Achilles - only affected if the sciatic and/or posterior nerve(s) are afflicted, along with possible intercurrent associated spinal root involvement
  d. Diagnostic testing
    i. Nerve conduction studies will not only confirm the presence and degree of sensory and/or motor involvement, but the nature (pathophysiology) in terms of the process being either primarily axonal (predominantly decreased conduction amplitudes with normal or slightly diminished conduction velocities) or demyelinating (predominantly decreased conduction velocities with grossly normal amplitudes) in nature
    ii. EMG studies - Will reflect the relative degree of denervation of muscles within the affected neural distributions. Acute findings: Activity at rest, including fibrillation potentials, positive sharp waves, etc. Chronic findings: Decreased recruitment patterns, typically associated with increased polyphasic potentials during minimal voluntary contraction
    iii. Nerve Biopsy
      (a) The sural is usually the nerve of choice
      (b) Will reveal whether demyelination or axonal processes predominate
      (c) May confirm a vasculitic process
      (d) In a suspected or clinically appreciable hypertrophic process (such as leprosy), biopsy will reveal characteristic "*onion bulb*" findings on myelin layered with fibrosis

          iv. Blood chemistries, serology and hematology may be indicated depending on the suspected etiology

          v. Synovial analysis may also be indicated depending on the suspected etiology

   e. Treatment

          i. Correction of any reversible underlying conditions

          ii. Physical therapy to decrease pain and enhance function

          iii. Possibly foot-and/or ankle-foot orthoses depending on presentation

          iv. Surgical intervention if contractures, ulcerations, or osseous deformities develop

3. Mononeuropathy Simplex - Involvement of a single nerve and its terminal branches

   a. Forms (etiologies)

          i. Traumatic

             (a) Neuropraxia is a physiologic impairment of nerve function without structural damage, i.e., conduction block or slowing, although the axons remain intact

             (b) Axonotemesis is the physical interruption of axons, although the epineurium remains intact

             (c) Neurontomesis constitutes complete disruption of the entire nerve including the axons, connective tissue structures and epineurium

          ii. Chronic compression may result from the following

             (a) Biomechanical factors such as excessive pronation

             (b) Space-occupying lesions

             (c) Venous engorgement

             (d) A fracture fragment and/or dislocation

             (e) An inflammatory process such as: synovitis, tenosynovitis, etc.

             (f) Hemorrhage, fibrosis

          iii. Neoplastic (e.g., schwannoma); and

          iv. Vascular (e.g., ischemia)

   b. Symptoms - Initially symptoms are typically vague such as a fullness, tightness, or heaviness. Later symptoms can include paresthesias, numbness, burning, cramping, and weakness

   c. Clinical findings

          i. If a purely sensory nerve is involved, proprioceptive deficits will manifest initially, followed by deficits in sharp/dull discrimination

          ii. A positive Tinel's sign is indicative of nerve regeneration and may indicate early resolution of neuralgia in contrast to being a sign of progressing pathology in neuritis

          iii. Check for signs of underlying trauma, inflammation, edema, venous, and/or ischemic involvement. Additionally, hypertrophic musculoskeletal lesions should be identified, as well as pathomechanical conditions and space occupying lesions

   d. Diagnostic testing

          i. Nerve conduction studies: revealing either decreased conduction velocities consistent with a compression neuropathy (demyelinating process), or decreased amplitudes indicative of an axonal process (as seen in ischemic processes or in cases with axonal disease or disruption)

          ii. EMG studies will reflect denervation associated with motor nerve involvement of muscles within the distribution of the involved nerve

          iii. Vascular studies may reveal the presence of venous and/or arterial deficits causing the neuropathy

   e. Treatment

          i. If possible, treatment should be directed toward correcting any reversible under-

lying etiology
    ii. Physical therapy to decrease inflammation, improve range of motion, and strengthen muscles
   iii. Injections and aspirations if indicated
   iv. Orthoses
    v. Immobilization
   vi. Surgical decompression or nerve repair

4. Polyneuropathies - Impairment of multiple (two or more) noncontiguous peripheral nerves. The impairment is attributed to a common underlying etiology, usually toxic or metabolic. While the impairment may be unilateral at first (and initially involve only one nerve), involvement in a bilateral and symmetric fashion with progression of deficits from distal to proximal is seen as the disease progresses

  a. Forms
     i. Metabolic, e.g.:
      (a) Diabetes mellitus
      (b) Hypothyroidism
      (c) Amyloidosis
      (d) Uremia
      (e) Hepatic insufficiency
      (f) Porphyria
     ii. Infectious, e.g.:
      (a) HIV
      (b) Hepatitis
      (c) Leprosy
      (d) Infectious mononucleosis
      (e) Diphtheria
    iii. Neoplastic - Carcinoma – Myeloma
    iv. Inflammatory/Connective Tissue and/or Autoimmune
      (a) Rheumatoid arthritis
      (b) Systemic lupus erythematosus
      (c) Paraproteinemias
      (d) Gufflain-Barré syndrome
     v. Nutritional deficiencies
      (a) Alcoholism
      (b) Vitamin B_{12} deficiency
      (c) Chronic gastrointestinal disease
     vi. Toxic
      (a) Drug intoxications (i.e., isoniazid, vincristine, amitriptyline, dapsone, hydralazine, disulfiram, etc.)
      (b) Heavy metals and industrial solvents (i.e., arsenic, lead, mercury, thallium, methyl bromide, etc.)
      (c) Note that acute intoxication usually manifests with cortical obtundation—peripheral neuropathy is typically the result of chronic exposure
    vii. Hereditary
      (a) Charcot-Marie-Tooth disease
      (b) DeJerine-Sottas disease
      (c) Refsum's disease
      (d) Roussy-Levy syndrome
      (e) Tangier's disease

(f) A beta lipoproteinemia

b. Symptoms

    i. These typically consist of a "pins and needles" sensation, numbness, and/or burning sensation often evolving initially in either the digits, ball of the feet, arch, or dorsolateral aspect of the forefoot. As the condition progresses, the bilateral and symmetric pattern classically described as a "stocking-like" distribution becomes apparent. A similar presentation in both hands will ensue in a "glove-like" pattern

    ii. Distal bilateral and symmetric motor complaints such as cramping, weakness, and/or fatigue generally occur later in the process, although may predominate during the early phases of some conditions, particularly in hereditary disorders such as Charcot-Marie-Tooth disease

c. Clinical findings

    i. In sensory processes, many, if not most, polyneuropathies will initially present with involvement of the small fibers traveling within the posterior columns. Therefore, a deficit in proprioception at the level of the metatarsalophalangeal joints is often the first objective finding on examination. However, some studies have concluded that loss of the ankle jerk is the first objective manifestation of diabetic neuropathy. Deficits in pallesthesia, sharp/dull discrimination, and light touch may follow in a symmetric distribution. When present, symptom progression is invariably in a distal to proximal fashion

    ii. Motor findings may be the earliest manifestation of some types of neuropathies but usually lag sensory loss by some time. Motor findings initially take the form of decreased muscle tone, followed by progressive weakness, and ultimately atrophy

    iii. Additional clinical findings may reveal neurotrophic sequelae such as dystrophic skin and nails, bullae, ulcerations, and osteoarthropathy

    iv. Advanced motor sequelae may include contractures, cavus foot deformities, exostoses, calluses, ankle sprains, general instability, and possibly foot drop

    v. Palpable hypertrophic nerves are typically found in disorders such as: Charcot-Marie-Tooth disease Type I, Leprosy, and Refsum's disease

d. Diagnostic studies

    i. Nerve conduction studies

        (a) NCV can usually confirm the presence, degree, distribution, and pathophysiology (e.g., axonal vs. demyelinating) of polyneuropathy

        (b) The involvement of sensory and/or motor fibers can be confirmed, qualified, and quantified through NCV's

        (c) Prolonged latencies and decreased conduction velocities will indicate demyelinating processes

        (d) Decreased amplitudes will indicate axonal disease

    ii. Electromyographic (EMG) studies

        (a) Will reveal the relative acuteness (indicated by abnormal activity at rest) or chronicity (indicated by polyphasic potentials during minimal voluntary contraction and decreased recruitment patterns) of any denervation

    iii. Biopsy

        (a) The most specific study to determine the underlying etiology of suspected autoimmune, inflammatory, and genetic neuropathies

e. Treatment

    i. Should be directed to the correction of any reversible underlying conditions if

possible
   ii. Immunologic, antibiotic, and antiviral therapy may be effective in selected cases
  iii. Nutritional supplementation may be valuable
  iv. Physical therapy for analgesia, range of motion, and strengthening
   v. Orthoses (foot, ankle-foot, and patellar tendon bearing) if indicated
  vi. Wound care may be necessary if neuropathic ulcerations develop
 vii. Elective, reconstructive, and limb salvage surgery may be necessary depending on the severity and course of the disease

BIBLIOGRAPHY

Adams RD., Victor M. *Principles ofNeurology.* McGraw-Hill Inc., 1989.

Kandel ER., Schwartz JH. *Principles of Neural Science.* Elsevier Science Publishing Co., 1985.

Oh SJ. *Clinical Electromyography: Nerve Conduction Studies.* University Park Press, 1984.

Rowland LP. *Merritt - Textbook ofNeurology.* Lea & Febiger, 1989.

Schaumburg HH., Berger AR., Thomas PK. *Disorders of Peripheral Nerves.* F.A. Davis Company, 1992.

Weber, GA. *Clinics in Podiatric Medicine and Surgery Neurologic Disorders of The Lower Extremity I.* W.B. Saunders Company, 1989.

Weber, GA. *Clinics in Podiatric Medicine and Surgery Neurologic Disorders Affecting the Lower Extremity II.* W.B. Saunders Company, 1990.

CHAPTER 4
NEUROLOGY

1.   A patient presents with right-sided weakness in the peroneal musculature. There is also weakness in
      plantarflexion on the right. The tendoachilles and extensorplantar reflexes on the right are absent. Sensation
      is normal throughout. The responsible lesion is most probably located at which of the following sites:

      A.   The anterior spinal root
      B.   The posterior spinal root
      C.   The mixed spinal nerve
      D.   The common peroneal nerve

2.   A patient presents paresthesias in the distal-lateral right lower leg and dorsum of the right foot. There is
      right-sided weakness in the peroneal musculature. Strength in plantarflexion is normal bilaterally. The
      tendoachilles reflexes are normal bilaterally. The extensor-plantar reflex is downgoing bilaterally. All
      sensory modalities are impaired in the distal-lateral lower right leg and the dorsum of the right foot except
      in the first interspace. The responsible lesion is most probably located at which of the following sites:

      A.   The anterior spinal root
      B.   The posterior spinal root
      C.   The mixed spinal nerve
      D.   The common peroneal nerve
      E.   The superficial peroneal nerve

3.   A patient presents with paresthesias in the distal-lateral right lower leg and dorsum of the right foot.
      There is right-sided weakness in the peroneal musculature. There is also weakness of the right
      gastrocsoleal complex. All sensory modalities are impaired on the plantar lateral right foot. The
      tendoachilles and extensor-plantar reflexes are absent on the right. The responsible lesion is most probably
      located at which of the following sites:

      A.   The anterior spinal root
      B.   The posterior spinal root
      C.   The mixed spinal nerve
      D.   The common peroneal nerve
      E.   The superficial peroneal nerve

4.   A patient presents with paresthesias in the distal-lateral right lower leg and dorsum of the right foot. There
      is right-sided weakness in the peroneal musculature. There is also weakness of the right tibialis anterior and
      the long and short dorsiflexors of the right hallux and lesser digits. Strength in plantarflexion is normal
      bilaterally. The tendoachilles reflex is present bilaterally and the extensor-plantar reflexes are downgoing
      bilaterally. Sensation is impaired to all modalities in the distal lateral lower-leg and the entire dorsum of the
      right foot. The responsible lesion is most probably located at which of the following sites:

      A.   The anterior spinal root
      B.   The posterior spinal root
      C.   The mixed spinal nerve
      D.   The common peroneal nerve
      E.   The superficial peroneal nerve

5.   A patient presents with paresthesias of the distal-lateral right lower leg, lateral dorsum of the right foot and the central plantar skin. Muscle strength is everywhere normal. The tendoachilles reflexes are normal bilaterally. The extensor-plantar reflex is downgoing on the left but mute (absent) on the right. The responsible lesion is most probably located at which of the following sites:

        A.   The anterior spinal root
        B.   The posterior spinal root
        C.   The mixed spinal nerve
        D.   The common peroneal nerve
        E.   The superficial peroneal nerve

6.   A patient presents with right-sided unilateral feeling that his right leg is about to "give out". On physical examination you note that sensation is intact bilaterally, strength on manual muscle testing is intact bilaterally, and the quadriceps reflex is present on the left but absent on the right. No abnormalities of cerebellar function are noted. The responsible lesion is most likely:

        A.   In the dorsal root serving the involved territory
        B.   In the ventral root serving the involved territory
        C.   In the mixed peripheral nerve
        D.   In the white matter within the spinal cord
        E.   In the brain or brainstem

7.   A patient presents with right-sided unilateral feeling that his right leg is about to "give out". On physical examination you note that sensation is intact, strength on manual muscle testing is intact on the left but grossly reduced on the right in the quadriceps, adductors of the hip, and tibialis anterior. The quadriceps reflex is present on the left but absent on the right. No abnormalities of cerebellar function are noted. The responsible lesion is most likely:

        A.   In the dorsal root serving the involved territory
        B.   In the ventral root serving the involved territory
        C.   In the mixed peripheral nerve
        D.   In the white matter within the spinal cord
        E.   In the brain or brainstem

8.   A patient presents with right-sided unilateral feeling that his right leg is about to "give out". On physical examination you note that sensation is intact, strength on manual muscle testing is intact on the left but moderately reduced diffusely throughout the right lower extremity distal to the hip. The quadriceps reflex is present on the left and brisk to hyperactive on the right. The patient has difficulty performing rapid alternating movements with his left knee and ankle but not with the right. When he walks, the patient tends to veer toward the right. The responsible lesion is most likely:

        A.   In the dorsal root serving the involved territory
        B.   In the ventral root serving the involved territory
        C.   In the mixed peripheral nerve
        D.   In the white matter within the spinal cord
        E.   In the brain or brainstem

9. A patient presents with right-sided unilateral feeling that his right leg is about to "give out". On physical examination you note that sensation is intact on the left but grossly diminished over the anterior thigh, medial calf, and medial aspect of the right foot. Strength on manual muscle testing is intact on the left but the right quadriceps shows severe weakness. The quadriceps reflex is normal on the left but absent on the right. Proprioception is normal at the left knee but severely impaired or absent at the right knee. Proprioception is normal at the level of the first metatarsophalangeal joints bilaterally. The patient is able to perform rapid alternating movements of both ankles. The responsible lesion is most likely:

   A. In the dorsal root serving the involved territory
   B. In the ventral root serving the involved territory
   C. In the mixed peripheral nerve
   D. In the white matter within the spinal cord
   E. In the brain or brainstem

10. A patient presents with right-sided unilateral feeling that his right leg is about to "give out". On physical examination you note that sensation is intact on the left but grossly diminished over the superior lateral and lower anterior right thigh, and upper medial right calf. Strength on manual muscle testing is normal bilaterally. The quadriceps reflex is normal on the left but absent on the right. Proprioception is normal at the level of the first metatarsophalangeal joints bilaterally. The patient is able to perform rapid alternating movements of both ankles. The responsible lesion is most likely:

   A. In the dorsal root serving the involved territory
   B. In the ventral root serving the involved territory
   C. In the mixed peripheral nerve
   D. In the white matter within the spinal cord
   E. In the brain or brainstem

TRAUMA TO THE FOOT AND ANKLE

John H. Walter, Jr.
Larry R. Goss

INTRODUCTION TO FOOT AND ANKLE TRAUMA

I. **The importance of prompt, aggressive treatment of foot and ankle injuries, both isolated and those associated with multiple trauma, has long been recognized**
    A. **Awareness and recognition of foot and ankle trauma over the past 10 years has greatly increased**
    B. **It is estimated that each year, about 10%-15% of the population sustains some kind of foot and ankle trauma**
    C. **The spectrum of traumatic injuries** - lacerations, puncture wounds, sprains and strains, open and closed fractures, dislocations, burns, etc. - is vast

II. **The management of traumatic foot and ankle injuries, however, is often inadequate and can lead to serious secondary complications, such as chronic and/or permanent foot discomfort**

III. **Thus, a comprehensive knowledge of the range of presentations and proper treatment protocols should be mandated for any clinician that treats the lower extremity**

IV. **Ideally, the patient should be inspected during the "Golden Hour", the first 40 to 60 minutes after any traumatic injury to the foot and ankle, when secondary symptoms and findings are minimal to nonexistent**
    A. **The physical examination and diagnostic manipulations are easy and relatively pain free**
    B. **As time passes, the effects of trauma** - pain, dislocation, inflammation, and edema - become increasingly more pronounced
    C. **Since most trauma patients present hours to days after initial injury, the diagnosis and identification can be complex**

V. **This chapter provides outlined information for the proper diagnosis and treatment proto-cols of many traumatic foot and ankle injuries**

INITIAL ASSESSMENT AND MANAGEMENT OF THE TRAUMA PATIENT

I. **Rapid primary survey** (ABC's of a trauma patient)
    A. **Airway with C-spine control**
    B. **Breathing**
    C. **Circulation with hemorrhage control**
    D. **Disability, utilizing brief neurological exam (AVPU)**
        1. **A**lert
        2. Responds to **V**ocal stimuli
        3. Responds to **P**ainful stimuli
        4. **U**nresponsive
    E. Exposure via completely undressing patient

II. **Resuscitation of vital functions**
    A. **Ventilate and oxygenate**
    B. **Establish IV lines/fluids using two large bore catheters**
    C. **Initiate EKG monitoring**
    D. **Draw blood for cross and match**
    E. **Manage shock**
    F. **Manage life-threatening injuries first**
    G. **Priorities** (in order of urgency):
        1. Airway/asphyxia
        2. Hemorrhage
        3. Sucking chest wound
        4. Shock
        5. Splint fractures

III. **Detailed secondary survey**
    A. **Head-to-toe evaluation utilizing LOOK, LISTEN, and FEEL techniques**
    B. **Assess basic cardiac function**
    C. **Get laboratory studies:** Complete blood count (CBC), serum and coagulation profiles, arterial blood gases, and so forth
    D. **Appropriate radiologic evaluation**
    E. **Complete neurologic exam** (Glasgow Coma Scale [see below])

IV. **Definitive care initiated**
    A. **Obtain a thorough history and perform a complete physical examination**
    B. **Check and document neurovascular status**
    C. **Stabilize/splint/immoblize fracture(s)**
    D. **Care for local wound(s)**
    E. **Debride wound(s)**
    F. **Administer tetanus prophylaxis as necessary** (see section on Puncture Wounds)
    G. **Administer antibiotic prophylaxis, if indicated**

H. **Manage pain**

I. **Get appropriate consultations**

J. **Consider medical and legal issues, i.e., bullet removed**

V. **Glasgow Coma Scale**

   A. <u>**Eye opening**</u>   <u>**Score**</u>

      Spontaneous: 4

      To sound: 3

      To pain: 2

      No response: 1

   B. <u>**Best verbal response**</u>   <u>**Score**</u>

      Oriented: 5

      Disoriented: 4

      Inappropriate words: 3

      Incomprehensible sounds: 2

      None: 1

   C. <u>**Best motor response**</u>   <u>**Score**</u>

      Obeys command   6

      Response to pain:

         Localizes: 5

         Withdraws: 4

         Decorticate: 3

         Decerebrate: 2

         No response: 1

   D. **Patients with a score of 7 or less have poor prognosis of survival (< 30%)**

   E. **Patients with a score of 8-11 have > 50% prognosis for survival**

   F. **Patients with a score greater than 13 have good prognosis of survival (> 80%)**

VI. **General principles of managing acute, lower-extremity trauma**

   A. **Establishment of hemostasis and medical stability**

   B. **Patient history with tetanus immunization status**

   C. **Dermatologic examination**

   D. **Vascular examination**

   E. **Neurologic examination**

   F. **Musculoskeletal examination**

   G. **Laboratory tests**

   H. **Radiographic studies**

   I. **Classification**

   J. **Development of differential diagnosis**

   K. **Definitive diagnosis**

   L. **Initial treatment**

   M. **Definitive treatment**

VII. **Shock**

   A. **Shock management**

      1. Shock: Inability to provide adequate blood and oxygen to maintain the integrity of cell membranes

2. Mechanism of shock occurs when cardiac output is insufficient to fill the arterial tree and blood pressure is too low to give proper perfusion of tissues

3. Cell membranes deteriorate as a result of lysosomal enzyme damage

B. Traumatic etiologies of shock

1. Vasovagal
   a. From trauma of an accident

2. Hypovolemia (hemorrhagic)
   a. From severe blood loss or massive loss of fluid for the skin
   b. Usually result of extensive burns or severe trauma

3. Neurogenic
   a. From severe injury to spinal cord or the brain
   b. Associated with reactive peripheral vasodilation

C. General clinical presentation of shock

1. Tachycardia
2. Hypotension
3. Thready pulses
4. Collapse of peripheral veins
5. Oliguria
6. Hypothermia
7. Metabolic acidosis
8. Mental status change

D. Stages of shock

1. Non-progressive (early) stage
   a. Compensatory mechanisms result

2. Progressive stage
   a. Characterized by tissue hyperperfusion and onset of circulatory and metabolic imbalances
   b. Metabolic acidosis is a prominent finding
   c. Compensatory mechanisms are no longer adequate

3. Irreversible (late) stage
   a. Organ damage and metabolic disturbances are so severe that survival is not possible

E. Classes of hemorrhagic shock

1. Class I hemorrhage: Loss of 15% of blood volume or 750 mls; signs: minimal, with exception of slight tachycardia

2. Class II hemorrhage: Loss of 15%-30% of blood volume or 750-1,500 mls; signs: tachycardia, tachypnea, and hypotension

3. Class III hemorrhage: Loss of 30%-40% of blood volume or 1,500-2,000 mls; signs: marked tachycardia, tachypnea, hypotension and change in mental status

4. Class IV hemorrhage: Loss of more than 40% of blood volume or greater than 2,000 mls; signs: loss of consciousness, pulse, and blood pressure

F. Treatment of shock

1. Goal: To restore organ perfusion

2. Rapid primary survey: ABC's of a trauma patient
   a. Maintain airway by administering oxygen at 8-10 liter/minute

3. Assess physical status of patient
   a. Recognize the presence of the shock state
   b. Identify the probable cause of the shock state

4. No place for vasopressors in the management of traumatic shock
   a. Epinephrine will not help because patient is already vasoconstricted from the com-

pensatory epinephrine released by the adrenal glands
- b. Patient needs fluids and blood to restore proper cellular and organ perfusion
- c. If there is not enough time to type and cross match, give O-negative blood (i.e., universal donor)

G. **Acceptable fluids**
1. Crystalloid solutions
   - a. 5% dextrose in hypotonic saline (one fourth, one third, one half normal saline)
     - i. Prevents excessive fluid loss
     - ii. Promotes diuresis and prevents alkaloses
   - b. Lactated Ringer's solution (with or without 5% dextrose)
     - i. Restores normal fluid shifts
2. Colloid: Protein
3. Type O blood: Can safely be given to a patient in shock
   - a. Give O-negative blood to females who are in their child-bearing or pre-child bearing years
   - b. Give O-positive blood to post-menopausal females and all males
   - c. Incidence of transfusion reactions are extremely low
   - d. For a patient in mild shock, resuscitate with Ringer's lactate, using 3 cc's for every 1 cc of blood loss
4. Laboratory studies to check pH, pO_2, pCO_2, serum electrolytes, BUN, lactic acid, hemogloblin, and hematocrit
5. Measure urine output and volume (normal volume = 30 ml/hour)
   - a. If patient is making urine, he or she must be maintaining an adequate blood pressure
   - b. Persistent oliguria (< 25 ml/hour) for more than 2 hours will cause renal cell death
6. A Swan-Ganz catheter can be used to assess cardiac function and cardiac output; gives an accurate assessment of the amount of fluid patient needs
7. Definitive care can be administered when the patient is medically stable

BREAKS IN THE INTEGUMENT SYSTEM

I. **Definitions**

A. **Laceration:** Tearing of tissues, usually the result of a sharp object
1. Linear laceration: Usually shear force
2. Stellate laceration: Usually compression or tension

B. **Abrasion:** Rubbed/scraped area of the epidermal skin layer, usually the result of a slipping/sliding injury

II. **Classification of soft tissue injuries**

A. **Tidy wound:** Surgical incision, laceration
B. **Untidy wound:** Abrasion
C. **Wound with tissue loss:** Burn, avulsion
D. **Infected wound:** Establishment of constitutional signs and symptoms of infection

III. **Treatment of lacerations and abrasions**

A. **A thorough and careful history must be taken, which should include information about**
1. Mechanism of injury
2. Depth of penetration

3. Cleanliness of removal of mechanism
4. Site of injury (environment)
5. Time of injury
6. Any treatment received

B. Check tetanus immunization status *(see section on Puncture Wounds)*
C. Check neurovascular status
D. Evaluate anatomy of area for possible associated trauma to other, deeper structures
E. Palpate adjacent tendon, muscles, and joint functions
1. Flexion and extension, joint range of motion, and muscle strength bilaterally should be evaluated and documented

F. Examine wounds
1. Check for any sensory, motor, or vascular complications
2. Examine for any cardinal signs of infection or contamination

G. Take deep cultures of wound and gram stain if there is any concern that the wound is contaminated
H. Decontaminate the wound site via local wound principles
1. Mechanical scrub
2. Debridement of all necrotic tissue
3. Copious lavage with physiologic solution (i.e., diluted betadine or normal saline solution)
4. Lacerations: Primary repair with nonabsorbable sutures if less than 4-6 hours
5. Lacerations: Secondary intent healing if greater than 6 hours
6. Abrasions: Secondary intent healing
7. Cover with nonadhesive dressing

I. Oral antibiotic based on clinical scenario for 5-7 days

IV. Puncture wounds

A. Initial wound evaluation and treatment
1. Most common cause of complications following a puncture wound: inadequate primary care of wound
2. The goals of treatment in puncture wounds are twofold:
    a. Conversion of a contaminated or dirty wound to a clean wound
    b. Prevention of tetanus
3. When a patient presents with a pedal puncture wound, the following steps should be performed:
    a. Take a thorough and careful history, which should include information about the following:
        i. Mechanism of injury
        ii. Depth of penetration
        iii. Cleanliness of removal of mechanism
        iv. Site of injury (environment)
        v. Shoe gear and clothing worn when injury occurred
        vi. Time of injury
    b. If the patient presents for the first time a few days after the injury occurred, additional information is needed about the following:
        i. When the injury occurred
        ii. Whether any initial treatment was received
        iii. What the patient did to the wound following the injury
        iv. Whether there has been any exacerbation of symptoms
    c. Physical examination should concentrate on the location of the wound and the

direction of the wound tract
    i. Trauma to the neurovascular supply or damage to osseous structures must be evaluated
    ii. Adjacent muscles and tendons should be checked for function
    iii. If the patient presents a few days after injury, he or she should be checked for any cardinal signs of infection
d. Radiographs or xeroradiographs should be taken to rule out any retained foreign body that may be radiodense, which will also be a useful baseline study if osteomyelitis does occur
e. The wound should be debrided of any debris or necrotic tissue
f. Local or regional anesthesia may be necessary; if local is used it should not be infiltrated in the immediate area of the wound, but should be used proximally to achieve anesthesia without risk of spreading contamination
g. The wound should be probed to determine the depth of the tract, the presence of any deep foreign body, and the possibility of contact with bone or penetration of the deep fascia; if the deep fascia is penetrated, a more aggressive debridement must be carried out to prevent osteomyelitis
h. Aggressive cleansing should be performed with an antibacterial solution, such as iodoform, followed by copious irrigation with a physiologic solution
i. A deep culture and sensitivity of the wound should be taken for aerobic and anaerobic organisms when possible
j. The wound should be kept open with packing or a drain when possible
k. The patient should be instructed to do the following:
    i. Keep off the foot as much as possible
    ii. Elevate the foot
    iii. Soak the foot twice each day in an antimicrobial solution
    iv. Monitor oral temperature daily
    v. Monitor the progress of the wound closely
l. The use of prophylactic antibiotics is still controversial
m. It is recommended that prophylaxis be withheld only when the wound is clean and tidy
n. Tetanus prophylaxis should be administered according to the following guidelines

V. Tetanus prophylaxis

A. Unimmunized, uncertain, or incomplete immunization
1. Low-risk wound
    a. 0.5 ml of toxoid (Td), followed by complete immunization, and thereafter a booster every 10 years
2. Tetanus-prone wounds or wounds neglected > 24 hours
    a. 0.5 ml of toxoid (Td), plus 250-500 U tetanus immune globulin (TIG), followed by completion of immunization

B. Full primary immunization with booster within 10 years of wound
1. Low-risk wound
    a. No toxoid necessary
2. Tetanus-prone wound
    a. If more than 5 years since last dose, give one dose 0.5 ml of toxoid
    b. If less than 5 years since last dose, no dose is necessary
    c. If wound has been neglected > 24 hours, 0.5 ml of toxoid, plus 250-500 U TIG

   C. Full primary unimmunization but no booster doses or last booster dose > 10 years
1. Low-risk wound
   a. One dose Td (0.5 ml)
2. Tetanus-prone wound
   a. One dose Td (0.5 ml)
3. If wound has been neglected > 24 hours, one dose Td (0.5 ml), plus 250-500 U TIG

Table 1. Tetanus prophylaxis chart

Tetanus History		Unknown or < Three Doses	Three Doses	> 10 Years Since Last Booster	> 5 Years Since Last Booster
Clean Minor Wounds	Td[1]	Yes	No	Yes	No
	TIG[2]	No	No	No	No
All Other Wounds (Tetanus-Prone)	Td[1]	Yes	No	Yes	Yes
	TIG[2]	Yes	No	Yes	No
1 - Td = Tetanus toxoid 0.5 ml: For children under 7 years old, DPT vaccine is preferred to tetanus toxoid alone					
2 - TIG = Tetanus Immune Globulin 250-500 IU: Based on the severity and duration of the wound					

VI. Complications of puncture wounds

   A. Soft-tissue infections (cellulitis)
   B. Osteomyelitis
   C. Retained foreign body granuloma
   D. Premature epiphyseal closure
   E. Epidermal inclusion cyst
   F. Joint degeneration
   G. Residual deformity
   H. Septic arthritis with or without pyarthrosis

VII. Causative agents

   A. Cellulitis
1. Causative organism in 50%-60% of the cases: *Staphylococcus aureus*
2. Other causative organisms
   a. *Escherichia coli*
   b. *Klebsiella pneumonia*
   c. *Staphylococcus epidermis*
   d. *Streptococcus* species
3. Treatment of the soft-tissue infection
   a. Puncture wound should be opened and explored
   b. Any retained foreign body should be removed and any necrosis debrided

    c. If an abscess is present, surgical incision and drainage must be performed

    d. Wound should be packed open to prevent premature closure

  4. Antimicrobial treatment of cellulitis should be empirically directed at all of the common pathogens pending culture and sensitivity reports

  5. Cefazolin, a first-generation parental cephalosporin, is the drug of choice because of its coverage of all of the above organisms; below find lists of alternative antibiotics by organisms isolated

VIII. Organism antibiotic selection

A. *Staphylococcus aureus* (methicillin susceptible)
1. Semisynthetic penicillin
2. First-generation cephalosporin
3. Clindamycin
4. Vancomycin
5. Trimethoprim-sulfamethoxazole
6. Erythromycin

B. *Staphylococcus aureus* (methicillin resistant)
1. Vancomycin
2. Trimethoprim-sulfamethoxazole
3. Ciprofloxacin (high resistance)
4. Imipenem/Cilastatin (Primaxn)

C. *Streptococcus species*
1. Penicillin V
2. First-generation cephalosporin

D. *Escherichia coli*
1. Ampicillin
2. First-generation cephalosporin
3. Trimethoprim-sulfamethoxazole

IX. Osteomyelitis

A. This is the most difficult complication to manage

B. Upon surgical debridement and culture of infected bone, *Pseudomonas aeruginosa* is isolated in 90% of cases

C. Treatment of osteomyelitis is both medical and surgical in nature
1. Necrotic bone must be surgically debrided
2. Any coexistent soft-tissue abscess should be incised and drained
3. Antibiotic therapy should be continued for 4-6 weeks following definitive debridement

D. Antibiotic selection
1. Ceftazidime, 2 g q 12h IV
2. Ciprofloxacin, 750 mg q 12h p.o.
3. Levaquin 500 mg q day p.o. or IV
4. Aztreonam, 1-2 g q 8h IV

X. Bite wounds

A. In general, most bite injuries are contusions and not lacerations; their infection potential is low

B. Approximately 1-2 million bite wounds occur per year; the three most common types of wounds are from humans, dogs, and cats

1. 90% inflicted by dogs
2. 5% inflicted by cats
3. 2%-3% inflicted by humans

C. **Of the three most commonly seen bite wounds, human bites are usually the most severe and dangerous**
   1. Human bites usually produce more crush and shear, with greater resultant tissue damage than animal bites
   2. Microbacterial flora of a human bite is more extensive and pathogenic
   3. Human bite wounds are more contaminated than dog or cat bite wounds
   4. Initially, the wound may appear innocuous; but as the non-treated wound progresses into the second day, the patient may start to develop a rapidly spreading inflammation, lymphangitis, lymphadenitis, and even septicemia and bacteremia
   5. The crushed tissue from the bite wound is locally ischemic, which creates an excellent medium for bacterial growth
   6. The human oral cavity may contain as many as 42 species of bacteria
      a. Alpha-hemolytic *Streptococcus* sp.: The most common isolate from human bite
      b. Anaerobes: Bactericodes sp. is the most common genus isolated
      c. *Staphylococcus aureus* and *Staphylococcus epidemidis*
      d. *Eikenella corrodens* (a gram-negative capnophilic rod found in dental plaques) has been isolated in 15%-20% of human bite wounds
   7. Also of concern is the possible transmission of the HIV and hepatitis virus, which can be determined by testing the attacker
   8. Other microbes that have been reported are *Haemophilus* sp., spirochetes and *Mycobacterium* sp.

D. **Colony growth in animal bites is generally less than colony growth in human bite wounds, which makes human bites more prone to infection and generally more severe than an equivalent dog or cat bite**
   1. Some authors have stated that the teeth of dogs are considered clean, and a dog's saliva has antibacterial enzymes, which decreases the flora in the mouth
   2. Dog bite wounds are susceptible to infection because of direct inoculation of bacteria
   3. Dog and cat bites differ in that a dog bite is more of a crush-and-tear-type of injury that exerts 150-450 psi while the cat bite is more of a puncture wound with a greater tendency for infection
   4. A broad spectrum of bacteria may be isolated following animal bites
   5. The most commonly isolated organisms from cat bite wounds are the following (in order of frequency):
      a. *Pasteurella multocida* has been overemphasized as a major infectious agent in animal bites
         i. Recent studies show that Pasteurella is a more common infectious isolate in cat bites (approximately 50%) as compared to dog bites (20%-26%)
      b. *Staphylococcus aureus*
      c. *Staphylococcus epidermidis*
      d. *Streptococcus* sp.
   6. The more commonly isolated organisms from dog bite wounds are the following (in order of frequency):
      a. Enterobacteriaceae family
      b. *Pseudomonas* sp.
      c. *Staphylococcus aureus*
      d. *Pasteurella multocida*

e. *Bacillus sublis*

f. Beta *Streptococcus* sp.

g. Another organism that has been isolated in dog bites is DF-2, also known as *Capnocytophaga canimorsus*, which seems to have a predilection for patients that are asplenic, cirrhotic, or immunocompromised (diabetics)

7. Primary versus secondary repair is a matter of controversy in animal bites

a. Loose closure by adhesive strips followed by delayed repair has been recommended

8. Antibiotic therapy is also a controversial issue with dog and cat bites

a. Some authorities believe that no bite can be considered "clean" because of the accompanying inoculation of bacteria and that prophylaxis should be withheld only when a wound is very trivial

b. Others believe antibiotic prophylaxis should not be given because they decrease the normal flora and allow for more pathogenic organisms to survive

E. Treatment of bite wounds

1. When the skin is broken, there is risk of local wound infection or transmission of systemic disease

2. Tetanus prophylaxis should be performed

a. If it is recommended that all human bite wounds, which are tetanus prone and contaminated, should have the tetanus toxoid administered

b. If the history of the cat or dog wound is uncertain, if immunization is more than 5 years old, or if the wound is determined to be tetanus prone

3. Radiographs of the involved area should be obtained

4. Deep cultures (anaerobic and aerobic) should be taken; some authors say cultures of bite wounds offer little information because of the multiplicity of organisms found and the absence of an established infection

5. Local wound care should be thorough and aggressive, including

a. Copious irrigation with sterile saline or saline with diluted betadine

b. Irrigation of the wound has been shown to decrease infection significantly

c. Debridement of all necrotic wound edges

d. Open packing and application of a sterile dressing

6. Irrigation and debridement combined are much more effective than any amount or type of antibiotic treatment in preventing infection

7. Patients with an established major infection should be hospitalized and started on intravenous antibiotics

8. Signs of localized pus, devitalized tissue, joint penetration, or foreign body mandates a surgical incision and drainage

9. Elevation and immobilization until 72 hours after initial occurrence

a. Prompt application of cold packs helps to decrease swelling and pain

10. Therapeutic antibiotics are started after cultures are taken; the suggested antibiotics include the following

a. For cat bites: Dicloxacillin, penicillin, cephalexin, Ciprofloxacin, or Augmentin

b. For dog bites: Dicloxacillin, cephadrine, or Augmentin

c. Drug of choice for human bites: Augmentin

d. For penicillin allergy: Erythromycin or Bactrim

11. Antibiotic administration is a controversial issue and should be based on clinical findings and the most prevalent organisms found in the wounds

12. Animal bites may require rabies vaccination based on the description of the attack

13. If the risk of rabies is high, the wound should be irrigated with 1% benzalkonium chloride because of an apparent virucidal action against the rabies virus

14. Local health officials should be contacted immediately to determine further measures

F. **Assessment and treatment of rabies**
   1. The decision to initiate rabies treatment depends on the knowledge of the incidence of rabies with respect to the species involved and the local region
   2. The risk of acquiring rabies from domestic dogs or cats is small and varies according to region
   3. To find out the risk of acquiring rabies, consult your local county and state health departments
   4. If a wild animal, such as a skunk, raccoon, fox, bat, bobcat, or coyote bit the patient, then rabies prophylaxis is indicated because rabies is prevalent in these species
   5. Rabies should be suspected if the animal behaves unusually, such as unprovoked, wild animal attacking in daylight
   6. If the nature of the offending animal is unknown, the worst should be suspected and treated for rabies
   7. If the treatment is started and the animal is shown to be negative for rabies, treatment can be discontinued
   8. Antirabies immunization consists of a combination of antibody and vaccine
   9. RIG (rabies immune globulin, human) provides passive immunity, which persist for only a short time (half-life of 21 days)
      a. Dose is 20 IU/kg body weight or approximately 9 IU/pound of body weight
      b. CDC recommends that half the RIG is injected in the area around the wound
      c. The other half is given in the gluteal area
      d. It is suggested to use two syringes, not the same one
   10. HDCV (human diploid cell vaccine) provides active immunity
      a. Requires about 7-10 days to develop, but persist as long as a year or more
      b. Dosage is 1.0 ml IM in deltoid area (never gluteal) area
      c. A series of five injections are given over a course of one month
      d. The injection series is 1, 3, 7, 14, and 28 days following the initial bite
      e. The first dose should be given as soon as possible after exposure
      f. World Health Organization (WHO) currently recommends a sixth dose 90 days after the first dose

TREATMENT OF OPEN AND CLOSED FRACTURES

I. **Open fractures**

   A. **Definition**
      1. Open fractures are a surgical emergency, with possible complications of osteomyelitis and delayed/nonunion
      2. Open fractures are defined as any fracture that breaks the continuity of the skin and allows the underlying bone to be exposed to the external environment
      3. Goals in the management of open fractures are to restore alignment, restore function, and prevent infection
      4. An open fracture presents with a wide spectrum of soft-tissue injury combined with osseous disruption
      5. Etiology of open fractures is the result of internal to external force vector and/or external to internal force vector
      6. Of patients with open fractures, 30%-40% sustain polytrauma

B. Physical exam of open fractures
  1. Initial assessment of soft-tissue and skeletal injury
  2. Record mechanism of injury, when, and where it occurred
  3. Adequately describe the wound, including the following:
     a. Location
     b. Size
     c. Degree of soft-tissue loss and/or exposed bone
     d. Extent of contamination
     e. Description of any visible foreign material
  4. Evaluate skeletal involvement by assessing the following
     a. Location
     b. Stability
     c. Type of fracture
     d. Joint involvement

C. Classification of open fractures by Gustilo-Anderson - Types I, II and III
  1. Type I
     a. Defined as *wounds less than 1.0 cm* in diameter and clean (minimal contamination)
     b. Minimal soft-tissue involvement or muscle contusion
     c. No crush component
     d. Fracture is usually a simple transverse or short oblique with minimal comminution
     e. Commonly referred to as an inside/outside wound
  2. Treatment based upon AO principles for Type I Injuries:
     a. Antibiotics: Usually a first generation cephalosporin (Ancef)
     b. Debridement and irrigation
     c. Possibly internal or external fixation of the fracture
     d. Secondary closure and granulation
  3. Type II
     a. Defined as a *laceration 1.0 to 5.0 cm* without extensive soft-tissue damage, absence of flaps or avulsion, and a minimal crush component
     b. No significant functional disability
  4. Treatment based upon AO principles for Type I:
     a. Same as above for Type I, except that add antibiotic for gram negative coverage
  5. Type III
     a. Open fracture with extensive soft-tissue damage to the skin, muscle, and neurovascular structures (usually greater than 5 cm)
     b. Associated with high velocity or ballistic-type injuries and a severe crush component
     c. Type III open fractures include:
        i. High-velocity injury with extensive soft-tissue damage
        ii. Farm injuries, irrespective of wound size, with soil contamination
        iii. Open fracture with neurovascular compromise
        iv. Traumatic amputations or degloving injuries
        v. Open fractures greater than 8 hours old
     d. Type III is subdivided into the following three parts:
        i. Type IIIA: Adequate soft-tissue coverage of fractured bone, despite extensive soft-tissue lacerations or flaps; high-energy trauma regardless of wound size
        ii. Type IIIB: Extensive soft-tissue injury loss with periosteal stripping and bone exposure; usually associated with massive contamination
        iii. Type IIIC: Associated with arterial injury <u>requiring</u> repair
  6. Treatment based on AO principles for Type III:

    a. Therapeutic IV antibiotics: Usually antibiotic combinations (i.e., Penicillin, an aminoglycoside and Clindamycin)
    b. Debridement and irrigation
    c. Reduction of fracture and splint
    d. Internal fixation of the fracture 5-7 days post-occurrence
7. Basic principles of therapy for open fractures
    a. Antibiotics
    b. Operative debridement and irrigation of all nonviable tissues
    c. Fracture stabilization
    d. Wound coverage

D. Important information regarding open fractures
1. Open wound should be classified before and after debridement and secondary incisions
2. Considered *contaminated* up to 6-8 hours post-occurrence without treatment
3. Considered *infected* after 6-8 hours post-occurrence without treatment
4. Patient should be started on therapeutic antibiotics within 3 hours of the occurrence if possible; the antibiotic should be effective against both gram-positive and gram-negative organisms
5. Gram stain and appropriate cultures and sensitivities should be taken before any treatment is instituted; most common organisms cultured from open fractures are the following:
    a. *Staphylococcus aureus* - penicillinase producing (most common organism)
    b. *Klebsiella* species
    c. *Pseudomonas* species
    d. Enterobacter species
    e. Diptheroids
    f. Clostridia: Can cause gas gangrene or tetanus
6. Tetanus prophylaxis is essential
7. Adequate debridement of all necrotic skin, fascia, muscle, and bone within 24-48 hours post injury
    a. Debridement should be meticulous and systematic to remove all devitalized tissue
    b. All foreign debris should be removed from soft tissue and bone
    c. Only exceptions are shotgun pellets or bullets not jeopardizing a vital structure or not within a joint
8. Copious lavage and irrigation with a physiologic solution (e.g., warm physiologic saline, lactated Ringer's solution, antibiotic solutions)
    a. Lavage aids in the reduction of contamination and removal of foreign materials in the wound
    b. Type I injuries require 1-3 L and Type II-III injuries require 3-6 L of irrigation
    c. Pulsating jet lavage systems are recommended
9. Fracture stabilization of fragments is essential for preservation of remaining viable soft tissue
    a. Realigning and stabilizing fractures optimizes local wound conditions and helps to prevent infection
    b. When the bone is exposed to the outside environment, antibiotics should always be considered
    c. External fixation should be considered in severe traumatic injuries with multiple fractures
10. Amputation is indicated in severe degloving or crush injuries with neurovascular compromise

11. Appropriate wound coverage should be arranged
    a. Primary closure should be performed only in wounds that occur less than 8 hours before treatment and in wounds that display no evidence of contamination
    b. Delayed primary closure within 3-10 days is recommended in all wounds more than 8 hours old
12. Rehabilitation should be started early
    a. Physical therapy is essential in reducing morbidity
    b. Aids the patients return to a functional state

II. Closed fractures
A. Definition and classification of closed fractures
1. Defined as break in the continuity of a bone that does not communicate with the outside of the body
2. Closed fractures result from two types of trauma
   a. Direct trauma: Result from a blow of varying velocity (two types)
      i. Tapping fractures: Low-velocity blow with only minimal soft-tissue damage
      ii. Crush fractures: High-velocity blow, extensive soft-tissue injury and comminuted fractures
   b. Indirect trauma: Results from forces acting at a distance to the fracture site (several types)
      i. Traction fractures: Also known as avulsion fractures
      ii. Angulation fractures: Caused by a bending force in one plane against a long bone
      iii. Spiral fractures: Caused by rotational forces
      iv. Compression fractures: Results from impaction injuries
      v. Angulation and axial compression fractures
      vi. Angulation and rotational fractures

B. Evaluation of closed fractures
1. Determine type of fracture
   a. Transverse: Line of break is transverse in relation to the longitudinal axis of the shaft
   b. Oblique: Line of break is oblique in relation to the longitudinal axis of the shaft
   c. Spiral: Fracture line is two times longer than the transverse diameter of the bone in the central area of the fracture
   d. Comminuted: Fracture must consist of three or more fracture fragments
      i. Segmental fracture
      ii. Butterfly fracture
   e. Impaction: Compression with shortening
   f. Avulsion: A fleck or piece of bone
2. Determine the aggressiveness of the treatment regimen:
   a. Is the fracture stable or unstable? The following questions should be considered before treatment is begun:
      i. How much bone-to-bone contact is there?
      ii. Are the fragments well aligned?
      iii. Is the area subject to movement?
      iv. How extensive is the soft-tissue involvement?
      v. How much blood is being supplied to the fractured segment?
      vi. What kind of bone is involved in the fracture?
      vii. Is the fracture intra-articular or extra-articular?
      viii. Does the fracture involve primarily cancellous bone, cortical bone, or both?

C. Description of closed fractures
   1. Include the basic fracture relationships described by the mnemonic **"TOE LARD LAD"**
       T = Type of fracture
       O = Open or Closed
       E = Extra-articular or Intra-articular
              L = Length
              A = Angulation
              R = Rotation
              D = Displacement
                     L = Location
                     A = Alignment
                     D = Direction of the fracture line
       a. Type: short bone or long bone; cortical or cancellous bone
       b. Open fracture or closed
       c. Angulation: Medial or lateral, abducted or adducted, dorsiflexed or plantarflexed
       d. Rotation: Varus or valgus
       e. Displacement: Separation of the fragments
       f. Length: Shortened or lengthened
       g. Alignment: Poor, fair, good, or anatomic position of all fragments overall
   2. Note whether the fracture is intra-articular or extra-articular
   3. Describe the direction in which the fracture line is running
   4. Describe the overall appearance of the fracture as anatomical, good, fair, or poor alignment
   5. Do not describe fractures in adults as "through and through", "complete", or "incomplete"
       a. All adult fractures should be considered as "through and through," even though this may not be evident radiographically
       b. These terms give a false impression and information, which may result in less than adequate method of treatment
   6. When evaluating a fracture for rotation, remember what the normal anatomy looks like; this baseline will promote detection of any rotation of the fracture fragments
   7. In general, consider anatomical and good alignment fractures for conservative management and fair and poor alignment fractures for open reduction management

D. Treatment of closed fractures
   1. Begin approach with assessment of possible other life-threatening injuries; ABC's of trauma patient *(Do not forget to check for pedal pulses)*
   2. Obtain a thorough history:
       a. Time and nature of injury
       b. Mechanism of injury
       c. Location of injury
       d. Previous treatment
       e. Pertinent past medical history, current medications, and allergies
       f. Note when the last meal was eaten (in case must go to OR)
   3. Perform a complete physical examination
       a. Look for clinical signs of fracture, such as local swelling, ecchymosis, deformity, localized tenderness, impaired function, abnormal mobility, and joint crepitus
       b. Assess damage to adjacent soft tissue structures
       c. Check neurovascular status
       d. Test muscle strength bilaterally

      e.   Document joint range of motion

  4. Radiographic examination

      a.   Prior to sending the patient for radiographs, the injured part should be splinted

      b.   Obtain functional views (e.g., angle and base of gait) when possible

      c.   Order the standard foot (DP, lateral, and obliques) and ankle (AP, lateral, mortise, and obliques) radiographic views, and calcaneal axial when necessary

      d.   Bilateral views are not necessarily indicated in unilateral trauma (exception: epiphyseal fractures in children)

  5. After determining the location of the injury and looking at the individual patient's status, develop a treatment regimen tailored to the needs of the patient and keep in mind several factors:

      a.   Age

      b.   Stature

      c.   Medical status

      d.   Physical status

      e.   Vascular status

      f.   Mental status

  6. The basic premise of emergency treatment of a fracture is seen in the mnemonic **"RIICE"**

      a.   Rest

      b.   Ice

      c.   Immobilization

      d.   Compression

      e.   Elevation

E. Treatment of closed fractures

  1. Usually non-displaced fractures in good alignment and position can be treated conservatively

  2. Conservative treatment options include:

      a.   ACE wraps

      b.   Strappings (i.e., with various tapes, Coban, or Elastoplast)

      c.   Posterior splints

      d.   Jones compression wrap

      e.   Soft cast or zinc oxide strapping (i.e., UNNA's boot)

      f.   Removable cast boot (i.e., CAM walker)

      g.   Hard cast (i.e., fiberglass or plaster cast)

  3. Immobilization techniques should hold the correction of the fracture in normal anatomical alignment (there are two positions of immobilization):

      a.   **Rest:** Position of most comfort for the patient

      b.   **Function:** Preferred position, which duplicates the position that the joint usually functions

  4. A good rule of thumb, when dealing with closed fractures is to examine and immobilize the *joint above and the joint below* the fracture site, to prevent motion at the fracture site

  5. With displaced fractures in fair to poor alignment, closed reduction techniques should be considered; if the reduction is not likely or unsuccessful, then open reduction with or without internal fixation is required

  6. Closed reduction should not be attempted without local anesthesia or pain medications considerations in most cases

  7. There are three important steps to any closed reduction of a closed fracture or dislocation

      a.   The deformity should be increased to allow any interposed soft tissues to be released

        b.   Distal distraction of the fragments should be provided to reduce the bone-to-bone contact

        c.   The mechanism of injury should then be reversed reducing the fracture

    8. Post-reduction films should be taken after closed reduction and the part is splinted or casted in most cases

E. Complications of closed fractures

    1. Delayed union and nonunion

    2. Joint stiffness

    3. Malunion

    4. Neurovascular injury

    5. Shortening

    6. Infection

    7. Avascular necrosis

    8. Skin sloughing

    9. Complex regional pain syndrome

FOREFOOT TRAUMA

I. Phalangeal fractures and nail injuries

A. Distal phalangeal fractures are frequently a result of a crush injury to the toe

B. Typically, when these injuries occur there is also some type of nail, nail bed and/or nail fold injury involved

C. If a distal phalangeal fracture is noted on a radiograph with nail injury, the nail bed must be examined for the possibility of disruption, because of its close proximity to bone

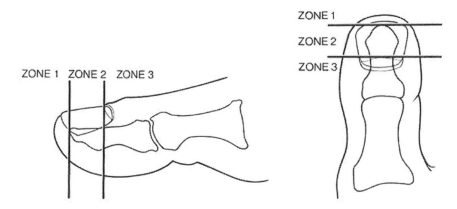

D. If a subungual hematoma present of greater than 25% of the nail plate, than the nail bed should be considered ruptured

E. Therefore, the digit must be anesthetized and the entire nail plate removed

F. If the nail bed is lacerated, the fracture is considered an open fracture and requires appropriate treatment *(see section on Open Fractures)*

G. The basic treatment for an open distal phalangeal fracture is local wound care, tetanus prophylaxis and antibiotic therapy

    1. Small exposed fracture fragments should be debrided and then the area is lavaged with sterile saline and covered with a non-stick dressing

    2. A surgical shoe is recommended for immobilization and protection even when sleeping

    3. Daily wound care should continue for 1 to 2 weeks

   4. Clean nail bed lacerations can be sutured
H. **Nail and distal tip injuries were classified by <u>Rosenthal</u> in 1983 for finger injuries** (this classification has been modified for the foot) •

II. **Rosenthal Classification** (1983): Nail injuries are divided into three zones:

A. **Zone I: Distal to the phalanx**
B. **Zone II: Distal to the lunula**
C. **Zone III: Proximal to the distal end of the lunula**
D. **Zone I Injuries:**
   1. This injury is described as minimal soft tissue loss, without exposed bone
   2. For zone I injury with soft tissue loss less than 1.0 cm, the injury should be cleansed and any necrotic tissue debrided
      a. This type of injury can usually be allowed to granulate closed by secondary intention
      b. The patient is allowed to ambulate in a surgical shoe to tolerance
   3. A zone I injury with soft tissue loss greater than 1.0 cm, skin grafting on an acute or delayed basis should be considered
      a. After cleansing and debridement of the injury, a split-thickness skin graft, as advocated and described by Newmeyer and Kilgore for the hand, is procured and placed over the defect on an acute basis
      b. This technique was described for use in fingertips and may not be effective where the injury is in a weight-bearing or contact area, because of poor graft durability
      c. In these regions, it is suggested to use *full thickness skin grafts* because of their increased durability
E. **Zone II Injuries:**
   1. Zone II injuries are complicated by exposed bone and substantial nail bed loss
   2. When determining the treatment for Zone II injuries, you have to consider the plane of amputation, for it will dictate the flap or graft you use
   3. You must evaluate the condition of the nail bed and whether augmentation will be successful or ablation of the nail bed is necessary
   4. You want to cover the defect with a flap that has adequate sensation and vascularity
   5. Treatment of these injuries requires appropriate debridement of any prominent bone and necrotic tissue
      a. After debridement, coverage of the tip of the digital and distal augmentation of the nail bed are usually achieved with a local adjacent neurovascular V-Y skin plasty (Atasoy or Kutler flaps)
      b. The *Atasoy flap* is a plantar V-Y advancement flap, while the *Kutler flap* is a biaxial V-Y advancement flap
F. **Zone III Injuries:**
   1. Zone III injuries are generally not amenable to initial definitive treatment in the ER or office, as compared to Zone I or II injuries
   2. The prognosis for nail bed survival in these injuries is poor and nail bed construction is usually not considered
   3. Debridement of these injuries usually is performed in the OR, followed by immediate or delayed revision of the distal aspect of the digit
      a. Primary amputation of the distal phalanx and ablation of the nail bed and nail matrix is usually performed in the OR
      b. Preservation of the distal interphalangeal joint and digital tendon function should be attempted

TURF TOE INJURY

I. Introduction
  A. **Turf toe is classically described as an injury to the great toe joint**
  B. **This type of injury is commonly experienced by athletes who play on artificial playing surfaces**
  C. **Oftentimes, athletes perceive the initial injury as either trivial or benign**
  D. **Symptoms of acute injury include pain, tenderness and swelling of the great toe joint**
  E. **Often there is a sudden acute onset of pain during push-off phase of running**
  F. **Usually, the pain is not enough to keep the athlete from physical activities or finishing a game**
  G. **This causes further injury to the great toe and will dramatically increase the healing time**
  H. **Up to 50% of turf toe injuries result in long-term morbidity**

II. Etiology of turf toe injuries
  A. **Playing on artificial turf that lacks cushioning and places extremely high amounts of stress on the great toe joint**
  B. **Lighter and more flexible shoegear is a rapid cause of the increasing numbers of turf toe injuries**
  C. **Activities such as football, basketball, soccer, field hockey and lacrosse show the highest incidence of injury to the great toe joint**

III. Mechanism of injury
  A. **There are two mechanisms of injury for turf toe:**
    1. The most common cause is *hyperextension* of the great toe joint
       a. The great toe is hyperextended and the heel is raised off the ground
       b. An external force is placed on the great toe and the soft tissue structures that support the great toe on the bottom are torn or ruptured
    2. The second mechanism is *hyperflexion* of the great toe joint (< 25%)
       a. In a hyperflexion injury, stress is placed on the top of the great toe
       b. Soft tissue structures that support the great toe on the top are torn or ruptured

IV. Classification
  A. **Grade I turf toe injury is considered to be mild and the supporting soft tissue structure that encompass the great toe are only sprained or stretched** (this is the most common type of injury)
    1. There is minimal swelling with mild local tenderness and usually no black and blue bruising evident
  B. **Grade II turf toe injuries are considered moderate in severity**
    1. They present with more diffuse tenderness, swelling, restricted range of motion and usually are mildly black-and-blue in appearance
    2. There is usually a partial tear of the supporting ligaments but no articular cartilage damage
  C. **Grade III injuries are considered severe in nature because of the considerable swelling, pain on palpation, restriction of range of motion, inability to bear any weight on the injured foot and diffuse black-and-blue appearance of the great toe**

    1. There are generally tears to the joint capsule, ruptured ligaments and possibly compression damage to the articular cartilage of the great toe

V. Treatment

  A. Treatment is usually centered on an individual basis and the severity of injury sustained

  B. The "RIICE" can be employed

  C. Use of a stiffer athletic shoe to resist motion of the great toe or the insertion of an orthotic to increase support of the great toe

  D. Strapping of the great toe to limit motion may allow a highly competitive athlete to return to activities quicker

  E. Non-steroidal anti-inflammatory drugs (NSAID) may be utilized for relief of minor pain as well as to decrease the inflammation of the injury

  F. Grade I injuries do well with strapping and usually only require a few days of rest

  G. Grade II injuries should adhere to the "RIICE" principles and usually require one to two weeks of missed practices and games

  H. Grade III injuries are more severe injuries and the healing process may take four to six weeks of recovery time from physical activities

  I. Sometimes, Grade III turf toe injuries do not heal appropriately with conservative care and result in chronic pain and instability

  J. Surgical reconstruction of the capsule, ligaments, and articular cartilage may be necessary to restore proper alignment and function in these extreme cases

SESAMOIDAL FRACTURES

I. Introduction

  A. With the increase of active sports programs, such as jogging, aerobics, long-distance running and race walking, injuries and fracture of the sesamoids have been increasing in frequency

  B. The etiology of sesamoidal fractures is usually a crush injury in which the sesamoids are crushed in the sagittal plane between the first metatarsal and the ground

  C. The onset of sesamoid injuries is usually insidious, with the patient being unable to recall any single traumatic event

  D. Biomechanical derangements predisposed to sesamoidal injuries include:

    1. Cavus foot

    2. Peroneus longus spasm

    3. Metatarsus primus equinus

  E. Typically, the patient with a sesamoid fracture presents with acute or chronic pain beneath the first metatarsal head

    1. The pain may be severe and the patient may guard against weight-bearing and dorsiflexion of the first metatarsophalangeal joint in acute injuries

    2. In acute injuries, edema and ecchymosis may or may not be present

    3. In chronic injuries, the pain usually increases with activity, dorsiflexion of the first metatarsophalangeal joint or in certain shoes

II. Diagnosis of a sesamoid fracture

  A. On physical examination, the pain is usually localized to the injured sesamoid(s) on direct palpation

B. Pain can also be elicited on dorsiflexion, abduction or adduction of the first metatarsophalangeal joint

C. If a sesamoid fracture is suspected at least three radiographic views bilaterally should be obtained (DP, medial oblique and sesamoidal axial)

D. Typically, a sesamoidal fracture is *transverse* or *comminuted* and the tibial sesamoid is the sesamoid most commonly involved, because of the increased load on it in the closed kinetic chain gait

E. With sesamoidal pain, you have to differentiate a fractured sesamoid from a bipartite sesamoid on radiographs

F. Listed below are some radiographic criteria that are suggestive of a fracture rather than a bipartite sesamoid
   1. No evidence of fracture on earlier/previous films
   2. Irregular, serrated, jagged line(s) of separation
   3. Longitudinally or obliquely oriented division lines
   4. Absence of similar findings on the contralateral film
   5. Bone callous formation
   6. Exaggerated space of fragment separations
   7. Anatomically abnormal fragment positions
   8. Multiple irregular fragments
   9. Interrupted peripheral cortices

G. If the radiographs are equivocal or if additional diagnostic information is needed, a Technetium-99 bone scans, CT, MRI or stress radiographs may be considered

H. In any case, if the radiographs suggest a possible fracture and the patient has symptoms, the injury must be treated as a fracture

I. Treatment of a fractured sesamoid is directed towards relieving direct and indirect pressure to the area
   1. This is accomplished by eliminating the first metatarsal from weight bearing by the use of a below the knee non-weight bearing cast extended beyond the toes, a weight bearing cast with an incorporated Dancer's pad, and/or hallux splint non-weight bearing (i.e., eliminates both direct and indirect pressures)

J. The problem with a sesamoidal fracture is that the area is highly avascular
   1. This accounts for the 80%-85% rate of non-unions to the area
   2. This result is acceptable, if the non-union is asymptomatic
   3. Should pain persist and conservative treatment fails, surgical excision of the sesamoids should be considered

K. One should be aware of *Ilfeld's disease*: Agenesis of one or both of the sesamoids

FIRST METATARSOPHALANGEAL DISLOCATION

I. Introduction

A. Traumatic dislocation of the first metatarsophalangeal joint are rare

B. Mechanism of injury: is a forced *hyperextension* of the first MTPJ (i.e., as a result of MVA)
   1. Other reported causes include: fall from height and Charcot joint disease

C. Clinically, the patient presents with a hallux that is dorsally subluxed at the MTPJ and a prominence of the metatarsal head is noted plantarly

D. Pain is elicited on palpation and attempted ROM of the joint

> **E.** **The extensor apparatus is in a contracted state, while the flexor apparatus is tightened due to the dislocation**
>
> **F.** **A classification was developed by _Jahss_ in 1980 based on two distinct radiographic patterns**

II. Jahss Classification (1980): for traumatic hallux dislocations

  A. Type I dislocation

    1. Dorsal dislocation of the proximal phalanx and sesamoids with the intersesamoidal ligament intact

    2. The sesamoids are unfractured and they remain generally apposed to the proximal phalangeal base

    3. In general, closed reduction treatment is usually _unsuccessful_, which attributed to the locked position of the metatarsal beneath the proximal phalanx and joint capsule

    4. This position is maintained by the soft tissue around the joint (abductor hallucis, adductor hallucis, flexor hallucis longus, and the collateral ligaments), therefore **open reduction** is required

    5. Adequate exposure of the joint can be provided through a dorsal linear incision

    6. After reduction, the foot is then splinted or put in a below the knee cast non-weight bearing for 3-4 weeks and then ambulation in stiff soled shoe to tolerance

  B. Type II dislocation

    1. Dorsal dislocation of the proximal phalanx and sesamoids with <u>rupture</u> of the intersesamoidal ligament

    2. There are two types (A and B)

      a. Type IIA: Dorsal dislocation of the proximal phalanx with wide separation of the sesamoids **without fracture** of either of the sesamoids

      b. Type IIB: Dorsal dislocation of the proximal phalanx with wide separation of the sesamoids **with a transverse fracture** of either of the sesamoids

    3. Radiographically, the proximal fragment remains in a normal position in relation to the adjacent sesamoid, while the distal fragment separates widely and is drawn distally into the joint space

    4. Acute Type II injuries may be reduced by closed reduction methods _(see section on Closed Reduction)_

    5. The foot is immobilized for 2-4 weeks non-weight bearing cast followed by weight bearing as tolerated

    6. With the type IIB injury, the distal fracture fragment or the whole sesamoid may need to be excised dependent on the symptomatology following closed reduction and immobilization

    7. A Type IIc was recently added and is described as a dorsal dislocation with fracture of both seasmoids

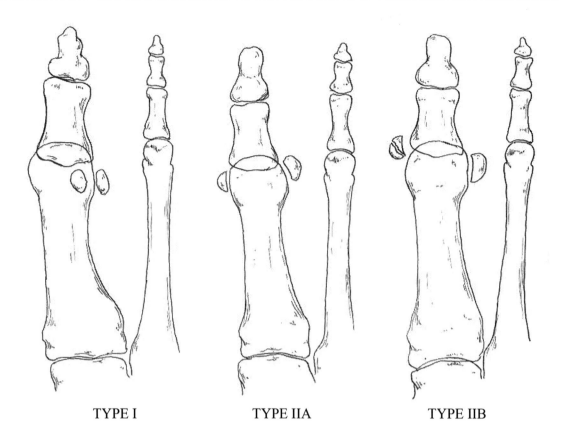

TYPE I   TYPE IIA   TYPE IIB

STRESS FRACTURES

I. Introduction

    A. Stress fractures have been described by a variety of terms, which include:
        1. March fracture
        2. Hairline fracture
        3. Fatigue fracture
        4. Insufficiency fracture
        5. Deutschlander's disease
        6. Bone exhaustion

    B. Stress fractures develop in bone without acute trauma
        1. They are generally secondary to microtrauma, which is usually a repeated submaximal strain upon the osseous structure
        2. This is commonly caused by overuse syndromes (i.e., usually exercise related injuries)

    C. Persons most commonly afflicted are athletes and military recruits

    D. Approximately 80% of all stress fractures occur in the lower extremity

    E. Listed below is the incidence in the lower extremity:
        1. Metatarsals - 20%
            a. 2nd metatarsal - 11% (most common)
            b. 3rd metatarsal - 7%
            c. 1st, 4th and 5th metatarsals - 2%
        2. Sesamoids, calcaneus, navicular, talus - 2%

3. Fibula and tibia - 24%

II. Diagnosis of stress fractures

A. **Radiographically, an acute stress fracture may be difficult to see on a plain radiograph**

B. **It may take 10-14 days or 30%-50% bone demineralization before there is radiograph evidence of a stress fracture, which is indicated by bone callus formation**

C. **Clinically, these patients will present with a diffuse pain, that can be localized to one specific point usually through palpation or the use of a tuning fork**

III. Treatment of stress fractures

A. **Treatment of most stress fractures is immobilization of part via below the knee cast, UNNA boot, or surgical shoe non-weight bearing for 4-6 weeks**

B. **You have to make sure the bone is immobilized in anatomical position, for it could be healed in a elevated position and cause transfer lesions**

C. **In six weeks, these fractures are usually clinically healed**

D. **This does not necessarily mean calcification on radiograph, but when you palpate or stress the site you get little or no movement and pain**

E. **In difficult cases, where there is equivocal findings on plain radiographs, other modalities such as Technetium-99 bone scans and CT scan are helpful in determining the existence of a stress fracture**

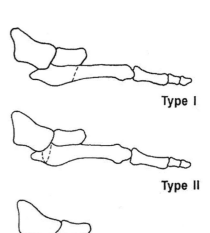

Type I

Type II

Type III

FIFTH METATARSAL BASE FRACTURES

I. Introduction

A. **Fractures of the base of the fifth metatarsal are among the most common of all skeletal injuries of the foot**

B. **They are commonly associated with inversion sprains of the ankle**

C. **Therefore, this region must be examined routinely after an inversion ankle sprain**

D. **Radiographically, these fractures can be seen on the lateral, medial oblique and DP views**

E. **There have been many different classifications developed for the fifth metatarsal base**

F. **The most commonly used one is the <u>Stewart</u> classification** (1960)

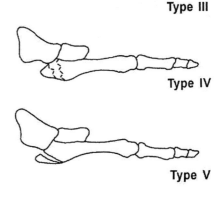

Type IV

Type V

II. Stewart Classification: 5th metatarsal base fractures

A. **Type I fracture**

1. ***This is the true Jones fracture!*** (this is the fracture that Jones originally described)

2. This fracture occurs between the epiphysis and diaphysis *(metaphyseal level)*

3. It is always an *extra-articular* oblique or transverse fracture
4. It is situated at the distal end of the articular capsule, above the intermetatarsal ligaments
5. The mechanism of injury is usually an internal rotation of the forefoot while the base of the fifth metatarsal remains fixed (the capsule is only stretched and the peroneus brevis takes practically no part in the injury)
6. Upon physical examination, extreme mobility of the shaft of the fifth metatarsal is found
7. This is a very unstable fracture and has a very poor blood supply (this fracture has a very high propensity to go onto delayed or non-union)
8. Because of the severe mobility of the fifth metatarsal shaft, the suggested treatment is a below the knee non-weight bearing cast for 4-6 weeks
9. Some authorities believe that CRIF is best option because of the decrease in non-union rates

B. Type II fracture
1. This is an *intra-articular* fracture of the fifth metatarsal base with usually one fracture lines at various locations in the base
2. This injury is the result of shearing force caused by the internal twisting of the forefoot while the peroneus brevis is contracted
3. Displacement of the fragments depends on the extent of the damage to the capsule and ligaments
4. The suggested treatment is a zinc oxide strapping (soft cast) or a below the knee non-weight bearing cast for 4-6 weeks
5. If the fracture is severely displaced and can not be closed reduced, ORIF is recommended

C. Type III fracture
1. This is an ***avulsion fracture*** of the base of the fifth metatarsal
2. This is the most proximal injury, where a small fragment is torn away
3. The fracture is *extra-articular* and the fracture line is usually at right angles to the long axis of the metatarsal base
4. The mechanism of injury is primarily a sudden sharp contraction of the peroneus brevis when the ankle is in plantarflexion
5. The suggested treatment is a zinc oxide strapping (soft cast) or a below the knee non-weight bearing cast for 4-6 weeks
6. If the fracture is severely displaced and can not be closed reduced, ORIF is recommended using either the tension band wiring technique or screw fixation
7. If the fracture fragment is too small for fixation and is severely displaced, excision of the fragment and reattachment of the peroneus brevis tendon is recommended

D. Type IV fracture
1. This is a *comminuted, intra-articular* fracture of the fifth metatarsal base
2. The mechanism of injury is similar to Type II, but in this case the fifth metatarsal base gets crushed between the cuboid and the ground/shoe causing the fragmentation
3. Since there is crushing, the trauma in this fracture is therefore at once direct and indirect
4. This fracture also has a high rate of delayed or non-union
5. The suggested treatment is a zinc oxide strapping (soft cast) or a below the knee non-weight bearing cast for 4-6 weeks
6. If the fracture fragments are severely displaced, bone grafting and ORIF may be required

E. Type V fracture
1. This is a fracture that occurs in children
2. There is a partial avulsion of the epiphysis with or without a fracture line or hairline crack as seen in type II
3. This fracture can also be classified as a Salter-Harris I

4. The suggested treatment is a zinc oxide strapping or a below the knee non-weight bearing cast for 3-4 weeks

REARFOOT TRAUMA
LISFRANC'S FRACTURE/DISLOCATION

I. **Introduction**

    A. **Lisfranc's dislocations are rare resulting in less than 1% of all fracture/dislocations of the foot and ankle**

    B. **The incidence is 1:50,000 people**

    C. **The severity may range from an occult subluxation to a severely malaligned fracture dislocation**

    D. **Approximately 20% of the time this fracture/dislocation is initially misdiagnosed, which may result in complications ranging from Lisfranc's arthritis to reflex sympathetic dystrophy to circulatory compromise**

    E. **Most commonly the injury is a result of major trauma** (i.e., motor vehicle accident)

II. **Midfoot anatomy**

    A. **The joints of the tarsometatarsal joints form an osseous "Roman arch" configuration across the foot from medial to lateral with the "keystone" of the arch being the recessed second metatarsal base**

    B. **This osseous configuration along with the ligamentous and surrounding soft tissue gives stability to the joint complex that is referred to as "Lisfranc's joint"**

    C. **The tarsometarsal joint is stabilized by numerous dorsal and plantar transverse and oblique ligaments as well as interosseous ligaments**

    D. **The most significant structure in this injury is the interosseous ligament that attaches the medial cuneiform to the second metatarsal base** (this ligament is better known as *"Lisfranc's ligament"*)

        1. Extends from the second metatarsal to the medial cuneiform in an oblique manner

        2. This ligament is key to the stability of the mortise

        3. Rupture or avulsion is necessary for fracture/dislocation of the second metatarsal

    E. **Ligamentous support:**

        1. Plantar ligaments are larger and stronger than dorsal ligaments

        2. No ligament joins the first and second metatarsals

        3. Secondary stabilizers are located plantarly

            a. Long flexor tendons

            b. Intrinsic muscles

            c. Plantar fascia

III. **Mechanism of injury**

    A. **The mechanism of a Lisfranc's dislocation is poorly understood, but two etiologies have been postulated: direct and indirect forces**

        1. Direct jnjury:

            a. Crushing injury to the forefoot and midfoot at or near the tarsometatarsal joint

            b. Usually results in severe soft tissue injury, osseous comminution, and neurovascular impairment

        c.   Usual mechanisms of injury are a vehicle running over the foot or industrial accidents

        d.   Must check for associated injuries

  2. Indirect injury:

        a.   Axial loading of the plantarflexed foot (i.e., twisting movement of the forefoot)

        b.   Usually occurs while playing contact sports

        c.   Plantarflexed foot is braced and is hyperplantarflexed by one's bodyweight or someone elses

        d.   Forefoot is trapped and forcefully plantarflexed and abducted on the cuneiforms and cuboid

        e.   This causes a fracture of the base of the second metatarsal base, medial cuneiform, or rupture of the Lisfranc's ligament resulting in a lateral displacement of the lesser metatarsals

        f.   Compression injuries to the cuboid may occur

IV. Diagnosis

A. Physical examination

1. Tenderness along the tarsometatarsal joint
2. Pain and crepitus with passive supination and pronation
3. Weight bearing is extremely difficult
4. Due to the nature of injury one must rule out dorsalis pedis injury and nerve involvement
   a. In grossly edematous feet, the use of a Doppler is required to find the pulses
   b. If there is neurovascular compromise, immediate reduction of the dislocation is required
5. Must rule out compartment syndrome

B. Radiographic evaluation

1. Often difficult to evaluate secondary to overlap in the region of injury
   a. Approximately 20% misdiagnosed
   b. If your radiographs are equivocal and you still suspect a Lisfranc's dislocation, a stress abduction radiograph should be performed under general anesthesia
2. DP view
   a. *"Fleck Sign"*: Avulsion from the plantar-medial aspect of the base of the 2nd metatrasal
   b. Incongruity with the medial edge of the first and second metatarsocuneiform joint
   c. Diastasis between the bases of the first and second metatarsals
      i. Normal space averages 1.3 mm
      ii. Diastasis averages 2-5 mm
      iii. This is the most consistent radiographic change
3. Medial oblique view
   a. Incongruity with the medial aspect of the third metatarsocuneiform joint and the fourth and fifth metatarsal-cuboid joint
4. Lateral view
   a. Dorsal or plantar dislocation of the metatarsals

C. Computed Tomography

1. Diagnostic exam of choice if surgery is considered
2. Produces images in a variety of planes
3. Images are free of overlap
4. Allows visualization of intra-articular fragments, interposed soft tissue structures, and plantar fragments

5. Should always be used if comminution is present

V. Classifications of Lisfranc's injuries

A. Quenu and Kuss Classification (1909)

1. Type 1: *Homolateral* or *convergent* dislocation of all five metatarsals together

2. Type 2: *Isolateral* dislocations in which one or two metatarsals are displaced from the others

3. Type 3: *Divergent* dislocations in which there is separation between the first and second metatarsals in both the sagittal and coronal planes

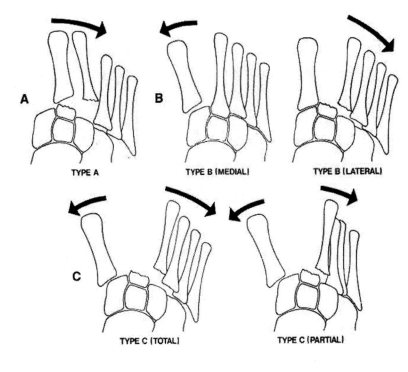

B. Hardcastle Classification (1982): (Modified by Myerson in 1986)

1. Type A: *Total incongruity* of the tarsometatarsal joint in any one plane or direction; displacement in either the sagittal (dorsoplantar) or transverse (lateral) direction

2. Type B1: *Partial incongruity* in which *medial* displacement affects the first ray in relative isolation

3. Type B2: *Partial incongruity* in which *lateral* displacement affect one or more of the lesser metatarsals

4. Type C1: A *divergent* pattern with the first metatarsal displaced medially and an *incomplete* number of lesser metatarsals displaced laterally

5. Type C2: A divergent pattern with the first metatarsal displaced medially and *complete* displacement of the lesser metatarsals laterally

VI. Closed treatment

A. Closed reduction is attempted in the absence of fractures under general anesthesia as soon as possible

B. Patient should be placed in a Jones' compression dressing if edema is too great for 3-7 days

C. Closed reduction is attempted by manipulation or Chinese finger traps

D. Involved metatarsals are percutaneously pinned into place

1. Percutaneous pinning is necessary to prevent a loss of reduction with decreased edema while healing

E. Patient is placed NWB in a short leg cast for 6-8 weeks

F. Post reduction radiographs are mandatory

G. **Aggressive physical therapy afterwards**

VII. **Open treatment**

A. **If the injury cannot be completely reduced or involves a fracture, open reduction is indicated**
B. **All interposed soft tissue and small intra-articular fragments should be excised**
C. **Large fragments are fixated with Kirschner wires, screws, and/or plates**
D. **Ligamentous repair should be attempted**
E. **Diastasis is reduced by placing a 3.5 or 4.0 mm screw obliquely from the medial cuneiform into the base of the second metatarsal**
F. **Patient is placed in a short leg cast NWB for 6-8 weeks**

NAVICULAR FRACTURES

I. **Introduction**

A. **Navicular fractures represent only 2.6% of all body fractures**
B. **The most common mechanism of injury is forced abduction with plantarflexion of the forefoot**
C. **Fractures are also caused by compression forces that impact the medial column against the head of the talus**

II. **Anatomy**

A. **Blood supply is a concern**
    1. Because of the amount of articular cartilage that is covering the surface area of the navicular, there is only a small area for vessels to enter and leave the navicular
    2. The navicular receives its blood supply dorsally from the DP artery, while plantarly from the medial plantar artery
    3. The tuberosity receives vessels from an arterial network formed by the union of the two source arteries
    4. Microangiographic studies show the medial and lateral thirds of the body have good blood supply, while the central third is relatively avascular
    5. As we age the number of arteries that supply the navicular decreases, therefore the risk of pseudoarthrosis and AVN increases

III. **Diagnostic modalities**

A. **Plain radiographs**
B. **Computed tomography**
C. **Magnetic resonance imaging**
D. **Bone scans: helpful in stress fractures**

IV. **Navicular classification: Watson-Jones classification (Goss & Walter modification)**

A. **Type I:**   **Fracture of the tuberosity**
B. **Type II:**   **Fracture of the dorsal lip**
C. **Type IIIA: Fracture of the body without displacement**
D. **Type IIIB: Fracture of the body with displacement**
E. **Type IV:**   **Stress fracture of the navicular**

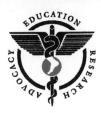

The American College of
FOOT & ANKLE ORTHOPEDICS & MEDICINE

OFFICERS
David Bernstein, DPM, FACFAOM, FACFAS
President
E-mail: dbernstein@acfaom.org
Seattle, WA

Craig Garfolo, DPM, FACFAOM
President-Elect
E-mail: cgarfolo@acfaom.org
Stockton, CA

Kirk Geter, DPM, FACFAOM
Secretary
E-mail: kgeter@acfaom.org
Washington, DC

Beth D. Jarrett, DPM, FACFAOM
Treasurer
E-mail: bjarrett@acfaom.org
Des Plaines, IL

Annemarie Edwards, DPM, FACFAOM, FACFAS
Past President *(ex officio)*
E-mail: aedwards@acfaom.org
Salt Lake City, UT

DIRECTORS
Denise B. Freeman, DPM, MSE, FACFAOM
E-mail: dfreeman@acfaom.org
Glendale, AZ

Robert S. Marcus, DPM, FACFAOM
E-mail: rmarcus@acfaom.org
Teaneck, NJ

Francine G. Schiraldi-Deck, DPM, FACFAOM
E-mail: fschiraldi@acfaom.org
Williamsport, PA

Elizabeth Weber-Levi, DPM, FACFAOM
E-mail: eweber@acfaom.org
Johnson City, NY

Norman Wallis, PhD
Executive Director
E-mail: nwallis@acfaom.org
Bethesda, MD

5272 River Road
Suite 630
Bethesda, MD 20816

1.800.265.8263
301.718.6505
Fax: 301.656.0989
Web site: **www.acfaom.org**
E-mail: info@acfaom.org

April 2005

Dear Reader:

On behalf of the American College of Foot & Ankle Orthopedics & Medicine, I am proud to present this fully revised *Review Text in Podiatric Orthopedics & Primary Podiatric Medicine (Second Edition)* to our profession. This textbook is the latest generation of a comprehensive review of what Podiatrists do the most during their day-to-day care of patients: practice medicine and orthopedics. It will prove to be an invaluable resource, not only for those studying for board certification examinations but also for students working hard to earn their Doctor of Podiatric Medicine degree and for practicing clinicians with years of experience.

This textbook is the synthesis of years of teamwork that started with the editors of the first edition. Dr. Bret Ribotsky, who recognized the need to update the text, initiated this latest edition during his presidency of the College. This was then carried forward by the work of this edition's three dedicated editors, Drs. John Walters, Anne Marie Edwards, and Larry Goss. Also, I extend a special 'Thank You' to Dr. Robert Baron, who, even after his term as ACFAOM's president had ended, doggedly pressed forward to keep this updated Review Text moving and financed. And, lastly, I would like to acknowledge the College's appreciation to Dermik Labs for underwriting the first printing of this new edition.

The process of this update began while I was still new to the ACFAOM Board of Directors and it has spanned across the terms of four presidents. I feel that I am the most fortunate of these presidents, as this second edition of the *Review Text in Podiatric Orthopedics & Primary Podiatric Medicine* came to fruition during my term.

David M. Bernstein, DPM, FACFAOM, FACFAS.
President

V. Navicular tuberosity fracture (Type I)

   A. Fractures of the tuberosity are relatively common as compared to the other types

   B. Mechanism of injury: Acute eversion of the foot, causing an avulsion type fracture

   C. This fracture is caused by increased tension placed on the tibialis posterior tendon

   D. These fractures are generally non-displaced because of the multiple soft tissue attachments to the tuberosity

      1. If the Type I fracture is severely displaced, you should suspect calcaneocuboid involvement, because the strong pronatory force will cause compression of the CCJ producing an occasional fracture of the cuboid and/or calcaneus

      2. The combination of a severely displaced fracture and compression fracture of the cuboid and/or calcaneus is referred to as the *"nutcracker syndrome"*

   E. Treatment:

      1. Typically it is recommended that the patient be placed in a soft cast or below-knee-cast for 4 weeks partial weight bearing. This area is highly susceptible to nonunion which may or may not be painful. If a symptomatic nonunion occurs, it is recommended that the fragment be removed and reattachment of the tibialis posterior performed

   F. It is important to differentiate the type I fracture from an accessory navicular

      1. Radiographically, they are differentiated based on three criteria:

        a. The accessory navicular is bilateral 90% of the time

        b. The fracture usually is sharp with jagged edges

        c. The accessory navicular has smooth rounded edges

VI. Navicular dorsal lip fracture (Type II)

   A. Fractures of the dorsal lip are the most frequent type of navicular fracture encountered, comprising 47% of all navicular fractures

   B. Mechanism of injury: *Plantarflexion* **of the foot followed by either** *forced inversion* **or eversion**

      1. Plantarflexion with eversion causes the dorsal tibionavicular ligament to become taut and avulses part of the dorsal cortex of the navicular

      2. During plantarflexion with inversion the talonavicular ligament becomes stressed and causes this avulsion

      3. The avulsed fragment usually contains articulate cartilage and therefore, the fracture is *intra-articular*

      4. These fractures are most commonly noted on the lateral radiograph and are located near the talonavicular articulation

   C. Dorsal lip fractures may be confused with two accessory ossicles that are found in the same area, the os supratalare and the os supranaviculare

   D. Treatment:

      1. Type II fractures are treated using a below-the-knee partially weight bearing cast for 4-6 weeks

      2. If the fragment is large and displaced, ORIF may be required, but is usually not necessary

      3. If late problems, such as a painful dorsal prominence occur, excision of the fragment is recommended

VII. Navicular body fracture (Type III)

   A. Are the least common of all navicular fractures

   B. Usually very severe injury

   C. Classified as either *non-displaced* **(Type IIIA) or** *displaced* **(Type IIIB)**

    D. **Mechanism of injury: direct** (crush injury) **or indirect** (fall from a height with the foot in a marked plantarflexion position at the moment of impact)

    E. **Always intra-articular and may involve the talus**

    F. **Conditions considered in the differential diagnosis of the navicular body fracture include bipartite tarsal navicular or lithiasis of the navicular**

    G. **Treatment:**
       1. Type IIIA fractures because of their non-displaced nature, even if they are comminuted, are treated with a below-the-knee walking cast for 6 to 8 weeks
       2. Type IIIB fractures are *not* satisfactorily managed by closed reduction
       3. They are, therefore, best managed by ORIF in a below-the-knee non-weight bearing cast for 6-8 weeks

VIII. Navicular stress fracture (Type IV)

    A. **Added to the Watson-Jones classification by Walter and Goss for completeness**

    B. **The occurrence of stress fractures of the navicular have been a commonly unrecognized condition, because of the lack of radiographic evidence and the often vague and diffuse pain associated with them**

    C. **Most of the patients that develop these injuries are athletes, most commonly track and field, whose pain increases with activity but decreases following activity**

    D. **The characteristic fracture, as found by Torg, is oriented in the sagittal plane and is located in the central one-third of the navicular**

    E. **The fracture is typically *intra-articular* and is usually found using either a bone scan or CT scan**

    F. **Treatment:**
       1. The early diagnosis of navicular stress fractures is the cornerstone of treatment
       2. If the fracture is non-displaced and uncomplicated, a below-the-knee non-weight bearing cast is used until radiographic union is noted (4-6 weeks)
       3. Fractures with displacement and nonunions require ORIF with or without bone grafting with below-the-knee non-weight bearing cast for 6-8 weeks

TALAR FRACTURES

    I. **Introduction**

      A. **Fractures of the talus are second in frequency of all tarsal bone injuries, but overall only represent 0.1% of all fractures**

      B. **Most of the talar fractures are avulsion or chip fractures from sites of ligamentous attachment**

      C. **Major fractures and dislocations are rare, and are often associated**

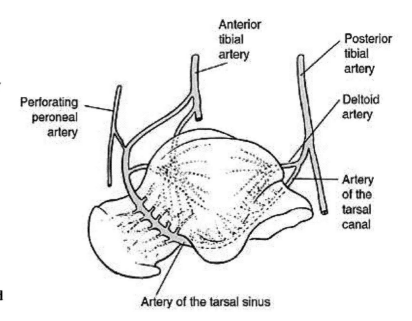

Anterior tibial artery

Posterior tibial artery

Deltoid artery

Perforating peroneal artery

Artery of the tarsal canal

Artery of the tarsal sinus

with ankle mortise injuries

D. Although fractures and dislocations of the talus are rare, their sequelae can be very serious

E. Injuries to the talus can result in substantial loss of motion and arthritic changes

F. Since the talus is covered by articular cartilage in three-fifths of its surface area, there is an increased risk of joint involvement in talar injuries

G. Talus has seven articular facets and no muscular attachments

II. Talar blood supply

A. With talar fractures, the biggest concern is the disruption of the vascular supply and the possibility of avascular necrosis

B. Two ways the talus is supplied: extraosseous and intraosseous

1. Extraosseous blood supply of the talus in order of importance is from the posterior tibial artery, the anterior tibial artery, and the perforating peroneal

2. All feed directly or indirectly into the periosteal network of vessels on the non-cartilagenous surface of the talus

3. The artery of the sinus tarsi and artery of the tarsal canal also supply the talus

C. The *posterior tibial artery* has calcaneal branches supplying a periosteal network over the posterior tubercle of the talus

1. One centimeter before the bifurcation of the posterior tibial artery into the medial and lateral plantar arteries, the *artery of the tarsal* canal is given off which passes anteriorly between the flexor digitorum and flexor hallucis longus to enter the tarsal canal posteriomedially

2. Just after its origin and before entering the canal, the *deltoid branch* is formed which supplies the rest of the medial side of the talus

3. As the artery moves anteriolaterally through the canal, it anastomoses with the artery of the sinus tarsi

D. Branches from the *anterior tibial artery*, supply the superiomedial surface of the talar neck

1. The *artery of the sinus tarsi* arises from an anasomotic loop between the lateral tarsal artery of the dorsalis pedis and form the perforating peroneal artery

2. It gives off a few branches to the talar head which may also branch directly from the lateral tarsal artery, and then enters the sinus tarsi giving branches to the talar body and finally anastomoses with the artery of the tarsal canal

3. This is the major blood supply to the body of the talus

E. The *perforating peroneal artery* is the last major artery supplying the talus

1. Small branches join with the calcaneal branches of the posterior tibial artery over the posterior tubercle of the talus

2. It also contributes to the plexus forming the artery of the sinus tarsi

F. The talar head is supplied superiomedially from the anterior tibial or dorsalis pedis arteries and inferiolaterally from the lateral tarsal artery, a branch from the sinus tarsi anatomosis, and directly from the artery of the sinus tarsi

G. The posterior tubercle is supplied by branches from its own periosteal network supplying only that area and the anterior trochlear surface of the talus is supplied by the arteries that enter the neck which also supplies a small portion of the middle one-third of the talar body

H. The major supply of the talar body is from the anastomoses inferiorly within the tarsal canal which gives off 4 or 5 branches

1. The vessel supplies almost all of the middle third of the talar body except for a small area

from the superior neck arteries

2. It supplies all of the lateral third except for the lateral aspect of the posterior facet and a small amount of the lateral edge of the trochlear part of the body

3. The deltoid branches enter the body on the medial side of the body and are also important

4. The sinus tarsi anastomoses send branches that enter the lateral anterior surface of the body to supply the lateral inferior aspect and most of the posterior facet

5. Therefore, trauma that can interrupt major nutrient supplies, especially the medial vasculature supplied by deltoid branches, along with the inferior arteries are more likely to cause avascular necrosis

III. Talar neck fracture

A. Accounts for 50% of all major injuries to the talus

B. Fractures of the talar neck are most commonly caused by motor vehicle accidents, airplane crashes and falls from heights

C. Anderson, in 1919, identified the mechanism of these injuries as a *hyperdorsiflexion* force exerted on the sole of the foot by the rudder bar of an aircraft upon impact, hence the term *"Aviator's astragulus"*

1. With this hyperdorsiflexion, the neck of the talus impacts against the anterior edge of the tibia, and a fracture line develops through the neck and enters the non-articular portion of the subtalar joint between the middle and posterior facets

D. The significance of these injuries is due to the frequency and severity of the long-term complications they produce

E. In 1970, Hawkins suggested a classification of vertical fractures of the talar neck

1. This classification was based on the radiographic appearance of the talus at the time of injury and he divided these talar neck fractures into three groups (Canale and Kelly in 1978 developed a fourth type that fits into the Hawkins classification)

2. Group I: Non-displaced talar neck fractures

   a. Only one of the three main sources of blood supply to the talus is interrupted (blood supply proceeding proximally from the talar neck)

   b. The talus remains anatomically within the ankle and the subtalar joint

   c. Fracture line usually transverses the talar neck for superiodistal to inferioproximal

   d. Treatment:

      i. The recommended treatment for Group I fractures is non-weight bearing for 6-12 weeks in a below-the-knee cast in neutral position until radiographic union is noted

      ii. The patient is then supported for another 2 to 5 months while ankle ROM exercises are performed

      iii. The prognosis for these injuries are good to excellent

3. Group II: Displaced talar neck fractures, with subluxation or dislocation of STJ

   a. The STJ dislocation occurs medially most commonly secondary to an inversion force

   b. If the subtalar dislocation is complete, the injuries are frequently open because of the thin subcutaneous layer of tissue

   c. At least two of the three sources of blood supply to the talus are interrupted

   d. Treatment:

      i. Closed reduction should be first attempted with type II injuries

      ii. If the post-reduction radiographs show good anatomical realignment, the patient is either casted or percutaneous K-wires are placed across the fracture and then casted in neutral position for 6-12 weeks

        iii. If closed reduction fails ORIF is required to gain anatomical alignment

4. Group III: Displaced talar neck fractures with associated dislocation of the talus from both STJ and ankle joints
   a. The talar body is often extruded posteriorly and medially and is thus located between the posterior surface of the tibia and the Achilles tendon
   b. The talar head maintains its normal relationship with the navicular
   c. All three of the main sources of blood supply to the talar body are damaged in Group III injuries
   d. The foot will adopt a position of slight eversion and lateral dislocation
   e. Greater than 50% of group III fracture-dislocations are open injuries
   f. Treatment:
      i. Although closed reduction is recommended by most authors, but it is usually not successful, some form of reduction is usually necessary to take tension off of the overlying skin to prevent ischemic changes, before ORIF is attempted
      ii. It is important to get early anatomical realignment to try to reestablish the talar blood supply
      iii. If the cartilage of the posterior talocalcaneal facet is denuded or severely damaged, primary
      iv. Subtalar joint arthrodesis is recommended
      v. Another option is a Blair fusion, which is a sliding bone graft from the anterior aspect of the talus into the remaining talar neck

5. Group IV: Displaced talar neck fracture from the STJ, ankle joint and dislocation of the talonavicular joint (Canale and Kelly in 1978 added this type)
   a. The most important factor is recognition of the talonavicular dislocation
   b. All three of the main sources of blood supply to the talar body are damaged
   c. There is high incidence of avascular necrosis with this type
   d. Open reduction with or without internal fixation is required for all Group IV injuries
   e. The casting and other options are the same as with the Group III fracture

F. **Because of the fragile nature of the blood supply to the talus and the great percentage that enter through the talar neck area, you must always be concerned of the possibility of avascular necrosis in talar neck fractures**
1. Avascular necrosis is the most serious complication following a talar neck fracture
2. There is a definite relationship between the severity of the injury and avascular necrosis, but the fate of the body of the talus following a fracture of the neck is unpredictable
3. Incidence of AVN and STJ arthritis after a talar neck fracture:

	AVN	STJ Arthritis
Group I	0%-13 %	RARE
Group II	20%-40%	60%-75%
Group III	75%-100%	80%-100%
Group IV	100%	100%

4. Staging of AVN of talus:
   a. Stage I: Increased density; no deformity
   b. Stage II: Increased sclerosis; moderate deformity of the talus
   c. Stage III: Severe deformity and sequestration
   d. Stage IV: Fragmentation of the talus
5. In cases of AVN, however, this subchondral atrophy is absent; thus the dome of the talus

appears radiopaque (dense) relative to the surrounding bones

    a.   The bones around the talar body does, however, do become osteoporotic (radiolucent) due hyperremia from the trauma and due to disuse from cast immobilization

  6.   Coltart and Hawkins cautioned against making the diagnosis of AVN of the talus based on the lateral radiograph alone, because the overlap of the lateral malleolus makes the talar dome appear dense on this view

G. Hawkins' sign

  1.   Hawkins noted that at approximately 6-8 weeks after injury, disuse osteopenia should be evident in the bones of the ankle and foot, surrounding the avascular tolar body, primarily because the patient is non-weight bearing

  2.   *"Hawkins' sign,"* indicates revascularization and early restoration of talar blood supply which will slowly reverse the radioopaque bone found with AVN of the tolar body

  3.   This radiolucency or subchondral atrophy that appears in the subchondral area of the dome of the talus is visualized on the AP radiograph

IV. Talar body fracture

A. Fractures of the body of the talus are extremely uncommon, representing approximately 1% of all fractures

B. Sneppen, in 1977, developed a classification based on the morphological types of talar body fractures with the goal of predicting a prognosis for each type (modified by DeLee in 1993)

C. Sneppen-DeLee classication of talar body fractures

  1.   Group I: Transchondral or compression fractures of the talar dome

    a.   These fractures have the same description, mechanism of injury, radiographic and physical appearance and treatment, as the Berndt-Harty fractures

  2.   Group II: Coronal, sagittal or horizontal shearing fractures involving the entire talar body

    a.   Includes fractures that involve the superior articular surface or trochlea of the talus

    b.   Group II fractures have two types:

        i. Type I: Coronal or sagittal shearing fractures (has three subtypes):

           (a) Type IA: Nondisplaced fractures

           (b) Type IB: Displacement only at the trochlear articular surface

           (c) Type IC: Displacement at the trochlear surface with dislocation of the subtalar joint

           (d) Type ID: Talar body fragments are dislocated from the subtalar and ankle joints

        ii. Type II: Horizontal shearing fractures (has two subtypes):

           (a) Type IIA: Nondisplaced

           (b) Type IIB: Displaced

  3.   Group III: Fractures of the posterior tubercle of the talus

    a.   Is a fracture of the posterior process of the talus and almost always involves the lateral tubercle

    b.   Fracture of the lateral tubercle is called a *"Shepherd's fracture"* named after F.J. Shepherd, who described this fracture in 1882

    c.   This is usually an oblique fracture that runs from anteriosuperior to posterioinferior through the lateral tubercle

    d.   It is very important to differentiate a Shepherd's fracture from an *"Intern's fracture,"* which is an os trigonum

    e.   On radiograph, a Shepherd's fracture and an Intern's fracture may be similar, it is your clinical findings that will differentiate the two (moving the great toe through

range of motion is painful in a Shepherd's fracture)
  f. Mechanism of injury:
      i. Two basic mechanism of injury have been described for this fracture:
          (a) Forced plantarflexion of the foot causing direct impingement of the posteriolateral process on the posterior tibial plafond
          (b) Excessive dorsiflexion causing avulsion of the posteriolateral process by increased tension of the posterior talofibular ligament
  4. Group IV: Fracture of the lateral process of the talus
      a. Fractures of the lateral process of the talus, account for 24% of all fractures to the body of the talus
      b. It is an intra-articular fracture that varies in size and shape
      c. The fracture line typically runs from superiolateral to inferiomedial in an oblique orientation
      d. Diagnosis is often difficult
  5. Group V: Crush fractures of the talar body
      a. Crush fractures of the body of the talus similar to those of Group II
      b. The difference is that the force progresses past the Group II Type ID fracture to cause impaction of the talus by the tibia into the calcaneus
      c. This fracture is usually highly comminuted and displacement is common
      d. Crush fractures to the talar body are the result of an extremely high-energy impact
      e. These fractures are usually associated with additional injury to the talus (i.e., talar neck or shear fracture), dislocation, open injuries, malleolar fractures, and other foot injuries

V. Osteochondral talar dome lesions (OTDL)

A. Represents an injury that results in a separation of a segment of articular cartilage in combination with a varying amount of subchondral bone of the talus is known as a chip fracture, a flake fracture, transchondral fracture, or an osteochondral fracture or defect

B. *Osteochondritis dissecans* is a term that specifically refers to a "chronic" condition in which a loose fragment of cartilage and necrotic bone has fractured from its ischemic subchondral bed

C. Clinical presentation:
  1. They are usually seen in the adult population, at an average age of 25 years, with a slight preponderance of males
  2. The common presentation is that of an ankle sprain, with the osteochondral fragment frequently missed because of low physician recognition and suboptimal radiographs
  3. Acute fractures are usually misdiagnosed as ankle sprains, while chronic pain is usually misdiagnosed as arthritis

D. Incidence of OTDL:
  1. Osteochondral injuries represent approximately 1% of all talar fractures
  2. Berndt and Harty found that 43% of these lesions are in the lateral aspect of the talus, while 53% are located on the medial aspect of the dome of the talus
  3. Approximately 75% of osteochondral fractures are initially misdiagnosed as sprained ankles
  4. Conversely, osteochondral fractures occur in 2%-6% of all ankle sprains
  5. It has been estimated that concurrent ligamentous injury occurs in 28%-45% of osteochondral injuries to the talar dome

E. Mechanism and location of OTDL:
  1. Most osteochondral fractures are traumatic in nature

2. Osteochondral fractures may occur on the medial or lateral aspect of the dome
3. The most common mechanism is an inversion or eversion injury of the ankle
4. Dorsiflexion and inversion result in anterolateral lesions

    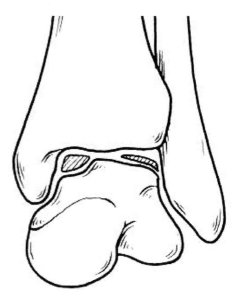

    a. The lateral lesions are all secondary to trauma (i.e., most often an inversion injury)
    b. Are typically shallow and wafer shaped
    c. They rarely heal spontaneously and are frequently associated with ongoing symptoms and later with degenerative changes
    d. In severe injuries, the lateral collateral ligaments may rupture
5. Plantarflexion and inversion result in posteromedial lesions
    a. With medial lesions, there is frequently no recognizable episode of trauma, and the lesions are usually deeper and cup or triangular shaped
    b. They produce fewer symptoms and frequently heal spontaneously
6. Those lesions on the medial aspect of the dome of the talus are usually located in the posterior third, while lesions in the lateral portion are most commonly located in the anterior and middle third of the talus

F. Classification of OTDL:
1. The radiographic classification of osteochondral lesions described by Berndt and Harty in 1959 remains the gold standard
2. In the Berndt-Harty classification:
    a. Stage I is a small area of compressed subchondral bone
    b. Stage II is a partially attached osteochondral fragment
    c. Stage III is a completely detached but non-displaced fragment remaining in the defect
    d. Stage IV is a completely detached and displaced osteochondral fragment loose in the ankle joint

G. Radiologic evaluation
1. Standard radiographs show an osteochondral lesion in approximately 70% of patients
2. Repeating the plain films after several months to delineate the development of subchondral sclerosis and make a diagnosis
3. If the radiographs are equivocal, the use of contrast studies, tomograms, bone scans, and CT and MRI are useful modalities to determine the location and extent of a osteochondral fracture of the talar dome
4. MRI and ankle arthroscopy are also choices

H. Treatment:
1. All stage I and II lesions, both medially and laterally, and acute and chronic, are usually treated with a below-the-knee non-weight bearing cast for 6 weeks or until radiographic union is evident
2. A medial stage III lesion is typically treated the same
3. If this conservative therapy fails, open arthrotomy using a transmalleolar approach or arthroscopy through the posteriomedial portal is suggested for either excision of the

fragment or ORIF of the fragment

4. Surgery is recommended on Stage III lesions of the lateral dome and all Stage IV lesions
5. Lateral lesions are accessed using either anteriolateral arthrotomy, or anteriolateral or anteriomedial arthroscopic portals
6. The fragments are either excised or ORIF using small AO screws, K-wires, or more recently, Orthosorb®
7. A good guideline for ORIF of a fragment is that it is at least one third of the medial or lateral dome, and the injury is acute
8. Patients are kept non-weight bearing for 8-12 weeks, depending on the size of the lesion, to allow adequate time for fibrocartilage ingrowth and healing of the malleolar osteotomy, in the case of medial lesions

CALCANEAL FRACTURES

I. **Introduction to calcaneal fractures**

   A. **Calcaneus is the most commonly fractured tarsal bone, constituting 60% of all major tarsal in**

   B. **Compromises only 2% of all body fractures**

   C. **The majority of fractures occur in males in their productive working years** (90% occur in males 40-49)

   D. **Most commonly as a result of a fall from a height** (75%-80% of these fractures occur from falls from a height greater than 3 feet)

   E. **About 7%-15% of all calcaneal fractures are bilateral and less than 2% are open fractures**

   F. **26% have associated extremity fracture**

   G. **10% have an associated spinal injury** (L1 most common)

   H. **2%-5% incidence of compartment syndrome**

   I. **Calcaneal fractures are frequently intra-articular and are more serious and disabling than the extra-articular fracture types** (Peter Essex-Lopresti and Carter Rowe, found that 75% and 56%, respectfully, were intra-articular fractures)

II. **Calcaneus anatomy**

   A. **Outer shell of thin cortical bone** (thicker at posterior tuberosity) surrounds cancellous medullary bone

   B. **The calcaneus has six surfaces: superior and inferior, medial and lateral, and anterior and posterior**

   C. **Neutral triangle: entrance of medullary vessels** (known as *"Ward's triangle"*)
      1. It lies just beneath the crucial angle of Gissane and carries the blood vessels to the medullary cavity of the calcaneus
      2. This area is considered to be the weakest portion of the calcaneus and is an area of concern in calcaneal fractures

   D. **Trabecular patterns:**
      1. Traction: Inferior surface
      2. Compression: Radiate from superior articular facets (also known as the *"thalamic"* portion of calcaneus)

III. **Diagnosis of calcaneal fracture**

   A. **Physical and clinical examination findings**

1. Varying degrees of edema and ecchymosis based on the severity of the fracture
2. Major fractures will produce severe edema and ecchymosis
3. Hematoma or bruising that extends to the sole of the foot is considered highly specific for a calcaneal fracture and is known as *"Mandor's sign"*
4. Often you will find that the injured heel is much wider than the unaffected contralateral heel
5. Fracture blisters and skin sloughing may be evident and occur in long-standing fractures
6. In children, they may present with a characteristic posturing with knee flexion and ankle equinus to avoid weight bearing
7. It is important that you also examine the patient's lumbar and cervical spine, head, wrists, knee and hip for any other possible injury incurred in the fall

B. Radiographic examination
1. Recommended three views are needed to evaluate a calcaneal fracture:
   a. DP of the foot: demonstrates the extent of involvement and displacement of the calcaneocuboid joint
   b. Calcaneal axial: widening of the calcaneus, disruption of the medial arch and displacement of the sustentacular fragment can be noted on this view
   c. Lateral view: serves to estimate *Bohler's tuberosity joint angle* and the *crucial angle of Gissane*
      i. Bohler's angle: formed by the intersection of two lines, one from the highest point of the anterior process to the highest point on the posterior articular surface and the other from the same point on the posterior articular surface to the most superior point of the calcaneal tuberosity
      ii. Crucial angle of Gissane: created by the subchondral bone of the posterior facet and the subchondral bone of the middle and anterior facets
      iii. Bohler's angle is typically between 25-40 degrees and the crucial angle of Gissane is between 120-145 degrees
      iv. In severe fractures involving the posterior facet and calcaneal tuberosity, Bohler's angle is significantly *decreased* (less than 25 degrees)
      v. The crucial angle of Gissane is usually *increased* in an intra-articular calcaneal fracture (greater than 145 degrees)
2. Other special views: (i.e., Broden and Isherwood views) can be used to evaluate the subtalar joint (specifically the posterior facet)
3. These special views are rarely used today because of the availability of CT scans
4. CT scans are essential to determine the extent of intra-articular fractures

IV. Radiographic classification

A. Most common radiographic classification is the <u>Rowe</u> classification (1963)
B. It is a more useful classification for extra-articular fractures of the calcaneus
1. Type I: (has three subtypes)
   a. Calcaneal tuberosity fracture (either medial or lateral)
   b. Sustentaculum tali fracture
   c. Fracture of the anterior process of the calcaneus
2. Type II: Is a fracture of the posterior superior aspect of the calcaneus (has two subtypes)
   a. Beak fracture
   b. Avulsion fracture at insertion of the Achilles tendon
3. Type III: Oblique fracture of the calcaneal body not involving the subtalar joint
4. Type IV: Fractures involving the subtalar joint
5. Type V: Central depression with varying degrees of comminution

C. **Rowe Type Ia fracture:** Calcaneal tuberosity fracture (either medial or lateral)
   1. Mechanism of injury: Usually the result of forceful heel strike in valgus or varus position shearing medial or lateral tuberosity
   2. Very rare as an isolated injury and usually extra-articular
   3. Treatment: Usually only closed reduction and casting is needed
D. **Rowe Type Ib fracture:** Sustentaculum tali fracture
   1. Mechanism of injury: Fall on inverted foot, talar shearing force causes fracture
   2. Usually intra-articular since middle facet is involved
   3. FHL and deltoid ligament support rarely allows for any displacement
   4. Calcaneal axial view best displays fracture
   5. Treatment:
      a. Usually only closed reduction needed (invert foot, plantarflex 1st MTPJ and apply digital upward pressure to sustentaculum tali)
      b. If non-displaced, the fracture is treated with a below-the-knee walking cast for 4-6 weeks with the foot casted in mild inversion to take stress off the fracture
      c. If closed reduction fails, ORIF of the fragment is recommended
      d. It is important in the treatment course of this fracture to start early ROM of the hallux to prevent adhesion of the flexor hallucis longus to the sustentaculum during healing
E. **Rowe Type Ic fracture:** Fracture of the anterior process of the calcaneus
   1. Mechanism of injury: (three etiologies)
      a. Inversion and plantarflexion: Avulsion of the anterior process by bifurcate ligament or calcaneal cuboid ligament
      b. Forced dorsiflexion with impaction (impaction against cuboid)
      c. Forefoot abduction against fixed rearfoot (usually supination)
   2. Can involve the calcaneocuboid joint if large
   3. Because of varying sizes and the proximity of the anterior process to the calcaneocuboid joint, this fracture may be extra-articular or intra-articular dependent on the size of the avulsion fragment
   4. Degan also classified these fractures:
      a. Type I: Undisplaced fracture, usually only involving the anterior process (extra-articular)
      b. Type II: Displaced fracture that does not involve the articular surface (extra-articular)
      c. Type III: Large, displaced fracture fragment that involves the calcaneocuboid joint (intra-articular)
   5. Os calcaneal secondarium can be confused with fracture
   6. Treatment:
      a. If non-displaced or small fragments, than 3-4 weeks NWB cast with early ROM
      b. If displaced, large fragments or involves greater than 25% of intra-articular fragment, than ORIF
      c. Excision of fracture fragment: usually after 1 year of conservative care
F. **Rowe Type II fracture** (Two types: beak and avulsion)
   1. Mechanism of injury: Avulsion fractures result of forceful contraction of Triceps Surae with foot in fixed or forced dorsiflexed position
   2. The fracture is typically oblique in nature and the fragment can vary in size and displacement
   3. Both fractures are extra-articular
   4. Some argue that "beak" fractures may not exist at all or may only be present in direct trauma situations
   5. Treatment:

a.   If non-displaced, than NWB cast immobilization for 6-8 weeks in equinus
b.   Should attempt closed reduction to maintain Achilles function
c.   If displaced or non-reducible, than ORIF is employed
d.   Displaced Type IIB fractures require ORIF followed by above-the-knee casting for 6-8 weeks

G. Rowe Type III fracture
   1.   Mechanism of injury: Usually fall from height
   2.   About 20% of calcaneal body fractures do not involve the calcaneocuboid or subtalar joint
   3.   This is an extra-articular fracture
   4.   Fracture often runs posterior-medial to anterior-lateral just behind the subtalar joint
   5.   Treatment:
       a.   If non-displaced fracture, cast immobilization NWB for 6-8
       b.   If displaced fracture, closed reduction or ORIF followed by 6-8 weeks of NWB casting

H. Rowe Type IV fracture: Body fracture involving the subtalar joint
I.   Rowe Type V fracture: Central depression fracture with various comminution patterns
J.   Rowe Type IV and V have been replaced by the classification system of Essex-Lopresti for intra-articular calcaneal fractures
K. Essex-Lopresti classification of intra-articular calcaneal fractures (contains two types):
   1.   Tongue type
   2.   Joint-depression
   3.   These fractures are classically differentiated by the location of the secondary fracture line and the shape of the fragments

V. Computed tomography classifications

A. Crosby and Fitzgibbons classification (1990)
   1.   Type 1: "Undisplaced", < 2 mm of diastasis or depression
   2.   Type II: "Displaced", > 2 mm diastasis or depression with no comminution
   3.   Type III: "Comminuted", severe comminution of the articular surface and the fracture fragments are small
   4.   Conclusion: all Type II and III fractures should have ORIF

B. Sanders classification (1992)
   1.   Based on axial and coronal images of calcaneal posterior facet at widest point
   2.   Addresses only intra-articular fractures
   3.   Lines A and B separate posterior facet into 3 fragments
   4.   Line C separates sustentacular fragment from tuberosity fragment
   5.   The lines are named A, B, C from lateral to medial
   6.   Four potential fractures exist:
       a.   Type I: All non-displaced intra-articular fractures, irrespective of the number of fracture lines
           i.   Usually require non-operative intervention
       b.   Type II: Are two part intra-articular fractures of the posterior facet
           i.   Three types exist: Type IIA, IIB, and IIC based on the location of the primary fracture line
           ii. ORIF has best functional result
       c.   Type III: Are three part intra-articular fractures that feature a centrally depressed fragment

       i. Three types exist: IIIAB, IIIAC, and IIIBC based on the location of the fracture lines

       ii. ORIF with bone grafting often required

    d. Type IV: Are four part fractures with a high degree of comminution

       i. Often more than four articular fragments exist

       ii. Primary arthrodesis or conservative care are treatment options

VI. Treatment of intra-articular calcaneal fractures

  A. There have been various methods described over the years for the treatment of intra-articular calcaneal fractures

  B. The various methods break down into four basic groups:

    1. Compression bandaging and early mobilization (non-reduction technique)

      a. Advantage: avoids pin tract infections and stiff joints secondary to prolonged immobilization

      b. Disadvantage: residual deformity not compatible with ambulation

    2. Closed reduction or semi-invasive reduction techniques with traction spikes or pins

      a. Included here would be the Essex-Lopresti method of closed reduction for tongue type fractures

      b. Advantage: quick and relatively easy to perform

      c. Disadvantage: does not address all of deformities present

    3. Open reduction with various methods of internal fixation (most commonly utilized for joint depression fractures)

      a. Advantage: can restore calcaneal height, width, and length

      b. Disadvantage: very difficult to accomplish with a high learning curve

      c. Sequence of intra-articular calcaneal fracture reduction:

        i. 4.0/5.0 mm Schantz Pin is inserted from medial to lateral in posterior body for 3 motion reduction

        ii. Restore height

        iii. Return to heel to valgus position

        iv. Medial translation

      d. Internal fixation devices

        i. Plates (2 types)

         (a) With arms: used to support posterior facet

          (1) Y-Montage plate

          (2) Calcaneal reconstruction plate

         (b) Without arms: no posterior facet support

          (1) One-third tubular plate

          (2) Pelvic reconstructive plates

          (3) Anterior cervical plate

          (4) H-plates

    4. Primary subtalar or triple arthrodesis

      a. Advantage: prevents need for another surgical procedure and period of immobilization in future

      b. Disadvantage: very difficult to correct all deformities present

VII. Post-operative care after ORIF

  A. Drain, if used removed POD #2

  B. 24-48 hours bedrest, ice and elevation

   C. **Two weeks posterior splint immobilization with early ROM if solid internal fixation achieved**

   D. **Followed by 8-12 weeks of non-weightbearing cast**

   E. **After adequate radiographic healing, 2-4 weeks of protected weightbearing**

   F. **Aggressive physical therapy and rehabilitation**

VII. **Complication of calcaneal fractures**

   A. **Subfibular impingement: from lateral wall blow out**

   B. **Peroneal tendon impingement**

   C. **Heel widening**

   D. **Malposition of heel and plantar fat pad**

   E. **Subtalar joint arthrosis**

   F. **Posterior facet malunion**

ANKLE INSTABILITY

I. **Introduction**

   A. **With respect to pain, disability and deformity, ankle sprains can be worse than ankle fractures**

   B. **Ankle sprains are among the most commonly misdiagnosed and mistreated foot and ankle injuries**

   C. **Approximately 2 million patients per year present to ER with ankle injuries, of which 60% are severely sprained**

     1. Inversion sprains account for 90%-95% of all ankle sprains

     2. Greater than 65% of the time the ATFL is injured

     3. When examing an inversion sprain, both medial and lateral ligamentous structures should be examined

   D. **Many non-fractured ankles with ligament instability go undertreated**

   E. **This can result is degenerative joint disease and chronic ankle instability**

II. **Anatomy of the ankle**

   A. **Osseous structures**

     1. The ankle is intrinsically stable due to the anatomic integrity of the distal tibia, which forms the roof and medial wall of the ankle joint

     2. The distal fibula forms the lateral wall of the ankle joint

       a. It also extends about 1.0 cm distally and posteriorly than the medial malleolus, thus limiting eversion

     3. The tibia and the fibula form the ankle mortise into which the talus fits

     4. The talus has limited motion in the frontal plane and uninhibited motion in the sagittal plane

     5. The talar dome has a greater width anteriorly than posteriorly; upon dorsiflexion, the talus fits snugly in the mortise, while upon plantarflexion, an increase in motion can be noted

   B. **Ligamentous structures**

     1. The ankle joint is secured by ligaments on the medial and lateral aspects of the ankle joint and also by the joint capsule

     2. The tibia and fibula are bound tightly together by the syndesmotic interval which is the

combination of the anterior, posterior inferior tibiofibular ligaments, and the interosseous ligament

3. The joint capsule surrounds the ankle joint and attaches the tibia, fibula, and talus, at their bone-cartilage interfaces

4. Anteriorly and posteriorly the capsule is redundant to allow for dorsiflexion and plantarflexion

5. The capsule is reinforced medially and laterally by collateral ligaments
   a. The lateral ligaments are inherently weaker than the medial collateral ligaments and may be subjected to more stress
   b. This explains why lateral ligamentous injury is more common than medial ligament injury

C. **Lateral collateral ligaments:** (ATFL, CFL, and the PTFL)
   1. Anterior talofibular ligament (ATFL)
      a. Usually the first ligament injured during an inversion injury
      b. It's formed by two distinct bands separated by an interval that allows the penetration of vascular branches
      c. The upper band is larger than the lower band
      d. The ligament *originates* from the inferior oblique segment of the anterior border of the lateral malleolus, it courses anteromedially and *inserts* on the talar body just anterior to the lateral malleolar articular surface
      e. It is an intra-capsular ligament
      f. The ligament is relaxed upon dorsiflexion and tight during plantarflexion
   2. Calcaneofibular ligament (CFL)
      a. Usually the second ligament injured during an inversion injury
      b. It *originates* from the lower segment of the anterior border of the lateral malleolus, the ligament courses posteriorly, inferiorly, and medially, and *inserts* on a small tubercle located on the posterior aspect of the lateral calcaneal surface
      c. It is an extra-capsular ligament
      d. Unlike the anterior talofibular ligament, the calcaneofibular ligament is relaxed upon plantarflexion and tight upon dorsiflexion
   3. Posterior talofibular ligament (PTFL)
      a. It's rarely found to be ruptured with inversion injuries
      b. It *originates* on the medial surface of the lateral malleolus from the lower segment of the digital fossa, it courses horizontally toward the lateral and posterior aspect of the talus in which it *inserts* on the posterolateral tubercle of the talus
      c. It is an intra-capsular ligament
      d. The ligament becomes more vertical upon dorsiflexion and prevents the talus from slipping backwards
   4. There is an angular relationship between the anterior talofibular ligament and the calcaneofibular ligament
      a. Normally, the angle between the two is between 70-140 degrees
      b. If the angle is above 120 degrees, ankle stability is reduced
      c. The CFL is oriented approximately 20-45 degrees posterior to the longitudinal bisection of the fibula when the foot is placed in a plantargrade attitude

D. **Medial collateral ligaments:** (Deltoid ligaments)
   1. Superficial ligaments
      a. Superficial tibiotalar ligament
         i. Origin is from the posterior part of medial surface of anterior and posterior colliculus

ii. It inserts on the anterior portion of the medial talar tubercle
 b. Tibiocalcaneal ligament
  i. Origin is the mid-portion of medial surface of anterior colliculus
  ii. It inserts on the medial boarder sustentaculum tali and merges with edge of the plantar calcaneonavicular ligament
 c. Tibionavicular ligament
  i. Origin is the anterior colliculus
  ii. It inserts on the dorsomedial aspect of the navicular and plantar calcaneonavicular ligament
2. Deep ligaments
 a. Anterior tibiotalar ligament
  i. Origin is the intercollicular groove and adjoining anterior colliculus
  ii. It inserts on the medial surface of the talus near the neck
 b. Posterior tibiotalar ligament
  i. Origin is the intercollicular groove and inferior segment of the posterior colliculus
  ii. It inserts on the medial surface of the talus and medial tubercle to the posterior third of the articular surface of the talar trochlea

III. Clinical presentation and evaluation

A. During the examination, ask questions such as:
1. If they heard or felt any "pop or snap"
2. Any previous history of ankle injuries
3. Check the neurovascular status
4. Note the degree of swelling, ecchymosis present or any other gross deformity
5. Ask if they can remember the mechanism of injury
6. Ask about any prior treatment
7. Prior to palpation or manipulations of the injured ankle, get radiograph
 a. Radiographs should include: AP, lateral, and mortise views
 b. Perform bilateral ankle examinations to compare the degree of motion
8. Palpate carefully and try to locate the point that hurts the most
9. MRI studies may identify total or partial tendon ruptures and soft tissue damage
10. CT studies will aid to rule out avulsion fractures or any other osseous deformity

IV. Ankle stability testing

A. Anterior drawer test: (also known as the *"Push-pull test"*)
1. Usually performed under anesthesia
2. Need to check both sides to prevent a false positive result
3. There are four methods to measure anterior ankle subluxation:
 a. Perlman method: Measure distance between the posterior lip of the tibia and the nearest portion of the talar dome
 b. Mortensson method: Calculating the perpendicular distance between the vertical lines drawn through the posterior lip of the tibia and the posterior tubercle of the talus
 c. Lindstrand method: Perpendicular distance between the centers of concentric circles of the joint surface of the tibia and the talar dome
 d. Kelikian method: Distance between the distal dorsal aspect of the talus at its articulation with the navicular and the anterior margin of the articular surface of the tibia
4. Greater than 5 mm from the contralateral ankle is considered a positive result

    5. When positive, an ATFL rupture is usually present
B. **Inversion stress test:** (also known as *"Talar tilt"*)
    1. Usually performed under anesthesia
    2. Need to check both sides to prevent a false positive result
    3. Greater than 10° is pathologic when compared to the contralateral ankle
        a. Laurin *et al*: Physiologic asymmetry rarely exceeds 10 degrees
        b. Anderson: Greater than 15° is indicative of ATFL and CFL rupture
        c. Anderson and Lecocq: Greater than 12° indicative of ATFL and CFL ligaments
        d. Rubin and Witten: 3-23° is normal
        e. Bonnin: 15-20° is normal
    4. Caution: inversion stress views may further damage the ligamentous structures and is contra-indicated in the presence of an ankle fracture
    5. Factors that influence an increase in physiological ankle stress results:
        a. Previous ankle trauma
        b. Subjects younger than 15 years old
        c. Marfan's syndrome
        d. Ehlers-Danlos syndrome
        e. Osteogenesis imperfecta
        f. Turner's syndrome
C. Ankle arthrography
    1. Radio-opaque contrast material is injected into the ankle joint (invasive technique)
    2. Due to its invasive nature, ankle arthrography carries with it certain risks (i.e., induction of a septic joint and allergy to contrast material)
    3. Has been replaced by MRI

V. **Predisposing factors for inversion ankle trauma**

A. **Fixed calcaneal varum**
B. **Tibial varum**
C. **Rigid plantarflexed first ray**
D. **Forefoot valgus**
E. **Phasic overactivity of the tibialis posterior and anterior tibial tendons**
F. **Ankle varus**
G. **Uncompensated ankle equinus deformity**
H. **Peroneal muscle weakness**
I. **Previous inversion ankle trauma**
J. **Congenital weakness of the AFTL**
K. **Limb length discrepancy**

VI. **Ankle sprain classifications**

A. **O'Donoghue classification**
    1. Type I: (single tear) tear of the anterior talofibular ligament (ATFL) only
    2. Type II: (partial rupture) tear of the ATFL and the calcaneofibular ligament (CFL)
    3. Type III: (complete rupture) tear of the ATFL, CFL, and PTFL
B. **Leach classification** (also known as the "anatomical classification")
    1. Grade I: ATFL sprain
    2. Grade II: ATFL and CFL sprain
    3. Grade III: ATFL, CFL and PTFL sprain
C. **Dias classification**

1. Grade I: partial rupture of CFL
2. Grade II: rupture of the ATFL
3. Grade III: complete rupture of ATFL, CFL, and PTFL

D. **Rasmussen (1984) classification**
1. Stage I: rupture of ATFL
2. Stage II: rupture of superficial anterior fibers of PTFL
3. Stage III: rupture of CFL
4. Stage IV: rupture of deep posterior fibers of PTFL

E. **AMA standard nomenclature system**
1. Grade I: ligaments only stretched (no instability and only *mild* pain and tenderness with little or no swelling)
2. Grade II: ligaments are partial torn (slight to moderate instability and *moderate* pain, tenderness, swelling and hemorrhage)
3. Grade III: ligaments completely torn (significant instability and *marked* pain, tenderness, swelling and hemorrhage)

F. **Jackson classification** (also known as the *"clinical classification"*)
1. Mild sprain: minimal functional loss, no limp, minimal or no swelling, pin-point tenderness, pain with reproduction of the mechanism of injury
2. Moderate sprain: moderate functional loss, unable to toe-rise or hop on the injured ankle, limp present, localized swelling and ecchymosis, pin-point tenderness, pain with reproduction of the mechanism of injury
3. Severe sprain: diffuse and severe tenderness, swelling, ecchymosis and pain, unable to ambulate on ankle

G. **Henry classification** *(clinical classification)*
1. Group I: Mild injury, tenderness over the ATFL, negative anterior drawer sign, talar tilt sign < 5 degrees
2. Group II: Moderate injury, tenderness over ATFL and CFL, negative anterior drawer sign, talar tilt < 15 degrees
3. Group III: Severe injury, lateral ankle swelling, ecchymosis and pain, positive anterior drawer sign, talar tilt > 15 degrees
4. Group IV: Chronic problems, positive anterior drawer sign and talar tilt > 15 degrees

H. **Mann and Coughlin classification** (related to treatment)
1. Type I: Stable ankle by clinical testing - treat symptomatically only
2. Type II: Unstable ankle with positive anterior drawer sign and/or positive talar tilt results
   a. Group 1: Non-athlete or older patient - use functional treatment
   b. Group 2: Young and very active
      i. Type A: negative stress radiograph - treat functionally
      ii. Type B: talar tilt > 15 degrees; anterior drawer > 1.0 cm - treat by open surgical repair
      iii. Type C: all of Type B criteria with 2 mm or more of anterior displacement of the calcaneus on the talus - treat by open surgical repair

VII. Differential diagnosis of an ankle sprain

A. **Base of the 5th metatarsal fracture** (Jones' fracture)
B. **Anterior process of the calcaneus** (Degan fracture)
C. **Osteochondral talar dome lesion** (Berdnt-Hardty)
D. **Avulsion fracture of the calcaneus** (Rowe Type II fracture)
E. **Shepherd's fracture** (Sneepen-DeLee Group III posterolateral process of talus)
F. **Maisonneuve fracture** (Weber Type C high fibula fracture)

G. **Tibial plateau fracture** (Pilon fracture)
H. **Fibula fracture** (Weber classification)
I. **Cuboid fracture** (*"Nutcracker effect"*)
J. **Peroneal tendon subluxation** (Rim sign of fibula)
K. **Peroneal tendon rupture**
L. **Talar fracture**
M. **Ligamentous damage**
N. **Sinus tarsi avulsion tear**

VIII. Conservative treatment of acute ankle sprains

A. **Mobilization techniques**
   1. ACE or strapping to support the ligaments
   2. Want to limit exogenous motion
   3. Allows for immediate ROM in the sagittal plane motion, but not the frontal plane
B. **Immoblization**
   1. Ankle braces or air cast
   2. Soft casts
   3. Posterior splints
   4. Jones' compression cast
   5. Walking boots
   6. Casting immobilization (plaster or fiberglass) 4-6 weeks WB or NWB followed by ROM therapy
C. **RIICE principle**
D. **NSAID's**
E. **Acute pain medication**
F. **Aggressive physical therapy**

IX. Surgical repair of chronic ankle sprains

A. **Single ligamentous repair**
   1. *Broström procedure*
      a. Reconstructs the ATFL
      b. Simple direct repair
   2. *Broström-Gould procedure*
      a. Reconstructs the ATFL with local structures (i.e., inferior extensor retinaculum)
   3. *Evans procedure*
      a. Used peroneus brevis tendon, split tendon in half, leave half intact at insertion of 5th metatarsal base
      b. Drill hole proximal-posterior to distal-inferior
      c. Establish strut between 5th metatarsal base and tip of fibula
   4. *Nilsonne procedure*
      a. Used peroneus brevis tendon, split tendon in half, leave half intact at insertion of 5th metatarsal base
      b. Anchored to tip of fibula
   5. *Watson-Jones procedure*
      a. Used peroneus brevis tendon and detach entire tendon proximally
      b. Pass PB through fibula, around neck of talus, and anchor to lateral fibula
   6. *Lee procedure*
      a. Modification of Watson-Jones

                b. Use a trephine plug
        B. **Double ligamentous repair**
            1. *Chrisman-Snook procedure*
                a. Uses peroneus brevis tendon
                b. Anchored to calcaneus and fibula with a trephine plug
            2. *Elmslie procedure*
                a. Utilizes piece of fascia lata
                b. Figure-of-eight type repair
                c. Two drill holes: one in fibula and one in talus
            3. *Modified Elmslie procedure*
                a. Same as original Elmslie except uses peroneus longus tendon graft
                b. Same as original figure-of-eight

ANKLE FRACTURES

I. **Eponyms:**
    A. **Pott's fracture** (1768) is transverse fracture of the fibula 5.0 to 7.5 cm above the distal end and associated with a tear of the deltoid ligament and lateral subluxation of the talus secondary to valgus injury (bimalleolar fracture)
    B. **Cotton Fracture** (1915) is described as a trimalleolar fracture
    C. **Dupuytren fracture** (1819) is a fracture of the fibula about 6.0 cm (2 1/2 inches) proximal to its tip accompanied by a rupture of the syndesmosis and either a fracture of the medial malleolus or a tear of the deltoid ligament (PER Stage III)
    D. **Maisonneuve fracture** (1840) is a spiral fracture of the fibula that occurs as high as the proximal third
    E. **Cowtail fracture** is an anterioposterior tibiofibular PER fracture involving rupture of the interosseous membrane with an associated high fibular fracture
    F. **Bosworth fracture** is a bimalleolar fracture; posterior displacement of fibula and Volkmann's fracture
    G. **Tillaux fracture** is an avulsion fracture of tubercle of Chaput of the tibia
    H. **Wagstaffe-Léfort fracture** is an avulsion fracture of the fibula
    I. **Frost fracture** is pediatric triplane fracture with the combination of a Salter Harris type II lateral view and Salter Harris type III (Tillaux fracture on AP view) of the distal tibia

II. **Classifications of ankle fractures**
    A. **Two purposes for classifying ankle fractures:**
        1. Understand mechanism of injury by looking at specific pattern of injury to bone and soft tissue
        2. Understanding mechanism so can reverse the injury via closed reduction
    B. **Three classification schemes are commonly employed when dealing with ankle fractures**
        1. *Danis-Weber classification (simpliest)*
        2. *Cedell classification*
        3. *Lauge-Hansen classification* (most common used)

III. **Danis-Weber classification**
    A. **Based on the level of the fibular fracture**

B. **Serves as a guide to the management by the level of the fibular fracture corresponding to the severity of the ligamentous injury**

C. **Easier to use over the telephone but not that good for guiding treatment or comparing fractures academically**

D. **Three types of fractures:**

1. **Danis-Weber A:**
   a. Fibula fracture is located ***below*** the level of the syndesmosis level
   b. Lateral ligament type injury (ruptured of calcaneofibular ligament)
   c. Intact ATFL intact because fracture below
   d. Good stability at ankle joint, because syndesmosis is intact
   e. Treatment:
      i. If non-displaced, only cast immobilization need
      ii. If displaced, tension-banding or screw fixation
      iii. NWB 6-8 weeks until radiographic healing

2. **Danis-Weber B:**
   a. Fibula fracture ***at*** the level of the joint
   b. Fracture of the fibula is located at the syndesmosis level
   c. Most common type of ankle fracture
   e. Implies syndesmosis usually disrupted, however may rupture syndesmosis (anterior tibiofibular ligament)
   f. 30% anterior tibiofibular ligament intact
   g. Unstable fracture if syndesmosis is ruptured
   h. Treatment:
      i. Medial side determines if needs ORIF (if < 2.0 mm no disruption medially)
      ii. 1-2 interfragmenting screws
      iii. Fibular plate placed on traditionally placed laterally
      iv. Need to suture syndesmosis

3. Danis-Weber C:
   a. Fibula fracture ***above*** the level of the joint
   b. Syndesmosis is disrupted
   c. Fracture above (proximal) to syndesmosis anywhere on fibular shaft
   d. Treatment:
      i. Always needs fixation
      ii. Very unstable fracture due to syndesmosis rupture
      iii. Must perform the **"hook test"**
      iv. Transyndesmosic screw (aka *"transfixation"*)

IV. **Cedell classification**

A. **Type A:**
   1. Anatomic alignment of ankle mortise
   2. No displacement
   3. Treatment: conservative NWB casting 4-6 weeks until radiographic healing

B. **Type B:**
   1. Good alignment of ankle mortise
   2. Less than 2.0 mm of displacement

C. **Type C:**
   1. Poor alignment of ankle mortise
   2. Greater than 2.0 mm of displacement

    D. **Type A and B usually only conservative treatment**
    E. **Type C usually needs ORIF**

V. Lauge-Hansen classification

    A. **Accurately predicts mechanism of injury in 95% of ankle fractures**
    B. **Only 5% of ankle fractures do not fit into this classification system**
    C. **Most common classification of ankle fractures**
    D. **Two word classification system:**
        1. First word = *"**position**"* of foot at time of injury
        2. Second word = *"**motion**"* of foot at time of injury
    E. **Five basic patterns of injury:**
        1. Supination-adduction
        2. Pronation-abduction
        3. Supination-eversion (SER)
            a. Most common type
            b. Occurs about 60% of time
        4. Pronation-eversion (PER)
        5. Pronation-dorsiflexion
            a. Least common type
            b. Occurs in less than 5% of injuries
    F. **Supination-Adduction:**
        1. Weber type A (below level of syndesmosis)
            a. No disruption of syndesmosis
            b. Best prognosis of any ankle fracture
        2. Mechanism of injury:
            a. Inversion ankle sprain injury
            b. Begins on lateral side of ankle
            c. Involves *"**uniplanar**"* inversion motion at ankle joint (not triplanar motion at STJ)
            d. Position = inversion (supination) motion at the ankle joint
            e. Motion = foot is adducting on leg or being driven up toward the medial malleolus
            f. Adduction refers to foot *"**adducting**"* on leg (drive toward medial malleolus)
            g. Injury occurs without disruption of syndesmosis
            h. Foot supinated (inverted) at time of injury and foot motion is adducting or inversion toward midline of body
        3. Two stages of Supination-Adduction
            a. Stage I: Occurs at the level of the fibula (Weber Type A fracture)
            b. Two things can happen:
                 i. Transverse fracture of distal fibula **(Hallmark fracture)**
                ii. Rupture of lateral collateral ligaments noted by increased clear space laterally
            c. Stage II:
                 i. Vertical fracture of tibial medial malleolus **(Hallmark fracture)**
        4. Treatment:
            a. Usually no ORIF is needed
            b. NWB cast immobilization for 4-6 weeks, until radiographic healing
    G. **Pronation-Abduction:**
        1. Weber Type B fracture of the fibula
        2. Eversion injury (uniplanar eversion at ankle joint)
        3. Foot pronated time of injury (body is on medial side)

4. Injury begins on medial side of the ankle
5. Foot *"abducted"* to leg (motion of foot)
6. Disruption of the syndesmosis (at level of syndesmosis)
7. Three stages of Pronation-Abduction
   a. Stage I: (two presentations)
      i. Transverse fracture of medial malleolus
      ii. Rupture of deltoid ligaments evidenced by increased medial clear space
   b. Stage II
      i. Partial or complete rupture of anterior and posterior tibiofibular ligaments
   c. Stage III
      i. Short oblique fibular fracture **(Hallmark fracture)**
      ii. AP view: fracture begins at joint line on medial side of the fibula then goes high on lateral side of fibula (short oblique)
      iii. Lateral view: fracture looks like transverse fracture
      iv. Hallmark fracture is a *"bend type"* fracture

H. Supination-Eversion (SER):
1. Most common ankle fracture due to this mechanism
2. Weber Type B fracture of the fibula
3. Foot position: supinated (inverted) at time of injury
4. Motion of foot: external rotation (not eversion)
5. External rotation of talus about a *"medial axis"*
6. Clinically picture:
   a. Flexion of knee
   b. Foot planted on ground
   c. Knee buckles
   d. Leg internally rotates
   e. Talus externally rotates
   f. Patient almost *"sits down"* on ankle
   g. Example: sliding into second base
7. Clinical mechanism:
   a. Get inversion of forefoot, external rotation of talus with slight dorsiflexion
8. Injury pattern:
   a. Begins *"antero-lateral"* at margin of the tibia and fibular syndesmosis, goes through fibula, around, behind ankle and ends at the medial malleolus
9. Four stages of SER
   a. Stage I begins antero-laterally
      i. Disruption of distal anterior tibio-fibular ligament
         (a) Avulsion fracture of tubercle of Chaput on this tibia *("Tillaux fracture")*
         (b) Avulsion fracture of the fibula *("Wagstaffe-Lefort" fracture)*
   b. Stage II: **(Hallmark fracture)**
      i. Short spiral oblique fibular fracture that begins "at" level of ankle joint
      ii. Weber Type B fibula fracture
   c. Stage III:
      i. Posterior malleolus disruption
      ii. Either osseous or soft tissue injury
      iii. Osseous:
         (a) Avulsion fracture off posterior malleolus *("Volkmann's fracture")*
      iv. Soft tissue:
         (a) Rupture of posterior tibiofibular ligament

       d. Stage IV:
          i. Talus not constrained so talus hits medial malleolus (transverse direction)
          ii. Transverse medial malleolar fracture
          iii. Rupture of deltoid ligaments evidenced by greater medial clear space

I. Pronation-Eversion (PER):
1. Mechanism of injury:
   a. External rotation about *"lateral axis"*
   b. Example: patient stepped into a hole
      i. Foot everts, foot planarflexed as fall into hole, and get external rotation force
   c. Foot position: pronated (everted) at time of injury
   d. Foot motion: external rotation of talus about a *"lateral axis"* with slight plantarflexion
2. Instability of syndesmosis is the most important aspect of this injury
3. Four Stages of PER:
   a. Stage I: get medial disruption with either:
      i. Avulsion fracture of medial malleolus (transverse)
      ii. Rupture of deltoid ligaments evident by medial clear space
   b. Stage II
      i. Disruption of distal anterior tibiofibular ligament
      ii. Tillaux fracture: avulsion piece from tubercle of Chaput
      iii. Wagstaffe fracture: avulsion piece from fibula
   c. Stage III: talus externally rotates about lateral axis pushes on fibula
      i. High fibular fracture **(Hallmark fracture)**
      ii. Rupture of the interosseous membrane
      iii. Fibular fracture begins ***above*** the syndesmosis
      iv. Weber Type C fibula fracture
      v. Fibular fracture is usually short oblique, but may be spiral or butterfly
   d. Stage IV: posterior disruption of posterior malleolus with either:
      i. Volkmann's fracture
      ii. Rupture of distal posterior tibiofibular ligament
      iii. May have a ***"Maisonneuve fracture"*** or high fibular fracture

J. Pronation-Dorsiflexion:
1. Least common type of Lauge-Hausen classification
2. Four stages of pronation-dorsiflexion:
   a. Stage I: fracture of medial malleolus
   b. Stage II: fracture of anterior tibial tip
   c. Stage III: supramalleolar fracture of fibula
   d. Stage IV: transverse fracture of posterior aspect of tibia

PILON FRACTURE

I. Introduction to Pilon fractures:

A. Pilon = hammer/Plafond = ceiling (French terminology)

B. To be considered a tibial pilon fracture, there must be a fracture line traversing the weight-bearing articular surface of the distal tibia
1. Get impaction injury of the anterior tibia, as well as a fracture of the distal fibula
2. Occurs more commonly in skiing accidents

C. **Differs from ankle fractures for several reasons:**
1. Mechanism of injury
   a. Tibial plafond fractures are caused predominantly by axial loading, whereas ankle (malleolar) fractures are caused predominately by rotational forces
   b. Rapid rate of loading in pilon fractures
2. Axis of motion of the talus
   a. In pilon fractures there is proximal displacement of the talus
   b. In ankle fractures there is translational displacement of the talus
3. Risk of complications is higher
   a. Much greater soft tissue injury in pilon fractures
   b. Higher rate of osseous comminution
D. **All tibial plafond fractures are severe injuries**
1. Two distinct and separate mechanisms of injury exist:
   a. Low energy:
      i. Usually produced by rotational forces
      ii. Pronation-dorsiflexsion mechanism
      iii. Minimal comminution
      iv. Common in sporting injuries, such as skiing ("boot-top fracture")
   b. High energy:
      i. Produced by axial compression forces
      ii. Usually numerous comminuted fragments
      iii. Common in MVA and falls from heights
E. **Position of foot:**
1. If dorsiflexed foot = causing large anterior fracture fragment
2. If plantarflexed foot = large posterior fragment exist
3. If neutral positioned foot = Y-shaped fracture with anterior and posterior fragments

II. **Incidence of Pilon fractures**

A. **Extremely rare fractures**
B. **Pilon fractures account for less than 1% of all lower extremity fractures**
C. **They account for 7-10% of all tibia fractures**
D. **20-25% occur as open fractures**
E. **Males are more commonly affected**
F. **They occur over a broad age range**
G. **However, uncommon in children and in elderly patients**
H. **Average patient age is 35 to 40 years**

III. **Clinical Examination:**

A. **Because of the high-energy nature of these fractures, a full-body examination by a general surgeon is recommended**
B. **Associated injuries are high (30-50%)**
C. **High degree of soft tissue injury**
D. **Internal organs are at risk (liver, kidney, spleen)**
E. **Diagnostic modalities:**
1. Standard radiographs are necessary for fracture fragment evaluation
2. Computed tomography (CT) is required for surgical reconstruction
3. If possible 3-D reconstructions are extremely helpful

IV. **Classification of Pilon fractures**

    A. **Rüedi and Allgöwer's classification** (1979) (three types based on the degree of comminution of the articular surface):

        1. **Type I:** fissure fracture without significant articular displacement

        2. **Type II:** fissure fracture with significant articular incongruity

        3. **Type III:** compression fracture with displacement of WB cancellous portion of tibial

    B. **Müller** (AO/OTA) (1990):

        1. Divided into three groups: extra-articular, partial articular and completely articular

           a. *Type A*: extra-articular

               i. **A1:** metaphyseal simple

               ii. **A2:** metaphyseal wedge

               iii. **A3:** metaphyseal complex

           b. *Type B*: partial articular

               i. **B1:** pure split

               ii. **B2:** split-depression

               iii. **B3:** depressed multi-fragment

           c. *Type C*: complete articular

               i. **C1:** articular simple, metaphyseal simple

               ii. **C2:** articular simple, metaphyseal multifragment

               iii. **C3:** multifragmentary

    C. **Ovadia and Beals** (1986): 5 types

        1. **Type I:** intra-articular fracture, not displaced

        2. **Type II:** minimally displaced articular fracture

        3. **Type III:** displaced articular fracture with severe large fragment

        4. **Type IV:** displaced articular fracture with multiple fragments and large metaphyseal defect

        5. **Type V:** displaced articular fracture with severe comminution

V. **Treatment options**

    A. **Closed reduction with cast immobilization**

    B. **Skeletal traction**

    C. **Calcaneal traction, femoral distractor, monoframe**

    D. **Limited fixation with external fixation**

    E. **External fixation**

    F. **Open reduction and internal fixation**

    G. **External fixation with delayed internal fixation**

COMPARTMENT SYNDROME

I. **Introduction**

    A. **Compartment syndrome results from elevated tissue pressure in a closed osteofascial space**

    B. **Compartment syndrome is defined when the interstitial pressure within a non-yielding myofascial compartment exceeds capillary hydrostatic pressure within that compartment, resulting in ischemia of neuromuscular tissues**

    C. **Tissue pressure increases, producing capillary collapse and blood perfusion below what is needed for tissue viability**

D. As a result of the inelastic nature of the structures contained within the osteofascial compartment, the pressure is incapable of being dissipated

E. Eventually, vascular occlusion and myoneurial ischemia result

F. This syndrome was first described by Volkmann, hence the name *"Volkmann's ischemia contracture"*

II. Etiology of compartment syndrome

A. In the leg: Usually encountered after blunt or penetrating trauma

B. Of the foot: Usually associated with crushing injuries, such as multiple metatarsal fractures, tarso-metatarsal joint dislocations, and calcaneal fractures

C. Suspicion of compartment syndrome should be entertained in all patients who present with foot injuries involving elements of crushing, multiple fractures, or dislocations

D. Crush injuries with large, open wounds can also result in compartment syndrome and do not constitute decompression because it is an open wound

E. Other known causes: Arterial embolism, chronic exertion activities, overuse syndromes, tight cast immobilization, tendon ruptures, major fracture/dislocation, and certain surgical procedures

F. Because compartment syndrome is a progressive clinical entity, patients who are suspected of having this must be constantly monitored

G. To ensure venous drainage, do not elevate the questionable extremity above the level of the heart, as this could compromise the arterial blood flow to the extremity

H. Do not apply circumferential dressings or casts that would constrict the extremity

III. Compartment anatomy of the foot and leg

A. The most common compartment of the leg to be involved in compartment syndrome is the anterior compartment; the deep posterior compartment is the second most common

B. Identified osteofascial compartments of the foot that could be involved in compartment syndrome of the foot:

1. Medial compartment
   a. The abductor hallucis and flexor hallucis brevis muscle bellies as well as the flexor hallucis longus, peroneus longus, and posterior tibial tendons
   b. Bordered dorsally by the inferior surface of the first metatarsal shaft, medially by an extension of the plantar aponeurosis, and laterally by an intermuscular septum

2. Central compartment
   a. Contains the flexor digitorum brevis muscle belly, flexor digitorum longus tendons, the lumbricales, the quadratus plantae muscle belly, the adductor hallucis muscle belly, the peroneus longus tendon, and the posterior tibial tendon
   b. Bordered inferiorly by plantar aponeurosis; medially and laterally by intermuscular septae; and dorsally by osseous tarsometatarsal structures, interosseous ligaments, and fascial expansions

3. Lateral compartment
   a. Contains the abductor digiti quinti muscle belly and the flexor digiti quinti muscle belly
   b. Bordered dorsally by the fifth metatarsal shaft, medially with an intermuscular septum, and laterally by the plantar aponeurosis

4. Interosseous compartments: Some sources consider four separate interosseous compartments, one between each of the metatarsals
   a. Contains interosseous muscle bellies

    b.   Bordered by the interosseous fascia and the metatarsal shafts

IV. Diagnosis of compartment syndrome

    A.   The diagnosis of compartment syndrome is a clinical diagnosis and is based on signs of nerve and muscle ischemia; the six P's have been classically used to diagnose compartment syndrome

        1. Pain
            a.   The hallmark of muscle and nerve ischemia
            b.   Described as pain out of proportion to that expected from a particular type of injury
            c.   Usually described as a deep, throbbing, unrelenting pressure that does not respond to immobilization
            d.   Will slowly get progressively worse; exception: exercise-induced compartment syndrome, which resolves when exercise is stopped
        2. Pain with stretch
            a.   With stretching movement of the involved compartment, severe pain will be elicited
        3. Paresthesia
            a.   Sensory deficit: One of the most reliable physical findings in compartment syndrome
            b.   As compartment pressure increases, anesthesia results as a result of nerve compression
        4. Pulses present: Do not use pulses to indicate absence of compartment syndrome
            a.   Increased compartment pressure is usually not enough to compress a major artery
            b.   Pulses in the compartment are usually palpable until very late in compartment syndrome
        5. Pressure
            a.   A tense, swollen compartment is usually one of the earliest objective findings
        6. Paresis
            a.   Muscle weakness, which is often hard to assess
            b.   May be the result of muscle guarding or nerve involvement

V. Measurement of intracompartmental pressure

    A. Techniques to measure intracompartmental pressure
        1. Needle manometer method
        2. Infusion technique
        3. Wick catheter and slit catheter techniques

Wick Catheter

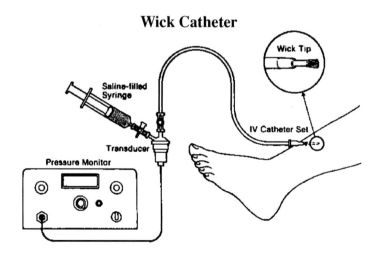

        a. Most commonly used

        b. Slit catheter is modification of the wick catheter and has the advantage of being less prone to coagulation

        c. Can be used to constantly monitor the pressure in the compartment

           i. Stryker intra-compartmental pressure monitor system

              (a) Pocket-sized, quick, easy-to-use, and contemporary machine

              (b) Results are accurate and reproducible

B. Normal compartmental pressure in the foot: 0-5 mmHg

C. When the intracompartmental pressure increases to 30 mmHg or greater after 8 hours, a fasciotomy is recommended

VI. Treatment of compartment syndromes

    A. Decompression via fasciotomy

    B. Decompression of all compartments, not just the suspected one

    C. Debridement of all necrotic tissue during the fasciotomy

    D. Stabilization of all fractures via internal and external fixation

    E. Fasciotomy incisions are left open and covered with a dressing

    F. Debridement of the wound again in 24-48 hours and irrigation of the incision sites with copious lavage

    G. Later closure of the incisions by delayed primary closure or skin grafting, if needed

    H. Many different incisional approaches (usually surgeon's preference is used)

VII. Complications of compartment syndromes

    A. Permanent loss of function

        1. Functional changes in muscle that become permanent after 2-4 hours of ischemia

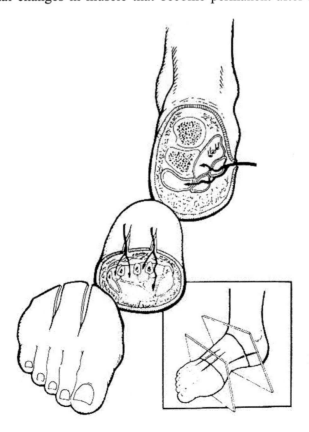

2. Contractures begin to develop after 12 hours of ischemia
3. Neurological changes begin to occur 30 minutes after ischemic changes occur
4. Increased postischemic swelling occurs after 3 hours of ischemia
5. Myoglobinuria can occur secondary to muscle necrosis

B. Myoneural necrosis
C. Structural deformities
   1. Clawfoot deformities
   2. Digital contractures
   3. Dropfoot deformities
D. Functional impairment
   1. Muscle stiffness
   2. Muscle atrophy
E. Sensory changes
F. Chronic pain
G. Sequalae secondary to vascular embarrassment

TENDON INJURIES

I. Definitions

  A. Tenosynovitis: refers to irritation of a tendon sheath secondary to either inflammatory or mechanical etiology
   1. Inflammatory tenosynovitis presents with a tender tendon and a distended sheath
   2. It is commonly seen in rheumatoid arthritis and other collagen vascular diseases
   3. Mechanical tenosynovitis occurs secondary to overuse, bone friction, and biomechanical abnormalities
   4. The presence of local tenderness or clicking of the tendon upon active motion can diagnose this syndrome
  B. Paratendonitis: refers to inflammation surrounding tendons that do not have sheaths
   1. This is caused by and condition that causes an inflammatory reaction adjacent to a tendon
  C. Stenosing tenosynovitis: refers to an inflammatory condition that causes triggering of tendon as it passes through a localized area of sheath constriction
  D. Tendonitis: is an inflammation of the tendon itself
   1. It is caused by trauma, tumor, or ossification with the tendon

II. Classification of tendon injuries

  A. Direct injury
  B. Indirect injury
  C. Spontaneous rupture
  D. Sublimation/dislocation
  E. Iatrogenic injury

III. Traumatic etiologies of tendon injuries

  A. Laceration (open)
  B. Crush (closed)
  C. Puncture/gunshot
  D. Stretching force applied to contracting muscle

    E. **Extremely forceful contraction**

    F. **Avulsion from osseous insertion**

    G. **Pathological** (tendon disease)

    H. **Corticosteroid injection**

    I. **Intra-operative complication**

IV. Diagnosis of acute tendon trauma

    A. **Obtain thorough history**
1. Mechanism of injury
2. Prior injury
3. Previous treatments

    B. **Extensive clinical examination in systematic manner**

    C. **Imaging studies**
1. Plain films
2. Tenography
3. Sonography
4. Magnetic resonance imaging

V. Specific tendon injuries

    A. **Tibialis anterior**
1. Mechanism of rupture: Strong, plantarflextory force on contracted muscle
2. Clinical diagnosis
   a. Tendon usually ruptures 1-2 cm proximal to insertion
   b. Partial loss of dorsiflexion
   c. Dropfoot or steppage gait
   d. Palpable bulbous enlargement at anteromedial ankle
   e. Pain, edema, and ecchymosis
3. Treatment
   a. Conservative: NWB-BK cast with foot dorsiflexed to neutral and inverted 3-6 weeks
   b. Surgical: End-to-end repair with 0 or 2-0 non-absorbable sutures or free tendon graft from EDL or a split portion of tibialis anterior tendon

    B. **Extensor hallucis longus**
1. Mechanism of rupture: Rare, but result of sudden plantarflextory force on extended hallux (i.e., stub toe in hole while running barefoot)
2. Clinical diagnosis
   a. Inability to dorsiflex hallux
   b. Palpable bulbous enlargement
   c. Loss of tented appearance at first MTPJ due to loss of extensor hood
   d. Pain, edema, and ecchymosis
3. Treatment
   a. Conservative: Short, soft cast with hallux dorsiflexed and ankle at 90 degrees for 4-6 weeks
   b. Surgical: End-to-end repair with 2-0 or 3-0 non-absorbable sutures

    C. **Extensor digitorum longus**
1. Mechanism of rupture: Ruptures of the lesser digits are extremely rare
2. Clinical diagnosis
   a. Partial loss of dorsiflexion
   b. Dropfoot

   c. Palpable bulbous enlargement

   d. Pain, edema, and ecchymosis

  3. Treatment

   a. Conservative: Usually successful with NWB-BK cast with foot dorsiflexed 4 weeks

   b. Surgical: End-to-end repair with 2-0 or 3-0 non-absorbable sutures or free tendon graft from a split portion of TA

D. Tibialis posterior

  1. Mechanism of rupture

   a. True spontaneous ruptures are rare

   b. Most commonly due to chronic or acute stress in a degenerative tendon

   c. Chronic tenosynovitis

   d. Sequelae of pes planovalgus deformity

   e. Most common site of rupture: Behind the medial malleolus (low vascularity)

  2. Surgical classification of lesion types of ruptured tibialis posterior *(Funk classification)*

   a. Group 1: Insertion avulsion

   b. Group 2: Midsubstance tear about medial

   c. Group 3: Incontinuity longitudinal tear without complete rupture

   d. Group 4: Tenosynovitis without visible disruption

  3. MRI classification *(Conti classification)*

   a. Type IA: 1-2 longitudinal splits in the PT tendon without degeneration

   b. Type IB: Multiple longitudinal splits and fibrosis without tendon degeneration

   c. Type II: Narrowing of the PT tendon, longitudinal splits, and tendon degeneration

   d. Type IIIA: Diffuse tendon swelling with uniform degeneration

   e. Type IIIB: Complete PT rupture

  4. Clinical diagnosis

   a. Collapse of medial longitudinal arch

   b. Poorly localized medial pain, with usually no recollection of trauma

   c. Positive "Jack test": Inability to invert heel on heel rise

   d. "Too many toes" sign from posterior view

   e. Inability to stand or rise on toes

   f. Possible edema and ecchymosis

  5. Treatment

   a. Conservative: NWB-BK cast with foot plantarflexed, adducted, and inverted 4-6 weeks, then WB cast for 2-4 weeks

   b. Surgical: Depends on the location and type of injury

    i. Avulsion: Reattachment to navicular using 0 or 2-0 non-absorbable sutures, absorbable sutures, or soft-tissue anchoring systems

    ii. Midsubstance tear: Interposition of FDL is used to anastamose with remaining tp stump or suture into drill hole into navicular

    iii. Incontinuity tears: Debridement, synovectomy and intubulation

    iv. If all soft-tissue procedures fail, then talonavicular fusion up to triple arthrodesis

E. Flexor digitorum longus

  1. Mechanism of rupture: Rare

   a. Most commonly from laceration

   b. Occurs with strong, dorsiflexory force of ankle or MTJ

  2. Clinical diagnosis

   a. Usually minimal symptoms

   b. May feel enlargement of tendon along its course

   c. Popping sensation of hallux

       d. Loss of IPJ plantarflex against resistance

       e. Pain, edema, and ecchymosis

   3. Treatment

       a. Conservative: NWB-BK cast with hallux plantarflexed 3-6 weeks

       b. Surgical: End-to-end Bunnell type repair with 2-0 or 3-0 non-absorbable sutures, followed by NWB for 3-4 weeks

F. Peroneal tendons

   1. Mechanism of rupture

       a. Strong tendon contraction against an actively inverted foot

       b. Longitudinal rupture occurs when PB splits the PL tendon as it gets caught between the cuboid and lateral malleolus during forced dorsiflexion

       c. PL tendon can tear as a result of an enlargement of the peroneal tubercle during sudden inversion

       d. Can cause peroneal tendon subluxation

   2. Clinical diagnosis

       a. Variable levels of pain

       b. Decreased active pronation against resistance compared to contralateral side

       c. Inability to palpable PB in the fibular sulcus

       d. Edema and ecchymosis

   3. Peroneal tendon subluxation classification *(Eckert and Davis classification)*

       a. Grade I: The superior peroneal retinaculum (SPR) and periosteum are stripped off the lateral malleolus by the dislocating peroneal tendons

       b. Grade II: A portion of the fibrocartilagenous ridge of the posterior aspect of the fibula is avulsed with the retinaculum

       c. Grade III: A fragment of cortical bone is avulsed with the retinaculum

   4. Treatment

       a. Conservative: NWB-BK cast with foot in neutral position for 4-6 weeks

       b. Surgical: End-to-end repair with 2-0 or 3-0 non-absorbable sutures or peroneal anastomosis

G. Achilles tendon

   1. Anatomy

       a. Gastrocnemius plus soleus make up the Achilles tendon

       b. Inserts into posterior 1/3 calcaneus

       c. Rotates medially into insertion

       d. Powerful plantarflexor of ankle joint

       e. Inverts the ankle joint

       f. Plantaris medial and anterior to TA

       g. Sural nerve and lesser saphaneous vein lateral

       h. Retrocalcaneal bursa between calcaneus and TA

   2. Achilles tendon blood supply

       a. Muscle belly: proximal tendon

       b. Tendon-bone junction: distal tendon

       c. Mesotendon: provides major blood supply

       d. *"Watershed Area"*: 2-6 cm proximal to TA insertion

   3. Mechanism of rupture

       a. Usually degenerative process

          i. Poor vascularity from inactivity

          ii. Langergren and Lindholm stated an increased susceptibility to TA rupture following prolonged inactivity of tendon

          iii. Watershed area is most susceptible due to pre-existing decreased vascularity

    b. Trauma: Direct or indirect trauma

          i. Partial or total rupture

          ii. Posterior fibers first

          iii. Anterior fibers last

          iv. Plantaris is rarely, if ever, torn

          v. Direct trauma

              (a) Laceration

              (b) Direct pressure

          vi. Indirect trauma

              (a) Violent dorsiflexion against plantarflexion at ankle joint

              (b) Knee forcefully extended while foot is dorsiflexed

    c. Predisposing systemic factors

          i. Rheumatoid arthritis

          ii. Tuberculosis

          iii. Gout

          iv. Hyperparathyroidism

          v. SLE

          vi. Scurvy

          vii. Hyperbetalipoproteinemia

    d. Steroid Use

          i. Local steroid injection or chronic systemic use

          ii. Weakens collagen cross-linking

          iii. Directly related to dose, type and frequency

    e. Miscellaneous: Fluoroquinolones use

4. Clinical diagnosis

    a. Tendon usually ruptures 2-6 cm proximal to insertion (i.e., watershed area)

    b. Audible pop or snap heard by patient at time of injury

    c. Feels like someone hit them in back of calf

    d. Stabbing pain in back of leg

    e. Positive Thompson-Doherty test: Calf is squeezed while patient is prone, and no significant plantarflexion results (long flexes will produce minimal flexion)

    f. Patient unable to rise on toes (Jack's test)

    g. Positive Copeland test: sphygmomanometer around calf, knee flexed 90 degrees, ankle plantarflexed, cuff inflated to 100 mmHg, no ankle dorsiflexion noted

    h. Positive Obrian's test: 4 needles placed at varying increments along Achilles tendon, when squeezed the distal needles do not move

    i. Pain, edema, and ecchymosis

    j. Palpable gap or defect in tendon with palpation

    k. Loss of heel inversion

    l. High retraction of calf muscle belly (i.e., ball-like)

    m. Abnormal passive dorsiflexion

    n. Decrease manual muscle testing

    o. Apropulsive gait

5. Classification of Achilles tendon ruptures *(Kuwada classification)*

    a. Type I: Partial rupture of the Achilles tendon

    b. Type II: Complete rupture of the Achilles tendon with < 3.0 cm gap

    c. Type III: Complete rupture of the Achilles tendon with a 3.0-6.0 cm gap

    d. Type IV: Complete rupture of the Achilles tendon with > than 6.0 cm gap

6. Treatment
   a. Conservative: NWB-BK gravity equinus cast 4-8 weeks
   b. Surgical:
      i. End-to-end repair with 0 or 2-0 non-absorbable sutures
      ii. Plantaris tendon as graft
      iii. Gastromemius aponeurosis flaps to repair defect
      iv. Fascia lata as graft
      v. Bone-anchoring systems

VI. Types of tendon repair techniques

A. The best results are obtained after early primary repair of complete tendon injuries

B. It is generally accepted that a primary repair may be carried out up to three weeks after acute laceration

C. Repair of tendons usually requires an intratendinous grasping suture for proper re-approximation of the tendon ends

D. Examples include: Kessler, Bunnell, Nicoladoni, Mason-Allen, Pulvertaft and Krackow techniques (includes modified techniques)

1. Kessler suture: box type suture
2. Bunnell suture: figure-of-eight type suture
3. Nicoladoni suture: intratendinous suture
5. Mason-Allen suture: horizontal mattress type suture
6. Pulvertaft suture: Fish mouth anastomosis
7. Krackow suture: interlocking technique (strongest suture technique for tendon repair)

PRINCIPLES OF WOUND AND BONE HEALING

I. Types of wound closure

A. Primary closure (first intention)
1. Closure of a wound in layers
2. Approximation of layers with sutures, staples, or steri-strips

B. Secondary closure (second intention)
1. Closure of a wound by the process of contraction
2. Preferred method of closure in infected wounds

C. Tertiary closure (delayed primary closure)
1. Closure of a wound in the presence of infection or contamination
2. Three to ten days later, after the infection has cleared, the wound is sutured by primary closure

II. Phases of wound healing

A. Substrate phase (inflammatory phase)
1. Also known as the *"exudative"* or *"lag"* phase
2. Lasts from the first day of wounding through the fourth day
3. Three components:
   a. Vascular reaction: Vasoconstriction, followed by vasodilation
   b. Hemostatic reaction: Vessel reaction, platelet aggregation, fibrin and clot formation
   c. Cellular reaction: Cells include PMNs, lymphocytes, macrophages, and masts cells

   B. **Proliferative phase** (fibroblastic phase)
      1. Also called the *"connective tissue"* phase
      2. Occurs from the fifth day through the twentieth day of wound healing
      3. Several components
         a. Epithelization period (four stages)
            i. Mobilization: Loosening of basal cells from dermal attachments
            ii. Migration: Fibroblasts prominent
            iii. Proliferation: Collagen synthesis
            iv. Differentation: Restoration of cellular function
         b. Wound contraction period
         c. Connective tissue repair period
   C. **Remodeling phase** (differentation phase)
      1. Also known as the *"resorption"* phase
      2. Occurs from the twenty-first day to the first year of wound healing

III. **Factors that interfere with wound healing**

   A. **Age**
   B. **Inadequate perfusion**
   C. **Infection**
   D. **Edema**
   E. **Poor nutrition**
   F. **Vitamin deficiencies**
   G. **Steroid medications**
   H. **Compromised host**
      1. Diabetes mellitus
      2. Venous stasis
      3. Collagen vascular diseases
      4. HIV

IV. **Treatment of nonhealing soft-tissue wounds**

   A. **Debridement of all necrotic soft tissue and bone**
   B. **Control of infection**
   C. **Control of metabolic state**
   D. **Nutritional support**
   E. **Avoidance of trauma**
   F. **Aggressive local wound care**
   G. **Intermittent compression and elevation to eliminate limb edema**
   H. **Revascularization of ischemic wound**

V. **Phases of bone healing**

   A. **Inflammation**
   B. **Induction**
   C. **Soft callus**
   D. **Hard callus**
   E. **Remodeling**

VI. **Complications of bone healing**

   A. **Malunion**

1. Misalignment of the fracture fragments along any of the three cardinal body planes
2. Caused by inadequate reduction, immobilization and/or fixation

B. Nonunion (see below)

C. Delayed union (see below)

D. Pseudoarthrosis

E. Avascular necrosis

F. Infection

VII. Nonunion versus delayed union

A. Nonunion
1. Cessation of healing, usually over 9 months of no healing on serial radiographs
2. Incapable of biologic reaction

B. Delayed union
1. Inability of a fracture to heal within an acceptable time period
2. Three serial radiographs that show no healing after 3-9 months is generally accepted

VIII. Classification of nonunions by Weber and Cech

A. Hypervascular: Most common type (90%) and capable of biological healing (three types)
1. Elephant type: Severe hypertrophy of callus formation and has best chance for healing
2. Horse hoof type: Moderate hypertrophy of callus formation
3. Oligotrophic type: Minimal hypertrophy of callus formation

B. Avascular: Only 10% and incapable of biological healing (four types)
1. Torsion wedge type: Butterfly fragment with unilateral healing (type of pseudoarthrosis)
2. Comminuted type: Numerous gapped fragments
3. Defect type: Loss of bone substance across entire span of bone with no osseous integrity
4. Atrophic type: Bones have undergone osteogenic reabsorption and have rounded edges

IX. Causes of nonunions

A. Inadequate reduction or immobilization

B. Inadequate internal fixation

C. Severe trauma to local soft tissue and blood supply in fracture site area

D. Infection with secondary osteomyelitis

E. Loss of bony substance

F. Distraction of bony fragments

G. Compromised host

H. Anemias

I. Anticoagulant therapy

J. Patient non-compliance

X. Treatment of nonunions

A. Surgical resection of fibronecrotic bony edges with rigid internal fixation

B. Bone resection followed by bone grafting with stable internal fixation

C. Rigid immobilization

D. Electrical bone stimulation (either internal or external)

E. Serial radiographs

F. Nutritional support

G. Avoidance of trauma

XI. Types of bone grafts (two types)

    A. Autogenous: From the same person

        1. Preferred for nonunions

        2. Advantages: More viable cells and immunological compatibility

        3. Disadvantages: Increased OR time, second surgical site, and donor site morbidity

        4. Four types

            a. Cancellous bone graft

                i. Provides largest amount of viable cells and heals quickly but are fragile

                ii. As healing occurs, graft appears radiodense initially

                iii. Preferred for nonunions, especially avascular nonunions

            b. Cortical bone graft

                i. Provides strength and stability, but incorporates more slowly than cancellous grafts

                ii. As healing occurs, graft appears radiolucent initially

                iii. Allows for secure attachments for fixation devices

            c. Corticocancellous bone graft

                i. Combine strength of cortical bone with the rapid osteogenic capabilities of cancellous bone

                ii. Iliac crest: Most common donor site

            d. Free vascularized graft

                i. Involves a graft in which the nutrient artery is intact to be anasfomosed to donor artery

    B. Allograft: From the same species

        1. Considered implants because the tissue contains primarily non-viable cells

        2. Many disadvantages: Primarily graft rejection as a result of immuno-incompatibility

        3. Three types

            a. Fresh allograft

            b. Freeze-dried allograft or *"lyophilized graft"*

                i. Process that removes 95% of moisture in graft

                ii. Infinite shelf life

            c. Artificial allograft

                i. Example is "coralline hydroxyapatite"

XII. Phases of bone graft healing

    A. Vascular ingrowth: Occurs during the first and second weeks

    B. Osteoblast proliferation: Osteoprogenitor cells differentiate into osteoblasts

    C. Osteoinduction: Process in which nonosseous tissue is induced to produce bone

    D. Osteoconduction: Also known as *"creeping substitution,"* the process by which the bone graft acts as a conduit or scaffold for migration of new bone

    E. Graft remodeling: Lasts for several months and results in reformation of the graft

XIII. Bone-grafting techniques

    A. Onlay: Utilizes autogenous cortical bone graft to bridge a nonunion

        1. Can be fixated with plates, screws, or wires

        2. Phemister described a technique that was not fixated and the graft was placed subperiosteally

    B. Inlay: Process by which a window or slot is formed and the graft is placed into it

    C. Sliding: Graft from long bone in which approximately half the diameter in width is used and moved forward across the recipient site

BURNS AND FROSTBITE INJURIES

I. **Introduction**

    A. **Thermal injury to the lower extremity, and, more specifically, to the foot and ankle, is relatively uncommon**

    B. **Thermal destruction of skin may result in severe local and systemic physiologic alterations**

    C. **The majority of minor burns may be treated on an outpatient basis, but the foot requires special consideration**

    D. **A thorough understanding of the pathophysiology of burn wounds, classification of burn levels, treatment options, and possible complications of burn wounds is necessary**

II. **Assessing extent of burn injuries**

    A. **"Rule of nines"**

        1. Most common method but has limited accuracy

        2. Used to determine burn injury extent

        3. Divides the body regions into general percentages

        4. Each lower extremity is considered 18% of the body surface, with each foot approximately 2.5%

    B. **Burn charts of Lund and Browder**

        1. Provides more accurate method to assess burn injury

        2. Burn charts relate age to body size

        3. Modified scales are used for children because the head and extremities of children constitute different percentages of total body surface from those of adults

        4. In children of less than 5 years, the head accounts for nearly 18% and the lower extremities are about 13% each

III. **Classification of burn injuries**

    A. **Burns can be broadly divided into minor, moderate, and critical burns:**

        1. Critical burns require specialized care facilities with highly trained professionals

        2. Many minor and moderate burns may be treated on an outpatient basis

    B. **Previously, burns were classified as first-, second-, and third-degree, based primarily on injury depth**

        1. First degree: Erythema without blistering

            a. Very superficial burn caused most commonly by prolonged sunbathing

            b. Characterized by discomfort and erythema only, with no other evidence of tissue damage

            c. Epidermis heals within a few days and the outer injured cells peel off without scarring

        2. Second degree: Erythema with blistering

            a. Deeper but still superficial injury

            b. Characterized by blister formation where the superficial epidermal layers are devitalized

            c. Characteristically very painful and hypersensitive to temperature and air currents

            d. Epidermal regeneration is prompt because the basal layers remain viable

            e. Usually heal spontaneously in 14 to 17 days unless exposed to infection or excessive drying

        3. Third degree: destruction of full thickness of skin and deeper tissues with sensation loss

a. Most severe burns that contain totally destroyed skin and appendages
b. Skin appears pale white or charred and is characterized by a translucent, inelastic, hard, leathery eschar
c. Injury is avascular with thrombosed dermal blood vessels
d. Wound is insensitive to all but deep pressure
e. Burns cannot heal spontaneously and require skin grafting

C. More recently, burns have been classified by thickness:
1. Partial thickness: Includes first- and second-degree burns
2. Full thickness: Corresponds to third-degree burns

D. General guidelines have been established for determination of minor, moderate, and critical burns

IV. General guidelines to burn categories

A. Minor burns
1. Second degree burn: Less than 10%-15% of the total body surface area is burned
2. Third degree burn: Less than 5% of the total body surface area is burned

B. Moderate Burns
1. Second degree burn: Involves 15%-25% of total body surface area
2. Third degree burn: Involves 10% of the total body surface area

C. Critical Burns
1. Second degree burn: Involves more than 30% of the total body surface area
2. Third degree burn: Involves more than 15%-20% of the total body surface area and critical body parts of face, hands, feet, or perineum
3. Burns complicated by respiratory tract injury, major soft-tissue injury, or fractures
4. Electrical burns
5. Chemical burns involving greater than 30%-40% of body surface

V. Etiology of lower extremity burn injuries

A. Exposure to flame
B. Contact burns
C. Scald burns
D. Electrical injuries
1. Cutaneous damage to the foot is common; entry wounds appear dry and depressed, and exit wounds appear irregular and raised
2. Deeper destruction includes myonecrosis with eventual gross demarcation between viable and nonviable tissue
3. The severity of tissue damage depends on several factors:
    a. Voltage
    b. Duration of contact
    c. Location of the entrance and exit wounds with respect to each other
    d. Current flow through the tissues

E. Chemical burns
1. Resultant tissue damage can be attributed to agent strength, concentration, quantity, duration, extent of penetration, and mechanism of action

VI. Treatment of burns

A. Initial management of severe burns consists of establishment and maintenance of an

adequate airway, institution of intravenous fluids, and advanced life support (ABC's of trauma patient)
   B. **Assess the extent and depth of injury**
   C. **Local wound care assumes priority only after stabilization of the injured person**
   D. **Initial and continued treatment plan depends on category of burn injury**
   E. **Basic principles of burn wound management are cleansing, debridement, and dressing**
      1. May need a peripheral nerve block or oral analgesic to control the pain
      2. Cut body hair in the region to remove contaminating hair
      3. Cleanse the area gently with surgical soap (or detergent) and water
      4. Debride all nonviable and devitalized tissue or skin
      5. Leave small blisters less than 2.0 cm in diameter intact
      6. Debride or drain blisters larger than 2.0 cm in diameter because they rupture easily and can become infected
      7. Leave small burns exposed or cover with a nonadherent dressing, base decision on their location and depth
      8. Decrease abrasion and pain with dressing
      9. Wash and dry exposed burn every day
   F. **Topical antimicrobial agents are indicated in all moderate and major burns**
   G. **Tetanus prophylaxis is mandatory in all but first degree burns**
   H. **Primary goals**
      1. To promote rapid epithelialization
      2. To prevent secondary bacterial colonization

VII. **Complications of burns**

   A. **Inadequate initial therapy may result in considerable functional impairment**
      1. Contracture of skin surface
      2. Hypertrophic scars from prolonged swelling and pain
      3. Infection
      4. Vascular damage
      5. Motor and sensory loss
      6. Discoloration of skin surface pigmentation
      7. Joint contraction
      8. Peripheral nerve damage
      9. Neural damage

VIII.   **Summary of burn injury**

   A. **Certain critical areas of the body, such as the feet, require special hospital care to maintain their functional capabilities**
   B. **In severe or major burns, the burn would only assume primary importance after the patient's airway is stabilized and fluid replacement is initiated**
   C. **Formulation of a treatment plan is then based upon the location, extent, and depth of the burn injury**
   D. **Local wound care consists of cleansing, debridement of all necrotic tissue, and dressing**
   E. **Tetanus prophylaxis is mandatory in all second-degree and greater burn injuries**
   F. **Treatment goals are prevention of dehydration and infection so that rapid wound closure is achieved**
   G. **When indicated, topical antimicrobial and/or enzymatic debridement agents are employed**

H. **Systemic antibiotics are only indicated when an uncontrolled invasive sepsis has been confirmed**

I. **Burns to the lower extremity and foot require special care and footwear, which are necessary during wound maturation and for months or years afterwards to prevent skin or graft breakdown or the occurrence of contractors**

J. **Watchfulness and follow-up are essential for proper wound care and successful healing**

IX. Frostbite injury

A. Predisposing factors in frostbite

1. Environmental factors
   a. Duration of exposure
   b. Wind chill factor
   c. Wetness
   d. Attitude
2. Individual factors
   a. Age
   b. Nutritional status
   c. Physical and mental condition
   d. Alcohol and smoking habits

B. Types of frostbite injuries

1. Frostnip
   a. Mildest form of frostbite
   b. A reversible superficial injury with symptoms of blanching and numbness of the skin
   c. Results from short exposure to freezing temperatures (below 32° F) for a very short duration of time (less than 30 minutes)
   d. The condition is not painful upon rewarming
2. Chillblains
   a. Also known as *"pernio"*
   b. Defined as repeated exposure to above freezing temperatures (above 32° F) in the presence of high humidity
   c. Classic symptoms in the foot are red, itchy lesions usually found on the dorsum of the foot
   d. Women are affected more often than men
   e. Two types
      i. Acute pernio
         (a) Caused by acute exposure to moist, cold, above freezing temperatures in the presence of high humidity
         (b) Symptoms: Slight edema, bluish discoloration of the skin, and intense itching
         (c) Rarely hemorrhagic pupura
         (d) Condition usually resolves without scarring of the skin
         (e) Treatment: Supportive, including elevation of the involved extremity, protection from additional exposure, and application of moisturizing lotion to the affected areas
      ii. Chronic pernio
         (a) Caused by repeated exposure to cold above freezing temperatures in the presence of high humidity
         (b) Symptoms: Red, painful, itchy cutaneous lesions and hyperpigmentation of area

(c) Treatment: Same as acute pernio, with the exception of possible late sympathectomy

(d) The sequelae: Scarring, fibrosis, and skin atrophy

3. Trench foot
   a. Also known as *"immersion foot"*
   b. Trench foot and immersion foot are considered the same condition by some, but there is a difference: Trench foot is caused only by cold and dampness, but immersion foot does not result without immersion in water
   c. Etiology of trench foot and immersion foot: Prolonged exposure (greater than 12 hours) to cold, above freezing water, usually at temperatures between 32° F and 50° F
   d. For both, clinical presentation is divided into three phases:
      i. Early phase, also known as *"vasospastic ischemic"* phase, in which affected extremity is usually pale and blue, pulses are present but reduced, and there are areas of patchy anesthesia
      ii. Postimmersion hyperemic phase
         (a) Vasodilation occurs
         (b) Foot is red, swollen, and hot to touch
         (c) No sweating in the affected extremity
         (d) Possible ecchymosis, ulceration, or gangrene
         (e) Patchy anesthesia replaced by intense, burning pain
      iii. Late vasospastic ischemic phase, in which the extremity is cold, painful, and stiff, and paraesthesia occurs

4. High-altitude frostbite
   a. A variant of true frostbite because of its differing pathogenically
   b. Results from extremely cold, below freezing temperatures (-40° F to -62° F) that cause actual freezing within minutes accompanied by intense vasoconstriction

C. **Pathophysiology of frostbite**
   1. Many theories describe the mechanism of frostbite injury
   2. Mechanism is now believed to be a combination
      a. Direct freezing of tissues
      b. Sequelae of vasomotor responses
      c. Intravascular response phenomenon

D. **Pathophysiology of frostbite mechanism**
   1. Prefreeze phase
      a. Blood vessel constriction in addition to dilation of veins
      b. Prolongation of this phase results in leakage of fluids due to congestion
   2. Freeze-thaw phase
      a. Extracellular crystal formation results in ruptured cell membranes
      b. If frostbite injury is halted at this stage, tissue damage may be reversed
   3. Vascular stasis phase
      a. Results from chronic venous dilation and arterial spasm
      b. Progression of this stasis leads to arteriovenous; shunting and tissue hypoxia
   4. Ischemic late phase
      a. Results from prolonged vascular occlusion and hypoxia with neural damage

E. **Classification of frostbite:** There are two widely utilized classifications of frostbite. Orr and Fainer developed a classification after the Korean war that consisted of four degrees. This classification was later challenged by Washburn, who believed that the former classification could only be applied retrospectively unless the patient was seen before rewarming took place. Washburn therefore devised a simpler two-part classification known as superficial and deep

1. Orr and Fainer classification of frostbite injuries
    a. First degree
        i.   Characterized by erythema, edema, and a white firm plaque of the involved part
        ii. No blister formation and no necrosis in this stage
    b. Second degree
        i.   Characterized by areas of erythema, edema, and blister or bleb formation (i.e., hallmark lesion)
        ii. Spontaneously healing without any late sequelae
    c. Third degree
        i.   A full-thickness injury with a hemorrhagic blister
        ii. Varying levels of necrosis but no loss of the affected part
    d. Fourth degree
        i.   Most severe degree of frostbite, with complete necrosis and loss of the affected part
        ii. Deep cyanosis without blister or edema formation
        iii. No revascularization is possible and often results in amputation of the affected part
2. Washburn classification of frostbite injuries
    a. Superficial
        i.   Defined as a cold-induced injury to the epidermis and dermis
        ii. Clinically seen as a white and frozen injured part that still has resilience when palpated
    b. Deep
        i.   Defined as damage to deeper tissues, including bone and tendon, which leaves the injured part stiff and without resilience when palpated

F. Clinical recognition of frostbite
1. The degree or extent of cold injury depends on several factors
    a. Length of exposure
    b. Ambient temperature during the exposure
    c. Wetness
    d. Wind velocity
    e. Kind, if any, of protective covering the patient wore during exposure
2. Early changes, if any, may be minimal
3. When first seen, the extremity may feel hard and "woody" and may appear pale or slightly purplish
4. There will be a decrease in capillary filling time and a delay in the usual blush following digital pressure
5. Within 24 hours, blisters begin to develop, swelling occurs, and more reddish-purple discoloration appears
6. After several days, the blisters enlarge and become hemorrhagic, and the "line of destruction" may begin to form
7. Within a few weeks, if the frostbite was severe enough, black eschar develops and demarcation becomes more pronounced

G. Adjuncts to Diagnosis
1. Limited value in determining the extent of tissue damage
2. Radiographs may show bony changes late in the course of frostbite
3. Angiography may help in deciding the point of demarcation

4. Thermography and radioactive evaluation of circulation are indicated
5. Bone scintigraphy
   a. Technetium-99 bone scan can aid in the assessment of tissue viability
   b. Scan can be used within 24-48 hours after injury and then repeated within 7-20 days
   c. Nonviable tissues will appear as a defect in perfusion, with viable tissue that is hyperemic showing increased soft tissue uptake and indistinct vascular structures
   d. With two periods of scanning, the physician will see the results of conservative treatment and the level of amputation, if necessary

H. **Principles of frostbite treatment**
1. Treatment of hypothermia takes precedence over that of the cold injury and may conflict with it
   a. Take body temperature rectally; if below 94° F, then treatment is necessary
   b. Treat severe hypothermia with heated peritoneal dialysis and administration of heated intravenous fluids, heated extracorporeal circulation, or heated inspired air
2. Tissue fares better if it is brought through the thawing process as rapidly as possible, which decreases the time during which the cells can be damaged by dehydration
3. The majority of damage results from ischemia gangrene, and, therefore, the goal is to restore and maintain blood flow. Rapid thawing has been shown to be the best treatment, it should never be done over an open flame or a heated object
4. The extremity should be submerged in a large vessel of hot water between 100° F or 110° F (i.e., between 38° C and 40° C) for 30-45 minutes
   a. The water should be swirled and the temperature checked and maintained constantly
   b. Hot water should never be poured directly on the extremity
   c. If the patient is already thawed on presentation, the extremity should not be heated in water
5. Vasospasm can be treated with reserpine or phenoxybenzamine hydrochloride to produce, in effect, a "sympathectomy"
   a. Especially effective if the frostbite is seen several days after it has been thawed, but is still having symptoms
   b. Symptoms will diminish immediately upon injection
6. Anticoagulants, such as heparin, and drugs which decrease platelet aggregation, such as aspirin, should be used during the first 30 minutes of treatment
7. After rapid thaw, all patients should be hospitalized
8. Topical creams such as aloe vera and silver sulfadiazine, can be very beneficial if used daily
9. Patients must avoid trauma to the area, avoid tight shoes, and expect at least 8 weeks of symptomotology
10. Patient should be notified that he or she will always have an increased susceptibility to frostbite
11. Physical therapy is very beneficial to frostbitten feet; used after demarcation of frostbite and then postoperatively can much improve the range of motion of the involved joint

I. **Complications of frostbite:** Ervasti studied over 900 cases of frostbite and reported on the complications
1. Cold sensitivity (82%): Most common complication
2. Skin color changes (73%)
3. Hyperhidrosis (58%)
4. Pain with use (39%)
5. Local skin changes (36%)

6. Hypoesthesia (23%)
7. Pain at rest (16%)
8. Phantom pains (10%)
9. Transitory numbness (5%)
10. Hyperesthesia (3%)

J. Summary of frostbite injury
1. Prevent infection
2. Wait for demarcation to indicate the level of surgical debridement
3. Cease smoking because of secondary affect of increased peripheral vasoconstriction
4. Use daily whirlpool baths, which are the mainstay of treatment; the water should be tepid (100° F); with an antiseptic soap for 20 minutes twice daily
5. Leave blisters intact, if possible
6. Apply aloe vera or silvadene cream twice daily
7. Prevent additional trauma with bedrest and elevation of the affected part
8. Administer tetanus prophylaxis, which is essential
9. Antibiotics are not indicated prophylactically
10. Prevent compartment syndrome with a fasciotomy to alleviate extreme edema
11. Control pain with analgesics
12. Avoid early amputation by waiting for demarcation (6-8 weeks)

NERVE AND VASCULAR INJURY

I. Nerve injury

A. Introduction
1. In every soft tissue injury which requires medical attention, clinical examination should include concern for a nerve lesion and great care during treatment of the wound
2. Of soft-tissue injuries, 4.5% contain some type of nerve damage
3. After complete severance of a nerve by a sharp object, spontaneous healing is rare; the exception occurs occasionally in small nerve trunks, such as digital nerves near the interphalangeal joint
4. The generally accepted rate of recovery after a nerve injury is 1-2 mm a day

B. Classification of nerve injuries
1. The most commonly used classification of traumatic nerve injuries is by Seddon:
   a. Neuropraxia: Contusion-or compression-type injury
      i. Temporary conduction blockade without transection of the axons
      ii. Etiology: Secondary to localized ischemic demyelination
      iii. Motor fibers more greatly affected than sensory fibers
      iv. Electrophysiologic responses are normal
      v. Recovery is usually spontaneous but can last hours to weeks
   b. Axonotmesis: Crush-type injury or partial tear from laceration
      i. Interruption of axons and myelin sheath while the endoneural fibers remain intact
      ii. Etiology: Compression and stretch of varying degrees
      iii. Wallerian degeneration of the distal nerve fibers results
      iv. Electrophysiologic responses are identical to those of denervation
      v. Recovery is nearly complete without surgical intervention but may take months
   c. Neurotmesis: Laceration injury with complete disruption of the nerve
      i. Complete transection of a nerve fiber, including the nerve sheath

          ii. Etiology: Injuries with a sharp object

          iii. Most severe form of nerve injury

          iv. Spontaneous regeneration or recovery is impossible

          v. Surgical repair is the treatment of choice

     d. Another commonly used classification is by Sunderland, in which five degrees of injury, which are defined by increasing severity and produce a loss function, are described

          i. First degree

            (a) Blockade of nerve conduction without axonal injury

            (b) Corresponds to neuropraxia

          ii. Second degree

            (a) Incomplete injury to axons

               (1) Corresponds to early stage of axonotmesis

               (2) Commonly seen in chronic compression syndromes, such as tarsal tunnel syndrome

          iii. Third degree

            (a) Injury to axons and endoneural connective tissue with preservation of perineurium

            (b) Corresponds to late stage of axontmesis

            (c) Commonly seen after blunt trauma

            (d) Development of fibrosis and scarring of nerve

          iv. Fourth degree

            (a) Injury to axons, endoneural tissue, and the perineurium

            (b) Corresponds to preneurotmesis

            (c) Preservation of the continuity of the nerve can be seen macroscopically

            (d) Seen after severe blunt trauma or incomplete transection of a peripheral nerve

          v. Fifth degree

            (a) Defined as complete severance with dehiscence of the nerve stumps

            (b) Corresponds to actual neurotmesis

            (c) Recovery is impossible

  2. Types of Nerve Surgery

     a. Neurolysis

          i. Process of releasing nerve from adhesion or scar tissue

          ii. Indicated in first-, second-, and third-degree injuries

     b. Neurorrhaphy

          i. Joining together of transected nerve via sutures

          ii. Indicated in fourth- and fifth-degree injuries

II. Vascular injury

A. Introduction

  1. Arterial injuries can vary from tiny punctures in the vessel wall to complete transections

  2. Numerous conditions, such as severe dislocations, puncture wounds, gun shots, and so forth, cause arterial injuries

  3. Most arterial injuries are not isolated to the adjacent nerve; tendon and venous structures are frequently involved

  4. Prompt diagnosis and repair of arterial lacerations enhances survivability of distal structures

B. Diagnosis of arterial lacerations

1. Arterial injury should be suspected with any deep, penetrating wound located along the course of a vascular bundle, particularly if there is abundant bleeding
2. The extremity distal to the injury may appear with signs of pallor, mottled cyanosis, and a delayed capillary refill time
3. The region usually displays a decrease in temperature as compared to the opposite extremity
4. Pulses may be decreased or absent
5. Diminished sensation and muscle strength distal to the injury may result

C. Treatment of vascular injury

1. Restoration of adequate arterial flow must be completed within 6 to 12 hours
2. Presence of good blood flow to the skin does not insure adequate perfusion to nerve and muscle tissue
3. Initial control of bleeding should be performed using direct pressure only
4. Surgical repair is the treatment of choice if the dorsalis pedis or posterior tibial arteries are involved, recommended sutures are 6-0 or 7-0 polypropylene or braided polyester in a simple interrupted fashion
5. If only one distal artery is severed and there is no evidence that distal regions are ischemic, the severed vessel may be ligated

PEDIATRIC INJURIES

I. Fractures

A. Introduction

1. Epiphyseal fractures can result in significantly different consequences from adult fractures
2. Presence of the epiphysis and apophysis, the failure of pediatric bone in both tension and compression and the relative increase in the child's haversian canal system compared with that of the adult, predisposes the pediatric patient to a specific subset of unique fracture patterns
3. Epiphyseal fractures can create premature epiphyseal arrest with resultant deformity in length and angulation of a child's limb
4. The dread complication of serious disturbance of growth is usually predictable and, in certain circumstances, can be prevented
5. An epiphysis may be displaced at the moment of injury and then return to its normal position, in which case clinical examination is likely to be of considerable importance in recognizing the nature of the injury
6. Thus, knowledge of the prognosis for a given injury to the epiphyseal plate in a particular child is of considerable importance to the podiatric physician, who has the dual responsibility of treating the child and advising the parents

B. Types of epiphyses

1. Pressure epiphysis:
   a. Articular in nature
   b. Located at the end of the long bones and transmit pressure through the joint
   c. Provide for rapid longitudinal growth of long bones
2. Traction epiphysis or apophysis:
   a. Nonarticular in nature

      b. Serve as sites for muscle attachment and are subjected to tremendous pressures

      c. Provide shape and contour of bone

C. Anatomy of the physis

  1. Physis

      a. Also known as *"epiphyseal plate"* or *"growth plate"*

      b. A radiolucent, cartilaginous plate located between the metaphysis and the epiphysis in a long bone

      c. Trauma of the physis is commonly known as an epiphyseal plate injury, which is a misconception because it is not the epiphysis, but rather the physis, that is damaged, which results in growth arrest

  2. Growth plate has three components:

      a. Cartilaginous zone (three subdivisions)

         i. Zone of growth: Contains the dividing and the resting cells

        ii. Zone of maturation: For calcification

      iii. Zone of transformation: For ossification

      b. Bone or the metaphysis: Assists in bone formation, and bone remodeling

      c. Fibrous components consisting of the ossification zone of Ranvier and the perichondral ring of LaCroix

D. Classification of physeal injuries

  1. The Salter-Harris classification for physeal injuries is the most widely used

      a. Based on the mechanism and relationship of the fracture line to the growing cells of the physis and on the prognosis of the disturbed growth plate

      b. Salter-Harris classification

         i. Type I: Epiphysis is completely separated from the metaphysis without any bony fracture

        ii. Type II: Fracture through the physis transversely exiting through the metaphysis on the side opposite the site of the initiating fracture that creates a triangular fragment (also known as *"Thurston-Holland sign"*)

      iii. Type III: Intra-articular fracture extending from the joint surface through the epiphysis to the physis and then extending along the plate to its periphery

      iv. Type IV: Intra-articular fracture extending from the joint surface through the epiphysis across the physealplate and through a portion of the metaphysis

        v. Type V: Severe, crushing injury and compression force of the physeal plate

      vi. Type VI (Rang's addition): Peripheral bruise or injury to the perichondral ring or its associated periosteum at the edge of the physis, causing an angular deformity

  2. Poland's classification of physeal fractures is classified into four distinct types based on the radiographic appearance of the fracture

      a. Type I: Pure and complete separation of the physis from the epiphysis

      b. Type II: Partial separation of the physis from the epiphysis with the fracture extending through the diaphysis

      c. Type III: Partial separation of the physis from the epiphysis with the fracture extending through the epiphysis

      d. Type IV: Complete separation of the physis from the epiphysis with the fracture extending through the epiphysis

E. Treatment and prognosis of physeal injuries based on Salter-Harris classification

  1. Type I injuries

      a. A weightbearing, short leg cast is applied for 3-4 weeks if injury is nondisplaced

      b. A rule of thumb for physeal healing in pediatric patients is to allow half of the time that it would normally take for adult bone to heal in that region

      c.   If injury is displaced, close, reduce, and apply a weightbearing shortleg cast for 3-4 weeks

      d.   Radiographs will reveal a pexiosteal reaction

      e.   The prognosis for the physeal plate is excellent with a Type I injury

2.   Type II injuries

      a.   Most common physeal plate injury

      b.   The fracture extends transversely along the physis and then exits through the metaphysis on the side opposite the site of the initiating fracture

      c.   Fracture pattern creates a triangular-shaped metaphyseal fragment that is referred to as the *"Thurston-Holland sign"* or the *"flag sign"*

      d.   The periosteum is torn on the convex side of the fragment while the concave side remains intact

      e.   If the fracture is nondisplaced, the patient may be placed in a shortleg, WB cast for 4-6 weeks

      f.   If the fracture is displaced as a result of the intact periosteal hinge, the fracture is generally closed and reduced via reversing the mechanism of injury

      g.   After reduction, the patient is placed in a long-leg, NWB cast with the knee flexed for 4 weeks

      h.   The patient should have post-reduction radiographs to assure adequate reduction

      i.   After 4 weeks, the patient is placed in a short leg walking cast for 2 weeks

      j.   The prognosis is excellent because the growing physeal cartilage cells remain with the epiphysis

      k.   There is a 5% risk of premature closure resulting in angulation deformities in Type II injuries

3.   Type III injuries

      a.   Rare injuries

      b.   An intra-articular fracture that begins at the joint surface of the epiphysis and progresses through the secondary ossification center until it reaches the physis

      c.   The fracture then turns 90 degrees and extends through the plate to the periphery

      d.   If the fracture is nondisplaced, a short-leg cast is applied for 4-6 weeks, with the initial 3-4 weeks NWB

      e.   If the fracture is displaced, up to 2 mm is acceptable for closed reduction

      f.   Injury requires accurate reduction in order to restore the smooth joint surface

      g.   Open reduction with internal fixation may be required to reduce the fracture adequately

      h.   It is acceptable to place smooth K-wires perpendicular to the physis and across the physis; these K-wires are removed in 4 weeks

      i.   Care must be taken when using screws or threaded K-wires across the physis because of the potential to compress the physis and create angulation deformities

      j.   There is also concern about the possible interruption of the blood supply to the free fragment in the injury

      k.   The prognosis is good if the blood supply to the fragment is intact

4.   Type IV injuries

      a.   An intra-articular fracture that extends from the joint surface through the epiphysis across the physeal plate and through a portion of the metaphysis

      b.   A nondisplaced fracture is treated with a nonweightbearing, longleg cast for 4 weeks with a weightbearing, short-leg cast for 2 additional weeks

      c.   If the fracture is displaced, ORIF with smooth K-wires or a 4.0 min cancellous screw placed perpendicular to the fracture in the epiphysis and metaphysis

      d. Prognosis is poor; Type IV injuries yield a high incidence of premature closure of the physeal plate with a resultant angulation deformity

  5. Type V injuries

      a. An uncommon injury, resulting from a very severe, crushing force applied through the epiphysis to one area of the physeal plate

      b. There is no physeal fracture or displacement in this injury, so it is impossible to diagnose it when it occurs

      c. A nonweightbearing cast is applied for 3 weeks

      d. The prognosis is very poor; and premature closure of the physeal plate is common with a resultant angulation deformity

  6. Type VI injuries

      a. Rare injuries

      b. Nonweightbearing cast is applied for 4-6 weeks

      c. High risk for premature closure of the growth plate and a resultant angulation deformity; in addition, this trauma to the perichondral ring may result in the formation of a solitary osteochondroma

F. Complications of physeal injuries

  1. Premature closure of physeal plate

  2. Growth arrest

  3. Angulation deformity

  4. Progressive bone shortening

  5. Degenerative joint disease

  6. Painful ambulation

G. Osteochondrosis in the pediatric foot

  1. A noninflammatory disturbance affecting the epiphysis or epiphyses that begins in childhood as a degenerative or necrotic condition

  2. Affects the primary or secondary centers of growth

  3. Etiology: Unknown, but the most accepted belief is that it results secondary to a vascular disturbance (i.e., infarct) to the ossification center, then collapses under strain, pressure, or tension during a time of greatest developmental activity

  4. Radiographic appearance of osteochondrosis is seen in three stages:

      a. Necrotic stage: Relative sclerotic appearance to area

      b. Regenerative stage: Increased fragmentation

      c. Remodeling stage: Complete bony replacement of the necrotic cortex and marrow

H. Types of Osteochondrosis

  1. Talus: Diaz disease

  2. Cuneiforms: Buschke's disease

  3. Fifth metatarsal base: Iselin's disease

  4. Sesamoids: Treve's disease

  5. Accessory tarsal navicular: Haglund's disease

  6. Navicular: Kohler's disease

  7. Second metatarsal head: Freiberg's disease

  8. Calcaneal apophysis: Sever's disease

SUMMARY

The diagnosis and treatment of foot and ankle trauma can present a challenge to any podiatric physician. This chapter stresses the importance of a thorough awareness and implementation of fundamental and rational management principles. The initial examination should cover the basic tenets of emergency medicine:

I. **Establishment of hemostasis and medical stability**

II. **Accurate patient history and physical examination: To elicit the mechanism of injury and extent of injury, tetanus immunization status, evaluation of dermatologic, neurovascular, and musculoskeletal systems**

III. **Establishment of a diagnosis with proper classification; and**

IV. **The institution of an effective primary treatment plan: standard principles are utilized to minimize complications, restore normal function and alignment, and promote rapid healing**

BIBLIOGRAPHY

Adelaar RS: The treatment of tarsometatarsal fracture-dislocation, Instr Course Lect 39:141, 1990.

Altman ML, Hutton SJ: Late neuropathic sequelae of cold injury. J Foot Surg 26:213-216, 1987.

Anderson LD: Injuries of the forefoot, Clin Orthop 122:18, 1977.

Bandyk DF: Vascular injury associated with extremity trauma. Clin Orthop 318:117-124, 1995.

Banerjee B, Das RK: Sonographic detection of foreign bodies of the extremities, Br J Radiol 64(758):107-112, 1991.

Benirschke SK, Sangeorzan BJ: Extensive intraarticular fractures of the foot: surgical management of calcaneal fractures, Clin Orthop 291:128-134, 1993.

Boas RA: Complex regional pain syndromes: symptoms, signs, and differential diagnosis. In Jänig W, Stanton-Hicks M, editors: Reflex sympathetic dystrophy: a reappraisal, Progress in pain research and management, vol 6, Seattle, 1996, IASP Press, p 79.

Böhler L: Diagnosis, pathology and treatment of fractures of the os calcis, J Bone Joint Surg 13:75, 1931.

Brostrom L: Sprained ankles. VI. Surgical treatment of "chronic" ligament ruptures, Acta Chir Scand 132:551-565, 1966.

Brown JE: The sinus tarsi syndrome, Clin Orthop 18:231-233, 1960.

Burton EM, Amaker BH: Stress fracture of the great toe sesamoid in a ballerina: MRI appearance, Pediatr Radiol 24:37-38, 1994.

Capasso G, Maffulli N, Testa V: Rupture of the intersesamoid ligament of a soccer player's foot, Foot Ankle 10:337-339, 1990.

Carter TR, Fowler PJ, Blokker C: Functional postoperative treatment of Achilles tendon repair, Am J Sports Med 20:459-462, 1992.

Cetti R, Christensen S, Ejsted R, et al: Operative versus nonoperative treatment of Achilles tendon rupture: a prospective randomized study and review of the literature, Am J Sports Med 21:791-799, 1993.

Colton AM, Fallat LM: Complex regional pain syndrome, J Foot Ankle Surg 35(4): 284-296, 1996.

Conklin MJ, Kling TT: Careful management of pediatric ankle fractures. J Musculoskel Med 9: 43-59, 1992.

Corey SV, Cicchinelli LD, Pitts TE: Vascular decompression: The critical element in forefoot crush injury. JAPMA 84: 289-296, 1994.

Corey SV: Puncture wounds of the foot. Update: Reconstructive Surgery of the Foot and Leg. The Podiatry Institute, 1992.

Crouch C Smith WL: Long term sequelae of frostbite, Pediatr Radiol 20(5): 365-366, 1990.

Dameron TB: Fractures and anatomic variations of the proximal portion the fifth metatarsal, J Bone Joint Surg 57A: 788-792, 1975.

Dellacorte MP, et al: The acutely painful foot and ankle (Part 1). Emerg Med 46-64, 1994.

Dellon AL: Wound healing in nerve. Clin Plast Surg 17: 545-570, 1990.

Ebraheim NA, Mekhail AO, Salpietro BJ, et al: Talar neck fractures: anatomic considerations for posterior screw application, Foot Ankle Int 17:541-547, 1996.

Edlich RF, Drake DB: Repair of lacerations: Wound preparation. Hosp Med 42-45,1995.

Edlich RF, Langenburg SE: Office repair of lacerations: Evaluating the wound. Hosp Med 56-59,1994.

Faciszewski T, Burks RT, Manaster BJ: Subtle injuries of the Lisfranc joint, J Bone Joint Surg 72A: 1519, 1990.

Fealy MJ, Ladd AL: Reflex sympathetic dystrophy: early diagnosis and active treatment, J Musculoskel Med, March 1996, pp 29-36.

Fitzgerald J, Michael E: Protocols for lower extremity trauma. J Foot Ankle Surg 34: 2-11, 1995.

Fritz RL, Perrin DH: Cold exposure injuries: prevention and treatment, Clin Sports Med 8(1): 111-126, 1989.

Giordano CP, Koval KJ, Zuckerman JD, et al: Fracture blisters, Clin Orthop 307:214-221, 1994.

Gudas CJ, Cann JE: Nonunions and related disorders. Clin Pod Med Surg 8: 321-331, 1991.

Gudas CJ Sports-related tendon injuries of the foot and ankle. Clin Pod Med Surg 3: 303-317,1986.

Gustilo RB, Anderson JT: Prevention of infection in the treatment of one thousand and twenty-five open fractures of long bones, J Bone Joint Surg 58B: 453, 1976.

Gustilo RB, Meakow RL, Templeman D: The management of open fractures. J Bone Joint Surg 72(A) 299-303,1990.

Hallock G: Cutaneous coverage for the difficult wound of the foot, Contemp Orthop 16:19, 1988.

Harper MC: Ankle fracture classification systems: a case for integration of the Lauge-Hansen and AO-Danis-Weber schemes, Foot Ankle 13:404-407, 1992.

Hart TJ, Napoli RC, Wolf JA: Diagnosis and treatment of the ruptured Achilles tendon. J Foot Surg 27: 30-39, 1988.

Hawkins LG: Fractures of the neck of the talus, J Bone Joint Surg 52A: 991-1002, 1970.

Healey KM, Danis, KM: Treatment of open fractures. Clin Pod Med Surg 12: 791-800, 1995.

Heckman JD, Champine MJ: New techniques in the management of foot trauma. Clin Orthop 240: 105-114, 1989.

Hidalgo D, Shaw W: Reconstruction of foot injuries, Clin Plast Surg 13:663, 1986.

Hunter JC, Sangeorzan BJ: A nutcracker fracture: cuboid fracture with an associated avulsion fracture of the tarsal navicular, AJR Am J Roentgenol 166:888, 1996.

Inaba AS, Zukin DD, Perro M: An update on the evaluation and management of plantar puncture wounds and Pseudomonas osteomyelitis, Pediatr Emerg Care 8(1): 38-44, 1992.

Johnson KA: Tibialis posterior tendon rupture, Clin Orthop 177:140-147, 1983.

Karlin JM: Management of open fractures. Clin Pod 2: 217-231, 1985.

Knapik JJ, Reynolds KL, Duplantis KL, et al: Friction blisters: pathophysiology, prevention and treatment, Sports Med 20(3): 136-147, 1995.

Krych SM, Lavery LA: Puncture wounds and foreign body reactions, Clin Podiatr Med Surg 7(4): 725-731, 1990.

Kucan JO, Bash D: Reconstruction of the burned foot, Clin Plast Surg 19(3): 705-719, 1992.

Kuwada GT: Diagnosis and treatment of Achilles tendon ruptures. Clin Pod Med Surg 12: 633-651,1995.

Kvist M: Achilles tendon injuries in athletes, Sports Med 18:173-201, 1994.

Lauge-Hansen N: Fractures of the ankle: analytic historic survey as the basis of new experimental, roentgenologic and clinical investigations, Arch Surg 56:259, 1948.

Leach RE, Schepsis AA: Acute injuries to ligaments of the ankle. In Evarts CM, editor: Surgery of the musculoskeletal system, vol 4, New York, 1990, Churchill Livingstone, pp. 3887-3913.

Mahan KT, Kalish SR: Complications following puncture wounds of the foot. JAPA 72: 497-502,1982.

Malkin LH: Reflex sympathetic dystrophy following trauma to the foot, Orthopaedics 13(8), 1990.

Mann RJ: Human bite injuries. J Musculoskel Med 6:112-139,1989.

Manoli A, Fakhouri AJ, Weber TG: Concurrent compartment syndromes of the foot and leg. Foot Ankle 14:339-342, 1993.

Milione VR, Kanat IO. Burns: A review of the pathophysiology, treatment, and complications. J Foot Surg 24: 373-382, 1985.

Moed BR, Thorderson PK: Measurement of intracompartmental pressure: A comparison of the slit catheter, side-ported needle, and simple needles. J Bone Joint Surg 75-A: 231-235,1993.

Motoki DS, Mulliken JB: The healing of bone and cartilage. Clin Plast Surg 17: 527-540, 1990.

Mueller JJ: Ruptures and lacerations of the tibialis posterior tendon. JAPA 74: 109-119, 1984.

Myerson MS: Experimental decompression of the fascial compartments of the foot: The basis for fasciotomy in acute compartment syndromes. Foot Ankle. 8: 308-314, 1988.

Myerson MS: Management of compartment syndromes of the foot. Clin Orthop 271: 239-248,1991.

O'Donoghue DH: Treatment of injuries to athletes, ed 3, Philadelphia, 1976, WB Saunders.

Oloff LM, Jacobs, AM: Fracture nonunion. Clin Pod Surg 2: 379-401, 1985.

O'Neill JA: Burns: Office evaluation and management. Primary Care 3: 351, 1976.

Orva S, Hulkko A: Delayed unions and non-unions of stress fractures in athletes, Am J Sports Med 16:378-382, 1988.

Perlman MD, et al: Traumatic classifications of the foot and ankle. J Foot Surg 28:551-583, 1989.

Pulla RJ, Pickard LJ, Carnett TS: Frostbite: an overview with case presentations, J Foot Ankle Surg 33(1):53-63, 1994.

Reinherz RP, et al: Recognizing unusual tendon pathology at the ankle. J Foot Surg 25:278-283,1986.

Resnick CD, Fallat LM: Puncture wounds: Therapeutic considerations and a new classification. 29: 147-153, 1990.

Richardson EG: Injuries to the hallucal sesamoids in the athlete, Foot Ankle 7:229-244, 1987.

Rockett MS, Gentile SC, Gudas SJ, et al: The use of ultrasonography for the detection of retained wooden foreign bodies in the foot, J Foot Ankle Surg 34(5): 478-484, 510-511, 1995.

Rogers LF, Campbell RE: Fractures and dislocations of the foot. Sern Roentgen 13: 157-166,1978.

Rorabeck CH, Caastle TS, Hardie R, et al: Compartment pressure measurements: an experimental investigation using the slit catheter, Trauma 21:446-449, 1981.

Rosen JS, Cleary JE: Surgical management of wounds. Clin Pod Med Surg 8: 891-907, 1991.

Rosenberg ZS, Cheung Y, Chass MH, et al: Rupture of posterior tibial tendon: CT and MR imaging with surgical correlation, Radiology 169:229-235, 1988.

Rosenberg ZS, Feldman F, Singson RD: Peroneal tendon injuries: CT analysis, Radiology 161:743-748, 1986.

Rowe CR, Sakellarides H, Freeman P, Sorbie C: Fractures of os calcis: a long-term follow-up study of one hundred forty-six patients, JAMA 184:920, 1963.

Rude C: Management of closed fractures. Clin Pod 2: 199-215, 1985.

Sabharwal H, Mitra A: The initial evaluation and treatment of lower extremity trauma. Trauma 10: 108-116, 1993.

Salter RB, Harris R: Injuries involving the epiphyseal plate. J Bone joint Surg 45-A: 587-622,1963.

Sammarco GJ: Peroneal tendon injuries: foot and ankle injuries in sports, Orthop Clin North Am 25:135-145, 1994.

Sammarco GJ: The Jones fracture, Instr Course Lect 42:201-205, 1993.

Sammarco GJ: Turf toe, Instr Course Lect 42:207-212, 1993.

Sanders R, Fortin P, DiPasquale T, Walling A: Operative treatment in 120 displaced intra-articular calcaneal fractures: results using a prognostic computed tomography scan classification, Clin Orthop 290:87, 1993.

Sanford JP: Bites from pet animals. Hosp Pract 79-87, 1993.

Sangeorzan BJ: Foot and Ankle Joint Trauma. Orthopaedic Trauma Protocols. Chap. 28, pp.339-368, 1993.

Sartoris DJ: Diagnosis of foot trauma: The essentials. J Foot Ankle Surg 32: 539-549,1993.

Scheller AD, et al: Tendon injuries about the ankle. Clin Orthop 11: 801-811, 1980.

Schoen NS, Gottlieb LJ, Zachary LS: Distribution of pedal burns by source and depth, J Foot Ankle Surg 35(3): 194-198, 1996.

Schwab RA, Powers RD: Conservative therapy of plantar puncture wounds, J Emerg Med 13(3):291-295, 1995.

Scurran BL: Fractures in children. Clin Pod 2: 365-377, 1985.

Seligson D, Gassman J, Pope M: Ankle instability: evaluation of the lateral ankle ligaments, Am J Sports Med 8:39-42, 1980.

Shereff MJ: Fractures of the forefoot, Instr Course Lect 39:133-140, 1990.

Smith GH: Measurement of the intracompartmental pressures of the foot. J Foot Surg 29: 589-592,1990.

Smith T: Pedal dislocations. Clin Pod 2: 349-363, 1985.

Smith TF, Vito GR: Subluxing peroneal tendons. Clin Pod Med Surg 8: 555-577, 1991.

Stanifer E, Wertheimer S: Review of the management of open fractures. J Foot Surg 3 1: 350-354,1992. 99. Stewart IM: Jones fracture: fracture of the base of the fifth metatarsal, Clin Orthop 16:190-198, 1960.

Tepelidis NJ, Karstetter K: Management of acute trauma. Clin Pod Med Surg 8: 757-770, 1991.

Van Hal ME, Keene JS, Lange TA, et al: Stress fractures of the sesamoids, Am J Sports Med 10:122-128, 1982.

Verdile VP, Freed HA, Gerard J: Puncture wounds to the foot, J Emerg Med 7(2): 193-199, 1989.

Walter JW, Goss LR, Rockett MS: Penetrating wound trauma to the foot and ankle complex. The Lower Extremity. Vol. 5(2), 1-15, 1998.

Walter JW, Goss LR: Metatarsal fractures. McGlamery's Comprehensive Textbook of Foot and Ankle Surgery. Editors Banks, AS, Downey, MS, Martin, DE, Miller, SJ. 3rd edition. pp. 1775-1791, 2001.

Wilson EC, Phillips HO, Gilbert JA: Plantar flexion injuries of the ankle, Clin Orthop 306:97-102, 1994.

Yablon IG, Heller FG, Shouse L: The key role of the lateral malleolus in displaced fractures of the ankle, J Bone Joint Surg 59:169, 1977.

CHAPTER 5
TRAUMA TO THE FOOT AND ANKLE

1.   In a patient who sustains polytrauma, at what stage would you draw blood for type and cross?

    A.   Rapid primary survey
    B.   Resuscitation of vital function
    C.   Detailed secondary survey
    D.   Definitive care initiated

2.   In the management of the polytrauma patient, a complete neurological examination, such as the Glasgow Coma Scale, would be included in what stage?

    A.   Rapid primary survey
    B.   Resuscitation of vital functions
    C.   Detailed secondary survey
    D.   Definitive care initiated

3.   Place the following in the correct order the following conditions in a patient who sustained polytrauma.

    1. Hemorrhage
    2. Sucking chest wound
    3. Asphyxia
    4. Splint fractures
    5. Shock

        A.   3, 1, 2, 5, 4
        B.   1, 2, 3, 4, 5
        C.   5, 3, 2, 1, 4
        D.   2, 1, 3, 5, 4

4.   Using the Glasgow Coma Scale, a score of 6 has what percentage of survival?

    A.   No change of survival
    B.   Less than 30%
    C.   Greater than 50%
    D.   100% change of survival

5.   Class III hemorrhagic shock is defined as?

    A.   Loss of less than 15% of blood volume
    B.   Loss of 15-30% of blood volume
    C.   Loss of 30-40% of blood volume
    D.   Loss of greater than 50% of blood volume

6.   Which of the following statements is **FALSE** concerning shock management?

    A.   Give O positive blood to females in their child bearing years
    B.   Give O positive to males
    C.   The universal donor blood is O negative blood
    D.   There is no place for vasopressors (epinephrine) in the treatment of shock

7.   A 36 year-old patient presents to the ER 36 hours after stepping on a fishhook. He is unsure of his tetanus
        status. What is the proper regimen?

        A.   No treatment is needed
        B.   0.5 ml of toxoid and 250 units tetanus immunoglobulin
        C.   250 units tetanus immune globulin (TIG)
        D.   500 units tetanus immune globulin (TIG)

8.   The most common organism that causes Osteomyelitis after a puncture wound is?

        A.   Pseudomonas aureginosa
        B.   Escherichia coli
        C.   Staphylococcus aureus
        D.   Klebsiella pneumonia

9.   Which of the following is not appropriate treatment for a P. aureginosa infection?

        A.   Aztreonam 1-2 grams Q8h
        B.   Levaquin 500 mg QO/IV
        C.   Clindamycin 900 mg IV Q6h
        D.   Ceftazidime 2 grams IV Q12h

10.   Which of the following statements if **FALSE** concerning bite wounds?

        A.   Most bite wounds are caused by dogs
        B.   The most dangerous of bite wounds is caused by humans
        C.   The most common organism to cause infection in dog bites is Pasteurella multocida
        D.   Tetanus prophylaxis should be considered in all bite wounds

11.   The most common isolate from human bites is **Eikenella Corrodens**.

        A.   True
        B.   False

12.   Rabies prophylaxis using the HDCV (Human Diploid Cell Vaccine) is given:

        A.   1, 2, 7, 14, and 28 days after the initial bite
        B.   3, 6, 9, 18, and 36 days after the initial bite
        C.   5, 10, 20, 40, and 80 days after the initial bite
        D.   Single dose that is given near the bite wound

13.   An open fracture with a 7.0 cm laceration, extensive soft tissue damage, exposed bone and arterial injury
        would be classified as?

        A.   Gustilo-Anderson Type I
        B.   Gustilo-Anderson Type II
        C.   Gustilo-Anderson Type IIIA
        D.   Gustilo-Anderson Type IIIC

14.   Open fractures are considered **infected** up to 6 to 8 hours post occurrence without treatment.

        A.   True
        B.   False

15.   Which is the correct order in closed reduction of fractures?

        1.   Distal traction on the fracture fragments
        2.   Reversing the mechanism of injury that produced the fracture
        3.   Traction along the long axis of the bone to increase the deformity
        4.   Post-reduction radiographs

                A.   1, 2, 3, 4
                B.   4, 1, 3, 2
                C.   3, 1, 2, 4
                D.   2, 3, 4, 1

16.   Using the Rosenthal classification for nail and distal tip injuries, a Zone I injury corresponds to:

                A.   Distal to the phalanx
                B.   Distal to the lunula
                C.   Proximal to the distal end of the lunula
                D.   Amputation at the IPJ

17.   A nail bed rupture should be considered when a subungual hematoma involves how much of the nail plate?

                A.   5%
                B.   10%
                C.   15%
                D.   25%

18.   A patient who sustains a lawnmower injury of his great toe and requires a plantar V-Y advancement flap for closure is termed:

                A.   Kutler flap
                B.   Atasoy flap
                C.   Newmeyer flap
                D.   Kilgore flap

19.   The most common mechanism of injury for a turf toe injury is:

                A.   Hyperextension
                B.   Hyperflexion
                C.   Hyperpronation
                D.   Hypersupination

20.   Biomechanical derangements that predispose a sesamoidal injury include all of the following except:

                A.   Cavus foot type
                B.   Peroneus longus spasm
                C.   Pronated foot type
                D.   Metatarsus primus equinus

21.   Which of the following is not a radiographic sign that suggests a fractured sesamoid rather than a bipartite sesamoid?

        A.   Irregular separation line
        B.   Bone callus formation
        C.   Interrupted peripheral cortices
        D.   Similar findings on a contralateral film

22.   What is the classification of a great toe dislocation that has a dorsally dislocated proximal phalanx and sesamoids with an intact intersesamoidal ligament and without a sesamoid fracture present?

        A.   Jahss Type I dislocation
        B.   Jahss Type IIA dislocation
        C.   Jahss Type IIB dislocation
        D.   Jahss Type III dislocation

23.   The most common location of stress fractures in the lower extremity is:

        A.   Metatarsals
        B.   Navicular
        C.   Calcaneus
        D.   Fibula and tibia

24.   What type of fifth metatarsal base fracture represents an extra-articular avulsion fracture of the epiphysis that is seen in children?

        A.   Stewart Type II
        B.   Stewart Type III
        C.   Stewart Type IV
        D.   Stewart Type V

25.   Regarding the Stewart classification, which of the following classifications does not match up?

        A.   Type 1 = True Jones fracture
        B.   Type 2 = Extra-articular with one or two fracture lines
        C.   Type 3 = Avulsion fracture of the 5th metatarsal base
        D.   Type 4 = Comminuted, extra-articular fracture

26.   In a tarsometatarsal fracture/dislocation, the LisFranc's ligament may rupture, where is the structure anatomically located?

        A.   Connecting the first metatarsal base and second metatarsal base together
        B.   Between the medial cuneiform and the base of the second metatarsal
        C.   Plantar to the first metatarsal and medial cuneiform
        D.   Connecting the medial cuneiform to the middle cuneiform

27.   What is the most commonly fractured tarsal bone?

        A.   Talus
        B.   Calcaneus
        C.   Navicular
        D.   Cuboid

28.   What is the classification of a tarsometatarsal fracture/dislocation that has partial incongruity with an isolated medial displacement of the first ray?

       A.   Hardcastle Type A
       B.   Hardcastle Type B1
       C.   Hardcastle Type B2
       D.   Hardcastle Type C1

29.   What is the most common type of navicular fracture?

       A.   Fracture of the tuberosity
       B.   Fracture of the dorsal lip
       C.   Fracture of the navicular body
       D.   Stress fracture of the navicular

30.   The "**Nutcracker syndrome**" is most commonly associated with what type of navicular fracture?

       A.   Watson-Jones Type I
       B.   Watson-Jones Type II
       C.   Watson-Jones Type IIIA
       D.   Watson-Jones Type IV

31.   A Watson-Jones Type IIIB fracture corresponds to:

       A.   Fracture of the navicular tuberosity
       B.   Dorsal lip fracture of the navicular
       C.   Non-displaced navicular body fracture
       D.   Displaced navicular body fracture

32.   The deltoid artery branch, which supplies the talar body, is derived from what primary artery?

       A.   Anterior tibial artery
       B.   Perforating personeal artery
       C.   Posterior tibial artery
       D.   Artery of the sinus tarsi

33.   What is the classification of a displaced vertical talar neck fracture with associated dislocations of the subtalar joint and ankle joint?

       A.   Hawkins' Group I fracture
       B.   Hawkins' Group II fracture
       C.   Hawkins' Group III fracture
       D.   Hawkins' Group IV fracture

34.   A partially detached osteochondral fragment of the talus is classified as a:

       A.   Berndt-Harty Stage I
       B.   Berndt-Harty Stage II
       C.   Berndt-Harty Stage III
       D.   Berndt-Harty Stage IV

35.   Which of the following statements is **TRUE** concerning talar fractures?

    A.   The "Hawkins' sign" is best visualized on a lateral radiograph
    B.   In a Hawkins' Group I fracture two of the three primary blood vessels supplying the talus are interrupted
    C.   The treatment of choice for a Hawkins' Type 1 is ORIF
    D.   The presence of the Hawkins' sign indicates restoration of the talar blood supply and represents a sign of viability

36.   Which of the following statements is **FALSE** concerning the Hawkins' sign?

    A.   Represents a sign of viability
    B.   Represents subchondral atrophy due to hyperemia
    C.   Usually seen on lateral radiograph
    D.   Typically seen on radiograph between 6 to 8 weeks

37.   Which of the following statements is **TRUE** concerning osteochondral talar dome lesions?

    A.   Osteochondritis dissecans is an acute condition involving a loose fragment of cartilage and necrotic bone
    B.   A Berndt-Hardy State 3 lesion is completely detached yet remaining in the defect
    C.   According to Berndt-Hardy, medial defects occur more often than lateral defects
    D.   Plantarflexion and inversion results in anterolateral lesions

38.   A fracture of the lateral talar process is classified as:

    A.   Sneppen Group I
    B.   Sneppen Group II
    C.   Sneppen Group III
    D.   Sneppen Group IV

39.   What percentage of patients with a calcaneal fracture sustains an injury to the spine?

    A.   1%
    B.   10%
    C.   30%
    D.   50%

40.   Which of the following statements is **TRUE** concerning calcaneal fractures?

    A.   Bohler's angle is between 25-40 degrees while the crucial angle of Gissane is between 125-140 degrees
    B.   The crucial angle of Gissane is decreased in a calcaneal fracture
    C.   A Rowe 2a involves the Achilles insertion
    D.   A Rowe 1c is an avulsion fracture of the calcaneal tuberosity

41.   An os calcaneal secondarius is often confused for what type of fracture?

    A.   Rowe Type Ia
    B.   Rowe Type Ib
    C.   Rowe Type Ic
    D.   Rowe Type Iia

42.   Regarding the Sanders classification, which of the following statement is correct?

        A.   This classification is based on axial and coronal CT images of the posterior calcaneal
                facet
        B.   Three lines break up the posterior facet into three fragments staring from medial to lateral
        C.   It addresses only intra-articular talar fractures
        D.   All are correct statements

43.   A patient who sustained a calcaneal fracture had a CT scan which revealed a five-fragment intra-articular
        calcaneal fracture that was non-displaced, what would the Sanders' classification correspond to?

        A.   Type I
        B.   Type II
        C.   Type III
        D.   Type IV

44.   Which of the following represents the proper sequence of calcaneal fracture reduction?

        A.   Return heel to valgus position, insert Schantz for reduction, restore height, medial translation
        B.   Insert Schantz pin for reduction, restore height, return heel to valgus, medial translation
        C.   Medial translation, insert Schantz pin for reduction, restore height, return heel to valgus
        D.   Restore height, insert Schantz pin for reduction, medial translation, return heel to valgus

45.   Which of the following is **NOT** a lateral ankle ligament?

        A.   Anterotalofibular ligament
        B.   Calcaneofibular ligament
        C.   Posterotalofibular ligament
        D.   Tibiocalcaneal ligament

46.   Which of the following statements is **FALSE** concerning lateral ankle instability?

        A.   A positive anterior drawer sign is greater than 5 mm when compared to the contralateral side
        B.   A positive talar tilt sign is greater than 10 degrees when compared to the contralateral side
        C.   A positive anterior drawer sign is indicative a torn ATFL and CFL
        D.   A positive talar tilt is indicative of a tear of both the ATFL and CFL

47.   Which of the following is **NOT** a Weber and Cech avascular non-union type?

        A.   Oligotrophic type
        B.   Defect type
        C.   Atrophic type
        D.   Torsional wedge type

48.   What would a Weber C ankle fracture correspond to?

        A.   Fibula fracture is located **below** the level of the syndesmosis level
        B.   Fibula fracture **at** the level of the joint
        C.   Fibula fracture **above** the level of the joint
        D.   Any fracture of the medial malleolus

49.   What is the **HALLMARK** fracture of a Supination-Adduction ankle fracture?

    A.   Transverse fibula fracture below the level of the ankle joint
    B.   High fibula fracture
    C.   Vertical fracture of the medial malleolus
    D.   Both A and C are correct

50.   What is a Wagstaffe-Lefort fracture?

    A.   Avulsion fracture of tubercle of Chaput of the tibia
    B.   Avulsion fracture off the fibula
    C.   Spiral fracture of the fibula that occurs as high as the proximal one-third
    D.   Transverse fracture of the fibula 5.0 to 7.5 cm above the distal end and associated with a tear of the deltoid ligament and lateral subluxation of the talus

PHYSICAL MEDICINE AND REHABILITATION, ORTHOTICS, AND PROSTHETICS

James B. McGuire

DEFINITIONS

I. Physical Therapy: That branch of medical science devoted to the study and application of various physical modalities or agents in the treatment and restoration of human neuromusculoskeletal dysfunction

II. Physical Therapist: A licensed health professional educated and trained to plan and administer prescribed physical therapy treatment programs designed to restore function, relieve pain, and prevent disability following disease, injury, or loss of a body part

III. Physical Therapist Assistant: A licensed health professional educated and trained to administer physical therapy services under the direct supervision of a licensed physical therapist

IV. Physical Medicine: The application of various physical modalities, agents, and therapeutic exercises by a licensed physician or physical therapist in the treatment and restoration of human neuromusculoskeletal dysfunction. The practice of physical medicine and rehabilitation involves the medical examination and evaluation of the disabilities of injured or disabled patients, the administration of physical medicine modalities or treatments, the prescription and medical supervision of physical, occupational, and other forms of therapy, the training of the handicapped person in ambulation and self care, and medical supervision and coordination of other rehabilitation procedures

V. Members of the Rehabilitation Team:

Physician: M.D., D.O., D.P.M.

Physical, Occupational, Recreational Therapist

Therapist Assistant

Speech Therapist

Social Worker

Nurse, Nurse Educator

Psychiatrist, Psychologist

Dietician

Clergy

Family

DOCUMENTATION IN PHYSICAL MEDICINE

I. Plan of Care Includes:

A. Detailed History
B. Physical Examination
C. Physical Assessment, Diagnosis, Prognosis
D. Establishment of Short Term Goals
E. Establishment of Long Term Goals
F. Treatment Program to Reach Stated Goals Including: modalities, exercise, etc.
G. Time Table for Completion
H. Discharge Planning

II. The Physical Medicine Record Must Include:

A. Initial History and Physical Examination
B. Plan of Care as Outlined Above
C. Daily Soap Notes or Flow Chart
D. Weekly Summary and Goal Revision
E. Discharge Note and Plan

III. Definitions

A. "A Physical Medicine Treatment consists of a planned program to relieve symptoms, improve function, and prevent further disability for individuals disabled by chronic or acute disease or injury."[3]
B. "...payment is prohibited for medical services that are for prevention, palliation, research, or experimentation. Palliation is generally defined as relieving or easing pain temporarily."[3]
C. Physical Medicine Services must be:
   1. Restorative - There must be the expectation that the patient's Condition will Improve significantly in a Reasonable and Predictable period of time
   2. Related to a Written Treatment Plan
   3. Reasonable in Amount, Frequency, and Duration
   4. Requiring the Judgement, Knowledge, and Skills of a physician or physical therapist

to perform the services

5. Records must show <u>Objective Measures</u> to document improvement
6. Reviewed <u>Periodically (Weekly)</u> to show progress

IV. The Physical Therapy Prescription must include:

A. Diagnosis
B. Date of injury or surgery
C. Surgery performed or history of injury
D. Precautions or contraindications to therapy
E. Modalities or services requested
F. Timetable for reevaluation (# weeks of therapy)
G. Physician signature and degree
H. Physician license #

PHYSICAL MODALITIES, CONDITIONS COMMONLY TREATED, AND FREQUENCY OF USE IN PODIATRIC MEDICINE (TABLE 1)

Modality	Condition	Frequency
1. Superficial heating modalities		
a. Infared	Pain	Rare
1. Lamps	muscle spasm	
2. Bakers		Rare
3. Monochromatic light stimulation		Occasional
b. Hydrocollator packs	Pain, spasm Fibrosis Stable contusion > 48 hrs. Superficial tendonitis Myositis, fasciitis Reflex vasodilatation of the lower extremity	Occasional
c. Paraffin	Pain, spasm Contracture Distal, small joint chronic synovitis Tendonitis, fasciitis, myositis	Occasional: Hygiene problems with repeated use of paraffin have reduced the use of this once commonly used modality
d. Fluidotherapy	Pain, spasm Distal joint, chronic synovitis Contracture Tendonitis	Frequent: No hygiene problems as in paraffin

Fasciitis, myositis
Stable contusion > 48 hrs.
Chronic edema
Osteoarthritis
Rheumatoid arthritis
Wound or ulcer healing

e.	Whirlpool, contrast baths	Pain, spasm Distal joint, chronic synovitis Contracture Tendonitis, fasciitis, myositis Chronic or acute contusion Chronic or acute edema Osteoarthritis Rheumatoid arthritis Pre-exercise warm-up Wound or ulcer debridement	Frequent
f.	Pool therapy	Limited weight-bearing exercise Buoyancy-assisted exercise Viscosity-resisted exercise	Frequent

2. Deep heating modalities

a.	Ultrasound	Pain, spasm Contracture Loss of connective tissue, distensibility Chronic tendonitis, Synovids, fasciitis, or myositis Myofascial trigger points Phonophoresis of selected medications (Cortisone most common) Osteoarthritis Rheumatoid arthritis Injection dispersal (Pulsed Mode)	Frequent
b.	Diathermy microwave short wave	All of the above except phonophoresis and dispersal of injections	Rare <u>Multiple precautions and cotraindications:</u> Acute inflammation and bleeding, fluid collections in tissues

Ischemia or insensitivity
Joint effusion
Excessive sweating
Moist dressings
Exposure to gonads
Boney prominences
Epiphyses in children
Pacemakers
Metal implants or jewelry

3. Cryotherapeutic modalities

a.	Ice:
	packs
	massage
	immersion
	cold compression
	units
		Pain, spasm
		Acute or Chronic:
		  Contusion,
		  Hematoma, tendonitis
		  Synovitis, fasciitis
		  Myositis
		  Myofascial trigger points
		  Sprain, strain, fracture
		  Post operation pain or
		    Edema
			Frequent

b.	Cold spray
	ethyl chloride
		Myofascial trigger points
		Spasticity: Contact-Relax
		  technique
		Pre-injection topical
		  anesthetic
			Frequent

4. Ultraviolet
2000 - 4000 A
UVC 2000 - 2900 A
UVB 2900 - 3200 A

UVA 3200 - 4000 A
PUVA Therapy
exposure
UVB and C most

Folliculitis
Dermatitis

Ulcer asepsis
Tinea pedis
Psoriasis
2%-5% Coal Tar Ointment

Methoxalen and UVA
  common

Rare
Complicated Dosing
MED <u>minimal erythemal
dose</u> - 24 hours post
exposure

1st Degree E.D. 2.5 X
  MED
2nd degree E.D. 5 X
  MED
Lamp height 30 in.

Perpendicular to skin 5
  seconds longer for each
  consecutive exposure
Protective eyewear
Multiple Complications
Porphyria, Pellegra,
Lupus erythematosis
Sarcoidosis, herpes
Herpes simplex
Xeroderma pigmentosa

		Acute eczema or psoriasis
		Renal or hepatic insufficiency
		Diabetes, hyperthyroidism
		Advanced arteriosclerosis
		Pulmonary tuberculosis

5. Low power or cold laser — Myofascial trigger points / Pain / Wound healing — Rare: unproven efficacy

6. Intermittent compression devices / Non-segmental, segmental — Acute or chronic / Lymphedema — Occasional

7. Electrical stimulation — Pain, spasm / Improve ROM / Tissue healing / Enhance muscle training / Muscle reeducation / Edema reduction by muscle pump — Frequent

   a. Alternating (biphase) current stimulators — — Frequent

   1. NMES: (Neuromuscular Electrical Stimulation) H-Wave Time-modulated AC (Russian Stimulation) — Edema reduction by muscle pump / Prevent muscle atrophy

   2. TENS: (Transcutaneous Electrical Nerve Stimulator)

   3. TEAM: (Tannenbaum Electro Analgesia Method)

   4. IF: (Interferential Stimulation)

   5. MENS: (Microcurrent Electrical Nerve Stimulation)

   6. FES (Functional E-Stim) — Dynamic bracing (heel activated doriflexor stimulation)

b. Direct (Galvanic) Current Stimulators	Same as above	Frequent
1. HVPC: High-volt pulsed current		
2. LVPC: Low Volt Pulsed Current (rarely used today)		
3. LIDC: Low-intensity direct current	Ulcer healing Bone healing Iontophoresis of selected ions	
c. Surface Electrode EMG	Muscle re-education	Occasional
d. E-stimulation for pain control:- Preferred modalities		Frequent
1. TENS: Biphasic pulsed AC, traditional, limited use		
2. TEAM: High frequency, biphasic, amplitude modulated, burst mode stimulator		
3. H-Wave: Exponentially decaying, biphasic wave stimulator		
4. IF: Questionable efficacy for pain control		
e. Diapulse Induction E-Stim	Wound healing Reduce inflammation	Occasional

V. PHYSIOLOGIC EFFECTS OF HEAT AND COLD

A. Effects of Heat

Increased local superficial temperature
Increased local metabolism
Vasodilitation
Increased blood flow
Increased leukocytes and phagocytosis
Increased capillary permeability and edema formation
Increased lymphatic and venous drainage
Increased metabolic waste production
Increased nerve conduction
Increased elasticity of connective tissue
Analgesia

Decreased muscle tone
Decreased muscle spasm

B. Effects of Cold
Decreased local temperature
Decreased metabolism
Vasoconstriction, initially
Decreased blood flow, initially
Decreased nerve conduction
Decreased delivery of leukocytes and phagocytes
Decreased capillary permeability
Decreased lymphatic and venous drainage
Decreased muscle excitability
Anesthesia
Reflex vasodilatation - Hunting response

C. Mechanisms of Heat Transfer and examples
1. Conduction – hot/cold pack
2. Convection - whirlpool
3. Radiation - infrared lamp
4. Energy Conversion - ultrasound
5. Evaporation - ethyl chloride spray

VI. DEEP HEATING MODALITIES

A. Ultrasound (figure 1)
1. Components
    a. High frequency generator

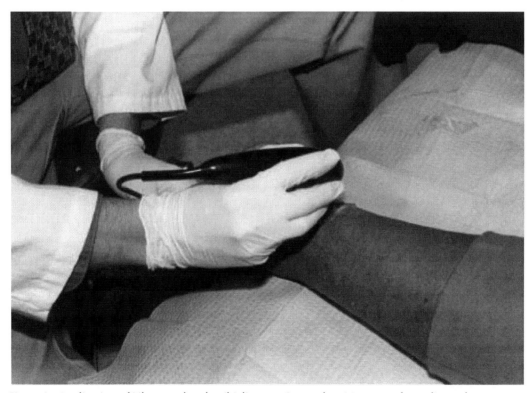

Figure 1: Application of Ultrasound to the tibialis posterior tendon. Note use of coupling gel

      b. Oscillator

      c. Transformer

      d. Coaxial cable

      e. Transducer – Applicator

2. Peizoelectric effect

    Mechanism of ultrasound generation:

        Electrical to mechanical energy conversion. Alternating current passing across a quartz or synthetic crystal produces an alternating compression and expansion of the crystal and generates a high frequency sound wave

3. HEAT transfer by energy conversion:

        Mechanical (sound) energy is converted to heat energy. Vibration of the transducer produces high frequency inter-mollecular friction within the target tissue

4. Therapeutic Ultrasound Frequency 0.75 - 3.0 Mega Hertz MHZ

    1.0 MHZ ultrasound - absorbed in deeper tissues, penetrates 3-5 cm

    3.0 MHZ ultrasound - absorbed in superficial tissues, penetrates 1-2 cm

5. Physiologic Effects

      a. Thermal - see Sect. V A. Effects of Heat

      b. Non-Thermal

          i. Cavitation - expansion and contraction of gas bubbles within the tissues

            Stable cavitation - positive therapeutic effects

            Unstable cavitation - tissue damage

         ii. Accoustic steaming - unidirectional movement of fluids along cell membranes

        iii. Non-thermal effects increase cell permeablity and may stimulate tissue healing Increase sodium and calcium ion permeablity

            Increase fibroblastic activity

            Increase protein synthesis

            Improve tissue regeneration

            Increase blood flow in chronically ischemic tissues

            Increase bone healing

            Improved healing non-union fractures phonophoresis

6. Transmission of Ultrasound Energy[10]

      a. Requires a mechanical medium or coupling agent

         i. Ultrasound gel

         ii. Underwater ultrasound

      b. Absorption is dependent on Tissue Impedance or the resistance of a tissue to the flow of ultrasound energy. Referred to as Attenuation of ultrasound energy

      c. Highest energy absorption is found in peripheral nerve tissues, then bone, then muscle, then fat. Lowest absorption occurs in blood or plasma. Potential for nerve damage exists if over irradiated

      d. Energy is reflected at tissue interfaces. The greater the difference in impedance between two interfacing tissues, the greater the reflection. 15%-40% at the soft tissue-bone interface. 1% at the soft tissue-fat interface. 100% at soft tissue/air interface

      e. A Hot Spot or Standing Wave is produced when the transmitted wave meets a reflected wave within the tissues. The Periosteum is a common site and produces what is commonly referred to as a "periosteal bone burn"

7. Continuous vs. pulsed ultrasound

      a. Pulsed ultrasound increases the mechanical effects of ultrasound within the tissues

b. The duty cycle of the ultrasound is usually expressed as 20%, 50%, or 100% (continuous)

$$\text{Duty Cycle} = \frac{\text{On Time (Pulse Duration)}}{\text{On Time + Off Time (Pulse Period)}} \times 100\%$$

c. Continuous ultrasound or use of the 100% duty cycle increases thermal effects within the tissues

8. Effective Intensity[8]

a. Expressed in <u>Watts/CM²</u> or <u>Total Watts.</u> Total Watts measures machine output and does not take into account the surface area of the transducer or applicator

b. Range 0.25 - 3.0 W CM²[4] Watts per cm² measures energy per unit area and is consistent from transducer to transducer

c. Temporal average intensity (used with pulsed ultrasound)

Duty cycle x Intensity in w/cm divided by 100

$$\frac{(50\% \times 2.0 \text{ w/cm}^2)}{100} = 1.0 \text{ w/cm}^2$$

This equals the effective intensity of the ultrasound delivered in a specific treatment and explains why you have to double the intensity of 50% pulsed ultrasound to deliver the same amount of energy as 100% or continuous ultrasound if both are applied for the same period of time

9. Dosage

a. Determined by intensity and duration of treatment

b. Dependent on:
   i. Tissue impedance
   ii. Depth of target tissue
   iii. Presence or absence of fat
   iv. Proximity of bone
   v. Area of tissue to be treated

c. Recommended dosages generally range between 2-3 minutes for each area 1 1/2 times the size of the transducer diameter, i.e., if the diameter of the transducer is 2 cm the effective treatment area is 3 cm in diameter. The treatment for an area 6 cm in diameter should last between 4-6 minutes[3]

d. Average treatment time for most foot applications is 6-8 minutes

10. Phonophoresis[4]

a. Utilizing ultrasound energy to drive medications through the skin into the subdermal tissues

b. Common medications used in phonophoresis
   i. Hydrocordsone
   ii. Dexamethasone
   iii. Salicylates
   iv. Lidocaine

c. Maximum recorded depth of penetration 5-6 cm

d. Both pulsed or continuous ultrasound can be used. Pulsed ultrasound may be preferred because of its greater mechanical effects [3]

e. Method of Application: First, rub medication into the skin completely then use regular coupling agents. Creams are poor transmission agents because they are air filled emulsions and should not be used as coupling agents or alone for phonophoresis

11. Contraindications and precautions[11,12]

a. Acute hemorrhage or hematoma - may cause vasodilation and interfere with clot formation. Hot spots may develop in areas of excess fluid accummulation

    b. Acute inflammation - increased vasodilation may aggravate areas of inflammation and increase local edema and tissue metabolism

    c. Thrombophlebitis - ultrasound may dislodge thrombi and increase risk of an embolus

    d. Peripheral vascular disease - patients have an inability to dissipate heat, which may result in tissue damage

    e. Impaired sensation - titration of dosage and prevention of hot spots depends on intact sensation

    f. Epiphyseal areas - irradiation of epiphyses may cause local tissue damage and early calcification

    g. Over metal or silicone implants - metal implants dissipate heat well and can be irradiated with caution. 3.0 Mhz preferrable because of shallow penetration. Silicone implants absorb ultrasound energy and may over-heat if irradiated excessively

    h. Malignancy - may increase risk of metastasis

    i. Over eye, heart, testicles, or pregnant uterus

B. Diathermy - limited use in the foot

    1. High frequency electromagnetic energy

        a. Thermal effects - see Section IV A

        b. Amount of heating depends on:

            i. Current density

            ii. Tissue resistance

            iii. Time on

            iv. Pulsed vs. continuous

    2. Short wave

        a. High frequency radio waves

            27.12 MHz wave length 11 meters

            13.56 MHz wave length 22 meters

        b. Alternating electrical and magnetic fields produce heating in the tissues by manipulation of dipole molecules. Conversion of electrical to magnetic to heat energy

        c. Selective heating of subcutaneous fat limits its use in some areas

        d. Electrodes

            i. Airspace capacitor electrodes

            ii. Pad electrodes

            iii. Induction coil electrode

            iv. Drum electrode

        e. Contraindications: short and microwave diathermy

            i. Fluid filled areas or organs

            ii. Excess perspiration

            iii. Moist wound dressings

            iv. Menstruation

            v. Gonadal exposure

            vi. Over boney prominences

            vii. Cardiac pacemakers

            viii.Metal jewelry

    3. Microwave diathermy

        a. High frequency (2456 MHz or 915 MHz) short wave length electrical field generator. Little magnetic effect

    b. Tissue heating by conversion of electrical energy to heat in the target tissues secondary to vibration of dipole molecules within the electrical field

    c. Single head applicator or electrode beams energy toward the tissues

    d. Selective heating of fat or tissues with high water content also seen with microwave

    e. Contraindications - same as for shortwave

VII. SUPERFICIAL HEATING MODALITIES

  A. Hydrotherapy (figure 2)

     1. Physiologic effect: See Sect. IV. Effects of Heat and Cold

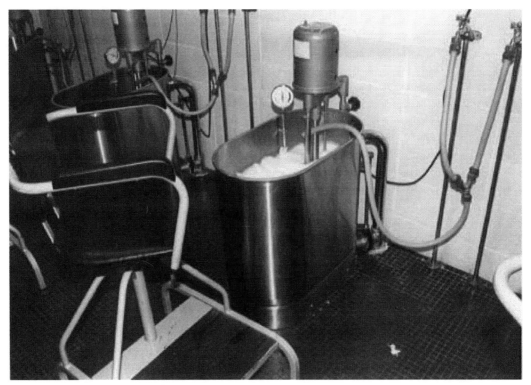

Figure 2: Foot and Ankle Whirlpool

     2. Physical properties of water

       a. Cohesion, viscosity - used to increase resistance to movement within the water and facilitate exercise

       b. Buoyancy, specific gravity - used in buoyancy-assisted movements to reduce resistance on the moving limb

       c. Hydrostatic pressure - used to facilitate the movement of fluids within the limb and help in the reduction of edema

       d. Mechanical effects

          The physical properties of water are used in therapeutic pool exercises to reduce weight bearing (**Buoyancy**) and resist (**Cohesion**) or assist (**Buoyancy**) motions performed in the water. Edema reduction can be achieved by deep immersion using the **Hydrostatic Pressure** effect. Ulcer debridement is performed utilizing the **Mechanical Effects** of moving water

     3. Heating or cooling occurs by conduction and convection

      a. Whirlpool temperatures[4]
- i. Cold 55°-65°F
- ii. Cool 65°-80°F
- iii. Tepid 80°-90°F
- iv. Neutral 92°-96°
- v. Warm 96°-98°F
- vi. Hot 98°-104°

Maximum Whirlpool Temperature Should Not Exceed 115°F

4. Scalding occurs at approximately 118°-120°F
5. Duration of treatment 20-30 minutes
6. Whirlpool additives and cleaning agents
   a. Chloramine-T (Chlorazene™) the preferred additive 100-200 ppm
      Less tissue irritation than Povidone-Iodine
      Equal disinfectant ability
   b. Sanizene™ the preferred surface disinfectant
   c. Povidone - iodine solution or surgical scrub also used as additive and surface disinfectant. Iodine sensitivity and cellular damage in granulating wounds may be a problem
7. Contraindications, precautions
   Peripheral vascular disease - inability to dissipate heat
   Loss of sensation - inability to report overheating or cold damage
   Acute inflammation - heat worsens acute conditions, particularly edema
   Vasospastic disorders, Raynaud's - cold triggers vasoconstriction
   Extreme hypersensitivity to aggitation
   Extremes of age: infants, aged have a decreased ability to dissipate heat

B. Fluidotherapy
1. Superficial heater
2. Dry heat utilizing suspended cork particles in a moving airstream
3. Provides heat, massage, desensitization
4. Slower heat transfer than water allows use of higher temperatures 110°-125°F
5. Sanitary - may be used with open wounds as limb is covered with stockinette or a plastic sleeve during treatment

C. Monochromatic Infrared Radiation - Anodyne™ (figure 3)
1. Stimulates the RBCs and cells of the endothelial lining of the microvasculature to release Nitric Oxide NO into the blood stream
2. Reduces local tissue inflammation
3. Promotes wound healing

VIII. ELECTROTHERAPY

A. Types of Current
1. AC alternating or biphasic current
2. DC direct or monophasic current - Also referred to as Galvanic current
3. Pulsed polyphasic current

B. Physiologic Response to Electrical Currents[10]
1. Excitation of nerve cells
2. Changes in membrane permeability
3. Protein synthesis
4. Fibroblastic and osteoblastic stimulation

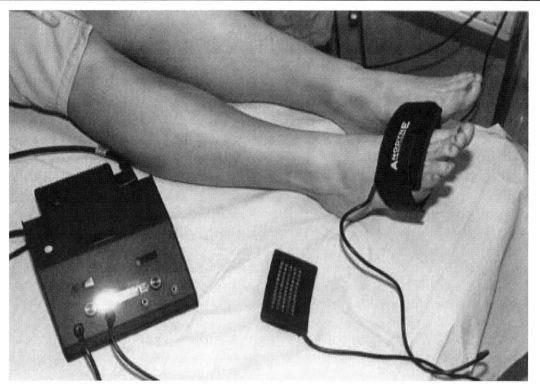

Figure 3: Anodyne infrared stimulator

    5. Changes in microcirculation
    6. Smooth and skeletal muscle contraction
    7. Tissue healing
    8. Increase joint mobility
    9. Enhance muscle fiber recruitment
   10. Muscle pumping action to improve lymphatic and venous flow
   11. Analgesic effects[10]
       a. Peripheral via gate and central biasing theories of Melzak and Wall
       b. Central via endogenous opioid theory of castel
   12. Gate theory of pain control
      Stimulation from A-Beta fiber afferents can result in a relative dampening or
      blocking of pain impulses carried by A-Delta and C afferents via their action on the
      substantia gelatinosa and the transmission cells within the spinal cord
   13. Central biasing theory
      Descending efferent fibers from the central nervous system (thalamus and brainstem)
      are able to block pain transmission of A-Delta and C fibers by its action on the
      substantia gelatinosa. Explains how emotion or previous experience may modify
      pain perception
   14. Castel endogenous opioid theory
      Ascending stimulation from A-Delta and C fibers via stimulation of the
      periaqueductal grey region of the midbrain and the raphe nucleus in the pons and
      medulla results in descending stimulation of serotoninergic and enkephalinergic
      interneurons which have an inhibitory effect on the transmission cells blocking the
      transmission of pain

C. Clinical Uses of Electrical Stimulation
    1. Produce muscle contraction by direct muscle stimulation or stimulation of the

innervating nerve
2. Pain control by peripheral or central mechanisms
3. Enhance tissue healing of wounds or ulcers
4. Enhance bone healing
5. Iontophoresis - movement of ionically charged medications across the skin using the polar effects of galvanic or continuous direct current stimulators
   Example: Phoresor 110 by Iomed

D. Direct Current Stimulators (figure 4)

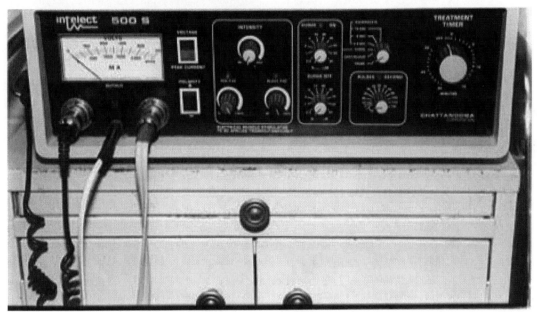

Figure 4: High volt pulsed galvanic stimulator

1. Biggest difference between DC and AC is DC's ability to cause chemical changes in the tissues
2. Medical galvanism[12] - the polarity effects of direct current stimulators allowing the accumulation of charged ions under each pole or electrode of the stimulator
3. Cathode: The <u>negative pole</u>. Usually the <u>active electrode</u> for muscle stimulation. <u>Sodium hydroxide</u> accumulates at this electrode producing an <u>alkaline reaction</u>, which results in <u>sclerolysis</u> or softening of tissues and is the mechanism of production for what is commonly referred to as the <u>galvanic burn</u>
4. Anode: The <u>positive pole</u>. Usually the <u>indifferent electrode.</u> <u>Hydrochloric</u> acid accumulates at this electrode producing an acidic reaction which results in sclerosis or hardening of tissues
5. Overall effect of any electrical stimulation depends on: [10]
   a. AC vs. DC
   b. Tissue resistance to current flow, impedance
   c. Current density or size of electrode
   d. Frequency of the current
   e. Intensity of the current
   f. Duration of the current
   g. Polarity of the active electrode
   h. Placement of the electrodes
6. Bacteriostatic effect may be seen under either the anode (+) or cathode (-) at different

intensities. Both electrodes have a bacteristatic effect at 5-10 <u>milliamps</u>. Only the cathode at 1.0 <u>milliamp</u> or less. Used in the treatment of infected ulcers

7. Enhanced bone or soft tissue healing is seen under the anode (+) at an intensity of 200-400 Milliamps. Low intensity stimulators are commonly employed in implantible stimulators used to enhance bone healing in delayed or non-union situations

8. Iontophoresis
   a. Quantity of ions transferred is dependent on the duration and current density measured in milliamp-minutes
   b. The stimulator must produce a continuous direct current at a constant voltage
   c. An important safety feature is an auto shutoff if skin impedance drops below a set limit because of the likelihood of a Galvanic burn
   d. Positive ions commonly used:
      i. Copper .... Fungicidal
      ii. Dexamethasone .... anti-inflammatory
      iii. Hyaluronidase ...... edema reduction
      iv. Lidocaine .... analgesic
      v. Zinc .... ulcer healing
   e. Negative ions commonly used:
      i. Acetate .... dissolve calcific deposits
      ii. Chlorine .... sclerolytic to scars
      iii. Citrate .... anti-inflammatory
      iv. Hydrocortisone .... anti-inflammatory
   f. Multipolar solutions used with alternating polarities:
      i. Tap water - reduce hyperhidrosis
      ii. Ringers - ulcer treatment

9. High volt pulsed stimulators or high volt galvanic stimulators
   a. High voltage 2000-2500 milliamps
   b. Short pulse duration 15-20 microseconds
   c. Increases the comfort of galvanic stimulation
   d. Increases depth of penetration
   e. Can be used for Neuromuscular E-Stim (NMES)

E. Alternating Current Stimulators (figure 5)
   1. Interferential current:
      a. Amplitude modulated AC
      b. Produced by the intersection of two circuits of slightly different frequency within the tissues
      c. Constructive and destructive interference produces a 3rd current or <u>beat frequency</u> within the tissues equal to the difference between the two frequencies, i.e.,
         Circuit A - Circuit B = Beat Frequency
         4000 hz-3900 hz = 100 hz
      d. Most effective for:
         i. Deep tissue stimulation
         ii. Pain relief
         iii. Tissue healing/osteogenesis
         iv. Neuromuscular stimulation
   2. Neuromuscular Electrical Stimulators (NMES)
      a. Interferential
      b. HVGS high volt galvanic stimulation
      c. Russian stimulation or time modulated AC stim (painful)

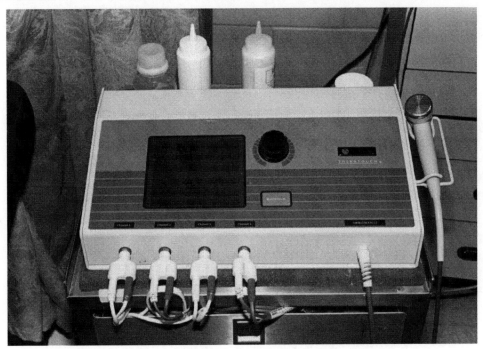

Figure 5: Combination Ultrasound and four channel electrical stimulator

      d. H-Wave-exponentially decaying biphasic wave
          Very comfortable stimulation
          May help in diabetic neuropathy
      e. Uses:
          i. Enhancement of muscle contraction during exercise
          ii. Muscle reeducation after inactivity or injury
          iii. Prevention of muscle atrophy during cast immobilization
          iv. Edema reduction by muscle pump action
3. Electrical Stimulation for Pain Control
      a. See Table 1, Section 7D
      b. Recent evidence has shown that pain control with TENS may be very limited
      c. Electrode placement is crucial to the success of any electrical stimulator used for pain relief
          i. Dermatome, Myotome
          ii. Trigger points
          iii. Peripheral nerve distribution
          iv. Accupuncture points
4. TEAM - Tannenbaum ElectroAnalgesia Method
    High Frequency, bi-phasic, amplitude modulated, burst mode stimulator
    May control pain better than traditional TENS
5. Functional Electrical Stimulation FES
      a. Use of electrical stimulation to replace bracing. Ex. foot switch activated, tibialis anterior stimulation at heel strike to prevent foot drop
6. Induction coil stimulation - Diapulse™ (figure 6)
      a. Electromagnetic induction of an electrical field in the sub-cutaneous tissues
      b. See Table 1, Section 7 E

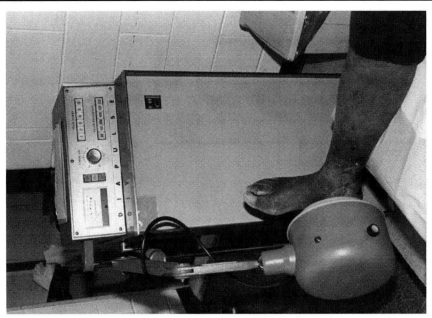

Figure 6: Diapulse induction coil electrical stimulator applied for healing of a venous stasis ulcer

IX. THERAPEUTIC EXERCISE AND MANUAL THERAPIES

A. Methods of Assessment

1. Range of motion - goniometric measurement
2. Manual muscle testing (table 2)
3. Myometric measurement - devices used to quantify force of contraction
   Example: Nicholas muscle tester
4. Isokinetic testing - recording robotic exercise devices
5. Functional testing - task specific proficiency. Example: number of toe raises to test ankle plantarflexion strength
6. Balance and coordination assessment
7. Sensory testing

Table 2.

Polio Foundation	Lovett	ROM	Resistance
5	Normal	Full	Normal
4	Good	Full	Moderate
3	Fair	Full	Against gravity only
2	Poor	Full	Gravity eliminated
1	Trace	No-motion	Palpable contraction
0	0	No-motion	No contraction

B. Passive Range of Motion PROM (figure 7)

1. Therapist performed movements
2. Includes: simple ROM, stretching techniques, joint mobilization, joint manipulation

C. Active Assisted ROM (figure 8)

Therapist assisted active movements

D. Active ROM

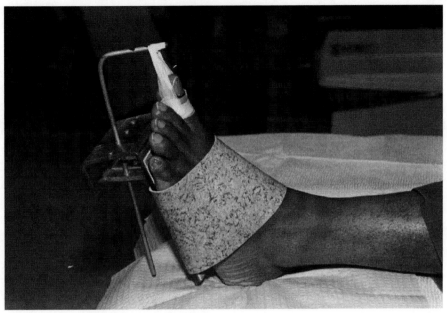

Figure 7: Passive stretching using the Whitney traction device

1.   Patient controlled movements
2.   <u>Open chain movements in</u> the lower extremity - proximal limb stable or fixed, distal limb free, non-weight bearing
3.   Closed <u>chain movements</u> in the lower extremity - distal limb stable, proximal limb free, weight-bearing (figure 9a and b)

E.   Progressive Resistive Exercises
1.   Increasing loads applied to the musculoskeletal system in a controlled manner
2.   Isometric exercise
   a.   Same length = iso + metric
   b.   Muscle increases tension while maintaining a fixed length

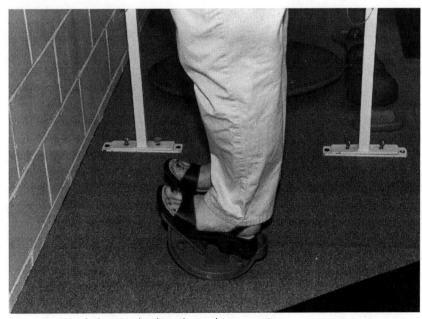

Figure 8: Weight bearing heel cord stretching exercises

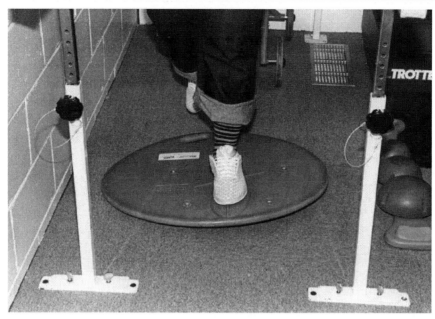

Figure 9a: Biomechanical Ankle Platform System closed chain exercise

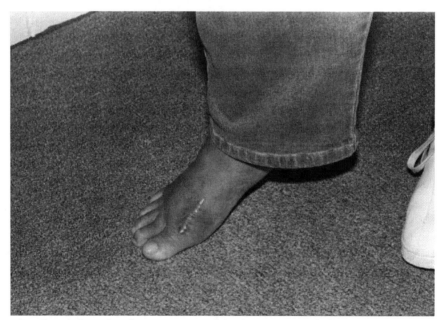

Figure 9b: Closed chain dorsiflexion exercise of the first metatarsophalangeal joint

      c. No joint motion occurs
3. Isotonic exercise
      a. Same weight = iso + tonic
      b. Muscle length and tension varies throughout a motion against a fixed or constant load. Example: Free weights
      c. Joint motion occurs with isotonic exercise (figure 10)
4. Isokinetic exercise
      a. Same speed = iso + kinetic
      b. Muscle length varies throughout a motion at a constant speed against a variable resistance

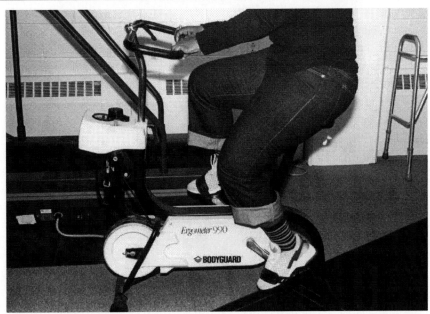

Figure 10: Cycling for progressive strengthening and improved range of motion

  c. Robotic or mechanical exercise devices. Examples: Biodex, Cybex, Kincom
   i. Calls for a maximal muscle contraction at each speed tested
 5. Types of muscle contraction
  a. Concentric - a shortening contraction. Example: Gastroc-Soleus ankle plantarflexion at propulsion
  b. Eccentric - a lengthening contraction. Example: Gastroc-Soleus slowing of the forward progression of the tibia during midstance
  c. Isometric - a stabilizing contraction where no joint motion occurs and there is no change in muscle length

F. Advanced Closed Chain Exercises
 1. Proprioceptive neuromuscular facilitation exercises
  a. Exercises that incorporate joint, skin, and balance input to produce improvement in motor output emphasizing balance and stability
  b. Includes:
   i. Stretching techniques
   ii. Manual exercise techniques
   iii. Biomechanical Ankle Platform System (BAPS) and other closed chain exercise devices
 2. Plyometrics
  a. Rapid eccentric loading of the musculoskeletal complex incorporating ballistic stretch and rapid muscle response
   Example: jumping activities
 3. Functional Progression Principle
  Ordered progression of motion, weight bearing and strength gains
  Example: cycling to walking to lunges to jogging to running to cutting to jumping
 4. SAID principle: Specific Adaptation to Imposed Demands. Muscle training specific for the sport or activity utilized during the training. Crossover from one sport or activity to another is often poor

G. Manual Therapies
 1. Massage

    a. Effleurage - light stroking motions, superficial

    b. Petrissage - deep, kneading of muscles and soft tissues

    c. Friction - localized, specific aggressive manipulation of soft tissues. Frequently utilized with scar tissue, fibrosis, or in myofascial release techniques

    d. Percussion - tapping or hitting of involved tissues. Deep. Commonly used in respiratory therapy

    e. Vibration - shaking of tissues. Helps induce relaxation. Also used in respiratory therapy

2. Accupressure - deep forceful manipulation of specific accupuncture points along established Meridans delininated by tradition for subjective relief of pain or symptoms

3. Myofascial release - a technique utilizing massage, tissue mobilization, cold spray, and stretching to release areas of muscle spasm or myofascial adhesion producing definable patterns of local and referred pain

4. Joint mobilization

    a. Joint play: Small passive movements available to a joint in the loose-pack or relaxed position. Necessary for normal movements. Grade I-IV oscillations are gentle pain free movements used to gradually improve and increase joint and soft tissue mobility. Oscillations are gently controlled to and fro or rocking motions designed to slowly stretch contracted tissues. They are graded based on the force utilized and the distance moved

    b. Gentle <u>pain free</u> movements designed to increase joint play, eliminate restrictions, and maximize joint motion

5. Joint manipulation

    a. Grade V oscillations

    b. Small amplitude, quick thrust movements designed to break adhesions or restrictions limiting pain free mobility

    c. The typical "Chiropractic" manipulation

H. Pool Therapy

1. Utilization of the physical properties of water to enhance exercise

2. Buoyancy - used to reduce weight stress on the lower extremities and enhance exercises assisted by limb floatation

3. Viscosity - used to increase resistance during certain movements and provide mild resistive exercise

4. Specific gravity and increased hydrostatic pressure with increasing depth - used to aid in edema reduction and proximal migration of fluids during exercise

5. Superficial heat - watch for systemic heating effects because of amount of body surface area heated

X. AMBULATORY AIDS

A. Crutches

1. Types: standard, lofstrand, platform

2. Crutch fitting

    a. Crutch tips 2" forward of and 6" outside of the toes

    b. Crutch tops 2" (three finger breadths) below the axilla

    c. Elbows flexed 20°

3. Crutch gaits: 2 point, 3 point, 4 point

4. Non, partial, full-weight bearing

    5. Elevations: stairs, curbs, ramps
       a. Uninvolved foot leads when ascending
       b. Involved foot leads when descending

B. Walkers (figure 11)
    1. Types: standard, folding, rolling, platform, reciprocal, kneeling
    2. Fitting: walker height is set so that the elbows are flexed 20°
    3. Gait patterns: step/hop to, step/hop through.

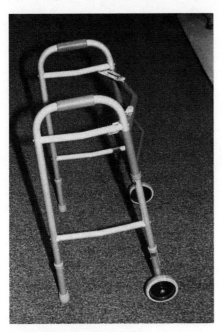

Figure 11: Wheeled Walker

C. Canes
    1. Types: standard, ortho-ease, adjustable
    2. Fitting: cane height is adjusted so that the elbow is flexed 20° when standing with the cane comfortably at your side
    3. Gait: use on the side <u>opposite</u> the injury. Cane and involved limb move together
    4. Weight reduction = none
       a. Used for balance only. The cane increases your base of support (BOS)

D. Wheelchairs
    1. Frames
       a. Rigid - lighter more stable
       b. Folding - heavier easier to transport and store
    2. Wheels - rear
       a. Mag - heavy, durable
       b. Spokes - lighter, less durable

    3. Tires
       a. Hard rubber
       b. Pneumatic
       c. Pneumatic with inserts
    4. Handrims
       a. Large/small diameter
       b. Thick
       c. Knobby
    5. Casters - front wheels
       a. Large - outdoor
       b. Small - indoor
    6. Seat cushions
       a. Foam
       b. Contoured foam
       c. Gel filled
       d. Foam with gel insert
       e. Air-filled villous

XI. ORTHOSES USED IN REHABILITATION

A. Definitions
    1. <u>Orthosis</u> - a device used to mechanically assist, restrict, or control function of the

musculo-skeletal system

2. <u>Foot orthosis</u> - a mechanical intermediary between the foot and the shoe
3. <u>Shoe fitter</u> - a person trained in the sizing and dispensing of proper fitting footwear
4. <u>Pedorthist</u> - a professional certified in the manufacture, dispensing, and adjustment of foot and foot and ankle orthoses prescribed by a licensed physician
5. <u>Orthotist</u> - a professional certified in the manufacture, dispensing, and adjustment of upper extremity, lower extremity, and spinal orthoses prescribed by a licensed physician
6. <u>Prosthetist</u> - a professional certified in the manufacture, dispensing, and adjustment of prosthetic devices prescribed by a licensed physician

B. **Materials** [6]
   1. Leather - earliest orthotic material
      a. Functional or accommodative depending on thickness or number of layers laminated together
      b. Thickness measured in: Inches, millimeters, irons, ounces
   2. Steel
      a. Rarely used for foot orthoses today
      b. Used for brace components and shoe shanks
   3. Aluminum
      a. Used for brace components
      b. Lightweight
   4. Rubber
      a. Latex - natural rubber strengthened by vulcanization
      b. Rubber butter - latex rubber & wood, cork, leather, or the moldable synthetic materials
      c. Commercially available cork & latex combinations
         Cushion Cork
         Korex™
         Orthocork™
         Thermocork™-heat moldable
      d. Synthetic rubbers solids or foams available
         i. Styrene-butadiene rubber (SBR) open cell multiple durometer
         ii. Nickleplast - multiple durometer
         iii. Spenco closed cell neoprene
         iv. Lynco open cell neoprene
   5. Open cell = conforming, accommodative, will bottom out. Closed cell shock absorption, protective, will <u>not</u> bottom out
   6. Polyurethane foam
      a. Thermosetting - not heat moldable
         i. Injected or poured into a mold under heat and pressure
         ii. Commonly used for running or walking shoe insoles
      b. Open or closed cell available
      c. PORON, PPT™ shock absorbing
         Open cell foam - even though it is open cell its density prevents it from bottoming out or compressing so it essentially behaves like closed cell foam
      d. Vylite™- closed cell polyurethane
      e. Orthofeet System™ - in-office manufactured polyurethane device
      f. Alimed D-soles™ commercially produced urediane/plastzaote combination
         i. Diabasole™ commercially produced poron/plastzaote combination

7. Polyolefins
   a. Polyethylenes
      i. Polyethylene Foams - accommodative. Will deform over time. Can be used to produce a temporary functional device
      ii. Plastazote™ #1 soft, #2 firm, #3 rigid
      iii. Evazote™ 1 durometer available
      iv. Peliteg™ 4 durometers
      v. Aliplast™ 6 Soft - 10 firm, XPE rigid
   b. Polyethylene Thermoplastics
      i. High Density – Ortholen™
      ii. Ultra High Density - Sub-Ortholen™ will deform or fracture over time when compared with polypropylene
      iii. Low Density – Aquaplast™ low temperature molding (hot water can be used to soften Aquaplast). Little use in foot orthoses. Commonly used in hand orthoses
   c. Polypropylenes
      i. High density thermoplastic
      ii. Excellent memory - will not deform if thickness appropriate for the patient's weight
      iii. Superform™ polypropylene with a nylon mesh laminated to the material to increase strength
      iv. Carbon flex - carbon impregnated polypropylene used to increase strength of the material
      v. Polypropylenes are usually posted with EVA or ethylene vinyl acetate. EVA comes in variable durometers, and can be a fairly noncompressible material depending on its durometer
8. Rohadur™ copolymer of methymethacrylate and acrylonitrile, also known as Thermolast II
   a. No longer manufactured by the Rohm and Haus Corp. in Germany
   b. Rigid control - posted with polymethylemethacrylate or ethylene vinyl acetate (EVA)
   c. The original material chosen for the Root functional orthosis
9. Polydur™
   a. A fairly recently developed acrylonitrile designed to be a replacement for Rohadur
   b. Rigid, unbreakable, heat moldable
10. Carbon graphite acrylic
    a. Graphite laminated with liquid resin
    b. TL-61™ earlier version
    c. TL-2100™ present version has improved strength and durability
    d. Tough, resilient, heat, moldable, may crack if not appropriately supported in heavy patients
11. Fiberglass
    a. Cannot be heat molded
    b. Rarely used today
12. Viscoelastic devices
    a. Sorbothane™ - a commercially produced polyurethane derivative
    b. Viscolas™
    c. Viscohte™

       d. Superior shock absorption, sticky, will bottom out over time

13. Silicone Copolymers
    a. Reicken's PQ™ variable durometer depending on the ratio of silicone copolymer to hardening agent. Superior shock absorption and accommodation. Difficult to use in orthotic construction
    b. Silipos™ sheeting and prefabricated pads - commercial use of silicone polymer technology

14. Polyvinyl Chlorine PVC
    a. Naugehyde - topcover

15. Polyamide (nylon)
    a. Cambrell - topcover

16. Silicone mold digital orthoses - use of silicone polymer technology to produce digital shields and orthoses
Examples:
    a. Moldable Podiatric Compound MPC™
    b. Berkoplast™
    c. Accumold™

17. Smart gel technology
Coploymer gels developed that respond to heat, light, pressure, and electrical current to change consistency and durometer

C. Foot Orthoses

1. Protective insoles
    a. Tissue supplement concept - utilizes shock absorbing, cushion materials such as those mentioned below to substitute for loss of natural padding
    b. Over the counter - protective insoles are commonly available in an OTC form
    c. Custom fitted - pads or accommodations are added to the insole to improve fit and its protective characteristics. Cut to fit and adjusted in the podiatrist's office
    d. Common materials: Spenco™, PPT™, Plastazote™, polyurethane™, Viscolas™, Laminates of various materials

2. Accommodative orthoses
    a. Dynamic molding - orthoses that gradually shape themselves to the foot utilizing body heat and the pressure of weight bearing
    b. Thermolding - orthoses that are shaped to the foot or a cast of the foot after they are heated to improve their malleability
    c. Custom fitted devices - usually they are manufactured from a prefabricated shell or orthoses that can be modified by the practitioner to customize the fit of the device
    d. Apertures, pads, bars, flanges
    e. Custom made devices - orthoses manufactured from a positive plaster cast or directly molded to the patient's foot
    f. Total contact molded insoles used in the treatment of diabetics, ulcers, neuropathy or PVD are examples of custom made devices
    g. Common materials: Plastazote, SBR, EVA, Nickleplast

3. Functional orthoses
    a. Rigid devices
        i. Root functional orthosis - a custom made orthosis fabricated from a rigid shell material molded to a neutral position off-weight bearing cast of the foot. Forefoot and rearfoot intrinsic or extrinsic posting is utilized to correct for malalignments; identified in a thorough biomechanical exam. This is a dynamic

device functioning in all three phases of gait; heel strike, midstance, propulsion

   ii. Roberts, Whitman, Schaeffer - three of the first orthotic designs used to control abnormal foot biomechanics. These have generally been replaced by the custom-made root functional device but are still available through many labs and in some OTC models

  iii. UCBL - developed at the University of California Biomechanics Lab for treatment of the flexible flat foot. It is fabricated around a weightbearing impression of the foot and utilizes a deep heelcup with long, high medial and lateral flanges to restrict pronation. Frequently used with cerebral palsy or other neurological conditions

  iv. Blake Inversion - originally developed to counteract marked pronatory forces encountered in running. Utilizes a significantly inverted standard off-weight bearing cast to produce a heel cup inverted 15° to as much as 75°. Requires significant arch fill to produce a device contoured to the patient's arch

   v. Kirby-Skive - a technique developed to produce an inverted heel similar to the Blake inversion orthosis without altering the natural arch contour and FF to RF relationship captured in the NP cast

  vi. Gait Plates, In-toe, Out-toe - rigid devices with extended medial or lateral anterior margins used to alter a child's gait to achieve a more cosmetic appearance. An elongated lateral margin induces out-toe and an elongated medial margin induces in-toe by forcing the child to adjust their angle of gait

 vii. Heel Stabilizers - rigid orthoses that utilize a deep heel cup with or without medial or lateral flanges to affect control of pronation by controlling calcaneal inversion and eversion

viii. The first ray cut-out - developed to address the need for independent first ray motion in propulsion. Commonly used with hallux limitus, functional hallux limitus, and hallux abducto valgus patients

  ix. DSIS Dynamic Stabilizing Innersole System - a combination of the UCBL deep heel cup with a varus offset or inversion of 5° to improve frontal plane control of the rearfoot. A deep midline cutout is utilized to encourage independent first and fifth ray motion

   x. OTC Pre-formed Orthoses (custom fitted) - because of the large variety of OTC devices now available and their relative economy preformed devices are commonly utilized to treat a wide variety of biomechanical imbalances in children and adults

b. Semi-Rigid devices

   i. It depends on thickness of many materials whether the material is rigid (4-6 mm polypropylene) or semi-rigid (2mm)

  ii. Direct mold orthosis - heat molded semi-rigid orthotics fabricated by directly molding the material to the weightbearing or semi-weight bearing foot

  iii. Custom fitted OTC - as there are numerous rigid devices available OTC there are also many semi-rigid materials to choose from

  iv. Laminated orthoses - combinations of variable durometer materials to achieve a device with properties of both materials utilized. Example: A rigid polypropylene shell with an accommodative plastazote top cover

    (a) Whitney CMO

      A semi-rigid laminated functional device emphasizing sagittal plane balancing as essential for the control of triplaner imbalances related to the anterior, posterior, or combined cavus foot deformities

(b) Sport orthoses - utilize lamination of various materials to provide accommodation, functional control, and shock absorption needed for specific sport conditions

D. Shoes[9]

1. Terminology

Bal - A front laced shoe with a V-shaped throat where the quarters are stitched or continuous with the vamp or upper part of the shoe over the metatarsals

Blucher - A front laced shoe where the quarters are not attached to the vamp distally to allow the throat to open wider for fitting. Standard on the "Oxford" shoe

Ball - The width of the sole at the metatarsal heads. Collar - the narrow strip of material or padding stitched around the top line or opening of the shoe

Brannok device - A measuring tool used to determine shoe size and width

Break - The crease or fold formed at the vamp of the shoe from dorsiflexion of the MPJ joints at push off

Combination last - A shoe form or last that deviates from standard proportions

Cookie - A longitudinal arch pad

Counter - The heel cup stiffener or reinforcing material. May be extended medially or laterally

Elevation - material added to the sole or plantar aspect of the shoe for leg length discrepancies

Flare - A widening of the shoe sole or heel

Goodyear welt - A shoe making process where the upper, inner, and outer soles are joined together by stitching

Goring - Elastic material inserted in the upper to allow the shoe to expand and accommodate the foot. Heel height - measurement from the ground up to the heel seat measured in eighths of an inch

Heel elevation - Material added to the heel for a limb length discrepancy or equinus position

Thomas heel - A heel with an elongated anteromedial aspect

Heel seat - The part of the sole on which the foot rests

Inflare or Inlast - A shoe last where the distal portion has more medial than lateral surface area. Curves inward or medially. The opposite of an out flare

Innersole - The material upon which the sole rests

Instep - Portion of the upper over the midfoot

Iron - Used to measure the thickness of the sole equal to 1/48 of an inch

Lace stay - Portion of the upper containing eyelets or lacing

Last - A wooden or plastic model around which a shoe is made

Last Systems - Method of sizing last dimensions

Length - Dimension on the center of the last from toe point to heel point

Levy mold - Full length contoured inlay

Metatarsal bar - A rubber leather or synthetic piece of rounded material applied externally to the sole or internally to the innersole with its apex just behind the metatarsal heads

Molded shoe - A custom made shoe using a plaster cast or the foot as a last

Outersole - The portion of the shoe that contacts the ground

Platform - An elevated sole

Rocker bar or sole - An angulated sole with its apex just behind the metatarsal heads which promotes a rocking action and eliminates the toe break at push off

Shank - The stiff inflexible area of the shoe between the heel and the ball

Toe box - Reinforced area of the shoe designed to protect the toes and maintain the shape of the shoe

Thomas heel – heel with the medial aspect extended out under the navicular

Vamp - The forepart of the shoe over the metatarsal shafts

2. Shoe types, styles - running, walking, tennis, crosstrainer, oxford, loafer, chukka, pump, mule, hiking

3. Orthopedic shoe – reinforced heel counter, steel shank, Blucher closure, Thomas heel

4. In-depth shoes - specially designed shoes to allow for increased toe room and a removable inner sole for an orthosis. Type covered under the Medicare Diabetic Shoe Bill

    Example: P.W Minor Extra Depth™, Drew™

5. Custom molded shoes – Used for odd sized or unusually shaped feet that cannot be accommodated in standard lasted footwear

E. Ankle-Foot Orthoses (AFO)[1,2]

1. Shoe attachments[2]

    a. Stirrup - a "U" shaped shoe attachment plate riveted to the steel shank of the shoe; used with metal braces

    b. Split stirrup - an attachment plate which allows the shoe to be removed from a double upright metal brace so the patient can wear alternative styles. Rectangular channels accept the flat steel arms of the two uprights

    c. Caliper - a round tube attached by a plate to the steel shank of the heel of the shoe which accepts the caliper ends of rounded steel uprights. Pivot is distal to the anatomical ankle joint causing motion of the brace on the foot and leg. Rarely used today

    d. Shoe insert - attachment of a double upright brace to a molded plastic shoe insert. Allows patient to change shoes freely. Replaced today by the Molded Ankle Foot Orthosis (MAFO)

    e. Scott-Craig reinforced solid stirrup - a "U" shaped shoe attachment plate with an angled reinforcement bar used with heavy patients

2. Double upright orthosis - The classic double upright brace with a fixed or movable ankle joint. Depending on the type of ankle joint the brace can provide free ankle motion, "stopped" or restricted motion, dorsiflexion assist, or knee movement control

    a. Ankle joints

        i.   Free - a simple free swinging hinge with no stops or restriction to motion

        ii. Solid - a fixed ankle joint providing no motion

        iii. Single Klenzak ankle joint uses a posterior spring within the joint to provide dorsiflexion assist in addition to a stop or pin that can be set to restrict plantarflexion ability

        iv. The double action ankle joint provides both dorsiflexion and plantar flexion range of motion utilizing adjustable pins or stops. When spring assist is used in the double action ankle joint it has been referred to as a double Klenzak

3. T-Straps for ankle varus/valgus control - leather restraining straps attached to the medial or lateral aspect of the shoe and running across the malleolus and up to the opposite upright to provide frontal plane support for excessive ankle varus or valgus

4. MAFO Molded Ankle Foot Orthosis - An AFO molded out of polypropylene[1] The most commonly used AFOs today

    a. Advantages - cost, cosmesis, light weight, interchangeable shoes, comfort, biomechanical foot support, varus/valgus control

    b. Custom made - fabricated from a cast of the patient's foot and leg

    c. Custom fitted - a pre-fabricated brace adjusted to fit each individual patient

   d. Solid MAFO - no ankle motion or slight motion allowed by the flexibility of the plastic itself
   e. Articulating MAFO - a MAFO with an ankle joint added to the device
       i. Replaces single & double upright braces
       ii. Common ankle joints utilized
           (a) Oklahoma joint - round plastic joints that can incorporate a plantar flexion stop or a dorsiflexion assist
           (b) Gillet joint - rubberized ankle joints that can be used to provide a free ankle, plantar flexory stop or dorsiflexion assist
           (c) PSA posterior spring assist - a spring loaded pin added to the posterior aspect of the MAFO to provide dorsiflexion assist to an otherwise free ankle joint
           (d) PAS posterior adjustable stop - a plantarflexion restriction stop added to the posterior aspect of the MAFO to allow for free dorsiflexion and limited plantarflexion in gait. Similar to the PSA without the spring
           (e) CAM joints - articulations that restrict motion to a predetermined arc set by small plastic or metal cams inserted into the joint itself
           (f) Gaffney joints - a metal free ankle joint. Heavy when compared to the Oklahoma
5. Tone reducing AFO or TRAFO: a MAFO utilizing a specifically molded foot plate with elevations and depressions strategically placed to reduce or enhance spastic tone to improve gait in CP, stroke, or other neurologic patients
6. Patellar tendon bearing braces
   a. Molded calf section - a polypropylene leg section intimately molded to the tibial condyles, patellar tendon, and popliteal space to cylindrically support the leg transferring weight from the patient's foot and ankle to the more proximal limb
   b. 40% weight reduction is the maximum you could expect
7. SACH modification
   a. Solid ankle cushion heel - concept
   b. Concept borrowed from prosthetic feet
   c. A variable durometer heel for the shoe is used to absorb shock at heel strike and provide a roll into midstance

F. Knee-Ankle Foot Orthoses (KAFO)[1,2]

Multiple knee bracing systems can be added to the AFO as already presented to improve knee stability in gait

G. Ischial Weight Bearing Brace (IWBB)

A KAFO that utilizes a high thigh shell with a proximal seat similar to those used in above knee prosthetics to transfer weight away from the foot, ankle, and knee to the proximal thigh and ischial tuberosity
1. A 70% weight reduction is the maximum you can expect from an IWBB under ideal conditions

H. Sport Knee Bracing[2]

Most commonly used for anterior cruciate ligament (ACL) and posterior cruciate ligament (PCL) injuries
1. Utilizes medial and lateral supports with mechanical joints and various limb suspension systems to provide anterior/posterior, medial/lateral, and rotational support for the affected knee joint
2. Most common braces:
   a. CTI™

    b. Lennox Hill™
    c. Edge™
    d. Donjoy™
    e. OMNI™
    f. Townsend™

I. Gait Training with Orthotic Devices:

An important aspect of physical medicine is evaluating the fit and proper function of lower extremity bracing including training in donning and doffing procedures and the proper use of the devices in gait and activities of daily living (ADL)

XII. LOWER EXTREMITY PROSTHETICS[1,2,7]

A. Level of Amputation

1. Digital
2. Ray or segment
3. Trans metatarsal
3. Lisfranc's - at the metatarsal cuneiform or cuboid joints
4. Chopart - at the mid-tarsal joint
5. Boyd - transcalcaneal osteotomy
6. Symes ankle disarticulation - may involve preservation of a portion of the talus or calcaneus; or a remodeling of the distal tibia and fibula
7. Below knee (BK) - the function of the prosthesis depends on the length of the tibia preserved in the amputation
8. Knee disarticulation - a difficult amputation to fit because of the type and level of the knee joint required for ambulation
9. Above knee (AK) - the function of the prosthesis also depends on the length of the femur preserved
10. Flip disarticulation/hemi pelvectomy - very difficult to fit and extremely difficult to learn to ambulate

B. Partial Foot Amputation Prosthetics

1. Short shoe - a custom molded shoe designed to provide an exact fit for the residual limb
2. Partial toe filler - an addition to an in-shoe orthosis used to take up space made by an amputated digit, ray, or entire forefoot
3. Shoe in shoe - a close fitting leather boot with a partial filler for the amputated segments which is inserted into a patient's own foot gear
4. MAFO with toe filler - the MAFO provides some medial and lateral stability and an anterior lever arm for the transmetatarsal, Lisfrancs, or Chopart amputation. Requires a rocker-soled shoe in order for it to work effectively
5. UCBL with toe filler - a short MAFO which eliminates the need for a rocker sole because of the free ankle joint
6. Lange silicone partial foot - a cosmetic replacement for the portion of the foot removed. Made out of silicone and pulled onto the residual limb. Not as functional as partial fillers. Hot. Skin occluded by the silicone

C. Prosthetic System Additions

Modifications needed to improve the function of a prosthetic

1. SACH Heel: A multidurometer compressible heel incorporated into the heel of an artificial foot or added to the heel of a shoe where a partial foot amputation prosthesis is being used. Functions like a heel roller

2. Heel elevations on either side may be needed to provide a level pelvis and a normal posture

3. Rocker bottom sole - used to provide a heel toe gait where you want to reduce distal pressure on a ray or transmetatarsal amputation or where a fixed ankle MAFO or brace has been used in conjunction with a partial filler. May be accompanied by a SACH or heel roller

4. Patellar tendon bearing addition to a MAFO or double upright brace may be used to reduce weight on a fragile residual limb

D. Symes Prosthesis

Uses the distal tibia and occasionally a portion of the calcaneus for a weight bearing surface. The natural flare of the malleoli are used for suspension of the prosthesis on the residual limb by means of a removable panel which allows entrance of the wide ankle into the prosthesis and then secures it snugly when it is replaced. Although this provides an excellent weight bearing surface for ambulation, the wide ankle is cosmetically unacceptable for many and the long prosthesis always requires a sole elevation on the opposite limb

E. Below Knee Prostheses [1,2,7]

1. Endoskeletal - this prosthesis uses an internal skeleton or pylon made of carbon fiber, plastic, aluminum alloy, or titanium to connect the residual limb socket and the prosthetic foot. It is covered by a soft, foam cosmetic skin which hides the structure. This is extremely light and is the preferred construction used today

2. Exoskeletal - a multilaminate prosthetic incorporating the socket and prosthetic foot in a single prosthesis. It is quite heavy and limited adjustments can be made after construction

3. Socket design and lining

    a. Patellar tendon-bearing socket (PTB)
        Allows transfer of 100% of the patient's weight to the residual limb. Triangular shaped socket with a flat posterior wall. Transfers weight to the medial and lateral tibial condyles, anteriortibial crest, and patellar tendon. Requires suspension by a suction socket, suspension sleeve, supracondylar cuff, waist belt, or thigh corset

    b. PTB Socket with a Supra Condylar Wedge PTB-SC
        Utilizes a wedge at the medial femoral epicondyle to make the socket self-suspending

    c. PTB Socket with Supracondylar/Suprapatellar Trimline PTB-SC/SP
        Suspension similar to PTB-SC. Used with short BK amputations when a corsetless suspension is desired

    d. PTB Socket with Joints and Corset PTB-J and C PTB socket with a hinged knee joint and thigh corset suspension. Maximum stability. Reduces weightbearing on the residual limb by up to 40%-60%

    e. Socket liners
        i. Hard socket - close fitting hard plastic
        ii. Soft socket - a soft insert made of polyethylene foam or silicone for protection and improved fit
        iii. 3-S silicone suction socket liner - A suction suspension system

F. Prosthetic feet [1,2,7]

1. Classification five types
    a. SACH foot
    b. Single-axis foot

     c. Multi-axis foot
     d. Solid ankle flexible keel foot
     e. Energy storing foot
  2. SACH foot
    Solid ankle cushion heel - a compressible heel allows for shock absorption at heel strike and roll-off for propulsion
  3. Single-axis foot
    A single mechanical axis with a combination of rubber bumpers or rigid stops to control ankle joint motion. Allows for quicker foot-flat for increased stability in gait
  4. Multi-axis foot
    Movement in all directions is permitted by a universal joint but limited by rubber bumpers or rigid stops. Improved shock absorption and stability on uneven ground. Examples: Greissinger Foot, Endolite Multiflex, SAFE II (Stationary Attachment Flexible Endoskeleton)
  5. Solid ankle flexible keel foot
    Lighter design. SACH heel with a flexible anterior keel. Improves shock absorption in late midstance. Examples: OttoBock, Kingsley Stored Energy (STEN)
  6. Energy storing effect
    Dynamic response feet. Utilize a spring keel of metal or graphite "leaf springs" to absorb energy during midstance and release it during propulsion to give the more active amputee a faster, more efficient gait. Examples: Seattle Foot, Carbon Copy II, Quantum Foot, Flex Foot

G. Knee Disarticulation Prostheses
  1. Endo vs. exoskeletal design - endoskeletal design provides a more cosmetically acceptable knee and is more functional than the older exoskeletal design that results in a long bulky prosthesis
  2. Socket design - similar to the Symes prosthesis. To accommodate the flare of the femoral condyles the socket may incorporate a removable window or an expandable inner liner
  3. Knee joints - the endoskeletal design requires a polycentric or "4-Bar Linkage" as other knee joints used with above knee amputations are too bulky and create a very long prosthetic limb with a joint that is too distal for proper function. The "4-Bar Linkage" allows for normal knee locking and swing with minimal added length and a better cosmetic appearance

H. Above Knee Prostheses[1,2,7]
  1. Socket designs
    a. Quadrilateral - a four sided total contact socket design with a flat, horizontal posterior shelf for ischial weight bearing, a narrow anterior to posterior dimension, and a wide medial to lateral dimension
    b. Narrow M-L or ischial containment socket - a total contact socket with an ischial shelf but with a narrow medial to lateral dimension. The narrow M-L socket includes lateral support for the greater trochanter and improves muscle control of the prosthetic limb allowing for more efficient ambulation at higher speeds in the active amputee
  2. Endo vs. exoskeleton
    Both are used today. Longer AK amputations require an exoskeletal design where shorter AK amputations do better with the endoskeletal prosthesis
  3. Knee joints
    A variety of knee joints are available for the AK prosthesis depending on the

patient's level of function. Single aids or polycentric, mechanical, hydraulic, or pneumatically controlled

    a. Hydraulic/pneumatic - not as commonly employed because of weight and expense. Examples: Mauch S-N-S, Endolite, Hydracadence

    b. Mechanical

        i. Single axis constant friction - rely on alignment for stability

       ii. Manual locking knee - can be manually unlocked for sitting, stiff knee in gait. Maximum stability

      iii. Weight activated stance control knee (SAFETY KNEE) locks on weightbearing to prevent buckling

      iv. 4-bar polycentric knee - instantaneous center of rotation allows for greater stability and improved symmetry in gait

  4. Foot design - all foot designs can be used with the AK prosthesis. Lightweight becomes more important with the AK than the BK prosthesis. See BK Prosthesis, Prosthetic Feet, Section 6

  5. Suspension mechanisms - the most common suspension is the suction socket. Pelvic belts with or without a hinged connection to the prosthesis or a light "Silesian belt" can be substituted in patients where the suction socket proves to be a problem

I. New Innovations in Prosthetic Design

  1. Robotics

  2. EMG control

J. Gait Training with Prosthetic Devices

Extensive training in prosthetic donning and doffing, stump care, and gait and balance are required to provide a fluid natural gait and a healthy stump. Ambulatory aids may be required for stability in older patients or those with additional neuromuscular impairment

REFERENCES

(1) Atlas of Orthotics: Biomechanical Principles and Application. American Academy of Orthopaedic Surgeons. C.V. Mosby Co., St. Louis, 1985.

(2) Braddon RL, et al. Physical Medicine and Rehabilitation. W.B. Saunders Co., Philadelphia, 1996.

(3) Department of Health and Human Services, Office of the Inspector General Report, March 1994.

(4) Helfand AE. Rehabilitation of the Foot. Clinics in Podiatry. W.B. Saunders Co., pp. 295-342, Philadelphia, 1984.

(5) Krusen FE, Kottke FJ, Ellwood PM. Handbook of Physical Medicine and Rehabilitation, 2 ed., W.B. Saunders Co., Philadelphia, 1981.

(6) Levitz SJ, Whiteside LS, Fitzgerald TA. Biomechanical foot therapy. Clin Pod Med Surg 5(3), pp. 721-736, 1988.

(7) Limb Prosthetics and Orthotics, J.E. Hanger, Inc., 1986.

(8) Michlovitz SL. Thermal Agents in Rehabilitation, 2nd ed. F.A. Davis Co., Philadelphia, 1990.

(9) PFA/BCP Desk Reference and Directory 1994/95. Pedorthic Footwear Association.

(10) Prentice WE: Therapeutic Modalities in Sports Medicine, 3rd ed. C.V. Mosby Co., St. Louis, 1994.

(11) Sammarco GJ. Rehabilitation of the Foot and Ankle. C.V. Mosby Co., St. Louis, 1995.

(12) Singer JM, Helfand, A.E. Physical Medicine and Rehabilitation for the Management of Foot Conditions. Hershey Board Certification Review Outline Study Notes. PA. Podiatric Medical Association. 1993.

CHAPTER 6
PHYSICAL MEDICINE AND REHABILITATION, ORTHOTICS, AND PROSTHETICS

1. If a patient is able to fully dorsiflex their ankle against moderate resistance the grade you would give them on a Polio Foundation muscle test is:

   A.   3
   B.   G
   C.   4
   D.   F +

2. The key elements that must be considered in developing a plan of care for a particular therapeutic modality:

   A.   Amount, Total modalities used, Intensity
   B.   Amount, Frequency, Duration
   C.   Frequency, Units of time, Intensity
   D.   Intensity, Duration, Settings

3. Treatments that ease pain temporarily are called:

   A.   Palliative
   B.   Restorative
   C.   Rehabilitative
   D.   Therapeutic

4. A licensed professional who provides physical therapy services under the direct supervision of a physical therapist is called:

   A.   Physical Therapy Aide
   B.   Physical Therapy Assistant
   C.   Therapeutic Assistant
   D.   Physical Medicine Assistant

5. In order for a physician to bill for Physical Medicine Services all the following must be part of the medical record except:

   A.   A thorough patient evaluation
   B.   A specific list of long and short term goals
   C.   A written treatment plan to reach stated goals
   D.   Specific contraindications to any modalities utilized
   E.   A time table for completion

6. The following deep heating modality selectively heats tissues that are high in water content resulting in the need for caution when using this modality over fluid filled organs or joint effusions:

   A.   Ultrasound
   B.   Shortwave Diathermy
   C.   Paraffin
   D.   Fluidotherapy

7.   All of the following conditions can be treated with ultrasound except:

        A.   Acute tibialis posterior tendonitis
        B.   Chronic tibialis posterior tendonitis
        C.   Plantar space abscess
        D.   Lateral ankle sprain
        E.   Scar adhesion

8.   Non-thermal effects of ultrasound are achieved through:

        A.   Cavitation
        B.   Acoustical streaming (microstreaming)
        C.   Excessive intermolecular friction
        D.   A and B
        E.   B and C

9.   The technique which uses ultrasonic energy to drive molecules through the skin is called:

        A.   Ultraphoresis
        B.   Iontophoresis
        C.   Sonography
        D.   Phonophoresis
        E.   Passive Transdermal Transmission (PTT)

10.   Which of the following is an example of a deep heating modality:

        A.   Whirlpool
        B.   Paraffin
        C.   Ultrasound
        D.   Fluidotherapy

11.   A professional certified in the manufacture, dispensing, and adjustment of upper extremity, lower extremity, and spinal orthoses prescribed by a licensed physician is called a:

        A.   Pedorthist
        B.   Orthotist
        C.   Prosthetist
        D.   Shoe fitter

12.   A foot orthosis developed for treatment of the flexible flat foot frequently used with cerebral palsy or other neurological conditions, fabricated around a weightbearing impression of the foot, utilizing a deep heel cup, and long high medial and lateral flanges to restrict pronation is called a:

        A.   Kirgy-skive orthosis
        B.   UCBL orthosis
        C.   Root functional orthosis
        D.   Blake inversion orthosis

13.   An orthotic ankle joint that uses a posterior spring within the joint to provide dorsiflexion assist in addition to a stop or pin that can be set to restrict plantarflexion ability is called a:

       A.   Gillette ankle joint
       B.   Klenzak ankle joint
       C.   Free ankle joint
       D.   Gaffney ankle joint

14.   A prosthesis that uses an internal skeleton or pylon made of carbon fiber, plastic, aluminum alloy, or titanium to connect the residual limb socket and the prosthetic foot and is covered by a soft, foam cosmetic skin which hides the structure is called:

       A.   Endoskeletal
       B.   Exoskkeletal
       C.   Patellar tendon bearing
       D.   SACH

Chapter 7

BIOMECHANICS

by Kendrick A. Whitney and Denise Freeman,
based on a chapter originally written by
Lester J. Jones

DEFINITIONS

I. The application of mechanical laws to the living structure (specifically to the human loco-motor system)

II. The study of the dynamic musculoskeletal system of the human being

BASIC TERMINOLOGY

I. **Cardinal body planes**
   A. Sagittal
   B. Frontal
   C. Transverse

II. **Motion**
   A. Pronation
   B. Supination
   C. Inversion
   D. Eversion
   E. Adduction
   F. Abduction
   G. Internal rotation
   H. External rotation
   I. Dorsiflexion
   J. Plantarflexion

III. Position
A. Pronated
B. Supinated
C. Inverted
D. Everted
E. Abducted
F. Adducted
G. Externally rotated
H. Internally rotated
I. Dorsiflexed
J. Plantarflexed

IV. Fixed positions
A. Adductus
B. Abductus
C. Elevatus
D. Varus
E. Valgus
F. Equinus (structural)
G. Calcaneus (structural)

V. Other terms
A. Hypermobility
B. Phylogeny
C. Anthropology
D. Ontogeny
E. Kinematics
F. Kinetics
G. Diarthrosis
H. Enarthrosis

ONTOGENIC DEVELOPMENT

I. Femur/tibia/fibula and foot
A. **Angle of inclination:** Frontal plane angulation
   1. Head and neck of the femur to the long axis of the femoral shaft: 160° at birth; 128° by adulthood
B. **Angle of declination:** Torsion within the shaft of the femur (transverse plane)
   1. Represented by the angulation of the head and neck of the femur to the femoral condyles
      a. At birth: 30°; 8°-10° by adulthood
   2. Represented by the angulation of the head and neck of the femur to the frontal plane
      a. At birth: 60° external; 8°-10° external at adult stage
   3. Antetorsion: Internal femoral torsion
   4. Anteversion: External femoral torsion
   5. Retrotorsion: External femoral position
   6. Retroversion: Internal femoral position

II. Malleoli

A. **The angular relationship of the malleoli to the frontal plane is 0° at birth**

B. **There is an external growth/twist/torque of 18°-23° true tibial torsion or 13°-18° of malleolar position that takes place in the transverse plane**

C. **Tibial varum:** Frontal plane inverted angulation of the lower leg to the ground in static stance

D. **Tibial valgum:** Frontal plane everted angulation of the lower leg to the ground in static stance

III. Rearfoot

A. **Relationship of the talus to the calcaneus**
   1. During fetal development there is frontal plane movement of the talus over the calcaneus from a more parallel position
   2. Talar head becomes less plantar-flexed relative to the body of the talus
      a. This is important for development of normal talo-calcaneal angulation; Cyma-line; talar declination angle, calcaneal inclination angle, and for normal midtarsal joint position

B. **Growth in length and width of metatarsal and phalanges from fetal development through birth to adulthood**
   1. There is a frontal plane torsion of metatarsals 1-5 in the direction of eversion
   2. Transverse relationship between the first metatarsal and lesser metatarsals
      a. During fetal development the first metatarsal is medially deviated by 50°
      b. At birth, the angle reduces to 6°
      c. This angulation increases to 7°-9° by age 4. If the angle increases beyond 7°-9°, the result will produce a juvenile hallux-abducto valgus and/or a metatarsus primus varus
      d. The lesser metatarsals are mildly adducted relative to the rearfoot and midfoot. At birth, this adductus is 25° and reduces to 15° to 18°

BIOMECHANICS OF THE LOWER EXTREMITY

I. Hip joint motion

A. **Diarthrosis**

B. **Enarthrosis:** Gliding, rotation, angulation, circumduction
   1. Permits motion in all three body planes
      a. Transverse plane: Internal/external range of motion (sagittal-frontal axis)
      b. Frontal plane: Abduction/adduction range of motion (sagittal-transverse axis)
      c. Sagittal plane: Flexion/extension/hyperextension (frontal-transverse axis)
   2. Mechanical axis of the hip: Center of hip to knee
   3. Axis of the femoral shaft: Greater to lesser trochanter relative to plane through femoral condyles

II. Knee joint motion

A. **Ginglymus:** 2° of freedom of movement

B. **Flexion-extension**

C. **Internal and external rotation**

D. **Transverse and sagittal plane motion**

   E. **Patella:** Increases lever action of the knee
   F. **Axes of motion**
        1. Transverse plane
        2. Frontal plane
        3. Gliding (flexion and extension)
             a. Important for mobility and stability of the knee joint
   G. **Rotation**
        1. Lateral femoral condyle rotates around medial condyle
        2. Rotation occurs between the tibia and meniscus
        3. Internal rotation: Lateral tibial condyle moves forward on lateral meniscus
        4. External rotation: Lateral condyle moves in reverse
        5. 5°-6° of transverse plane motion occurs with flexion and extension of the knee
        6. Greatest amount of transverse plane motion is observed with the knee at 90° of flexion
   H. **Non-weight-bearing:** Tibia rotates on femur; open kinetic chain motion
   I. **Weight-bearing:** Femur rotates on tibia; closed kinetic chain motion

III. **Ankle joint motion**

   A. **Diarthrosis:** Ginglymus joint (1° freedom of motion)
   B. **Articulation of the talus and the corresponding surfaces of the medial and lateral malleoli**
   C. **Demonstrates triplane motion:** Axis is oblique to all three body planes, but motion predominantly in sagittal plane

IV. **Subtalar joint motion**

   A. **Nature and quality of motion**
        1. Oblique hinge: Diarthrosis
        2. Triplane motion
        3. Motion from a fully pronated position to a fully supinated position describes an arc
             a. Two-thirds of the arc is in a supinatory direction from neutral position
             b. One-third of the arc is in a pronation direction from neutral position
   B. **Open kinetic chain pronation**
        1. Abduction
        2. Eversion
        3. Dorsiflexion
   C. **Closed kinetic chain pronation**
        1. Adduction
        2. Eversion
        3. Plantarflexion

V. **Midtarsal joint motion**

   A. **Oblique axis mostly dorsiflexion-plantar flexion/adduction-abduction with minimal inversion-eversion**
        1. Correlates with calcaneocuboid joint motion
   B. **Longitudinal axis mostly inversion-eversion with minimal dorsiflexion plantar flexion and adduction-abduction**
   C. **Both axes produce triplane motion**
   D. **Maximally pronated with dorsiflexion and abduction of the lateral column while**

allowing the medial column to seek its own level

    E. **As subtalar joint pronates, the midtarsal joint "unlocks" with resultant hypermobility of the first ray**

    F. **Locked midtarsal joint produces a rigid lever or rigid beam effect for forefoot stability necessary for efficient propulsion**

    G. **Unlocked midtarsal joint produces hypermobility necessary for forefoot adaptation to ground surface**

THE BIOMECHANICAL EXAMINATION

I. Hip joint range of motion

    A. Equal range of internal and external rotation in adults

        1. Should be the same with hips flexed or extended

            a. If different, check hamstrings or iliopsoas for tightness

    B. Total range of motion decreases with age

    C. Neutral position should align with frontal plane

II. Knee position

    A. Should align with frontal plane when hip joint and subtalar joint are neutral

    B. End range of motion 180°

        1. Residual flexion or hyperextension could indicate compensation for equinus

III. Ankle joint range of motion

    A. Dorsiflexion with knee extended 10° or greater

        1. Less than 10° indicative of equinus

    B. Dorsiflexion with knee flexed greater than 10°

        1. No change from knee flexed to extended position is indicative of a gastrosoleus or osseus equinus

    C. Plantar flexion 25°-30°

IV. Subtalar Joint Motion

    A. Ideal normal subtalar joint

        1. Normal rearfoot (example)

            a. 20° of inversion with supination

            b. 10° of eversion with pronation

            c. Perpendicular rearfoot (calcaneus to ground relationship) with the subtalar joint neutral and midtarsal joint pronated

        2. Subtalar varus, deformity (example)

            a. 25° of inversion with supination

            b. 5° of eversion with pronation

            c. 5° calcaneal inversion to the floor results with abnormal compensatory pronation

        3. Subtalar varus with tibial varum deformity (example)

            a. 25° of inversion with supination

            b. 5° of eversion with pronation

            c. 5° of tibial varum

d. Calcaneus is perpendicular to the ground when the subtalar joint is maximally pronated (compensated rearfoot varus)
    i. Poor visual indicator for abnormally pronated foot

4. Partially compensated rearfoot varus deformity (example)
    a. 30° of inversion with supination
    b. 0° of eversion with pronation
    c. 5° of tibial varum
    d. Calcaneus is 5° inverted to the ground when the subtalar joint is maximally pronated
        i. Poor visual indicator of abnormal foot pronation

V. Midtarsal joint

A. With subtalar joint pronation, the plantar plane of the forefoot becomes more everted than normal in relationship to the plantar plane of the heel because of the increase in range of motion in the midtarsal joint

B. With subtalar joint supination, the plantar plane of the forefoot becomes more inverted than normal in relationship to the plantar plane of the heel because of the decrease in range of motion in the midtarsal joint

C. Inverted forefoot to rearfoot (fixed): Forefoot varus

D. Everted forefoot to rearfoot (fixed): Forefoot valgus

E. Compensatory inverted position of forefoot to everted rearfoot: Forefoot supinatus

VI. First ray

A. Equal excursion of 5 mm above and below the level of the normal second ray

B. Plantar flexed first ray: Maximum dorsiflexion motion is below the level of the second metatarsal

1. Results in valgus relationship of forefoot to rearfoot (i.e., first through fifth metatarsals versus second through fifth metatarsals)

C. Rigid plantar-flexed first ray: Hallux hammertoe

1. Functions as *forefoot* valgus
2. Causes retrograde supination of midtarsal joint
3. If severe, may cause retrograde supination of subtalar joint
4. Associated with hallux hammertoe because of intrinsic dorsiflexed position (relative) of proximal phalanx to metatarsal
    a. Gives mechanical advantage of flexor hallucis longus; and extensor hallucis longus over flexor hallucis brevis and extensor digitorum (hallucis) brevis
    b. Interphalangeal joint plantar-flexes resulting in hammertoe

D. Flexible plantar-flexed first ray

1. Flexible forefoot valgus
2. Clinically, does not function plantar-flexed
3. May function at level of lesser metatarsals or above, if rearfoot is pronated or midtarsal joint is unlocked

E. First ray elevatus (metatarsus primus elevatus): Hallux limitus

1. Elevatus defined as a position in which the first metatarsal rests at a higher transverse plane level than metatarsals 2-5
2. Etiologies
    a. Congenital: First ray develops elevated resting position from birth
    b. Acquired: Long-standing pronation leads to hypermobile first ray, eventually osteoarthritic changes cause first ray to retain elevated position even during

non-weight-bearing
   c. Iatrogenic: Usually associated with base wedge osteotomies
  3. Sequelae to first ray elevatus include hallux limitus
    a. Other etiologies of hallux limitus include the following: Long first ray, long hallux, hypermobile first ray, trauma (especially intra-articular trauma to the first metatarsal phalangeal joint that leads to a displaced intra-articular fracture), sesamoid adhesions, and arthritis
  4. An elevated first metatarsal is usually associated with reactive rearfoot valgus during weight-bearing, which leads to excessively pronated foot
  5. Met primus elevatus may be associated with forefoot varus or simply with an elevated first ray with metatarsals 2-5 resting on a transverse plane position parallel to the supporting surface

VII. First metatarsal phalangeal joint

  A. Dorsiflexion: 65° required for active propulsion
  B. Plantar flexion: Stabilization against ground reactive force

VIII. Lesser metatarsophalangeal joint

  A. Dorsiflexion: 15° required for normal propulsion
  B. Plantarflexion: Stabilization against ground reactive force
    1. When proximal phalangeal stability is lacking, flexor stabilization with hammertoe formation results

GAIT ANALYSIS

I. Phases of gait

  A. Heel contact
  B. Forefoot contact
  C. Midstance
  D. Heel-lift
  E. Toe off
  F. Swing

II. Heel contact

  A. Hip joint extending
  B. Knee joint flexing
  C. Ankle joint plantar-flexing
  D. Subtalar joint neutral and pronating

III. Midstance

  A. Hip joint flexing
  B. Knee joint extending
  C. Ankle joint dorsiflexing
  D. Subtalar joint supinating
  E. Midtarsal joint pronating

PHASIC ACTIVITY OF LOWER EXTREMITY MUSCLES

I. **Hip adduction**
   A. **Heel contact to midstance**
   B. **Heel off to midswing**

II. **Hip abduction**
   A. **Late swing phase prior to heel off**

III. **Hamstrings**
   A. **Late swing to 25% stance**

IV. **Quadriceps femoris**
   A. **After heel contact to 25% stance**
   B. **Prior to toe off to early swing**

V. **Triceps surae**
   A. **15%-20% of stance to toe off**

VI. **Anterior leg muscles**
   A. **Swing to midstance**

VII. **Lateral leg muscles**
   A. **15%-20% of stance to toe off**

MUSCLE STRENGTH TESTING

I. **Five point system**
   A. **5:** Examiner cannot overcome force of muscle contraction
   B. **4:** Examiner can overcome force of muscle contraction with effort
   C. **3:** Examiner can easily overcome the contraction force of the muscles, but patient can overcome gravity resistance
   D. **2:** Patient cannot overcome gravity resistance but can move with gravity
   E. **1:** Patient cannot move against any resistance or no resistance, but muscle contracture is noted
   F. **0:** No muscle contracture is noted

LOWER EXTREMITY PATHOMECHANICS: COMMON CLINICAL FINDINGS

I. **Hip joint**
   A. **Asymmetric hip joint range of motion**

      1. Excessive internal to external range of motion
        a. Tight adductor musculature
      2. Excessive external to internal range of motion
        a. Tight abductor musculature
      3. Restricted range of motion unilaterally
        a. Consider unequal limb length
      4. Developmental or congenital hip dysplasia also a source of asymmetry

II. Knee joint

A. Genuvalgum
      1. Pronatory influence on subtalar joint and metatarsal joint

B. Genuvarum
      1. Should be clinically distinguished from tibial varum
      2. If excessive, forces subtalar joint to maximally pronated position

C. Genurecurvatum
      1. Should rule out compensation for limited ankle joint dorsiflexion
      2. Can be due to ligamentous laxity

D. Genuflexion
      1. Should rule out tight hamstrings
      2. Should rule out tight gastrocnemius

III. Ankle joint

A. Limited dorsiflexion secondary to
      1. Osseous equinus
        a. Flattened trochlear surface of talus
        b. Osteoarthritis/degenerative joint disease
      2. Tight gastrocnemius or gastrosoleus complex
        a. Evaluate ankle dorsiflexion flexed and extended to differentiate/isolate gastrocnemius tightness versus gastrosoleus tightness
      3. Functional equinus (pseudoequinus)
        a. Due to plantar-flexed forefoot
        b. Causes retrograde loading of ankle joint in closed kinetic chain, limiting anterior migration of leg in gait (i.e., closed chain dorsiflexion of ankle)

IV. Equinus: Fixed structural relationship of the leg to the foot whereby there is a lack of 10° of dorsiflexion of the ankle joint with the knees fully extended and locked, the subtalar joint neutral, and the midtarsal joint locked

A. Types
      1. Compensated: Normal heel off because of compensation at subtalar joint and midtarsal joint
      2. Partially compensated: Early heel off because of inadequate compensation at subtalar joint and midtarsal joint
      3. Uncompensated: No heel contact noted

B. Etiology
      1. Posterior muscle group contracture
        a. Clonic spasm
        b. Tonic spasm

        c. Accommodative shortening

    2. Congenitally short gastrocnemius muscle

    3. Congenitally short triceps surae

    4. Osseous ankle block

    5. Tight posterior ankle joint capsule

C. Mechanism of compensation

    1. Abducted gait

    2. Knee flexion

    3. Subtalar joint pronation, causing unlocking of the midtarsal joint, which results in dorsiflexion of the forefoot on the rearfoot

    4. Genurecurvatum: Posterior subluxation of the knee

    5. Decreased stride length

D. Gait analysis

    1. Compensated equinus

        a. Subtalar joint pronated at heel contact

        b. Midstance pronation with abduction of the forefoot on the rearfoot

        c. Foot lifts from the ground in two segments: The rearfoot lifts early, and then the forefoot lifts

        d. Toe off is apropulsive

    2. Partially compensated equinus

        a. Heel contact demonstrates an audible contact of the heel on the ground

        b. Heel off is early in midstance

        c. Resupination occurs late during propulsion

    3. Uncompensated

        a. Forefoot contact only

        b. Toe walking

E. Characteristics

    1. Compensated equinus: Pronated foot with flattened medial arch, unlocked to subluxed midtarsal joint, rocker bottom foot type, forefoot supinatus, and prone to hallux abductovalgus (H.A.V.) development

    2. Partially compensated: Mildly pronated foot, normal arch structure

    3. Uncompensated: Normal foot type, foot plantar flexed to the leg

    4. Ankle equinus: Solid abrupt end to the range of dorsiflexion motion at the ankle joint versus a spongy end to the range of motion in a soft-tissue equinus

F. Posterior muscle group contracture

    1. Produces an equinus deformity with clonic spasm

        a. Upper motor neuron lesion (e.g., cerebral palsy)

        b. Hypertonicity

        c. Hyperreflexia

        d. Functionally short muscle

    2. Tonic spasticity

        a. Inflammation of ankle and/or subtalar joint

        b. Fibrillation

        c. Reversible with rest

        d. Abnormal foot position may be relieved by forced opposition

    3. Contracture by accommodative shortening

        a. Loss of stretch stimulus

        b. Abnormal foot position

    4. Muscle imbalance with secondary contracture

> > a. Flaccid paralysis, spastic paralysis
> 5. Trauma
> > a. Loss of agonist-antagonist action of muscles
> > b. Myositic contracture

G. Signs and symptoms of equinus
1. Leg cramping
2. Painful aductovarus, fifth digits
3. Hallux abductovalgus
4. Retrocalcaneal exostosis
5. Postural fatigue
6. Plantar hyperkeratoses (diffuse)
7. Forefoot supinatus

V. Tibial varum: Inverted relationship of the tibia to the ground in static stance

A. Compensation
1. Ground reactive force everts heel relative to tibia
2. Eversion of the calcaneus to the perpendicular relationship to the ground

B. Partial Compensation
1. Caleaneus remains inverted to the ground with maximal subtalar joint pronation

VI. Rearfoot varus: Condition in which the sagittal plane of the posterior surface and plantar surface of the calcaneus are inverted to the weight-bearing surface when the subtalar joint is in the neutral position in standing angle and base of gait

A. Etiology. Lack of valgus torsion of the calcaneus

B. Uncompensated rearfoot varus
1. Foot remains inverted to the supporting surface
2. Insufficient eversion available in the subtalar joint to allow the medial column of the foot to purchase the supporting surface
3. Calcaneus remains inverted to ground

C. Compensated rearfoot varus
1. Eversion of the calcaneus to the perpendicular relationship to the supporting surface
2. Caused by ground reactive force at heel contact
3. Continued compensation remains in effect as long as 75% of the heel and forefoot are in contact with the supporting surface

D. Partially compensated rearfoot varus
1. Insufficient subtalar joint range of motion is available to evert the calcaneus to the perpendicular in relation to the supporting surface
2. Abductory twist occurs in gait in order to transfer weight to the medial aspect of the foot
3. A fairly stable foot type

VII. Forefoot varus: Fixed structural, congenital, osseous deformity in which the plantar plane of the forefoot is inverted to the plantar plane of the rearfoot with the subtalar joint in neutral position and the forefoot is maximally pronated about both midtarsal joint axes

A. Etiology
1. Ontogenetic
2. Inherited
3. Resulting from lack of valgus torsion of the head and neck of the talus as it relates to the body (most common reason)

4. Medial aspect of the forefoot fails to approach the horizontal plane and is therefore fixed in an inverted position

5. Lack of longitudinal torsion or valgus torsion of the calcaneus results in the cuboid calcaneal joint remaining in a plantar-flexed and inverted position

B. Forefoot supinatus:

1. Compensatory inverted position of forefoot to rearfoot due to excessively pronated rearfoot

2. Due to soft tissue contracture around talonavicular joint rather than osseous torsion

3. When placing subtalar joint in neutral position, medial forefoot will be reducible to ground, with spongy resistance

   a. Forefoot varus would not be reducible with same maneuver

C. Types of forefoot varus

1. Compensated forefoot varus

   a. Subtalar joint and midtarsal joint pronation sufficient to bring forefoot to ground

2. Partially compensated forefoot varus

   a. Maximum pronation of the subtalar joint with the forefoot still inverted to the ground

3. Uncompensated forefoot varus

   a. Forefoot in varus with no subtalar joint motion

D. Signs and symptoms of forefoot varus

1. Callus, plantar to the second, fourth and/or fifth metatarsal heads

2. Postural fatigue

3. Tailor's bunion

4. Adductovarus hammertoe deformities of the fourth and fifth digits

5. Hallux valgus deformity

VIII. Forefoot valgus: Fixed congenital osseous deformity in which the plantar plane of the forefoot is everted to the plantar plane of the rearfoot when the subtalar joint is in the neutral position and the forefoot is maximally pronated about both midtarsal joint axes

A. Plantarflexed first ray causing forefoot valgus

1. Acquired deformity

2. Muscle imbalance (intrinsic)

3. First metatarsal-cuneiform deformity

4. Peroneal longus muscle hyperactivity

5. Retrograde buckling of the hallux, creating plantar-flexed first ray

6. Weakness or absent action of the tibialis anterior muscle

      a. Peroneus longus dynamic imbalance creates a plantar-flexed first ray

7. Weakness of the gastrocnemius/triceps surae

8. Retrograde force from a hallux hammer toe deformity secondary to intrinsic muscle imbalance

B. Rigid forefoot valgus

1. Compensation by long axis supination and subtalar joint supination

2. During forefoot contact, the medial side of the foot contacts the ground giving rise to medial forefoot loading rather than normal lateral forefoot loading

   a. Can create tibial sesamoiditis owing to too much vertical stress on forefoot loading in this area

3. Abrupt supination around the midtarsal joint longitudinal axis and subtalar joint axis to bring the lateral forefoot in contact with the supporting surface in midstance

   a. Associated rapid external rotation with lateral deflection of the knee, places abnormal stress on the medial structures of the knee

   b. Stress placed on tensor fascia lata, creating strain in this area

  4. Propulsion with the foot in a laterally unstable supinated position

  5. Lateral digital propulsion, rather than propulsion by the hallux

  6. Foot and extremity recovery by swing phase pronation, producing a normal heel contact at the initiation of the next cycle in gait

C. Mobile forefoot valgus deformity

  1. Also called non-rigid forefoot valgus

  2. Normal heel contact

  3. Compensation by midtarsal joint longitudinal axis supination

  4. First ray moves dorsally, leaving second ray responsible for weightbearing with continued long axis supination until forefoot contact occurs

  5. First ray is hypermobile

  6. Propulsion is through the hallux, unlike the rigid form of forefoot valgus

  7. Calcaneus can be inverted, perpendicular, or everted depending upon the rearfoot deformity

IX. Limb length inequality

A. Structural

  1. Within the femur

  2. Within the fibula/tibia segment

  3. Combination of both

B. Functional

  1. Secondary to pelvic tilt (e.g., resulting from scoliosis)

   a. Lower side of pelvis creates functionally long limb

   b. Higher side of pelvis creates functionally short limb

  2. Secondary to abnormal pronation

   a. Unilateral forefoot varus

   b. Unilateral forefoot supination with compensated equinus

  3. Secondary to unilateral supinating deformities

   a. Forefoot valgus compensated by subtalar joint supination

   b. Severe rigid plantar flexed first ray

C. Compensation for structural limb-length discrepancy (long side)

  1. Increased subtalar joint pronation

  2. Relative decrease in height of pelvis on the same side owing to lower ankle-to-ground relationship from pronation

  3. Shoulder drop on same side

  4. Scoliosis (secondary)

  5. Head tilt towards long side (same side)

  6. Increased stance phase of gait on same side

  7. Increased single limb support time on same side

D. Compensation for structural limb-length discrepancy (short side)

  1. Increased subtalar joint supination (decreased pronation)

  2. Relative increase in height of pelvis on same side

  3. Increased shoulder height on same side

  4. Remainder of compensations opposite to those on long side

RADIOGRAPHIC BIOMECHANICAL EVALUATION

I.   **Talocalcaneal angle** (used as an index of relative foot pronation and supination)
    A. **Increases with pronation**
    B. **Decreases with supination**

II. **Talar declination angle** (is the estimation of the amount of plantarflexion of the talus)
    A. **Increases with pronation**
    B. **Decreases with supination**

III. **Calcaneal inclination angle** (is the determinate of the relative arch height)
    A. **Decreases with dorsiflexion of the forefoot on the rearfoot**
    B. **Increases with plantarflexion of the forefoot on the rearfoot**

IV. **Superimposition of the talus over the calcaneus**
    A. **Decreases with pronation**
    B. **Increases with supination**

V.   **Forefoot adductus** (is the relationship of the forefoot as compared to the rearfoot)
    A. **Decreases with pronation owing to unlocking of the midtarsal joint with abduction of the forefoot on the rearfoot**
    B. **Increases with supination**

VI. **Cyma line** (describes the relationship of the tabnavicular joint to the calcaneal cuboid joint on the sagittal plane)
    A. **Anterior displacement with pronation on AP (DP) and lateral view**
    B. **Posterior displacement with supination on AP (DP) and lateral view**

VII. **Talonavicular articulation**
    A. **Usually 70%-75%**
    B. **Percentage varies with position:** with the pronation the amount of articulation decreases, with supination it increases

VIII. **Cuboid Abduction angle** (estimates the amount of abduction the midfoot has on the rearfoot)
    A. **Increases with pronation**
    B. **Decreases with supination**

IX. **Pseudo Sinus Tarsi**
    A. **Seen in a pronated foot as a translucent area that occurs dorsal and distal to the sustentaculum tali**

X.   **Compensated rearfoot varus**
    A. **No evidence of subluxation**
    B. **Cyma line appears unbroken**
    C. **Pseudo sinus tarsi**

XI. **Uncompensated rearfoot varus**

    A. **Greater superimposition of the talus over the calcaneus and greater superimposition of the lesser tarsal and metatarsals**

    B. **All secondary to the inverted position of the entire foot**

    C. **No evidence of pronation subluxation**

XII. **Compensation for transverse plane deformities**

    A. **Abnormally high talocalcaneal angle**

    B. **Talus is anteriorly displaced and adducted on the calcaneus**

    D. **Severe anterior displacement of the Cyma line**

    E. **Severe increase in cuboid abduction angle**

XIII. **Compensated forefoot varus**

    A. **Frontal plane displacement resulting from subluxation of the talus on the calcaneus**

    B. **Decreased superimposition of the talus on the calcaneus**

    C. **Wedging of the navicular**

    D. **Flattening of the medial head of the talus**

    E. **Severely anteriorly displaced Cyma line resulting from compensation with subluxation of the midtarsal joint**

    F. **Compensation by midtarsal and subtalar joint pronation**

XIV. **Uncompensated forefoot varus**

    A. **No evidence of subluxation of the subtalar or midtarsal joints**

    B. **Excess superimposition of the lesser tarsal and metatarsals**

    C. **No evidence of abnormal superimposition of the tarsals**

XV. **Compensation for rigid versus mobile forefoot valgus**

    A. **Compensation by midtarsal and subtalar joint supination:** Rigid forefoot valgus

    B. **Compensation by midtarsal joint supination only:** Mobile forefoot valgus

    C. **If compensated by subtalar joint supination the talocalcaneal angle decreases and the calcaneal inclination angle increases**

    D. **If compensated by midtarsal joint, the talocalcaneal angle is normal with normal superimposition of the talus on the calcaneus**

XVI. **Compensated equinus** (talipes equinus)

    A. **Dorsiflexion of the *forefoot on* the rearfoot, giving a rocker-bottom appearance**

        1. "Nutcracker syndrome"

    B. **Loss of the calcaneal inclination angle**

    C. **Loss of the declination angle of the cuboid**

    D. **Adducted plantar-flexed and anteriorly displaced talus on the calcaneus**

    E. **Anteriorly displaced Cyma line**

    F. **Flattening of the trochlear surface of the talus**

    G. **Bony proliferation and narrowing of the ankle joint space**

    H. **Flattening of the medial aspect of the head of the talus**

    I. **Wedging of the navicular**

    J. **Increased talocalcaneal angle**

    K. **Abducted cuboid with subluxed midtarsal joint**

XVII. **Uncompensated equinus** (talipes equinus)

    A. **Plantar-flexed angle of the foot to leg**

    B. **Normal calcaneal inclination angle**

    C. **Normal talar declination angle**

MECHANICAL TREATMENT OF FOREFOOT FRONTAL PLANE DEFORMITIES

  I. **Compensated forefoot varus**

    A. **Treatment objective is to prevent the compensatory subtalar and oblique midtarsal joint pronation by supporting the forefoot in its inverted position, relative to the supporting surface**

    B. **Support the deformity with intrinsic posting on the positive cast or combination of intrinsic and extrinsic posting on orthoses**

  II. **Compensated forefoot valgus**

    A. **Treatment objective is to support the forefoot everted to the ground**

    B. **Support the forefoot with intrinsic posting on positive cast or combination of intrinsic posting and extrinsic posting on orthoses for desired correction to the deformity**

  III. **Plantar-flexed, first ray deformity**

    A. **Treatment objective is to support the plantarflexed position of the first ray**

    B. **First ray cut-out at medial distal edge of orthoses**

    C. **Reverse Morton's**

PATHOMECHANICS OF HALLUX ABDUCTO VALGUS DEFORMITY

  I. **Etiology**

    A. **Pronated subtalar joint**

    B. **Unlocked, unstable midtarsal joint**

    C. **Hypermobile first ray**

    D. **Dorsiflexed and inverted first ray**

    E. **Limitation in sagittal plane dorsiflexion of the hallux**

    F. **Lateral displacement and valgus rotation of the hallux**

    G. **Medial displacement of first metatarsal head resulting from retrograde force of the hallux**

    H. **Adaptation of the subchondral bone at the medial aspect of the first metatarsal head resulting from compression from the hallux**

    I. **Lateral displacement of the sesamoids caused by abduction and valgus rotation of the hallux**

    J. **Abductor hallucis becomes more plantar in relationship to the axis of the first ray, decreasing its abductory force on the hallux, allowing further valgus rotation of the hallux**

    K. **Plantar fascia begin to bowstring**

    L. **Flexor hallucis longus and flexor hallucis brevis gain a better mechanical advantage as a** result of the abducted position of the hallux

M. Continuation of this process leads to degenerative joint disease

N. Further degeneration leads to hallux limitus/rigidus/autofusion

PATHOMECHANICS

I. Hammer toes

    A. Biomechanical etiology: Abnormal pronation

        1. Subtalar joint abnormal pronation

        2. Midtarsal joint abnormal pronation

        3. Malfunction of the quadratus plantae, flexor digitorum longus, lumbricales, and interossei

        4. Secondary contracture of the flexor digitorum brevis and extensor expansion

        5. Weakness of the flexor digitorum longus

        6. Contracture of the extensor longus

        7. Secondary weakness of the flexor digitorum longus and flexor digitorum, brevis

        8. Lack of normal function of quadratus plantae owing to abnormal subtalar and midtarsal joint position, producing an adducting force on the lateral digits with flexion of the interphalangeal joint

    B. Flexor stabilization type of hammertoe deformities

        1. Occur as a result of the long flexors gaining mechanical advantage over the intrinsics

        2. The flexors fire earlier and longer to help stabilize the pronating hypermobile flatfoot

        3. The intrinsics cannot counter the deforming forces leading to hammertoe deformity

    C. Flexor substitution type of hammertoe deformities

        1. Occurs with weakness of the triceps surae

        2. May be congenital or a result of surgical over lengthening of the tendo achilles

        3. A high arched foot with a calcaneal type gait may be observed

    D. Extensor substitution type of hammertoe deformities

        1. Swing phase occurrence associated with weakness or over activity of the anterior crurals

        2. May occur secondary to pes cavus, EDL spasticity or ankle equinus conditions

    E. Regardless of the etiology of hammer toes, they all have the following in common

        1. Extension of the proximal phalanx

        2. Flexion of the PIPJ's

        3. Flexion of the DIPJ's

II. Tailor's bunion

    A. Etiology

        1. Abnormal subtalar joint pronation

        2. Unstable unlocked midtarsal joint

    B. Fifth ray

        1. Pronatory axis of motion

        2. Subluxation of the fifth ray

    C. Development

        1. With subtalar joint pronation, the calcaneus everts, thereby forcing the cuboid to be everted

        2. Continued stress produces lateral splaying of the fifth metatarsal shaft

        3. The abductor digiti quinti displaces plantarly, decreasing its adductory force along with varus rotation of the fifth digit

III. Retrocalcaneal exostosis

    A. Etiology

      1. Compensated subtalar varus

      2. Partially compensated subtalar varus

    B. Mechanism

      1. Irritation of the posterolateral border of the calcaneus against the shoe heel counter with eversion of the calcaneus to the vertical with heel contact pronation

      2. The calcaneus everts within the shoe during heel contact pronation

CAVUS FOOT CLASSIFICATION & COMPENSATORY PATTERNS

OVERVIEW

Pes cavus is characterized by feet exhibiting high vaulted medial longitudinal arches, clawed toes with the forefoot hyperdeclinated on the rearfoot. Classification of cavus feet are based on the locus of deformity with reference to the sagittal and frontal planes. The etiology of cavus foot types and conditions may include neuromuscular, congenital-hereditofamilial, and other traumatic or idiopathic causes. The most common neurological causes are Charcot Marie-Tooth and Cerebral Palsy, but many other conditions such as Friedrich's ataxia produce cavus foot types via progressive nerve degeneration and associated muscle imbalance. Neurogenic anterior cavus deformities generally involve the anterior crurals and lateral muscle groups while posterior cavus deformities result from a weakness or paralysis of the triceps surae musculature. While traumatic and neurogenic influences produce the most dramatic and severe cavus deformities, the much more prevalent and milder forms are hereditofamilial in nature. Classification and compensatory patterns produced by these cavus foot types will be covered

I. Cavus foot types

    A. Anterior Cavus

      1. Plantarflexion of the forefoot upon the rearfoot

      2. May occur at the Midtarsal, Lesser tarsal, or Lisfranc's joints (Fig. 1)

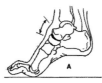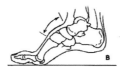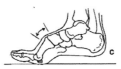

Fig 1., A., Midtarsal Cavus, B., Lesser Tarsus Cavus, C., Tarso-Metatarsal Cavus

      3. May be global in nature (rectus forefoot to rearfoot) or may have a more pronounced lateral or medial column component (Fig. 2). Lateral column cavus deformities are often termed *flexible* due to the compensatory pronation with weight bearing. Medial column cavus deformities may be referred to as forefoot valgus due to the everted relationship of metatarsals 1-5 relative to the rearfoot. Compensation generally occurs via STJ supination

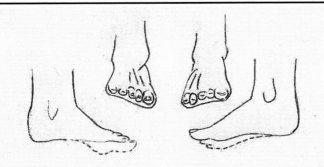

Fig. 2, Diagramatic representation of Medial and Lateral Column Cavus

4. Radiographic findings are consistent with the high STJ and MTJ axis orientations associated with anterior cavus foot types. Lateral views generally reveal high calcaneal inclination angles, increased metatarsal declination angles and decreased talar declination angles (Fig. 3). Dorso-plantar viewing demonstrate transverse plane compensations such as increased Kite's and cuboid abduction angles and splaying of the first and fifth rays

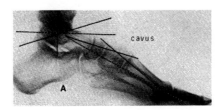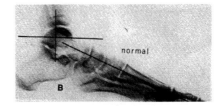

Fig. 3, Radiographic findings consistent with normal and cavus foot types (lateral views)

5. Most commonly is of congenital origin but may also be an acquired condition usually as a result of neurogenic induced muscle imbalance, i.e., Charcot Marie Toothe

6. Ground reactive dorsiflexion of the hyperdeclinated forefoot produces *pseudoequinus stress* (Fig. 4) and a compensatory posterior body imbalance

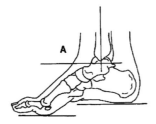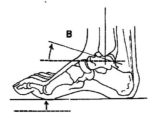

Fig. 4, Diagramatic representation of the etiology of Pseudoequinus Stress

7. Clinical findings may include clawtoes, anteriorly displaced sub-metatarsal fat pad, splay forefoot, prominent metatarsal heads and taught plantar fascia (Fig. 5)

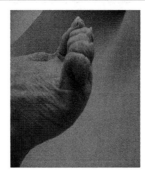
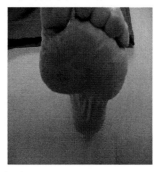

Fig. 5, Retracted toes, displaced fat pad and taught fascia associated with anterior cavus

8. Primary symptomatology may include metatarsalgia, plantar fasciitis/heel spur, neuritis/
    neuroma, posterior tibial tendinitis, achilles tendonitis, bunion and lesser digital
    complaints
9. Secondary symptomatic complaints may include calf, hamstring, or low back pain
    associated with the compensatory posterior body imbalance (Fig. 6)

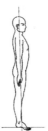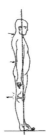

Fig. 6, Clinical representation of postural compensation for Anterior Cavus

10. Treatment should be focused at de-compensation of the sagittal plane deformity with
    appropriate heel elevation via optimal shoe and orthosis management. The orthosis
    should also include a deep heel cup and high medial and lateral flanges to help control
    transverse plane foot malalignments. Anterior cavus deformities with prominent medial
    or lateral column components will additionally require frontal plane orthosis posting

B. Posterior Cavus
1. Rearfoot Cavus
2. May be an isolated congenital deformity of the calcaneus or may occur secondary to
    ankle dorsiflexion conditions *calcaneus* producing posterior cavus
3. Clinical presentation will generally demonstrate a high arched foot with increased
    calcaneal inclination angle on lateral radiograph
4. Compensation generally occurs with STJ pronation and a forward shift of body balance.
    Digital contraction deformities may occur due to the anterior imbalance
5. Presenting symptomatology may include heel pain with possible bursal formation due to
    the prominent heel bone
6. Posterior cavus deformities may be distinguished from similar appearing foot-types such
    as rigid forefoot Valgus, with the use the Coleman Block Test to subtract the
    compensation for the plantarflexed first metatarsal (Fig. 7)

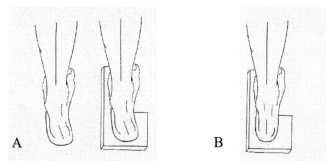

Fig. 7, Coleman Block Test, A., Posterior Cavus, B., Forefoot Valgus de-compensated with block test

C. **CalcaneoCavus**

1. CalcaneoCavus represents a combination deformity with posterior and anterior cavus components (Fig. 8)
2. The ankle joint is strongly dorsiflexed while the forefoot is markedly in an equinus attitude
3. The majority of calcaneo cavus deformities are associated with neurologic conditions in which weakness, paralysis, or dystrophy of the calf muscles will produce the deformity
4. Compensation occurs with dorsiflexion of the hyperdeclinated forefoot that produces a heightened plantar fascial and tendoachilles stress. Clawing of the digits also occurs as a result of the posterior imbalance

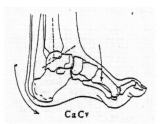

Fig. 8, Clinical and radiographic representation of CalcaneoCavus

FIRST RAY DEFORMITIES AND CONDITIONS

I. **Congenital First Ray Deformities**

A. **Metatarsus Primus Equinus**

1. The first metatarsal is structurally plantarflexed at the first metatarsal cuneiform joint (Fig. 9)
2. This deformity is also commonly referred to as a rigid forefoot valgus deformity due to the relative eversion of metatarsal segments 1-5 with frontal plane viewing
3. Compensation for this deformity is via subtalar joint supination producing a lateral imbalance tendency during stance and gait
4. Clinical presentation may include the presence of discrete submetatarsal head one and five lesions, dorsal first metatarsal-cuneiform joint exostosis, and retro calcaneal bump
5. Symptomatic presentation may include submetatarsal head one and five pain, sesamoiditis, lateral ankle sprain tendency, and dorsal and/or retrocalcaneal exostosis pain or irritation

6. Treatment should be focused at off-loading the plantarflexed first metatarsal via orthosis management with first ray or head cut-out. The orthosis may be further modified with a deep heel cup, extended flanges, and Valgus posting for enhanced support and control

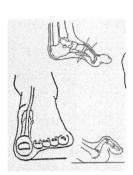
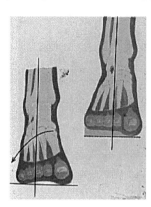

Fig. 9, Clinical and radiographic representation of Metatarsus Primus Equinus

B. Metatarsus Primus Elevatus

1. The first metatarsal is structurally dorsiflexed at the first metatarsal cuneiform joint (Fig. 10)
2. Compensation for this deformity is via STJ pronation with a shift of body weight forward and medial. This resultant anteromedial imbalance further elevates the first metatarsal leading to increased stress and jamming at the first metatarsophalangeal joint. Dorsiflexion required during the propulsive phase of gait will occur at the Hallux IPJ rather than the MTPJ
3. Clinical presentation may include a dorsal exostosis at the head of the first metatarsal, Hallux IPJ hyperextension, medial hallux "pinch" tyloma, and a submetatarsal head two tyloma
4. Symptomatology may include hallux limitus, plantar hallux pain and lesser metatarsalgia
5. Treatment may include the use of a Morton's Platform to bring the ground up to the structurally elevated first metatarsal. Neutral STJ positioned orthosis management to help control pronation may also be utilized. Rocker sole shoe modifications may also be beneficial to reduce first metatarsophalangeal joint pain

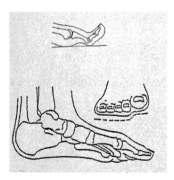

Fig. 10, Clinical and radiographic representation of Metatarsus Primus Elevatus

C. **Hypermobile First Ray**
   1. Limited first metatarsophalangeal joint ROM during gait (less than 65°) is termed *Functional Hallux Limitus* (FHL). Clinical presentation may include a dorsal exostosis at the head of the first metatarsal, Hallux IPJ hyperextension, medial hallux "pinch" tyloma, and a submetatarsal head two tyloma
   2. Treatment for *non-adapted* FHL may include neutral position orthosis management with modifications that may include a first metatarsal head cut-out with kinetic wedge (hallux prop) or a first ray cut-out. First ray repositioning with a plantarflexory force applied to the first metatarsal during orthosis casting may also be utilized to improve first ray position and function during gait

II. **Flexible vs rigid flatfoot deformities**
   A. **Both types have some or all of the following characteristics:** everted heel, abduction of the forefoot on the rearfoot, and collapse of the medial column (Fig. 11)

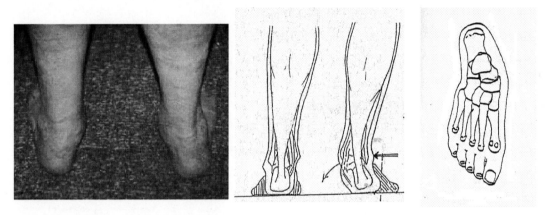

Fig. 11, Clinical and diagrammatic representation of calcaneal eversion and forefoot abduction

   B. **A flexible flatfoot implies that the deformity is easily reducible by manipulation, while a rigid flatfoot is not**

III. **Etiologies of flexible flatfoot**
   A. **Compensated forefoot varus**
      1. In order to bring the medial forefoot to the ground, the subtalar joint must pronate leading to eversion of the calcaneus and the foot. This unlocks the MTJ and allows for more MTJ pronation resulting in forefoot hypermobility
   B. **Compensated <u>flexible</u> forefoot valgus**
      1. In order to bring the lateral forefoot to the ground the MTJ can supinate without STJ motion or the STJ can pronate. Both lead to MTJ instability
   C. **Compensated equinus**
      1. Abnormal pronation of the STJ and MTJ occurs to compensate for the lack of dorsiflexion at the ankle (Fig. 12)

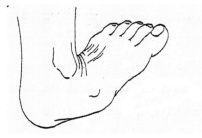

Fig. 12, Clinical appearance of compensatory malalignments associated with ankle equinus

D. Congenital talipes calcaneovalgus
  1. If not corrected with casting, the pronated position of the STJ will be propagated with weightbearing (Fig. 13)

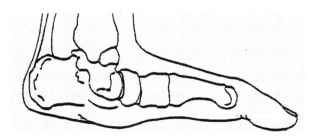

Fig. 13, Radiographic and clinical appearance of congenital talipes calcaneovalgus

E. Torsional abnormalities
  1. Adduction deformities can compensate by pronating the STJ and MTJ, which abducts the forefoot (Fig. 14 B)
  2. Abduction deformities can force the STJ into pronation because the body weight will fall medial ward to the line of progression (Fig. 14 A)

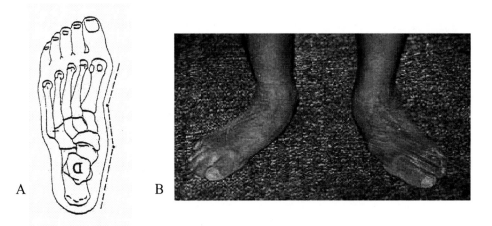

Fig. 14, A, Compensated metatarsus adductus **B,** Foot abduction secondary to external hip position

F. **Muscle imbalance**
   1. Weakness of the supinators of the STJ and MTJ can lead to a maximally pronated STJ
G. **Neurotrophic feet**
   1. In the early stages when lack of proprioception is most pronounced, the muscle tone appears inadequate to support the normal structures, which usually leads to pronation of the STJ
   2. A wide base of gait can lead to a medial shift in weightbearing leading to excessive pronation

IV. **Etiologies of rigid flatfoot**

   A. **Congenital convex pes valgus** (vertical talus)
      1. Dorsal subluxation of the navicular on the talus, which prevents reduction
   B. **Improperly corrected clubfoot**
      1. Leads to plantar subluxation of the tarsal-metatarsal bones
   C. **Tarsal coalitions with or without peroneal spasm**
   D. **Peroneal spastic flatfoot**
   E. **Trauma**
   F. **Neurotrophic feet**
      1. Persistent soft tissue imbalance can eventually lead to rigid subluxation of the joints

V. **Biomechanics of flexible flatfoot**

   A. **In weight bearing the STJ is maximally pronated** (the calcaneus everts, the talus adducts and plantarflexes)
   B. **This allows the MTJ to increase its range of motion because the axis of each joint is more parallel to each other**
   C. **As the forefoot attempts to bear weight, the MTJ is unable to stabilize the pronatory forces of the reactive force of gravity; hence, the normal osseous stability is lost**
   D. **This leads to a severe deforming force plantarly subluxing Choparts joint** (the Achilles is plantarflexing the rearfoot and the reactive force of gravity is dorsiflexing the forefoot)

VI. **Planal dominance**

   A. **The axis of the STJ averages 42 degrees from the transverse plane and 16 degrees from the sagittal plane. Deviation from this average axis can greatly affect motion around the STJ**
   B. **The more vertical the STJ axis, the greater will be the percentage of transverse plane motion** (adduction/abduction). **The more horizontal the STJ axis, the greater will be the percentage of frontal plane motion** (inversion/eversion). With the STJ axis 2/3 (60 degrees) elevated from the transverse plane, twice as much motion will be seen in add/abd as in inv/ev at the STJ. With the STJ axis 1/3 (30 degrees) elevated from the transverse plane, one will see twice as much inv/ev as add/abd
   C. **The more parallel the STJ is to the sagittal plane, the greater will be the percentage of frontal plane motion, and the more parallel it is to the frontal plane, the greater the percentage of sagittal plane motion.** Because the STJ deviates little from the sagittal plane (16 degrees), there is little dorsiflexion/plantarflexion at the STJ
   D. **In examining the range of motion of the joints of the foot the axis of motion can be estimated.** If eversion/inversion is the predominate motion, the axis will be more horizontal. If adduction/abduction is the predominate motion, the axis will be more vertical. If

dorsiflexion/plantarflexion is the predominate motion, the axis will lie closer to the frontal and horizontal planes

VII. Radiographic evaluation

A. When transverse plane is dominant
1. Increase in the dorsoplantar talocalcaneal angle
2. Increase in cuboid abduction angle
3. Decrease in forefoot adductus angle
4. Decrease in talonavicular congruency

B. When frontal plane is dominant
1. Widening of lesser tarsal area on DP view
2. Decrease in the first metatarsal declination angle
3. Decrease in height os sustentaculum tali
4. Increase in superimposition of the lesser tarsus on the lateral view

C. When sagittal plane is dominant
1. Increase in talar declination angle
2. Naviculocuneiform breach
3. Increase in lateral talocalcaneal angle
4. Decrease in calcaneal inclination angle

CASTING FOR FOOT ORTHOSES

I. Patient positioning

A. Suspension technique
1. Patient seated with knee slightly flexed to decrease external rotation force from the hip, which can cause a supination force on the foot when the examiner suspends the foot during the casting procedure
2. Application of plaster of Paris splint to the foot in a smooth bonding pattern
3. Grasping of fourth and fifth digits by holding with the thumb and index finger
4. Use opposite hand to grasp malleoli and stabilize the extremity against external rotation
5. Slight dorsiflexion and abduction of the forefoot on the rearfoot with the subtalar joint neutral, thereby locking the midtarsal joint
6. Evaluation of cast for accuracy of impression of the foot with the subtalar joint neutral and midtarsal joint locked

II. Other casting techniques

A. Vacuum casting: Biovac system (in shoe technique)
B. Prone casting
1. Good alternative for young children
2. Good for patients with high external hip position
C. Semi-weight-bearing casting for accommodative orthoses

BIBLIOGRAPHY

Canale S.T. Campbell's operative orthopaedics (Vol. 2). Mosby, St. Louis, 1998.

Philps JW. The functional foot orthosis. Churchill, Livingston, New York, 1990.

Root ML, Orien WA, Weed JH. Normal and abnormal function of the foot. Clinical Biomechanics Corporation, Los Angeles, 1977.

Root ML, Orien WA, Weed JH, and Hughes RJ. Biomechanical examination of the foot, Vol. 1. Clinical Biomechanics Corporation, Los Angeles, 1971.

Seibel MO. Foot function, a programmed text. Williams & Wilkins, Baltimore, 1988.

Sgarlato T. A compendium of podiatric biomechanics. College of Podiatric Medicine, San Francisco, 1971.

Grumbine N: The Varus Components of the Forefoot in Flatfoot Deformities, J Am Podiatr Med Assoc, 1987; 77(1): pp 14-20.

Whitney A, Green D: *Pseudoequinus,* J Am Podiatr Med Assoc, 1982; 72(7): pp 365-371.

Whitney A, Whitney K: Anterior Cavus Foot Problems. In : Jay R., Current Therapy In Podiatric Surgery, pp 230-241, Philadelphia, B.C. Decker, 1989.

Whitney K, McGuire J: Recognizing and Managing The Anterior Cavus Deformity, Podiatry Today, 1997.

Valmassy RL. Clinical biomechanics of the lower extremities, Mosby, St. Louis, 1996.

CHAPTER 7
BIOMECHANICS

1.   All of the following are true regarding the following lower extremity ranges of motion except:

        A.   Dorsiflexion of the ankle joint will generally be greater with the knee extended versus with the knee flexed
        B.   Hip joint range of motion in the transverse plane should have equal amounts of internal and external rotation in the adult
        C.   Ideal subtalar joint ranges of motion exhibit 20° of inversion and 10° of eversion in the frontal plane
        D.   Ankle joint plantarflexion is normally 25° - 30°
        E.   None of the above

2.   During the midstance phase of gait, all of the following lower extremity motions normally occur except which of the following:

        A.   Extension of the knee joint
        B.   Flexion of the hip joint
        C.   Supination of the subtalar joint
        D.   Supination of the midtarsal joint
        E.   None of the above

3.   All of the following are true regarding the femur except which of the following:

        A.   The head and neck of the femur are angulated 160° from the long axis of the shaft at birth
        B.   Femoral torsion of the femoral shaft in the transverse plane should be 30° at birth
        C.   Anteversion refers to external femoral torsion
        D.   Retroversion refers to external femoral position
        E.   None of the above

4.   All of the following are true regarding a lesser tarsus cavus foot type except which of the following:

        A.   Also referred to as a "hump foot"
        B.   Exhibits increased convexity over the dorsal midfoot
        C.   Dorsiflexion of the forefoot during stance may increase plantar fascial stress and strain
        D.   Treatment should include the use of low or negative heeled shoewear
        E.   None of the above

5.   Anterior cavus foot types may occur at all of the following locations of the foot with the exception of which of the following:

        A.   Lisfranc's joints
        B.   Midtarsal joints
        C.   Subtalar joint
        D.   Lesser tarsal joints
        E.   None of the above

6.   The most common etiology of forefoot varus is:

        A.   Failure of the normal valgus torsion of the calcaneus during gestation
        B.   Failure of the normal varus torsion of the calcaneus during gestation
        C.   Failure of the normal varus torsion of the talar head and neck during gestation
        D.   Failure of the normal valgus torsion of the talar head and neck during gestation
        E.   None of the above

7.   Which of the following most correctly describes the compensation pattern seen in a structurally long limb?

        A.   Shoulder drop away from long side
        B.   Head tilt towards long side
        C.   Relative height of pelvis on the long side is increased
        D.   Relative height of pelvis on the short side is decreased
        E.   None of the above

8.   Which of the following deformities would produce the lowest Talocalcaneal angle?
        A.   Equinus
        B.   Forefoot varus
        C.   Forefoot valgus
        D.   Rearfoot varus
        E.   None of the above

9.   Which of the following does not result in a rigid flatfoot?

        A.   Congenital talipes calcaneovalgus
        B.   Congenital conves pes valgus
        C.   Peroneal spastic flatfoot
        D.   Tarsal coalition
        E.   None of the above

10.   A subtalar joint axis that is elevated 60 degrees from the transverse plane would exhibit motion
        predominately in which plane?

        A.   Sagittal plane
        B.   Transverse plane
        C.   Frontal plane
        D.   Cardinal plane
        E.   None of the above

Chapter 8

SPORTS MEDICINE

updated for the 2004 edition by Franklin Kase and Howard Palamarchuk

ROLE OF THE SPORTS PODIATRIST

I. Evaluate and treat

II. Determine causative factors and correct them
  A. Prevent recurrent injury
  B. This role characteristic distinguishes sports podiatrist from general practitioner
  C. Understand the nature of athletes and the motives that drive them

ETIOLOGIES OF ATHLETIC INJURIES

I. Training errors
  A. **Technique**
    1. Perform efficiently to reduce injury
    2. Attention to training principles ("too much, too soon, not enough rest")
  B. **Attire:** Dependent on weather
    1. Cold weather: Use layers of clothing, caps, and mittens to conserve body heat
    2. Warm weather: Light, loose-fitting clothing (also drink adequate amounts of water to prevent dehydration and hypothermia)
  C. **Increasing activity level**
    1. Gradual increases to allow the body to adapt to new stress
    2. Adequate rest and recovery periods integrated into training
  D. **Surfaces and terrain**
    1. Hills versus flat ground
      a. Important in unidirectional activities, such as running, walking, and roller skating
      b. Hills increase demand on musculoskeletal system
        i. Only for experienced, well-conditioned athletes

          ii. To be avoided with any lower-extremity injury
              (a) Uphill stresses the hamstrings, low back, and Achilles tendons
              (b) Downhill stresses the heels, quadriceps, knees, and anterior compartments of the legs

2. Running
   a. Best surfaces: Compacted dirt and synthetic track

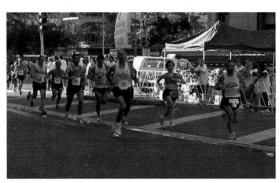

Figure 1.

   b. Worst surfaces: Concrete and sidewalk (cannot dissipate shock)
   c. Acceptable surface: Grass turf that is without ruts and if there is no ankle instability
   d. Preferable to concrete but not as good as track: Asphalt (Figure 1)
   e. Banked surfaces: Produce functional leg-length discrepancy (i.e., inside leg acts as long leg and outside (uphill) leg acts as short leg
      i. Compensate by alternating direction (i.e., 1-2 laps clock-wise and next 1-2 laps counter-clockwise)
      ii. Found in indoor and outdoor tracks and shoulders of streets with high crowns

3. Aerobic dance
   a. Best surfaces: Wood over airspace, heavily padded and carpeted concrete floors
   b. Worse surfaces: Carpet over unpadded concrete floor

E. Nutrition
  1. Well-balanced diet emphasizing all four food groups
  2. Vitamin and mineral supplements permissible, but not to substitute for nutritious meals
  3. Increased need for water, which must be consumed daily, including before, during, and after athletic activity; sport drinks contain low levels of carbohydrates and electrolytes and are acceptable substitutes for water when performing athletic activities
  4. Eating disorders can have a serious impact on the health of both female and male athletes

F. Competition versus recreation
  1. Recreational athletes – violate the principles of training
   a. More frequent and severe injuries
   b. Usually not on a regular exercise program
   c. Not well conditioned
   d. Not attuned to body's signals
  2. Competitive athletes – well coached and informed
   a. Less injury
   b. Focused on a specific sport
   c. Regularly exercise
   d. Attuned to body signals

II. Inadequate conditioning program: Warm-up, cool down, stretching, and strengthening

    A. Warm-up: Activity that precedes actual athletic activity to warm the body's core temperature

        1. Low-level exercise, such as walking, jogging or biking, followed by stretching all muscle groups to be used during the actual sports activity

        2. Warms and prepares muscles for the increased demands of sport; increases muscle elasticity

    B. Cool down: Activity that follows actual athletic activity

        1. Aerobic activity at a lesser intensity, 5-10 minutes after vigorous exercise

        2. Allows heart to return gradually to its pre-exercise pumping rate

           a. Reduces possibility of cardiovascular collapse

           b. Returns body to less stressed condition

    C. Stretching exercises

        1. Counteracts exercise-induced contracted muscles

        2. Enhances joint flexibility and allows body to withstand increased physical stress

        3. Should be performed daily, in addition to pre- and post-exercise, to maintain joint and muscle flexibility

        4. Should be eased into, held for 20-30 seconds, and gradually released

        5. Best if strain is avoided; should not be painful

        6. Avoid bouncing, which causes reflexive muscle contracture, and strain injury

    D. Strengthening exercises

        1. Protects joints from injury by maintaining adequate stability

        2. Improves musculoskeletal function

        3. Prevents body fatigue

        4. Should be performed on alternate days to allow sufficient muscle recovery – no more than three times a week

        5. Best if performed initially with the aid of an experienced person (e.g., trainer, physical therapist, exercise physiologist)

III. Shoe gear problems

    A. Athlete's most important equipment

    B. Universal principles in shoe selection

        1. There is no "best athletic shoe" for everyone

        2. Individual fit and comfort of the shoe to the foot are the most important factors in selection

        3. End of shoe should be a thumb's width from the longest toe

        4. Shoes should be measured to the feet at the end of the day, when the feet have achieved maximum size (i.e., normal swelling)

        5. Shoe requirements vary with the specific activities; even within a single sport (e.g., running), requirements vary between training and competing (e.g., a training shoe may be worn for racing, but a racing shoe may not be worn for training)

    C. Specific shoe characteristics

        1. Unidirectional sports (running, walking, jogging) require shoes that have more rearfoot stability and that tend to reduce excess lateral motion should have the following qualities:

           a. Firm, rigid, heel counter and support

           b. Midfoot stability and forefoot flexibility

           c. Rearfoot cushion

        2. Multi-direction sports (e.g., tennis, aerobic dance, and basketball) require shoes with more lateral flexibility, more forefoot cushion, and greater traction capability

D. Wear patterns
1. Running and walking
   a. Greatest at lateral heel and mid forefoot (Figure 2)
   b. Correspond to normal weight-bearing stress pattern
      i. Any variation of above indicates possible biomechanical abnormality
      ii. Severely worn shoes should be replaced
         (a) Shoe stability and cushion have been compromised
         (b) Greater risk of injury
   c. Should be replaced every 500 miles or 3 to 6 months
2. Other sports
   a. Variable wear patterns, depending on specific sport during which they are worn
   b. Should be replaced when they display excessive wear

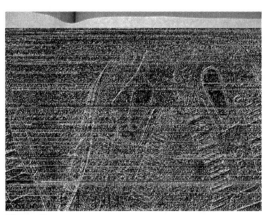

Figure 2.

IV. Biomechanical imbalances

A. Factors unique to running
1. Flight phase of running gait
   a. Both feet are off the weight-bearing surface simultaneously
   b. More prevalent as speed increases
   c. Three to four times body weight generated in lead foot at contact
2. Pendulum effect
   a. Functional varus angulation of the foot and leg to the ground
   b. Excessive lateral shoe wear results
   c. Excessive internal leg rotation and subtalar joint pronation results, predisposing athlete to an array of overuse injuries
   d. More significant in females because of typically wider pelvis (i.e., increase in Q angle)

B. Normal walking gait
1. Stance phase: 60% of gait; swing phase: 40% of gait
2. Heel-midfoot-toe contact
3. One foot always in contact with supporting surface
4. Foot moves from "mobile adapter," to "rigid lever"
5. Angle of gait approaches 15 degrees abducted from a line through the center of the body

C. Runner's gait
1. Phases of gait analogous to walking, with specific differences:
   a. Jogger or long distance runner has heel-toe contact, although in a shorter time period than walking

       b.   Sprinter exhibits a forefoot-toe type of gait (i.e., running on the toes and balls of feet)
          i.   Less shock-attenuation and body protection
          ii. Predisposition to impact-shock injury (stress fractures, etc.)
          iii. Should be performed by experienced or supervised runners
    2. Angle of gait could approach 0 degrees
    3. Double floatation phase of gait
       a.   Both feet off the ground simultaneously
       b.   Body weight increases at impact of contact foot
       c.   More prevalent as speed increases
       d.   Predisposition to impact-shock and overuse injury
       e.   Minor biomechanical imbalances may become significant liabilities, as compensation leads to injury
          i.   Short-leg syndrome
          ii. Forefoot varus and valgus

D. Multi-direction activity gait
    1. Usually no distinct swing and stance phase
    2. Excessive amounts of lateral motion
    3. Both feet usually in contact with the ground unless jumping or momentary single-limb support is required
    4. Angle of gait varies with specific activity

E. Abnormal gait in sports
    1. Related to biomechanical imbalances, including structural and functional components
    2. Related to musculoskeletal or neuromuscular pathology
    3. Related to other causes
       a.   Acquired or congenital musculoskeletal injury
       b.   Incorrect or poorly fitted shoegear
       c.   Degenerative joint disease and arthridities
       d.   Other metabolic underlying disease states

ROLE OF ORTHOSES IN THE PREVENTION AND TREATMENT OF ATHLETIC INJURIES

I. Types of orthoses used in sports

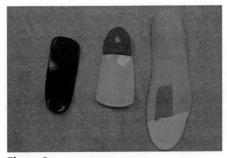

Figure 3.

A. Soft orthoses: Made from soft materials (e.g., Plastizote, Neoprene, EVA)
    1. Augment cushioning of shoe
    2. Provide additional protection to the foot

3. Accommodate painful areas or lesions
4. Can be used as a temporary orthosis while awaiting fabrication of permanent functional devices

B. Semi-rigid orthoses: Made from materials that partially deform under weight bearing (e.g., Polypropylene, Subortholen)

1. Reduce excessive pedal motion (pronation and supination)
2. Attenuate impact-shock to the foot
3. Useful in multi-directional activities (e.g., tennis, golf, aerobic dance)
4. Useful when "absolute functional pedal control" is not required

C. Rigid orthoses: Made from materials that do not deform under weightbearing loads (e.g., Polydur, carbon fiber composites)

1. Control feet around the neutral position (Root Biomechanics)
2. After complete sports history has been obtained and biomechanical examination has been performed, an accurate cast impression of plaster or foam must be taken (Figure 4)
3. Used in athletes whose overpronation results in compromised function, injury, and/or lack of optimum performance
4. Used most often in unidirectional sports (e.g., walking, running, race walking)

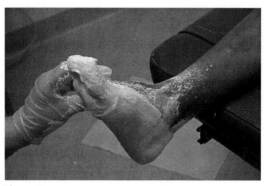

Figure 4.

II. Prescribing orthoses: Additional considerations

A. Posting: Generally enhances overall efficiency of orthotics

1. Rearfoot posts
    a. Used in sports in which greater control of the subtalar joint is necessary
    b. Because of pendulum effect, often used in runner's orthoses
    c. Usually allow for 4 to 6 degrees of subtalar motion
    d. May be rigid, (acrylic) with a medial grind off, or soft and compressible (EVA crepe) without a grind off
    e. In multidirectional sports, use less than 4 degrees of rearfoot posting to avoid lateral instability (ankle sprains)
    f. Rearfoot posts are generally designed to support the foot in a varus position; occasionally can be used to support the foot in, or place the foot in, a valgus position
2. Forefoot posts
    a. Used in sports in which increased forefoot control is necessary to support forefoot deformity
    b. Often used in sprinting and hurdling
    c. May be made from rigid or compressible materials (extrinsic post)
    d. Usually not necessary in most orthoses because of laboratory proficiency in intrinsic balancing of the forefoot to the rearfoot via manual or computer cast correction

e.   Enhances the effectiveness of flexible orthoses

B. Posting elevators
1.   Ensure that the posted orthosis clears the shank of the athletic shoe
2.   Must inform laboratory of shoe type in which orthosis will be worn
3.   Common shoes are ice skates, roller skates, bicycling shoes requiring elevator

C. Heel and sole lifts
1.   May be necessary in a structural limb-length inequality
2.   Also dependent on amount of limb difference and the type of sport activity
3.   Example: a walker with a three eighths to one quarter inch limb difference may not require any lift, but a runner with a three eighths to one quarter limb difference may require a lift to be added to both the orthosis and the midsole of the athletic shoe

D. Accommodations, extensions, and clips
1.   May improve function and/or enhance comfort
2.   Extensions and accommodations reduce pressure on painful lesions and provide additional cushioning to the foot and forefoot for balancing of painful pressure areas
3.   Augment atrophic soft tissue and reduce pressure on painful heels and forefoot metatarsalgia (e.g., horseshoe pad, metatarsal button)
4.   Added medial or lateral rear clips, deep heel seats, and rearfoot skives, enhance subtalar, ankle, and midtarsal joint stability; generally requires wearing athletic shoes with higher heel counters

ATHLETIC INJURIES: GENERAL CATEGORIES

Athletic injuries may be classified as acute traumatic, chronic, or related to overuse. In order to properly evaluate, diagnose and treat the injured athlete, it is necessary to understand the traumatic events and tissue responses that occur with each of these injuries

I.   **Acute traumatic injury occurs when a musculoskeletal tissue undergoes an abrupt stress beyond its normal physiologic adaptive capacity**

   A. Physiologic response
   1.   Acute inflammatory response: First 10 minutes to 72 hours following a traumatic event
      a.   Immediate vasodilatation of blood vessels, releasing histamine and other cellular mediators of tissue repair
         i.   Capillary permeability increases: edema, pain, erythema, and warmth
         ii. First line of treatment: Rest, ice, compression, and elevation (RICE) (Figure 5)

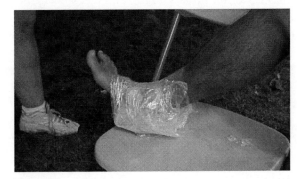

Figure 5.

(a) Allows earlier return to pain free function

(b) Reduces unpleasant effects of inflammation

iii. Nonsteroidal anti-inflammatory drugs (NSAIDS) may be beneficial, as they reduce the continued release of prostaglandin, a cellular element associated with the inflammatory phase

2. Repair phase: Second phase of inflammation, which lasts up to 6 weeks

a. Removal of waste products

b. Repair of injured tissues by collagen synthesis and deposition

c. Greatest vulnerability to re-injury, although athlete feels much better

i. Athlete should participate in non-stress-loading activities (e.g., bicycling, swimming)

ii. Athlete should participate in an active conditioning program

3. Remodeling phase: Third phase of inflammation, which lasts from 3 weeks to 12 months

a. Newly deposited collagen remodels to withstand anticipated physiologic stress demand on the tissues

b. These "new" tissues need to be protected; athlete should use protective braces, splints, tape, or wraps when participating in sports

II. **Chronic injury.** Associated with repetitive microtrauma, which produces a low-grade inflammatory response in the injured tissues over an extended period of time

A. **Initially perceived by athlete as an annoyance and not severe enough to cause modification or cessation of activity**

B. **Over time, athlete begins to compensate to avoid pressure on the injured area, which can affect other musculoskeletal tissues**

C. **Can result in eventual modification or cessation of activities**

D. **Continued nonattenuated. Microtrauma may lead to acute injury** (i.e., stress fracture)

E. **Important for athlete to be attuned to the body's warning signals to prevent injury**

F. **Can be prevented by examining and correcting etiology factors** (i.e., training errors, conditioning problems, shoe problems, and biomechanical dysfunction)

III. **Overuse injury:** Chronic athletic injury, which results from vigorous participation in athletic activities and for which the body's tissues have not, been adequately conditioned to accommodate the increased level of resultant stress (i.e., cyclic repetitive stress)

A. **Musculoskeletal tissues become overworked and overstrained as they attempt to meet the demand**

B. **Tissues fatigue, and the activity eventually ceases, which prevents further tissue injury**

C. **Injury prevention involves modifying training programs to lower demand, proper body conditioning, exercising on more yielding surfaces, wearing more supportive shoe gear, and wearing foot orthoses when appropriate**

D. **Injuries are often associated with excessive pronation for biomechanically dysfunctional feet**

E. **Examples of overuse injuries:** Plantar fasciitis, patellar-femoral syndrome, Achilles tendonitis, and shin splints (posterior tibial tendonitis and medial tibial stress syndrome)

IV. **Strains, sprains, fractures, and other bone injuries**

A. **Strains:** Injuries to the muscle or muscle-tendon units

1.   Mild: Athlete is aware of some discomfort but is able to continue sports activity without alteration; only ice is required
2.   Moderate: Level of discomfort requires athlete to modify, and even restrict some activity, treatment involves rest, ice, gentle stretching, and physical therapy
3.   Severe: Complete disruption of the muscle-tendon unit; athlete stops all athletic activity that requires use of that tissue as absolute rest of the injured part is the rule until partial repair of the injured tissue and new collagen deposition occurs

B. Sprains: Injuries to ligamentous tissue
1.   Grade I: Small tear in the ligament resulting in minor hemorrhage, local swelling, and joint pain; treatment is a short period of RICE followed by supportive splinting or taping when athletic activity is resumed
2.   Grade II: Substantial numbers of ligamentous fibers are torn, but, as a whole, ligament remains intact; joint function and stability may be compromised
   a.   Initial treatment: Absolute rest and non-weightbearing on injured extremity in addition to RICE
   b.   Thereafter, protected weightbearing and joint rehabilitation with physical therapy treatments for early joint mobilization and for restoration of adjacent muscle strength and prevention of loss of joint function and stability
   c.   Bracing and taping of the injured joint for 1-2 months on return to athletic activity (Figure 6)

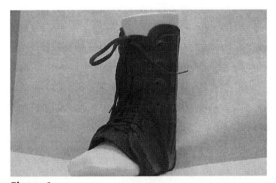

Figure 6.

3.   Grade III: Ligament is completely ruptured and incapable of providing any stability to the injured joint
   a.   Cast immobilization and non-weightbearing to injured extremity until partial healing occurs
      i.   If ankle is involved, it may be dorsiflexed in cast to increase resultant ankle joint stability
   b.   Surgical primary repair
      i.   Usually performed on a competitive athlete
      ii. Injury associated with a fracture or wide diastasis
   c.   Either treatment followed by protective weight bearing with a removable walking cast boot
   d.   Early joint mobilization as soon as partial restoration of joint stability has occurred
   e.   Aggressive physical therapy to increase surrounding muscle strength
   f.   Athletic activity is resumed once joint stabilization has been restored to maximum potential

      g.   Joint protection with bracing and splinting is used indefinitely when involved in sport

C. Bone contusion: Results from forceful stress on the bone, which causes interosseous hemorrhage but no violation of cortical continuity
1. Radiographs usually unremarkable
2. MRI can demonstrate it
3. Pain and swelling over bone are present
4. Treat with RICE, NSAIDS, and support

D. Cortical stress reactions: Occur when repetitive stress loads on bone produce accelerated remodeling and apposition bone growth without interosseous hemorrhage
1. Radiographs show cortical hypertrophy or thickening (Figure 7)
2. Rarely symptomatic and usually requires no treatment

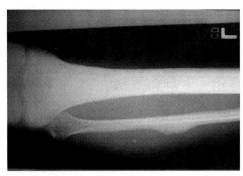

Figure 7.

E. Fractures: Complete disruption of the osseous tissue and violation of cortical continuity
1. Radiographs indicate site of fracture and may or may not indicate severity
2. Clinical findings include pain over the bone, inability to bear weight, swelling, gross deformity or angulation, partial or complete loss of use or motion
3. May require use of other imaging techniques for detection and/or visualization
    a.   CT scan: Used to see tarsal fractures
    b.   Bone scans: Used to pick up occult or stress fractures
    c.   MRI
4. Overt fractures in sports usually relate to collision or contact sports (e.g., football, hockey, and basketball)
5. Stress fractures result from repetitive stress loads on a bone that exceed the bone's physiologic adaptive capacity
    a.   Radiographs may not indicate site of fracture until after repair process has commenced and bone callus tissue has been produced, usually 2-3 weeks following injury
    b.   Clinical findings include pain, which increases with level of activity; swelling, and extreme tenderness over the site of injury
    c.   A Technetium 99 bone scan may be required to confirm presence of a stress fracture
        i. Important to perform in a competitive athlete, as treatment for a stress fracture differs significantly from a similar soft tissue injury
6. Treatment options
    a.   Unstable or displaced fracture
        i. May use open reduction-internal fixation with no weight bearing and cast immobilization

        ii. May use closed reduction with or without percutaneous fixation, and/or cast immobilization, non-weightbearing until radiographic evidence of bone healing is seen

    b. Stable fracture may only need compression wrap and splinting of injured extremity

    c. In any fracture, the athlete is generally precluded from weightbearing sports participation until adequate bone healing is observed radiographically, usually a minimum of 4-6 weeks

    d. Substitute aerobic activities are recommended to provide for, and maintain, good cardiovascular fitness (i.e., bicycling, swimming, or running in water)

V. Injuries requiring emergency treatment

A. Most sports-related lower-extremity injuries respond to RICE

1. Exceptions include compartment syndrome, which can result in an ischemic limb or an open compound fracture; both injuries require surgical intervention to prevent morbid injury to the athlete

B. Extreme thermal injury (e.g., heatstroke, frostbite) may result in death if immediate care and treatment are not received

1. Running in very humid, hot weather without adequate fluid replacement
2. Working out in frigid weather without adequate hand, feet, and head coverings
3. Water intoxication - drinking too much fluid leading to hyponatremia

VI. Specific injuries

A. Sesamoiditis

1. Etiology
    a. Plantar position of the sesamoid bones makes sesamoids vulnerable to injury
    b. Predisposing activities include ballet, sprinting, aerobic dancing, and tennis
    c. Associated with rigid, cavus feet or plantarflexed first ray
2. Evaluation
    a. Pain and swelling at plantar first metatarsophalangeal joint
    b. Pain and possible limitation of range of motion of first metatarsophalangeal joint
    c. Plantar flexion of the first metatarsophalangeal joint against resistance frequently elicits pain at the sesamoids

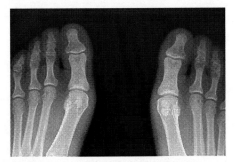

Figure 8.

    d. Radiographs may or may not show fracture of sesamoid; may be a bipartite sesamoid (Figure 8)
      i. Bonescan occasionally necessary to determine fracture of sesamoid
      ii. MRI: Occasionally needed to determine avascular necrosis or extent of fracture

3. Management
   a. RICE
   b. If no fracture, peri-sesamoidal injection of local anesthetic, steroid, and/or hyalu-ronidase
      i. Decrease inflammatory response
      ii. Decrease pain
   c. Provision for off-loading sesamoid bones
      i. Allow for relief of weight-bearing stress
      ii. Dancers' pads and tape
      iii. Heel platform shoes: Darco, IPOS
      iv. Orthoses: Accommodative or functional with appropriate first submetatarsal balancing
      v. Crutch ambulation, with or without weight bearing, boot or short-leg cast
   d. Physical therapy modalities: Used after initial inflammation decreases
      i. Ultrasound
      ii. Iontophoresis and phonophoresis, interferential current
   e. Surgical removal of injured sesamoid bone
      i. Performed only if conservative measures have not resulted in a comfortable gait and allowed the athlete to return to sports activity
      ii. May need only to remove part of the sesamoid bone
      iii. May require orthoses after surgery to properly balance the foot and prevent further pedal injury

B. Plantar fasciitis
   1 Etiology
      a. Inflammation of plantar fascia: Three bands of dense connective tissue that extend from the calcaneus to the forefoot and are seen on MRI as confluent with the distal fibers of the Achilles tendon
      b. Any pedal motion that places the plantar fascia in excessive stretch (i.e., extreme pronation) or a contracture (i.e. cavus or supinated foot)
      c. Related to running on hard, unyielding surfaces; overtraining; improper conditioning, especially failure to stretch the Achilles tendon and hamstrings; and excessive shoe wear
      d. Overstretching of the plantar fascia leads to a "traction enthesitis" and may result in formation of a "heel spur"
      e. Rigid cavus foot in which excessive load-bearing produces stretch on the plantar fascia (Figure 9)

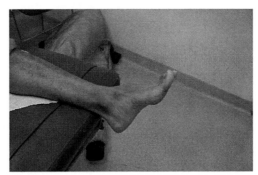

Figure 9.

      i. Athletic activity may lead to further strain of already tensioned stretched tissue

      ii. Inherent inability to absorb impact-shock at heel contact causes traumatic heel injury and plantar fasciitis

   f. Ankle joint equinus from gastrocnemius and/or soleus muscle tightness or from osseous blockage produces compensatory subtalar joint pronation, which produces hypermobility, placing increased tension on the plantar fascia

2. Evaluation

   a. Poststatic dyskinesia: Pain in heel on arising after being seated or lying down for prolonged period of time; in runner, pain is present at outset of run, diminishes as run continues, and recurs more intensely after run ends – especially after being non-weightbearing for awhile

   b. Tenderness along the course of the plantar fascia, especially at insertion to the calcaneus

   c. Pain may increase with ankle joint dorsiflexion as plantar fascia is stretched

   d. Possible swelling and warmth at calcaneal insertion

   e. Check plantar fascial bands for continuity and uniformity of thickness; eliminate possibility of fascial rupture or soft tissue mass (e.g., fibroma)

   f. Compression of body of calcaneus from medial to lateral elicits no pain; eliminates possibility of calcaneal stress fracture

   g. Radiographs, taken while bearing weight and in angle and base of gait, are necessary to evaluate biomechanical foot structure and function, and to determine the presence of osseous projections and any unusual causes of heel pain (e.g., cysts, systemic arthropathy, stress fractures, coalitions, and tumors)

3. Management

   a. Initial treatment: RICE

   b. Reduce acute symptoms and correct faulty etiology factors

      i. Supportive taping to reduce stress on plantar fascia (e.g., Low Dye, Campbell rest, stirrup)

      ii. Stretching exercises to increase calf muscle flexibility

      iii. NSAIDS

      iv. Trigger point injections (up to three) of local, short-acting or intermediate acting corticosteroid and local anesthetic

      v. Physical therapy, including deep massage, ultrasound, iontophoresis, and interferential stimulation

      vi. Appliances, including heel lifts, heel cups, horseshoe pads, and posterior night splints

      vii. Extracorporeal Shock Wave Therapy - pulsed shock waves delivered to heel up to 1,000 impulses at a session. Performed under local anesthesia. One to three treatments

   c. Evaluate training techniques and modify to reduce strain on plantar tissues

      i. Train on softer surfaces

      ii. Decrease level of intensity of training

      iii. Reduce distance, speed, and hilly terrain until injury is completely resolved

   d. Wear shoe gear with more heel support and good heel counter as well as adequate cushioning

   e. Replace excessively worn shoes immediately

   f. Use orthoses after determining biomechanical function and need

      i. Assess demands of sport, foot type, and desired objectives – combine with appropriate athletic shoe

g. Surgical intervention
   i. Consider it after 6-month trial of conservative care cannot return to a previous comfortable level of participation
   ii. Consider after elimination of all other causes of heel pain, except excessive plantar fascial tension or neuritic involvement
       (a) Rule out HLA B-27 arthridities
       (b) Rule out stress fracture or tarsal coalition (bone scan, CT, or MRI)
   iii. Performed in less than 8% of all heel pain cases
   iv. May involve soft tissue and/or bone
       (a) Plantar fasciotomy
       (b) Release of calcaneal or posterior tibial nerve entrapment
       (c) Heel spur resection; rarely necessary as symptoms not measurably improved over plantar fascial release without spur removal
   v. Need to use functional orthoses postoperatively

C. **Enthesitis:** Inflammation at the insertion of a connective tissue (e.g., tendon, ligament, or fascia) to bone
   1. Etiology
      a. Repetitive stress exerted on connective tissue leads to inflammation at insertion to bone, which is point of maximum strain
         i. Plantar fasciitis results from a "traction enthesitis" in which tension on the fascia results in inflammation at its attachment to the calcaneus
         ii. Achilles tendon enthesitis, results from continuous strain on a tight tendon during gait or athletic activity, resulting in inflammation and occasionally calcification at the posterior aspect of the calcaneus (i.e., retrocalcaneal heel spur)
   2. Evaluation
      a. Pain at the insertion of soft tissue to bone, which is aggravated by increasing activity
      b. Tenderness to pinpoint palpation at the heel insertion
      c. Stretching the tissue leads to an increase in discomfort at the enthesis
      d. Localized swelling, increased heat, and erythema occasionally found
      e. Radiographic findings include osseous projections, cortical hypertrophy, or increase in soft tissue density at the irritation – often a bursitis
   3. Management
      a. Immediate: RICE
      b. Partial immobilization with taping or bracing to reduce stress on the injured tissues, application of an Unna Boot
      c. Physical therapy modalities
         i. Ultrasound with or without steroid gel
         ii. Interferential stimulation
         iii. Gentle stretching and joint mobilization
         iv. Cross friction massage
         v. Night splints
      d. Correction of etiological factors
         i. Training modifications (e.g., avoidance of hills, smooth versus rough terrain, relaxed body positions)
         ii. Increase in flexibility exercises
         iii. Change to shoes that provide additional support, especially at the heel
         iv. Functional foot orthoses, heel lifts, and wedges

D. **Ankle sprains/strains:** Lateral stress is imposed on a joint that functionally moves primarily in the sagittal plane; the surrounding ligaments are stretched and/or torn, and inversion or eversion sprain results

1. Etiology
    a. Inversion sprains account for 85% of all ankle sprains and are the most common injury in sports
        i.   Ankle is in plantar flexed position and foot becomes inverted
        ii. Lateral collateral ligament becomes strained (grade I sprain)
        iii. If lateral force is more severe, collateral ligaments become partially torn (grade II sprain)
        iv. If excessive lateral force is present, complete rupture of collateral ligaments with possible fracture of the tibia and/or fibula (grade III sprain)
    b. Eversion sprains
        i.   Foot is everted, tibia is externally rotating, and a medially directed force is applied to ankle
        ii. Deltoid ligaments are primarily injured
        iii. Extreme force may cause severe damage to the tibiofibular ligament and interosseous membrane as well as fracture
            (a) May lead to diastasis and gross ankle instability
        iv. May be associated with fracture of one or both malleoli

2. Evaluation
    a. Pain around the foot and ankle joint, aggravated with weight bearing; limping often noted
    b. History of ankle being twisted or torqued, as in stepping into a pothole
    c. History of previous ankle injuries
        i.   Possibility of chronic ankle instability
        ii. Predisposition to ankle injury
    d. Swelling, tenderness, ecchymosis, erythema, and heat over medial and lateral aspects of ankle and foot
    e. Pain on attempted range of motion of subtalar and ankle joints
    f. Spasm of peroneal and/or posterior tibial tendons
        i.   Body's attempt to restrict motion of the injured joint
        ii. Protection mechanism
    g. Stressing the ankle anterior to posterior (Drawer Sign) and lateral to medial determines degree of ligamentous injury and instability
        i.   Stress testing should be performed bilaterally
        ii. Often helpful to take stress radiographs
    h. Radiographs of injured and contralateral extremities should be taken prior to any manipulation of the injured joints
        i.   Radiographs should include three views of the ankle (AP, MO, and lateral) and MO of the foot (i.e., rule out base of fifth metatarsal fracture)
        ii. May need lower leg films if high fracture is suspected

3. Management
    a. Initial: RICE for all three grades
    b. Grade I sprain
        i.   Usually resolves without further treatment
        ii. Supportive taping or bracing when participating in sports until athlete has no sense of discomfort
            (a) Over-the-counter ankle support
            (b) Strorngren-type ankle support (stabilizes ankle and subtalar joint)
            (c) Air splint

    c. Grade II sprain
        i. Moderate degree of swelling and inflammation
          (a) Initial compression is essential
             (i) Unna boot
             (ii) Jones compression wrap
             (iii) Venous heart wrap
       ii. Partial or full weightbearing to tolerance with protective foot gear
          (a) Wooden or Darco shoe
          (b) Removable double upright walking cast boot (e.g., Equalizer, CAM walker, Aircast)
      iii. NSAIDS
      iv. Once acute inflammatory response has abated, begin program to restore normal joint function
          (a) Range-of-motion exercises
          (b) Adjacent muscle strengthening
          (c) Biornechanical ankle proprioceptive system (BAPS) board to restore proprioceptive loss
          (d) Aerobic activity substituted to maintain cardiovascular fitness while protecting injured joint
             (i) Swimming
             (ii) Running in water (flotation vest)
             (iii) Bicycling
       v. Protective support or bracing of ankle on return to weightbearing athletic activity for 3-12 months
          (a) If any sign of ankle instability remains, ankle brace should be worn indefinitely
    d. Grade III sprain
        i. Nonsurgical treatment: Most common treatment in non-competitive athlete
          (a) Nonweight-bearing below-the-knee cast immobilization, followed by weightbearing cast immobilization for a period of 4-6 weeks
          (b) May be used for associated nondisplaced fracture
          (c) Once adequate repair of ligaments has occurred, begin program of joint restoration and rehabilitation
             (i) Intense physical therapy
             (ii) Adjacent muscle strengthening
             (iii) Range-of-motion exercises
             (iv) BAPS board to improve proprioceptive loss
             (v) Aerobic activity substituted to maintain cardiovascular fitness
          (d) Resumption of sports participation requires ankle bracing for indefinite time period
       ii. Surgical repair
          (a) Used if wide diastasis or displaced fracture
          (b) Used in competitive athlete, if possible
          (c) Primary repair in most ligamentous ruptures is controversial
          (d) If ankle is chronically unstable with recurrent ankle sprains, consider ankle stabilization procedure
          (e) Follow all ankle ligament surgery with immobilization, and institute physical therapy and rehabilitation as soon as is practical

E. Shin splints: Tendonitis/periostitis of the lower leg: defined by the American College of Sports Medicine as "pain and discomfort in the leg from repetitive running on hard surfaces or forcible use of the foot flexors; diagnosis should be limited to musculotendinous inflammations, excluding ischemic or fracture disorder"

1. Etiology
   a. Involves posterior tibial tendon and muscle and periosteal structures of the lower two thirds of the tibia. Soleus attachment is also a possible etiology
   b. Anterior tibial muscle and tendon less frequently involved (more related to compartment swelling)
   c. Overuse injury - not unique to runners
      i. Seen in any sport that involves running, jumping, sustained walking, or frequent directional changes (e.g., basketball, aerobic dance, football, tennis)
   d. Associated with inadequate conditioning
      i. Tight posterior musculature (i.e., calf muscles)
      ii. Weak anterior and posterior tibial muscles
      iii. Foot mechanics hypermobility and excess pronation
   e. Associated with poor training techniques, improper or defective shoe gear, and biomechanical dysfunction (e.g., excessive subtalar joint pronation secondary to a fully compensated forefoot varus)
2. Evaluation
   a. Tenderness along medial and/or anterior two thirds of the lower tibia (Figure 10)

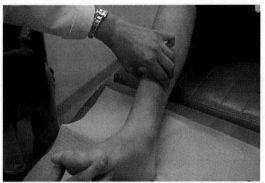

Figure 10.

   b. Pain increases with plantar flexion, inversion, or dorsiflexion of the foot against resistance
   c. Limitation of ankle joint dorsiflexion, resulting from tight calf muscles
   d. Moderate to excessive midstance subtalar joint pronation is often observed
   e. Running gait, in anterior shin splint syndrome, may reveal a foot slap at forefoot contact
   f. Plain radiographs of the lower legs are often unremarkable
   g. Radiographs of the feet often reveal abnormal biomechanical position
   h. Additional imaging studies may be needed occasionally to determine the presence of a tibial stress fracture
      i. Technetium 99 bonescan demonstrates focal uptake in all three phases in a stress fracture
      ii. Technetium 99 bonescan demonstrates diffuse, variegated uptake, in only one or two phases in shin splint syndrome (i.e., no fracture present) (Figure 11)
3. Management

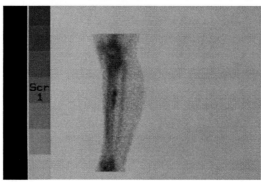

Figure 11.

    a. Immediate: RICE

    b. NSAIDS

    c. If no stress fracture, modify activity; do not necessarily discontinue activity but allow crosstraining

    d. Reduce stress on the musculoskeletal tissues of the lower leg
        i. Compressive wrap or sleeve around leg
        ii. Supportive taping of foot to decrease overactivity of the posterior tibial muscle

    e. Ice massage after workouts for first few weeks

    f. Physical therapy modalities of ultrasound, interferential stimulation, and iontophoresis may be of some benefit

    g. Correct faulty etiologic factors
        i. Work out on softer, yielding surfaces
        ii. Replace excessively worn shoe gear
        iii. Intensify conditioning program to include more stretching of posterior muscle group and strengthening of lower leg muscles
        iv. Use functional foot orthoses, as appropriate

    h. Surgery not indicated, except in acute compartment syndrome

F. Compartment syndrome

    1. Etiology: Increased pressure in one or more of the three compartments of the lower leg

        a. During exercise, the muscles of the leg, which are surrounded by an inelastic covering, expand as a result of increase blood flow
            i. If the sheath does not allow for expansion of muscle, tissue becomes compressed and squeezed
            ii. Intra-compartmental pressures increase

        b. May result from intense workouts
            i. Often responds to decreasing activity level and non-emergent measures
            ii. Need to adjust workouts to keep compartment pressures at a physiologic level

        c. If pressure in compartments increases where neurovascular structures are compressed, ischemia and paralysis to the lower extremity may result; **this is a medical emergency**

    2. Evaluation

        a. Pain along the lower leg, especially over the involved muscle groups
            i. May be severe and intractable; requires emergency treatment
            ii. May be mild to moderate; responds to conservative treatment and sports modification

        b. Leg may be tense, warm, and swollen

        c. Pulses and pedal neurologic sensation may or may not be intact

        i. Absent pulses and loss of pedal sensation and musculature function, including a "foot drop," indicates a major medical emergency

        ii. Requires aggressive, immediate treatment: fasciotomy

    d. Measurement of intra-compartmental pressures may indicate significant increase above normal

  3. Management

    a. RICE

    b. Non-emergency cases

        i. Stretching exercises

        ii. Training modifications, including decrease in exercise intensity

        iii. Shoe gear modifications, including more heel support and midsole cushion

        iv. Functional foot orthoses

        v. NSAIDS

        vi. Physical therapy modalities to decrease intra-compartmental pressure

          (a) Interferential stimulation

          (b) Dynawave

          (c) H-wave

        vii. Splinting or compression bracing of the leg when exercising

          (a) Neoprene sleeve

          (b) Cho-pat compartment brace

          (c) Coban wrap

    c. Emergency cases

        i. Surgery: fasciotomy and compartment release

          (a) Performed if clinical findings include intractable pain, pallor, pulselessness, loss of muscular function, or numbness, or in cases of chronic compartment syndrome, which is inhibiting performance of a competitive athlete

G. Iliotibial Band Syndrome

  1. Anatomy

    a. Iliotibial band: A thick band of fascia lata, originating from the iliac crest and progressing along the lateral aspect of the thigh

        i. Derives its insertion from both the tensor fascia lata. and gluteus muscle

        ii. Inserts onto the lateral tibial condyle at Gerdey's tubercle

    b. Iliotibial band: A lateral stabilizer of the knee

  2. Mechanism

    a. Repeated flexion and extension of the knee, which occurs with long distance running, causing rubbing of the band over the lateral femoral condyle

        i. Friction and inflammation

        ii. Acute bursitis

        iii. Lateral knee pain with burning sensation

  3. Common clinical presentation

    a. Bowlegged runners with pronated feet

    b. Running on banked surfaces

    c. Leg-length discrepancy

    d. Shoes excessively worn laterally

  4. Evaluation

    a. Pain on palpation at Gerdey's tubercle and along iliotibial band

    b. Pain when walking down stairs or running downhill

    c. Swelling and erythema may or may not be present

    d. Palpable click or snap with flexion and extension of the knee (i.e., Ober's Test)

5. Management
    a. Immediate: RICE
    b. Stretching and strengthening exercises
        i. Iliotibial band stretches (crossover toe touches)
        ii. Hamstring stretching and strengthening program
    c. Physical therapy modalities
        i. Phonophoresis with steroid gel
        ii. Ultrasound
    d. Training modifications
        i. Avoid hills until symptoms improve
        ii. Change directions every two laps on a banked track (i.e., clockwise to counter-clockwise)
        iii. Run on softer surfaces
        iv. Decrease athletic activity intensity
        v. Avoid high crowned roads
    e. Replace laterally worn shoes
    f. NSAIDS
    g. Correct biomechanical imbalance with custom orthoses
        i. May need varus or valgus; rearfoot post, depending on foot structure
        ii. If excessive subtalar joint pronation is present, use a varus rearfoot post
        iii. If rigid cavus foot with heel unable to reach perpendicular is present, consider valgus rearfoot post
    h. Steroid injection to Gerdey's tubercle occasionally necessary if unresponsive to other measures
        i. Need to check state license limitations
        ii. May require referral to orthopedist
    i. Surgery rare: Release or lengthening of iliotibial band

H. Chondromalacia patella (Patellofemoral Pain Syndrome)
    1. Definition
        a. Misnomer that describes anterior knee pain, attributable to multiple causes
            i. Patellofemoral dysfunction
            ii. Patellar subluxation
            iii. Patellar compression syndrome
        b. Overuse syndrome experienced by participants in almost every sports activity
        c. Pseudonyms for the condition include runner's knee and biker's knee
    2. Etiology
        a. Abnormal tracking of the patella in the femoral groove, usually the result of a weak vastus medialis muscle
        b. Related to increased Q angle and tight vastus lateralis and iliotibial band
        c. Aggravated by excessive internal leg rotation, associated with any deformity that may increase subtalar joint pronation (e.g., compensated forefoot varus), compensated rearfoot varus
    3. Clinical presentation
        a. Aching or soreness around or under the kneecap, which is aggravated by stair climbing or hill running
            i. Pain is usually medial but may be lateral
            ii. Squatting and kneeling aggravates pain
        b. "Movie theater sign": Pain in the knee after sitting with knees flexed for an extended period of time

c. Knee may occasionally feel as if it is "locking"
d. Patella is noted to track laterally on flexion-extension
e. Weakness of muscle tone in the vastus medialis
f. Commonly demonstrate pain to palpation along the posterior aspect of the patella, both medially and laterally
g. Patellar apprehension test: Lateral movement of the patella causes quadriceps contraction
h. Extending knee from 30° of flexion to full extension elicits pain
i. Compressing patella against femoral condyles produces pain (Clarke's Test)
j. Radiographs are rarely diagnostic (Sunrise view) (Figure 12)

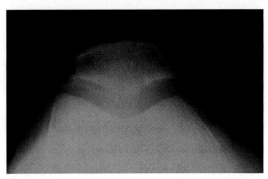

Figure 12.

4. Management
    a. Immediate: RICE
    b. Quadriceps-strengthening program
        i. Emphasize vastus medialis (last 10 degrees of knee extension)
        ii. Never flex knee beyond 40 degrees
        iii. Include isometric, isotonic, and isokinetic exercise
    c. Hamstring and Iliotibial band stretches
    d. NSAIDS
    e. Physical therapy modalities
        i. Muscle stimulator
        ii. Ultrasound or phonophoresis
    f. Reduce internal leg rotation
        i. Heel wedges
        ii. Prefabricated or custom foot orthoses
    g. Bracing in resistant cases
        i. Neoprene foam sleeve
        ii. Cho-pat knee strap
        iii. Horseshoe brace
        iv. Infra-patellar strap
    h. Training modifications
        i. Decrease or avoid hills, especially downhill, running
        ii. Shorten stride length
        iii. Decrease level of workout intensity
    i. Shoe gear with firm heel counters
    j. Surgery: Lateral retinacular release used only for extremely resistant cases in which pain interferes with daily activities

I. Children's Sports Injuries
1. Background
    a. Sports are an important part of child growth and development
    b. Develops good health and living habits as well as teaches sportsmanship and fair play
    c. Millions of both male and female children participate in organized sports daily
    d. Fastest growing injury rates in sports are now in youth sports
2. Children are not miniature adults
3. Cannot expect a child to handle the same training loads and stresses that an adult athlete undergoes
    a. "Little League Syndrome"
    b. Parent interference
    c. Children can be turned off to sport for life
    d. Parents try to train their children like the professionals-consequence can be serious injury
4. Child has no more time to be a child
    a. One endless season – no off-season or vacation time away from serious competition
    b. Youth sports violates every rule of training; especially rest intervals and age appropriate activity
5. Common injuries in Growing Children
    a. Acute injury
        i. ankle sprain
        ii. Probable growthplate injury. Salter – Harris Classification Grade One
        iii. Salter – Harris Grade Two – Serious injury that could result in permanent deformity
    b. Overuse Injury
        i. Increased participation has resulted in similar injury patterns as seen in adults
        ii. Growing pains
        iii. Rapid growth of bone exceeds the lengthening of muscles & tendons
        iv. Occurs during the growth phase of adolescence
        v. Results in excess traction or pulling on the open epiphyseal plates
    c. Eiphyseal Injuries (trauma)
        i. Epiphysis is 3 to 5 times weaker in structure than surrounding bone and tendon
        ii. Salter – Harris fracture type injuries
        iii. Tillaux fracture – external rotation with fracture of the distal tibial epiphysis anterior lateral fragment
        iv. Triplane fracture of distal tibia
        v. Stress fractures of metatarsal, tibia & fibula
    d. Calcaneal Apophysitis (Sever's Disease)
        i. Considered the model Overuse Injury
        ii. Ages 8 – 13 years old
        iii. Often bilateral – will resolve with time – visualized on x-ray (Figure 13)
        iv. Underlying biomechanical faults can result in apophysitis
        v. Self limiting condition – will resolve with time and supportive therapy
        vi. Use of taping, heel lifts, heel cups, ice packs, and physical therapy with gradual stretching of the heel cord
        vii. Limited play – play half a game rather than entire game
        viii. Cleated shoes with improper use can lead to apophyseal plate injury (Figure 14)
    e. Freiberg's Infraction
        i. AVN of second metatarsal or lesser metatarsal heads

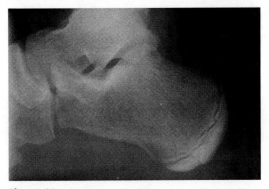

Figure 13.

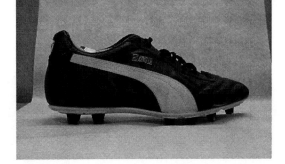

Figure 14.

      ii. Result in permanent deformity

      iii. Early diagnosis important

      iv. Protect area from further trauma – balanced orthotics

  f. Osgood-Schlatter's Disease

      i. Tibial tubercle – AVN

      ii. Jumping & ballistic sports

      iii. Telltale bump on knee

      iv. Orthopedic consult recommended

  g. Kohler's Disease

      i. AVN Navicular

      ii. Can result in navicular wedging deformity and upset of mechanical balance in feet

      iii. Early arthritic & degenerative changes

      iv. Use of orthotic support can help relieve stress on the navicular

  h. Legg-Calve-Perthes Disease

      i. AVN of the proximal femoral epiphysis

      ii. Referred pain to the knee

      iii. Can result in hip joint deformity and disability in later life

  i. Slipped Capital femoral epiphysis

      i. Again – referred pain to the knee

      ii. Limping gait, limb length discrepancy

      iii. Surgical correction with pinning necessary

BIBLIOGRAPHY

Pagliano j et al. Clinics in Podiatric Medicine and Surgery, vol. 3:4. W.B. Saunders Co., Philadelphia, 1986.

Clinical Symposia, vol. 45: 1. Ciba-Geigy, Summit, NJ 07901, 1993.

Subotnik SI. Podiatric sports medicine. Futura Publishing Co, Mount Kisco, 1975.

Subotnik SI, ed. Sports Medicine of the Lower Extremity 2nd ed. Churchill Livingstone, New York, 1999.

CHAPTER 8
SPORTS MEDICINE

1. The worst surface on which to run is:

    A. Grass
    B. Dirt track
    C. Sidewalk
    D. Asphalt

2. Which of the following are not primary etiologies of running injuries?

    A. Training errors
    B. Improper or inadequate conditioning program
    C. Biomechanical imbalances
    D. A high carbohydrate diet
    E. Shoe gear problems

3. All are characteristics of a running/walking shoe except:

    A. Firm, rigid heel counter
    B. Rearfoot cushion
    C. 2 inch or higher heel
    D. Midfoot stability

4. The second phase or repair phase of the acute inflammatory response following an injury lasts from:

    A. 1-7 days
    B. 2 weeks -11 months
    C. 3 days - 6 weeks
    D. 6 months - 12 years

5. All of the following treatments are considered appropriate for a grade II ankle sprain in a 55-year old recreational athlete, except:

    A. RICE
    B. Physical therapy
    C. Surgical exploration and restoration of the ankle ligaments
    D. Protective bracing and taping

6. Appropriate initial treatment for a first episode of sesamoiditis, without evidence of fracture, includes all of the following except:

    A. Off-loading sesamoid
    B. Accommodative or functional foot orthoses
    C. Steroid injection
    D. Surgical removal

7.   When there is inflammation at the site of insertion of a connective tissue to bone, it is called:

        A.   enteritis
        B.   collagenitis
        C.   enthesitis
        D.   entropy

8.   Shin splints most often involve which muscle-tendon structures?

        A.   peroneals
        B.   gastrocnemius-soleus complex
        C.   posterior tibialis
        D.   anterior tibialis

9.   The iliotibial band, which is implicated in lateral knee and hip pain, inserts into:

        A.   the femur
        B.   the popliteal fossa
        C.   Gerdey's tubercle at the tibia
        D.   the pes anserenus

10.   Clinical signs of chondromalacia patella include all of the following except:

        A.   positive movie theater sign
        B.   pain in the knee when squatting or kneeling
        C.   strong vastus medialis muscle tone
        D.   patella tracks laterally

Chapter 9

Surgical Criteria and Complications

by Elizabeth Weber and Robert Weber, based on a chapter originally written by Alan M. Warren

PERIOPERATIVE CARE

I. Healthy/Compromised Individuals

A. Podiatric Surgical Indications

1. Soft tissue
   a. Skin lesions
   b. Nail procedures
   c. Cyst removal
   d. Debridement of ulcers and gangrenous tissue secondary to:
      i. Ischemia
      ii. Venous return insufficiency secondary to:
         (a) CHF
         (b) Nonpatent valves
         (c) Varicosities
      iii. Pressure secondary to:
         (a) Poor shoe gear
         (b) Poor home/hospital care
      iv. Infection
      v. Diabetes
         (a) Autonomic neuropathy
         (b) Poor healing secondary to poor glucose control
2. Skin grafts
   a. Autograft
   b. Skin products & growth factors
3. Tendon procedures for biomechanical correction
4. Neuralgia relief
   a. Impingement release

      b.   Neuroma excision
5. Osseous Procedures
      a.   Relief of:
           i. Forefoot deformities
          ii. Rearfoot deformities
      b.   Osteomyelitis
      c.   Tumors
      d.   Amputations
6. Arterial Bypass
7. Compartment syndrome
8. Reconstruction
      a.   Trauma
      b.   Charcot foot

B. General Preoperative Protocol for Healthy Patient
1. Purpose
      a.   Patient safety
           i. Assure it is the correct patient
          ii. Correct operative limb
        iii. Address medical conditions & allergies
      b.   Surgeon medicolegal protection
2. 3 major areas of concern
      a.   Coagulation disorders
      b.   Drug history
      c.   Previous anesthesia complications
3. Elective surgery
      a.   Begins in surgeon's office, after non-surgical measures have been reasonably exhausted and surgical need has been confirmed
           i. First visit = inform patient
               (a) Explain procedure, anesthesia, preop diet & medications, & postop course including recovery time and ambulation
               (b) Answer all questions to patient satisfaction
               (c) Ask if all questions have been asked
               (d) Document
          ii. Second vist = Informed consent
               (a) Repeat explanations, and answer questions
               (b) Consent form
               (c) Schedule surgery date
               (d) Order pre-admission testing, antibiotic prophylaxis, crutch training
      b.   Medical Clearance from Primary Care Physician if patient has specific medical needs
      c.   Pre-Admission Testing
            i. History & Physical
          ii. Labs
               (a) Electrolytes
               (b) CBC with Differential
               (c) UA
               (d) Glucose
               (e) PT/PTT

(f) For general anesthesia, add pregnancy test for women in childbearing years and CXR if over 40 or Hx of smoking
   iii. ECG
   iv. CXR
   v. Creatinine Clearance if suspected kidney disease or diabetic
   vi. Blood typing and crossing if major sx or anticoag patient
  d. Admission to Hospital
    i. Outpatient surgeries
    ii. 23 hour observation for surgeries that are:
     (a) More disabling (i.e., Rearfoot, geater tissue dissection)
     (b) Greater pain control needed briefly
     (c) Medical condition warrants brief monitoring
    iii. Admission for several days
     (a) Patient unable to care for self
     (b) Sequence of more major surgery requiring longer monitoring amputation, etc.)
     (c) Major complications during surgery or in recovery room
  e. Interviews to assure patient safety
    i. Floor or SSU nurse
    ii. Preop-Holding nurse
    iii. Surgeon
    iv. Anesthesiologist/anesthetist
     (a) Airways
     (b) Drug interactions
     (c) Allergies
     (d) Cardio/pulmonary conditions
     (e) Antibiotic prophylaxis
    v. OR circulator
    vi. Surgeon Identification in OR (in some hospital protocols)
 4. Urgent / Emergent Surgery
  a. Stabilize & Obtain Medical Clearance
    i. In ER if emergency
    ii. On floor if medical conditions warrant delay
  b. Enough testing has usually been done to draw conclusions relating to surgical condition. Otherwise order any remaining tests, as in elective surgery
  c. All else is the same as for elective surgery

C. General Postoperative Protocol for Healthy Patient
 1. Begins in operating room
  a. Antibiotic prophylaxis
    Installation of drains to prevent hematoma
  b. Application of sterile dressings in a sterile manner to avoid unneccessary contamination
  c. Splinting / reinforcing digits, joints, & limbs
    i. Maintain surgical correction via immobility
    ii. Prevent rupturing of repaired ligaments, tendons, osseous corrections
    iii. Protect from outside injury
 2. Recovery in Post anesthesia care unit or Short stay unit prior to discharge or return to floor for 23 hour observation or several days of post op care
  a. Monitor vitals

    b. Nausea control

    c. Pain control

    d. Rest, ice, immobilization, compression, and elevation (RIICE)

    e. DVT prophylaxis
- i. Intermittant leg pumps on nonoperative leg
- ii. Early ambulation
- iii. ASA 81 mg
- iv. Heparin
- v. Dalteparin (Fragmin)
- vi. Enoxaparin (Lovenox)

    f. Protection of operative limb from trauma via wooden shoe
- i. Protect exposed pins / K-wires
- ii. Avoid dehiscence
- iii. Prevent disruption of vascular & osteoblastic healing process
- iv. Avoid disturbance of alignment of osseous corrections
- v. Avoid infections

3. Home Care

    a. Crutches or walkers:
- i. Help NWB & PWB status
- ii. Keep others at safe distance to avoid bumping or stepping on operative limb

    b. Ice for 48 hours

    c. Rest, ice, immobilzation, compression, and elevation (RIICE)

4. Postoperative office visits & exams

    a. examine condition of dressings, casts, postop shoes for cleanliness, dryness, intact condition as an indication of patient compliance

    b. examine incision sites and limb in general for vascularity, signs of infection, wound healing, and reduction of inflammation

    c. patient's general health and attitude

    d. Reapply dressings, splints, casts, boots

    e. Stress importance of NWB or PWB as necessary

    f. Commence physical therapy as warranted to encourage proper connective tissue production

II. Diabetic Patient

A. Goals

1. Avoid hypoglycemia

    a. Schedule early AM surgery slot so npo status is shortest and equilibrium is easier to maintain between insulin & glucose

    b. D/C chlorpropamide (Diabinese) 2-3 days prior to surgery because of its 60 hr. 1/2 life

2. Avoid ketosis (hyperglycemia)

    a. Generally, patient BS should be less than 200 mg/dL

    b. Increased BS impairs wound healing

    c. Can avoid with administration of IV glucose & insulin

    d. Chronic condition increases risk of postop infection

3. Avoid hyperosmolar state because reduced plasma albumin retards wound healing

4. Avoid hypokalemia inherent with too much insulin

5. Maintain good general nutritional health prior to surgery

B. Evaluation Studies

1. HbA$_{1C}$ glycosilated hemoglobin demonstrates blood sugar levels for past 3 months
2. BUN & Creatinine state the baseline preoperative renal status
3. SGOT is the preferred hepatic function test
4. Urinalysis
5. Frequent finger-stick glucose measurements help monitor BS easily even in outpatient settings

C. General protocols based on diabetic type and BS level

1. BS test 1 hr before and 1 hr after surgery via Accu√ fingerstick test
2. Hypoglycemia: postponing procedure is recommended
3. Diet-controlled
   a. BS < 200: no meds needed
   b. BS = 200: use IV regular insulin based on sliding scale
   c. Long, major procedures may require IV regular insulin and/or D5 1/2 NSS @ 125 ml/hr intraop. with BS checks every hour
4. NIIDM
   a. General suggestion
      i. IV insulin & glucose:
         (a) Piggyback separate bags thru single IV port
         (b) Allows separate flow rate control
         (c) Prevents overdosing of either glucose or insulin in event of undetected clogged IV port since both are through the same port
      ii. Npo after midnight, OR clear liquids up to 4 hrs prior to surgery (studies demonstrate increased gastric emptying with clear liquids so that 4 hours is sufficient)
   b. Protocol 1 for all short, minor procedures
      i. Early AM surgery best
      ii. Npo after midnight
      iii. D/C oral hypoglycemic morning of surgery (d/c chlorpropamide 2-3 days before)
      iv. No insulin – no glucose during surgery
      v. Reinstate med regimen when patient begins eating
   c. Protocol 2 for all short, minor or long, major procedures
      i. Npo after midnight
      ii. D/C oral hypoglycemics morning of surgery (d/c chlorpropamide 2-3 days before)
      iii. Perform Accu√ BS test
         (a) BS of 100-200mg/dL - IV lactate Ringer's solution or the house isotonic crystalloid
         (b) BS < 100 start IV D5 - NSS
         (c) BS > 200 start IV regular insulin according to sliding scale
      iv. Surgeries > 1 hr – introp Accu√
5. IDDM
   a. Protocol 1 for all short, minor procedures
      i. Npo after midnight
      ii. 1/2 patient's regular dose (reg & NPH SQ) morning of surgery
      iii. D5 1/2 NSS IV drip during procedure
      iv. 1/2 patient's regular dose (reg & NPH SQ) postop
      v. Administer IV regular insulin according to sliding scale as indicated by Accu√ 1 hr postop
   b. Protocol 2 for all short s/b and long procedures

      i. Best if early AM surgery

      ii. Hold all regular and NPH insulin AM of sx

      iii. Npo after midnight

      iv. Accu√ prior to surgery

         (a) BS < 250 mg/dL - Lactate Ringer's solution or house isotonic crystalloid

         (b) > 250 mg/dL - IV reg. Insulin based on sliding scale or patient's usual use; consider D5 1/2 NSS for long procedure

D. Unstable diabetics

  1. Should be hospitalized up to 3 days preop

    a. To normalize BS

    b. Obtain control with insulin management

  2. Consult PCP and/or internist

E. Severe diabetic autonomic neuropathy

  1. Results in resting tachycardia & orthostatic hypotension

  2. Increases the risk of gastroparesis & aspiration, consequently increasing the risk of sudden death

F. Sliding scale for basic postop BS management (mg/dL) subject to tailoring by internist (also used intraop)

  1. 150-199   2 units regular insulin

  2. 200-249   4 units "

  3. 250-299   6 units "

  4. 300-349   8 units "

  5. 350-399   10 units "

  6. >400   12 units "

G. Anesthesia Risk

  1. General anesthesia:

    a. Causes increased insulin demands

    b. Increased risk of silent MI

    c. Greater risk of nausea, vomiting

    d. Delayed postop food & oral med intake

  2. Spinal & local anesthesia preferred

H. Bleeding problems if patient is in early to mid stage diabetes because arteries are beginning to dilate secondary to decreased autonomic control

  1. Tourniquet use is a relative contraindication

  2. Epinephrine use is a relative contraindication

I. Postop pain may not be a problem in neuropathic individuals and can lead to problems with non-compliance & premature ambulation

III. Autoimmune Diseases

A. Complications due to therapeutic medical treatments for these conditions are covered in the section on specific medications

B. Rheumatoid Arthritis

  1. Prone to infections due to therapeutic immunosuppression – greater risk with Felty's syndrome of leukopenia & splenomegaly – give prophylactic antibiotics

  2. Anemia of chronic disease may impair healing

  3. Recurrant synovitis & pannus formation after synovectomy – give immunosuppressive drug postop

  4. Medication complications & recommendations (see section on specific medications)

    a. NSAIDs

        i. Many recommend d/c ASA 2 wks prior to surgery

       ii. D/C other NSAIDs 2-3 days prior to surgery if potential hemostasis problem suspected

     iii. Some recommend d/cing NSAIDs 7-14 days prior to surgery for safety

     iv. D/C herbals, especially St. John's Wort, 7 days prior to surgery b/c of bleeding complications

  b. Corticosteroids

    i. Supplement patient already on steroids

     (a) Minor procedures under local-sedation

       (i) Prednisone 15 mg po 6AM before surgery

       (ii) 15 mg po same afternoon

       (iii) 15 mg po next afternoon

     (b) Minor procedures under anesthesia:

       (i) Protocol 1:

          Hydrocortisone 100mg IV or IM evening before surgery

          100 mg prior to start of surgery

          100 mg q8h X 24h

       (ii) Protocol 2:

          Hydrocortisone 100mg IV or IM preop

          100 mg postop

     (c) Major procedures

       (i) Follow minor procedure protocol 1 above

       (ii) Administer hydrocortisone 100 mg q8h until stress of postop period has passed

       (iii) Tapering needed if usage longer than 3 days

    ii. Can increase microcirculatory constriction – avoid epinephrine in local anesthetics

    iii. Can increase risk of infection – give prophylactic antibiotics

    iv. Use local & spinal anesthesia where possible because they are less stressful & require less steroid supplementation

    v. Sedatives/tranquilizers can reduce steroid needs by reducing stress

  c. Immunosuppressive drugs

    i. Group #1: Includes chloroquine, gold salts, penicillamine, & methotrexate

     (a) Continue, but may adjust dose schedule perioperatively, according to patient needs

     (b) Use to prevent recurrent synovitis or pannus formation postop if performing synovectomy

    ii. Group #2: Includes cyclophosphamide, chlorambucil, 6-mercaptopurine & azothiopurine

     (a) Increase risk of infection – give antibiotics prophylactically

     (b) Delay wound healing

5. Stable arthritic patient on low-dose prednisone or NSAIDs can be predictably managed during surgery

6. Highest risk found in RA patients with:

  a. Advanced joint deformity

  b. Rheumatoid nodules

  c. High titer of rheumatoid factor

7. Increased incidence of fractures & trachea crush injuries during major surgery

  a. Atlantoaxial subluxation present in 40% of RA patients makes them subject to severe

neurological interruption upon marked flexion of the neck during anesthesia
   b. Consult anesthesiologist for preop evaluation
   c. Obtain preop flexion-extension lateral cervical neck radiographs
   d. Use cervical collar during surgery if > 4mm between anterior arch of 1ˢᵗ cervical vertebra & odontoid process
   e. Take care in moving patient
   f. Avoid elective surgery on patients with advanced subluxation that cannot be protected

8. Avoid joint surgery during arthritic flareups – outcome is more predictable in stable end-stage states

9. Seronegative spondyloarthropathies
   a. Includes Ankylosing Spondylitis, Reiters Syndrome, Psoriatic Arthritis, & Enteropathic Arthitis
   b. May be on NSAID therapathy (see medication section)
   c. Perform elective surgery between flareups
   d. Decreased chest expansion capacity increases risk of postop atelectasis & other pulmonary complications
   e. Anesthesia considerations:
      i. Intubation for general anesthesia can be more difficult secondary to cervical vertebrae deformity
      ii. Lumbar ankylosing complicates spinal administration
   f. Excessive periarticular fibrosis and joint stiffness can occur postoperatively in joint surgery

10. Gout
   a. Risk groups for postop gouty attacks:
      i. Previous gout patients
         (a) Local surgery trauma
         (b) Dehydration
         (c) Temporary interruption of uricosuric medication
      ii. Non-gout prone patients with higher risk
         (a) Those taking diuretics (e.g., Lasix)
         (b) Those on salicylates (elevate uric acid levels)
   b. Risk levels
      i. High risk:
         (a) Attacks within past year
         (b) Marked relief after test course of colchicine
         (c) Documented need for antihyperuricemic medication
      ii. Moderate risk:
         (a) Past episodes of acute monarthritis resembling gout clinically
         (b) Hyperuricemia during the acute episode (no joint aspiration for documentation)
         (c) Patients on diuretics (e.g., Lasix)
         (d) Patients on salicylates
      iii. Low risk:
         (a) Asymptomatic primary hyperuricemia
         (b) Asymptomatic hyperuricemia associated with drugs
         (c) Some primary medical state (leukemia tumor)
   c. Uric acid levels
      i. Normal range

        (a) Serum
           (1) Male
                2.4-7.4 mg/dL (conventional)
                or 140-440 _mol/L (SI)
           (2) Female
                1.4-5.8 mg/dL (conventional)
                or 80-350 (SI)
           (3) General rule: maintaining level below 6 mg/dL should prevent crystalization of urate
        (b) Urine > 600 mg of uric acid/day
     ii. Abnormals
        (a) Serum
           7-9 mg/dL (420 to 530 1/2M) = mild to moderate problem
        (b) Urine
           < 800 mg/day
             - Indicates undersecretion
             - Tx: uricosuric agents (probenicid)
           >800 mg/day
             - Indicates overproducer
             - Tx: allopurinal

  d. Treatment
     i. Perioperative management has not been standardized
     ii. Accepted protocols:
        (a) High risk pt:
           Colchicine 0.5 mg tid X 2-3 d prior to surgery
           Colchicine 0.5 mg tid X 4-5 days postop
        (b) Moderate risk pt: Same as high risk patients
        (c) Low risk pts: no treatment needed
     iii. Postop attacks treated same as any patient with acute gouty attacks
11. SLE
  a. Generally same risks as RA patient, including accompanying vasculitis
  b. Associated Raynaud's phenomenon – Epinephrine and ice are relative contraindications in foot surgery

IV. Peripheral Vascular Diseases
A. Functional vasospastic
  1. Raynaud's disease
B. Sclerotic
  1. Atherosclerosis
  2. Mönckeberg's
  3. Arteriolosclerosis
C. Progressing to occlusive organic
  1. Arteriosclerosis obliterans (ASO)
  2. Thromboangiitis obliterans (Berger's disease)
D. Arterial emboli
  1. Emergent condition, requiring immediate attention if collateral insufficient
  2. Ischemic pain
E. Diagnosis
  1. Clinical exam

      2. Non-invasive tests
         a. Segmental plethysmography
         b. Photoplethysmography
         c. Transcutaneous oximetry
            i. Not adversely affected by medial calcific sclerosis
            ii. Useful in predicting wound healing levels involving limb salvage or conservative amputation
         d. Doppler
            i. Conventional (measures velocity)
            ii. Laser (measures velocity) – sensitive indicator of cutaneous blood flow
            iii. Duplex (direct visualization of thrombus, in addition to flow characteristics)
            iv. Triplex (color) imaging
      3. Angiography – being replaced by duplex & triplex imaging

F. Prophylactic considerations
      1. Consult vascular specialist
      2. Delay elective surgery until bypass or sympathectomy performed, then perform as soon as possible while bypass is still patent
      3. For Raynaud's
         a. Elective surgery should be performed only in warm weather
         b. Patient should wear warm socks for 2 wks, minimum, prior to surgery
         c. Ice application is contraindicated after surgery

V. Cardiovascular Diseases

A. Hypertension
      1. Types
         a. Primary or Essential
         b. Secondary
            i. Renal disease
            ii. Endocrine disease
            iii. Oral contraceptives
            iv. Pregnancy
            v. Coarcation of the aorta
      2. Indicators
         a. BP
            i. Take 3 times to eliminate other factors such as stress
            ii. Take reading in each arm. Significant difference indicates certain disease states
         b. S_4 Gallop
            i. Most common finding
            ii. Left ventrical hypertrophy with systolic aortic ejection murmur
         c. Optic fundi – retinopathy indicates severity of disease
         d. Associated with peripheral vascular disease
      3. Preop & intra-op considerations
         a. Proper diagnosis & management with consultation even if symptom-free
         b. Continue htn drugs for periop period (except guanethidine)
         c. Preop evaluation of potassium blood levels
            i. Thiazides (eg., HCTZ) lower K levels
            ii. Patients on K-sparing drugs (e.g., spironolactone) less problematic
         d. Postpone elective surgery until adequate control is achieved for patients with BP < 160/90

e. Don't use epinephrine – patients very sensitive to vasopressors
4. Postop hypertensive episode
   a. Due to:
      i. Pain
      ii. Volume overload
      iii. Emergence exitement
      iv. Endotracheal tube
   b. Treatment
      i. Sublingual Procardia
      ii. Eliminate cause

B. Ischemic heart disease (angina pectoris, MI)
1. MI < 6 mo. : delay elective surgery
2. Continue routine meds, including beta-blockers, perioperatively
3. If npo, use nitroglycerin patch, or sublingual long acting nitrates
4. Order ECG
5. D/C ASA 2 weeks preop
6. D/C all NSAIDs 3 days preop except Celebrex and Mobic

C. Congestive heart failure
1. Tests to order preop
   a. CXR
   b. Electrolytes
   c. Digitalis levels
2. Well-controlled, stable CHF: no contraindication to surgery
3. Poorly-controlled CHF: delay elective surgery and get consult

D. Endocarditis
1. Risk increased for bacterial endocarditis:
   a. Synthetic valves
   b. History of rheumatic fever – damaged valve
   c. Mital valve prolapse
2. Foot & ankle procedures increasing risk of infection:
   a. Surgery in an infected limb
   b. Procedures > 90 minutes, especially with tourniquet
   c. Prosthetic implants
   d. Any major reconstructive surgery with extensive dissection
   e. Contaminated nail surgery
3. Most common organism is Staphalococcus aureus
4. Prophylactic antibiotic recommended:
   a. 1st generation cephalosporin or clindamycin
   b. Podiatric procedures on low risk patients do not require prophylaxis unless there is infected tissue

VI. Pulmonary/Respiratory Disease Patient
A. Goals
1. Avoid atelectasis
2. Avoid infection
B. Increased risk with
1. Smoking
2. Obesity
B. Preop management

1. Arterial blood gas study in patient with known pulmonary history
    a. If pCO_2 > 45 & pO_2 < 55, then patient requires pulmonary function studies & possible use of bronchodilators such as theophylline
2. D/C smoking at least 1 wk prior to surgery
3. Treat all respiratory infections prior to surgery
4. Use incentive spirometry to prevent atelectasis & consequent pneumonia
5. Administer heparin 5,000u SQ for prophylaxis of venous thromboembolic disease if patient has history of:
    a. CHF
    b. Idiopathic thrombophlebitis
    c. Other diseases in which venous stasis may occur
6. Use sequential compression devices preop, intra-op, & postop
7. Asthmatic patients
    a. Use local or spinal anesthesia
    b. Meds.
        i. Continue asthma meds up to 1 1/2 hr. prior to surgery with sip of water
        ii. Continue inhalant meds as prescribed by medical doctor up to 1 1/2 hrs. prior to surgery
        iii. Administer aminophylline
            (a) 800 mg in 500 cc D5W IV @ 20 cc/hr (5 cc/hr for children)
            (b) Adjust rate according to theophylline level

VII. Clotting Abnormalities

A. Preoperative tests
1. Platelet count
2. Bleeding time (especially if patient on ASA)
3. PT/PTT

B. Diseases
1. Von Willebrand's disease: give fresh frozen plasma
2. Hemophilia types (VIII, IX, XI)
    a. All have normal bleeding time & prolonged PTT
    b. Preoperative treatment
        i. Factor replacement
        ii. Fresh frozen plasma
        iii. Whole blood
        iv. Cryoprecipitate (4-6 units preop & the same postop)
        v. Lyophilized concentrate
    c. Must achieve level of 70-100% prior to surgery with minimum of 40% being attained for 10 days
    d. Increased incidence of Hep C & HIV: use caution
3. Vitamin K deficiency
    a. PT & PTT prolonged
    b. Give Vit K 10 mg SQ – normalizes patient in 8 hrs.

VIII. Sickle Cell Conditions

A. If suspected:
1. Order sickle-cell prep
2. Order Hemoglobin electrophoresis

    B. Anesthesia considerations
1. Avoid respiratory depression with narcotics & sedatives
2. Avoid hypoxia with general anesthesia

    C. Tourniquet use
1. Relative contraindication in sickle cell trait
2. Absolute contraindication in sickle cell disease

    D. Avoid hypoxia, dehydration & acidosis intraoperatively & postop

    E. Complications
1. Delayed healing
2. Increased incidence of wound dehiscence
3. Increased leg ulcerations
4. Increased bone infection (osteomyelitis usually caused by Salmonella)
5. Aseptic necrosis

IX. Alcoholic Patient

    A. 3-4 days of rehydration (helps to prevent DTs), vitamins, proper diet; no alcohol

    B. Blood tests
1. Serum albumin
    a. Normal = 3.4-5.4 g/dL
    b. This is a measurement of nutritional status for previous week
    c. Not a good indicator of nutritional status the day of surgery
2. Total lymphocytes
    a. $< 900mm^3$
    b. Measures response to stress
    c. Good indicator of nutritional status for the day of surgery

X. Patients on Certain Medications

    A. Asthmatic medications
1. Consider local or spinal anesthesia
2. Medication considerations
    a. Continue asthma meds up to 1 1/2 hours prior to surgery with sip of water
    b. Continue inhalant asthma meds, as prescribed by medical doctor, up to 1 1/2 hours prior to surgery
    c. Administer aminophylline
        i. 800 mg in 500 cc D5W IV @ 20 cc/hour (5 cc/hr for children)
        ii. Adjust rate according to theophylline level

    B. NSAID's
1. Many recommend d/c ASA 2 wks prior to surgery
2. D/C other NSAID's 2-3 days prior to surgery if potential hemostasis problem anticipated

    C. Corticosteroids
1. Used for asthma, COPD, Autoimmune diseases, malignancy
2. Indications for preoperative & introperative supplementation
    a. Suppress hypothalamus/pituitary axis (HPA)
    b. Need supplementation for any patient on oral corticosteroids within past year and if > 7.5 mg/day of prednisone used for longer than 1 wk prior to surgery
    c. Need 10 X normal levels of endogenous corticosteroids for increased physical & emotional stresses imposed by surgery
    d. No supplement needs for patient on intra-articular injections

3. Supplementation schedules
   a. Minor procedures under local sedation
      i. Prednisone 15 mg po 6 AM before surgery
      ii. Prednisone 15 mg po same afternoon
      iii. Prednisone 15 mg po next afternoon
   b. Minor procedures under anesthesia
      i. Protocol 1:
         (a) Hydrocortisone 100 mg IV or IM eve before surgery
         (b) Hydrocortisone 100 mg prior to start of surgery
         (c) Hydrocortisone 100 mg q8h X 24h
      ii. Protocol 2:
         (a) Hydrocortisone 100 mg IV or IM preop
         (b) Hydrocortisone 100 mg postop
   c. Major procedures
      i. Follow minor procedure protocol 1 above
      ii. Administer hydrocortisone 100 mg q8h until stress of postop period has passed
      iii. Tapering needed if usage longer than 3 days

D. Immunosuppressive Medications
   1. Side effects
      a. Increase bleeding time
      b. Bone marrow suppression
      c. Thrombocytopenia
      d. Increase risk of infection
      e. Consider prophylactic antibiotics
      f. Affects collagen synthesis
      g. Consider vitamin C supplementation
   2. Groups
      a. Group 1
         i. Methotrexate
         ii. Penicillamine
         iii. Gold salts
         iv. Chloroquine
      b. Group 2
         i. Cyclophosphamide
         ii. Chlorambucil
         iii. 6-mercaptopurine
         iv. Azothiopurine
   3. Protocol
      a. Continue, but may adjust dose schedule perioperatively, according to patient needs
      b. Use Group 1 drugs to prevent recurrent synovitis or pannus formation postop if performing synovectomy
      c. Give prophylactic antibiotics

E. Antihypertensive Medications
   1. Types of hypertension
      a. Essential (primary)
      b. Secondary
         i. Renal disease
         ii. Endocrine disease
         iii. Oral contraceptives

          iv. Pregnancy

          v. Coarctation of the aorta

2. Perioperative treatment

  a. Measure potassium levels and supplement as needed to prevent hypokalemia-associated cardiac arrhythmias

    i. K < 3.5 mEq: give oral replacement

    ii. Normal K = 4 mEq for patients on digitalis or diuretics

    iii. Normal values vary with each hospital; these are averages

  b. Don't use epinephrine - very sensitive to vasopressors

  c. For secondary hypertension - eliminate etiological factor if possible

  d. Continue medications (EXCEPT GUANETHIDINE)

  e. Take preoperatively @ 6 AM if med is normally taken in the AM

  f. Postpone elective surgery if BP is 160/90 or higher

3. Postoperative complications

  a. Acute elevations of BP can be due:

    i. Pain

    ii. Reaction to endotrachial tube

    iii. Volume overload

    iv. Emergence excitement

  b. Treatment

    i. Eliminate cause

    ii. Administer:

      (a) Sublingual Procardia - lowers BP quickly without dropping below normal

      (b) Sublingual nitroglycerine

      (c) Nitroprusside

      (d) Nitropatch

      (e) IV diuretics

4. Medications

  a. First-line drugs

    i. Diuretics - Thiazides

    ii. Angiotensin Converting Enzyme (ACE) inhibitors

    iii. Beta Blockers prevent angina

    iv. Calcium Channel Blockers

  b. Second-line drugs

    i. Loop diuretics - (Lasix) used when fluid retention is refractory to thiazides

    ii. Potassium-sparing diuretics - Aldactone

  c. Others

    i. Potassium channel blockers

    ii. Central sympathomimetics - Clonidine

    iii. Arteriolar dilators - hydralazine, Minoxidil

    iv. Alpha adrenergic blockers - Minipress

  d. Combinations

    i. Of above

    ii. Pharmacy-made

F. Anticoagulation Medications

1. Used for management of

  a. Ischemic heart disease

  b. Atrial fibrillation

  c. Mitral stenosis

      d. Transient ischemic attacks

      e. Prosthetic heart valves

      f. Perioperative prophylaxis to prevent DVT's

2. Types

      a. Heparin

           i. Inhibits intrinsic clotting pathway; interrupt thrombus formation, but do not actively dissolve the thrombus

          ii. Short-term therapy for prophylaxis against DVTs

        iii. Effects reversed with protamine sulfate

        iv. Types

             (a) Regular IV: unfractionated, low-dose (LDH)

                (1) Inc. risk of DIC

                (2) PTT's not used for prophylaxis monitoring

             (b) Low molecular weight (LMWH): enoxaparin

      b. Coumadin

           i. Inhibits extrinsic clotting pathway; interrupt thrombus formation

          ii. Long-term therapy for prophylaxis against DVT's after surgery

        iii. Dosage regulated according to PT

        iv. Effects reversed by

             (a) Vitamin K - delayed

             (b) Fresh frozen plasma – immediate

      c. Thrombolytic Therapy

           i. Dihydroergotamine

             (a) Venoconstrictive agent

             (b) Coadminister with LDH

             (c) Helps prevent valve destruction

          ii. Antithrombin III

             (a) Reduces associated bleeding complications

             (b) Supplemental use with LDH

      d. Aspirin

           i. D/C 2 wks prior to surgery to reduce bleeding complications

3. Presurgical management protocols with low suspicion of postop DVT episode

      a. Protocol 1

           i. Stop anticoagulants 3-6 days prior to surgery

          ii. Reinstate therapy postop 24 hrs.

      b. Protocol 2

           i. Stop coumadin 3 days prior to surgery & start heparin drip

          ii. Stop heparin drip 2-4 hrs. preoperatively

4. Presurgical management protocols with high index of suspicion for postop DVT episode

      a. Heparin protocol

           i. Initial SubQ bolus: 5000U 2 hrs prior to surgery

          ii. Administer 5000 U subQ q12h until patient is ambulatory or Administer a continuous IV drip of 800 U/hr

        iii. Maintain a PTT of 1.5-2 X base control

      b. Coumadin protocol

           i. Available in 5 mg tablets

          ii. Administer orally, 10mg/d X 3d in evening

        iii. Begin 24 hrs after initiation of heparin therapy when patient's condition is stable

        iv. Monitor qd AM via PT as outpatient, then phone patient for dose adjustments

v. Maintain a PT of 1.5-2 X base control for 24 hrs, then d/c heparin, which lengthens PT slightly

vi. Heparin is usually administered for at least 1 wk

vii. Preferable if patient is ambulatory before heparin is d/c'd

G. Antihyperglycemic Medications (See section on the diabetic patient)

XI. Anesthesia Complications

A. Malignant Hyperthermia

1. Frequency of occurence:
    a. 1 in 15,000 children
    b. 1 in 100 children with halothane & succinylcholine
    c. 1 in 50,000 to 150,000 adults

2. Early identification of susceptible individuals needed to prevent
    a. Genetic markers (chromosome 19)
    b. Increased masseter muscle rigidity in susceptible patients
    c. Increased incidence in children with strabismus
    d. Strongly suggested susceptibility in patients with repeatedly elevated CPK values who are related to a known susceptible individual
    e. Diagnostic tests
        i. Halothane-caffeine contraction test is 95% reliable
        ii. Phosphorus nuclear magnetic resonance spectroscopy is non invasive

3. Associated disorders – consult anesthesiologist
    a. Beckers dystropy
    b. Central core disease
    c. Duchenne muscular dystropy
    d. King-Denborough syndrome
    e. Myotonia congenita
    f. Neuroleptic malignant syndrome
    g. Osteogenesis imperfecta
    h. Periodic paralysis
    i. Schwartz-Jampal syndrome
    j. Sudden infant death syndrome

4. Triggering factors
    a. Volatile anesthetics such as Halothane, Isoflurane, Sevoflurane
    b. Depolarizing m. relaxants such as Succinylcholine
    c. Potassium salts
    d. Controversial agents such as ketamine, caffeine, curare, phenothiazines
    e. Possibly propofol

5. Clinical signs
    a. Respiratory & metabolic acidosis
    b. Increase in end-tidal CO_2
    c. Decrease in mixed venous oxygen
    d. Tachypnea
    e. Tachycardia
    f. Unstable blood pressure
    g. Cardiac dysrhythmias
    h. Cyanosis
    i. Mottling
    j. Muscle rigidity

  k. Sweating

  l. Fever

  m. Electrolyte abnormalities (increased Ca2+, increased K+)

  n. Rhabdomyolysis

  o. Myoglobinuria

 6. Differential diagnoses sharing common features

  a. Drug reactions

   i. Cocaine intoxication

   ii. Neuroleptic malignant syndrome

   iii. Radiologic contrast in the CNS

  b. Heat stroke

  c. Iatrogenic heating

  d. Pheochromocytoma

  e. Seizure

  f. Sepsis

  g. Thyrotoxicosis

  h. Transfusion reaction

 7. Treatment

  a. Primary measures the surgeon should know

   i. Treat immediately if malignant hypothermia suspected

   ii. Discontinue all triggering agents

   iii. Hyperventilate with 100% oxygen at high flow rates

   iv. Dantrolene: 2.5 to 10 mg/kg by IV push. Need help to mix. Repeat every 5 min if necessary until acidosis, HR & temp begin to correct

  b. Cancel surgery if possible or complete surgery expeditiously

  c. Secondary measures

   i. Begin cooling methods by all routes

   ii. Change breathing circuit and CO2 absorbers

   iii. Treat persistant or life-threatening dysrhythmias: procainamide IV

   iv. Treat life-threatening hyperkalemia: hyperventilation, NaHCO2, glucose/insulin, Ca++

   v. Treat metabolic acidosis: NaHCO3 based on arterhial blood gases & base deficit

   vi. Vasoactive & cardioactive agents only if necessary; avoid calcium channel blockers

   vii. Steriods?

   viii. Monitor vitals, urine, gases, coagulation, CPK, multiple body temp sites

B. Preoperative Hypothermia

 1. Increased susceptibility

  a. Very young and old

  b. Burn patients

  c. Spinal cord injury patients

  d. Trauma patients

  e. Alcohol intoxication patients

  f. Endocrine disorders

  g. Prolonged operative time

  h. Procedures involving body cavities

   i. Major vascular structures

   ii. Major blood loss

  i. Anesthetic agents

          i. Widen thermoregulatory thresholds
          ii. Vasodilator effects

2. Greatest rate of decrease to core temperature occurs immediately after induction of anesthesia
3. Complications
   a. Occur at core temps < 33.0° C & are reversible upon rewarming
   b. Metabolism & clearance of many drugs are altered & may alter cardiovascular, pulmonary & neurologic function
   c. Include:
      i. Dysrrhythmias
      ii. Increased blood viscosity
      iii. Platelet & coagulation abnormalities
   d. Shivering may increase oxygen consumption 300% to 800%
   e. Consequences of mild hypothermia usually are well tolerated by healthy adult patient
4. Means of maintaining normothermic state is to use forced-air warming system
5. Treatment of shivering
   a. Prevent hypothermia
   b. Supplemental oxygen
   c. Radiant heat
   d. Forced-air convective warming system
   e. CNS depressant drugs
      i. Chlorpromazine
      ii. Droperidol
      iii. Morphine
   f. Epidural narcotics
   g. Neuromuscular blocking agents

C. Bronchospasm

1. Most common cause of anesthesia-related morbidity & mortality
2. Frequency has decreased since use of monitors began - pulse-ox, capnometry
3. Principal clinical finding is wheezing
4. Treatment
   a. Inhaled volatile anesthetics (halothane, etc.)
      i. Induce bronchodilation
      ii. Attenuate constricting responses to a number of agents
   b. Halothane reduces coughing
   c. Ketamine recommended when patient actively wheezing
   d. Ketamine & aminophylline together may decrease seizure threshold & induce seizures – the role of aminophylline remains controversial
   e. Sympathomimetic drugs useful when patient is in spasm
      i. Administration can be po, IV, SQ, or inhaled route
      ii. IV epinephrine is drug of choice for severe allergic reactions associated with hypotension
      iii. Beta-2 predominant agonists preferred for bronchospasm
   f. Corticosteroid agents may produce immediate benefits
   g. Anticholinergic agents & Lidocaine may prevent or reverse bronchospasm

XII. Postoperative Complications

A. Non-compliance can cause many of the following problems if patient insists on:

1. Early weight-bearing when contraindicated

2. Over-energetic postop activity
3. Getting dressings wet
4. Bathing of surgical area when contraindicated
5. Allowing operative limb to depend too much and too long
6. Not wearing postop shoe when indicated
7. Bumping into doorways and furniture
8. Not using NSAIDs when indicated
9. Not using pain meds when indicated
10. Not reporting for followup exams

B. Infections

1. Clinical presentation
   a. Probable early infection
      i. Fluctuance with engulfed sutures
      ii. Disappearance of skin wrinkles
      iii. Scarlet or salmon-colored redness
      iv. Heat
      v. Slight drainage
   b. Obvious infection
      i. Raised cellulitis (erysipilas)
      ii. Wound necrosis
      iii. Vesiculation
      iv. Crepitation
      v. Tachycardia out of proportion to fever
      vi. Anaerobic infections may be severe:
         (a) Gas Gangrene – rare
         (b) Myonecrosis
         (c) Necrotizing fasciitis
         (d) Anaerobic cellulitis
   c. Pyrexia
      i. Many variables of normal due to:
         (a) Age
         (b) Activity level
         (c) Hormones
         (d) Ambient temps
         (e) Time of day
      ii. Regardless, normal range is consistent
         (a) 97.0-99.5° F
         (b) 36.2-37.5° C
      iii. Causes of postop fever
         (a) Wind = pulmonary causes
         (b) Water = UTI
         (c) Wound
         (d) Walk = phlebitis
         (e) Wonder drugs
2. Laboratory Assessment
   a. CBC
      i. $\geq$ 10K/mm^3 is significant
      ii. Shift to left = bacterial infex = band cells
      iii. Shift to right = viral infex = lymphocytes

        iv. Anemia may indicate infex due to hemolysis

    b. ESR

        i. Normal range (avg)

            (a) M - < 10 mm/hr

            (b) F - < 20 mm/hr

        ii. Sensitive but nonspecific

        iii. Best for following long course

    c. CXR – When symptoms suggest respiratory disease

    d. UA – When symptoms suggest urinary tract disease

    e. No lab test is infallible

    f. If white cell count decreases, but ESR remains increased, consider osteomyelitis

3. Culture and Sensitivity of any drainage

    a. Superficial and deep

    b. Aerobic and anaerobic

    c. Fungal cultures

    d. Acid-fast smears for mycobacteria

4. Probe for abcess with sterile, blunt instrument

5. Bone biopsy

    a. Best taken through a secondary incision

6. Consider fluctuance may be seroma or hematoma – see section on Vascular complications: hematoma

7. Facility for treatment

    a. Outpatient (or skilled nursing with home parental antibiotic therapy)

        i. Conditions

            (a) Temp $\leq$ 98.6-100 °F

            (b) CBC with diff and ESR are essentially normal

            (c) Limited or absent drainage

            (d) Local or no cellulitis without lymphadenitis

        ii. Treatment

            (a) Oral antibiotics 7 – 10 days average

            (b) Follow-up in 1-3 days

            (c) Infectious 'storm' should abate within 12-24 hours

            (d) Postinflammatory hyperpigmentation may persist for months to years

    b. In-hospital patient

        i. Conditions

            (a) If previous treatment protocol fails to resolve problem speedily

            (b) Organizing and indurated cellulitis threatening broad, nonsurgical areas

            (c) With or without low. ext. lymph node involvement

            (d) Bacteremic

            (e) Septic

            (f) Untrustworthy or noncompliant patient

        ii. Treatment

            (a) Consult Infectious Disease Internist

            (b) Blood cultures

               (1) Best if drawn during chills or spiking temps

               (2) Series of 3 or 4 drawings within 24 hrs

               (3) Blood is sampled from different extremities

               (4) Drawn upstream of any indwelling IV lines

               (5) When 6 blood cultures drawn within 2 days fail to elicit any organisms,

no further blood culturing is recommended

(c) Consider opening the wound, if not done before, and drain

(d) Confine patient to complete bed rest

(e) Mild elevation of infected part decreases passive spread of infex

(f) Apply moist heat to help coalesce and bring it to a head

(g) Whirlpool baths possibly

(h) X-rays if osteomyelitis suspected

(i) Consider bone biopsy

(j) Parental antibiotics

(1) Initial: Broad spectrum penicillinase-stable penicillin or 1st generation cephalosporin

(2) If MRSA is suspected - Vancomycin added or substituted

(3) Fine-tune after results of Gram's stain & cultures

(k) Eliminate distant foci of infection, particularly

(1) Skin

(2) Respiratory system

(3) Genitourinary system

(4) These previously undetected preoperative infections can treble the potential postop infection rate

8. Wound treatment

a. Opened

b. Cultured

c. Lavaged

i. Pulsatile jet spray

ii. Up to 2 liters

iii. Warmed physiological solution

d. Lightly pack with gauze

e. Inspect wound daily

f. Debride daily

i. Leave no necrotic tissue

ii. Leave no foreign debris

iii. Leave no dead spaces with tension on tissues

g. Irrigate daily if feasible

h. If left open:

i. Wet-to-dry dressings

ii. Gentle moist heat application

iii. Limb elevation

iv. Drain installation - leave in no longer than 2 days to prevent it from becoming a bacteriogenic focus

v. Leads to steadily improving phagocytic ability for up to 5 days because of delivery of more phagocytic cells

vi. Remember:

(a) Granulation tissue is still quite contaminated

(b) Bacteria ingested by phagocytes can still be viable

9. Osteitis or Osteomyelitis

a. Sequence infection surgical complication

i. Periostitis – pus under periosteal layer

ii. Osteitis – penetration of cortex

iii. Osteomyelitis – involves cortex and marrow

b. Diagnosis
  i. Early diagnosis is the key to successful tx
  ii. Modalities
    (a) CBC, ESR, CRP are all nonspecific indicators of inflammation
    (b) Bone scintigraphy
      (1) Useless after osseous surgery because normal postsurgical bone healing resembles osteomyelitis
      (2) Otherwise use with gallium
        - To determine if cellulitis or osteomyelitis
        - Gallium positive for both
        - Tc99 delayed phase positive for osteo, neg for cellulitis, generally
    (c) CT & MRI can locate abcesses in soft tissue and evaluate cross-sectional location and distribution of osteo
    (d) Plain radiographs
      (1) Should be taken if postop infex is suspected after surgery involving bone
      (2) These serve as baseline for comparison with subsequent films
      (3) Radiographic signs lag behind actual occurrence by 10-14 days – 30-60% of bone must be resorbed or destroyed before evident in X-ray
      (4) Normal postop osseous healing can look same as infection, radiographically
        - Rarefaction
        - Mild resorption at bone margin
        - Eventual new bone reaction
        - Periosteal reaction
      (5) Must judge by comparing X-rays to clinical and lab findings
c. Treatment
  i. Usually recalcitrant to treatment methods
  ii. Continuous closed-suction irrigation
  iii. Direct antibiotic infusion pump
  iv. Wound-packing with antibiotic-loaded cement beads, blood clots, or plaster of paris pellets
  v. Best to excise infected bone but save as much as possible when the removal will have a devastating biomechanical or physical effect

10. Gas gangrene
  a. Rare in civilian practice
  b. Few authoritative data for treatment
  c. Symptoms and signs of extreme toxemia
  d. Mortality rate lower if gangrene limited to distal portion of extremities
  e. Treatment – combination
    i. Antibiotics
      (a) Penicillin 1 million units q 3 h if infex is established
      (b) Tetracycline (if allergic to pcn) 500 mg q 6 h
    ii. Polyvalent antitoxin
      (a) Composed by British WWI
        (1) 7500 u of Clostridium welchii antitoxin
        (2) 3750 u of C. septicum antitoxin
        (3) 2500 u of C. novyi antitoxin
      (b) Initial dose of 50,000 u asap
      (c) Repeat q 12 h if patient unchanged

          (d) No good later

          (e) Some surgeons do not believe in it

       iii. Whole blood replacment (for anemia)

       iv. Hyperbaric oxygen therapy

          (a) Use as adjunct to above therapies

          (b) Full body compression chamber technique

          (c) @ 3 atmospheres of pressure

          (d) Patient breathes oxygen through mask for 1 1/2 hours

          (e) Decompressed over 35 minutes

          (f) Treat for 3 days

          (g) Increases oxygen tension in tissues 15X, theoretically

          (h) Delay surgery, tissue responds and can be salvaged

       v. Surgery

          (a) Debridement may be necessary while giving the other therapies time to take effect

          (b) Amputation may be necessary if infection is not confined to one muscle group

11. Wound dehiscence

   a. Causes

      i. Occult infection

      ii. Impending infection

      iii. Impaired wound healing

   b. Treatment

      i. Enteric or parental nourishment (if suspected neglect from inability or addictions)

      ii. Surgical debridement

      iii. Antibiotics

      iv. Plastic surgery consultation if needed

12. Sepsis – see fracture and fixation section

13. Tetanus – see fracture and fixation section

14. Fracture blisters – see fracture and fixation

15. When to close wound

   a. The idea of using serial cultures (3 negative) to confirm wound healing lacks legitamacy and makes sense only:

      i. If microbes are suspected to be evolving or changing

      ii. Wound care and antibiotic protocol are not progressing in right direction

   b. Daily CBC with re-equilibration of neutrophil/lymphocyte balance

   c. ESR should show a steady decrease

16. Closing the wound

   a. Secondary intention

   b. Delayed Primary

   c. Skin grafts

   d. Biologic equivalents

C. Fractures and fixation complications, can be applied to intentional surgical fractures and fixation

1. External fixation complications

   a. Disadvantages

      i. Meticulous pin insertion required to prevent pintract infection

      ii. Frame assembly can be difficult

      iii. Cumbersome and not very asesthetically pleasing

   iv. Fracture through pin tracts may occur
   v. Refracture after frame removal unless limb is adequately protected until the underlying bone can again become accustomed to stress
   vi. Expensive
   vii. Noncompliant patient may disturb appliance adjustments
   viii.Joint stiffness if across joint
  b. Complications
    i. Pin tract infection
     (a) Most common – 30% of patients
     (b) Colonization occurs in approx 100% of cases
     (c) Can be a minor inflammation remedied by local wound care
     (d) Superficial infection requiring
      (1) antibiotics
      (2) local wound care
      (3) occasional pin removal
     (e) Osteomyelitis requiring sequestrectomy
     (f) Prevention
      (1) Careful pin insertion technique
      (2) Meticulous pin care
      (3) Decrease possibility of pin motion
       - Threaded pins move less
       - Bulky dressing decrease motion of skin-pin interface
       - Topical antibiotics
       - Betadine-soaked dressing gauze
       - Reduction of skin-pin tension by adeqate skin release around the pin minimizes soft tissue necrosis and resultant infex
      (4) Most superficial infections resolve upon removal of pin
    ii. Sepsis
     (a) Infections in open fractures common
     (b) Treat aggressively:
      (1) Antibiotics
      (2) Repeated surgical debridements
     (c) Easier to treat osseous non-union in continuity than an unstable infected non-union (must treat infex first if occurs)
    iii. Tetanus
     (a) Prophylactic treatment with 250 units IM
     (b) According to following protocol devised by the Centers for Disease Control and Prevention

History of Absorbed Tetanus Toxoid	Clean, minor Wounds	All other Wounds[1]
Unkown or < 3 doses 3 or more doses	Td[2] / TIG Yes / No No[4] / No	Td / TIG[3] Yes / Yes No[5] / No

[1]Such as, but not limited to, wounds contaminated with dirt, feces, soil, saliva, etc; puncture wounds; vulsions; and wounds resulting from missiles, crushing, burns, and frostbite

[2]Tetanus toxoid and diphtheria tosoid, adult form. Use only this preparation (Td-adult) in children older than 6 years

[3]Tetanus immune globulin

[4]Yes if more than 10 yrs. have elapsed since last dose

[5]Yes if more than 5 yrs. have elapsed since last dose

---

    iv. Wound dehiscence – see infection section
    v. Fracture blisters or blebs
      (a) Cause
        (1) High energy trauma
        (2) Fractures adjacent to joints or areas of restricted skin mobility
      (b) Treatment
        (1) Do not deroof or incise
        (2) Avoid surgical incision through these areas
        (3) If possible, delay surgery and allow blebs to resolve: 10-14 days
        (4) OR – treat aggressively
          - Fx blisters resemble burns, histologically
          - Use burn tx protocol in surgery (sterile technique and silvadene ointment qd)
    vi. Neurovascular impalement: the following consequences have been observed
      (a) Vessel penetration
      (b) Thrombosis
      (c) Late erosion
      (d) Arteriovenous fistules
      (e) Formation of aneurysms
      (f) Most common L.E. injuries involve the anterior tibial artery and the deep peroneal nerve at the junction of the distal quarter of the leg
      (g) Use half-pins to reduce risk (penetrate skin, soft tissue on one side of bone, and both cortices, only)
    vii. Ankle Stiffness
      (a) Greater occurrence in stabilization of tibia fractures
      (b) Causes
        (1) Failure to dorsiflex ankle before pin insertion
        (2) Failure to encourage active jt. motion above and below fixator
        (3) Use of transfixion pins. Less problems with half-pins
        (4) Muscle impalement – muscles restrained from normal ROM

viii. Compartment syndrome
    (a) Increases in intracompartmental pressures of only several millimeters secondary to pin traversing compartment can result in full-blown syndrome
  ix. Refracture
    (a) Union due to rigid fixation is largely endosteal
    (b) With very little peripheral callus formation
    (c) De-stresses cortical bone
    (d) Results in cancellization of cortex
    (e) Refracture possible following fixation removal unless limb is adequately protected by crutches, supplemental casts, or supports

2. Internal fixation complications
  a. Repositioning can ream out bone center and lose holding power
  b. Too-early attempt to fuse bone in Charcot cases
  c. Screws
    i. Poor purchase
    ii. Can back out after surgery
  d. Staples - Splitting of bone

3. Delayed unions
  a. Definition – when healing has not advanced at the average rate for the location and type of fx
  b. Causes
    i. Rigid fixation, because
      (a) Eliminates macromotion at fx site
      (b) Eliminates impaction forces that allow cylic loading
      (c) Thus, eliminating the stimulation of callous formation
    ii. Not enough immobilization – new vessels are continually disrupted as soon as they are formed
    iii. Poor reduction leaving too large a fracture gap
  c. Treatment
    i. Cast
      (a) Immobilization
      (b) WB
      (c) Walking
      (d) 4-12 wks
      (e) Re-evaluate if not united:
        (1) Continue conservative tx
        (2) Or - treat as non-union
    ii. Electrical Stimulation – continue 6-8 months, at least, after surgery. See description in non-union section
    iii. Open reduction
      (a) Remove interposed soft tissue
      (b) Oppose widely separated fragments if poor reduction
      (c) Iliac bone graft with plat and screws
      (d) Medullary nailing in large, long bones

4. Non-unions
  a. Definition:
    i. Healing has ceased clinically or radiographically, and union is highly improbable
    ii. FDA def: when minimum of 9 months has elapsed since injury and the fx

shows no visible signs of healing for 3 months (experience shows this cannot be applied to every type of bone)

b. Types

    i. Hypervascular

        (a) Elephant foot: from insecure fixation or premature WB in a reduced fx whose fragments are viable

        (b) Horse hoof: from moderately unstable fixation with plate and screws

        (c) Oligotrophic: occur after major displacement of a fracture distraction of fragments, or internal fixation without accurate apposition of ends

    ii. Avascular

        (a) Torsion wedge

            (1) Intermediate fragment is decreased in blood supply

            (2) Intermediate fragment heels to one main frag but not other

            (3) Seen with plate & screw fix

        (b) Comminuted

            (1) Necrotic intermediate frag

            (2) Result from broken plate

        (c) Defect

            (1) Loss of frag of diaphysis of bone

            (2) Ends are viable

            (3) Gap

            (4) Occur after:

                - Open fractures

                - Sequestration of osteomylitis

                - Resection of osseous tumors

        (d) Atrophic

            (1) Missing intermediate fragment

            (2) Non-osteogenic scar tissue forms across gap

    iii. Causes unknown but more common when:

        (a) Open fracture

        (b) Infected

        (c) Segmental with impaired blood supply, usually to middle fragment

        (d) Comminuted by severe trauma

        (e) Insecurely fixed

        (f) Immobilized for an insufficient time

        (g) Treated by ill advised, unecessary open reduction

        (h) Distracted by either traction or a plate & screws

        (i) Soft tissue interposes

        (j) Presence of bone pathology such as neoplasms exists

c. Diagnosis

    i. Difficult

    ii. Modalities

        (a) Clinical – motion & pain at fx site

        (b) Plain x-rays- gold standard – deviation from normal progression of healing stages;

            (1) 1-4 days - inflammatory

            (2) 1-3 weeks - soft callus, radiolucent line widens

            (3) 3-4 weeks - hard callus

        (c) Stress fluoroscopy – does not show vascularity of bone ends

        (d) Bone scans – Tc99 – uptake stages:
- (1) Diffuse - 1st 4 weeks - fracture site adjoining bones
- (2) Biphasic – 4-12 weeks - fractured ends of bones
- (3) Coalescence – 2 years? – uptake at fracture site only

        (e) Tomograms – help visualize presence of trabeculation or a persistant fracture line

        (f) Computed Tomography
- (1) Best for midfoot & hindfoot
- (2) Can assess articulations & soft tissue impingements
- (3) Aids in determining extent of graft necessary
- (4) Aids in determining selection of appropriate fixation

e. Requirements of healing
- i. Adequate perfusion = oxygen
- ii. Nutrients
- iii. Cells
  - (a) Osteoblasts
  - (b) Osteoclasts
  - (c) Osteocytes

f. Treatment
- i. Proper reduction
- ii. Immobilization
- iii. Internal fixation
  - (a) Compression plating
  - (b) Interlocking nails
  - (c) Medullary nailing
- iv. External fixation
  - (a) Ilizarov frame
  - (b) Simple pin fixation for gradual distraction (1 cm/day for several days to restore length), then closed medullary nailing
- v. Bone grafting
  - (a) Adjunct: use internal fixation
  - (b) Or - without plates & screws – use only periosteom and peeling cortical bone shingles to retain
- vi. Electrical Stimulation
  - (a) General
    - (1) Must be adequately immobilized
    - (2) Must remove any synovial lining creating a pseudoarthrosis
    - (3) May be used for hypertrophic or atrophic
    - (4) Not affected by age, sex, nerve loss, number of failed operations, or length of disability
    - (5) Not for patients with pacemakers
    - (6) Gap ≤ 1 cm
    - (7) Gap ≤ 1/2 diameter of bone near non-union site
    - (8) Use 3-6 months
    - (9) Overall success rate = 80-90%
  - (b) Types
    - (1) Implanted devices
      - Constant direct current
      - Cathode implanted in non-union site and left in after healing occurs

- Anode & power pack placed in subQ tissues
  (2) Noninvasive inductive coupling device
   - Electromagnetic coil surrounds non-union site
   - Capacitive coupling device – 2 quarter sized electrodes are placed on skin on either side of non-union site, through holes in supportive cast
 (c) Radiographic changes seen in 1-2 months
  (1) Sharp, distinct bone margins become fuzzy and indistinct
  (2) Radiolucent line between frags takes on a smoky, cloudy appearance
 (d) Bone scan can be used to monitor for proper changes

g. Treatment of infected non-union
 i. 2 methods
  (a) Conventional: clear the infection, then fixate
   (1) Infection must be first completely cleared from bone and soft tissue
   (2) No draining sinus for 6 months
   (3) Follow with bonegraft
   (4) Follow with fixation
  (b) Active: rigid stability for healing of non-union, then clear infection
   (1) Infected tissue & bone are debrided initially, not overzealously
   (2) Exfix is applied
   (3) Bone grafts
   (4) Or - internal fixation if no drainage is noted
  (c) Remove residual sequestrae after osseous union has occurred
   (1) Malunions

h. Cause – same as nonunion – see nonunion section
i. Symptoms
 i. Prolonged swelling
 ii. Deformity
 iii. Joint stiffness and pain
j. Treatment
 i. Assuming osteotomy has been appropriately performed and fixated – immobilization in a postop shoe 3-4 wks to alleviate propulsive phase of gait is usually adequate for metatarsal, more if more proximal bones
 ii. NWB with crutches for several wks with forefoot cast or slipper works for long bones form which a cylinder of bone has been removed for shortening

D. Suture reactions
1. Types & characteristics
 a. Inflammatory = "reactivity" 1/2 foreign body response
  i. Males > females
  ii. Old > young
  iii. Longer incisions or wounds > shorter
  iv. General body sites > lower extremity
  v. Surgeon experience of less than 5 yrs. > Exp 5 or more yrs.
  vi. Thicker gauge suture > extra knot throws
  vii. Later adhesions not demonstrated to be related to inflammatory reaction
  viii.Natural materials > synthetic
  ix. Chromium slats added to gut for strength and duration can also invoke allergic reaction
  x. Patients have demonstrated physical rejection of lengths of polyglactin suture before full degradation. Self limiting problem, mostly

xi. In general, materials have not been demonstrated to be statistically significant factor in inflammatory reaction after multivariate analysis

xii. Some earlier research demonstrated absorbable material reactivity in following order:

(a) Greatest = gut & collagen

(b) Next = Polyglactin 910 (Vicryl)

(c) Next = Polyglyconate (Maxon)

(d) Least = Polydioxanone (PDS)

xiii. Nonabsorbable suture materials

(a) Natural = silk

(1) Greatest tissue reaction

(2) Swells when implanted

(3) Becomes encased with debris & infiltration by tissue growth

(4) More painful to remove than synthetic

(b) Synthetic

(1) Polypropylene and nylon give little trouble

(2) Polyester

- Coatings of teflon & silicone shed fragments that can cause inflammatory response

- Polybutilate coating bonds well to polyester & doesn't flake off = less problem

(c) Usually are removed from skin before causing major problems

(d) Use in deep tissue closure or tendon repair can present the occasional flare up

b. Infection

i. Males > Females

ii. 50 y.o. or older > younger than 50 y.o.

iii. Natural sutures > synthetics 2° inflammatory response

c. Wound dehiscence

i. Males > Females

ii. Younger than 25 y.o. > 25 y.o. or older

d. Discoloration

i. Dyed forms of synthetics may contribute to:

(a) Pigmentary changes

(b) Discolorations

(c) Scar discolorations

2. General rules for avoidance of problems

a. Delicate tissue handling

i. In grasping with forceps, hemostats, etc.

ii. In driving needles with accuracy and rotating wrist motion with needle curvature

b. Use less reactive suture material

c. Choose smallest suture gauge sufficient for the application

d. Needle choice appropriate for tissue and purpose

E. Vascular complications

1. Postop ischemic toe = white toe syndrome

a. Symptoms

i. Doesn't pink up

ii. Cold

iii. Increased pain from normal postop pain

    iv. Necrosis can occur in 3-6 hrs
   b. Cause
    i. Arterial insufficiency
     (a) Overaggressive dissection, vessel disruption
    ii. Or arterial spasm
     (a) Conditions such as Lupus or Raynaud's
     (b) Caused by
      (1) Pinning toe in dorsiflexed position
      (2) Over-lengthening, stretching vessels
   c. Treatment in basic order of execution
    i. Never let patient out of OR with white toe
    ii. Depend foot and flex knee
    iii. D/c ice if already using
    iv. Loosen bandage
    v. Press down on pin or wire if used
    vi. Remove pin
    vii. Remove tight sutures
    viii. Local block to area for sympathetic release
    ix. Apply warm compresses proximal to N-V bundle
    x. Apply vasodilatory patches proximal to N-V bundle
    xi. Vascular consult
 2. Blue toe syndrome
   a. Symptoms
    i. Toe pinks up upon torniquet release
    ii. Quickly becomes dark blue
    iii. Warm
    iv. Pain level normal for postop pain
    v. Can become gangrenous
   b. Cause
    i. Venous insufficiency, congestion of fluid in toe from disruption of too many vessels
   c. Treatment
    i. D/C ice
    ii. Make sure bandages are not too tight
    iii. Rest
    iv. Elevation
    v. Avoid
     (a) Ice
     (b) Nicotine
     (c) Caffeine
    vi. Usually OK in 24-48 hours
 3. Sausage toe syndrome
   a. Symptoms
    i. Excessive swelling which can be permanent
    ii. Heals with excessive fibrous tissue which is a heavier & less organized collagen type
    iii. Patient has less ROM
    iv. Can't wear regular shoe
   b. Cause = Overaggressive dissection

        i. Lymphatic disruption

       ii. Venous disruption

  c. Treatment

        i. Compression

          (a) Digital taping daily

          (b) Gauze between toes

          (c) Coban pieces

             (1) Wrapped around toe individually

             (2) Beginning distally

             (3) Working proximally

             (4) Overlapping each layer

          (d) Remove at night & milk out swelling

          (e) Silo pads and urethane in shoe can compress toe

       ii. Immobilization

      iii. Tube foam cushioning

4. Hematoma / seroma

  a. Seroma can act as fibrin clot and nidus of bacterial infection

  b. Hematoma, although a blood clot is avascular and becomes a good culture medium for bacteria

  c. Prevention

        i. Must close dead space

       ii. Must seal tie off vessels large enough to visualize lumen

      iii. Cauterize smaller vessels

      iv. Some recommend releasing tourniquet before suturing so that bleeding vessels can be seen and repaired, ligated, or cauterized

  d. Early removal

        i. Removal of one or more sutures and express

       ii. Or - Aspirate

  e. Tend to present with point tenderness without burgeoning infex

  f. Neglected hematoma

        i. Persistantly painful

       ii. Can take weeks or months to resolve

  g. Protocol for later removal

        i. Evacuate through original or secondary incision

       ii. Remove gently and thoroughly

      iii. Lavage gently and thoroughly

      iv. Close wound primarily if no other signs of infex are present

5. Dissecting hematoma

  a. Definition

        i. Hematoma has separated and filled the potential space between intact and viable dermis and overlying epidermis

       ii. Also, intradermal dissection

  b. Symptoms

        i. Dark appearance, looks like blue toe

       ii. Warm, initially, then gets cold

      iii. Sensation initially intact, then anesthetic

      iv. Consequent epidermal symptoms

          (a) Clear drainage

          (b) Macerated interspaces

(c) Blistering which will slough

(d) Nail may fall off (regrows eventually)

(e) Basal layer may be necrotic

(f) Increased risk of infection due to dead skin

    v. Live tissue (dermis) usually lies underneath

  c. Treatment

    i. Correct interpretation of symptoms is critical, rule out blue toe

    ii. Debridement of superficial layers of skin

(a) Inspection

(b) Ascertain extent of tissue involvement, whether deeper tissues are viable

    iii. Arterial doppler assessment of digital vessels

    iv. Later debridement which may result in tissue loss

F. Deep Venous Thrombis (DVT) can lead to Pulmonary Embolism (PE)

1. High frequency of occurrence

2. Potentially fatal if clot embolizes in pulmonary arteries

3. Classic clinical features

  a. Notoriously unreliable – only 50% of patients with evidence of DVT on venography have clinical signs

  b. Calf swelling and tenderness

  c. Elevated temperature

  d. Positive Hohman's sign

4. Risk factors

  a. Age

  b. Obesity

  c. Oral contraceptives

  d. Cardiovascular diseases

  e. Malignancy

  f. Leg trauma

  g. Immobility

  h. Pelvic surgery

5. 3 contributory factors (Virchow's triad)

  a. Venous stasis – pooling

  b. Vein wall injury – local

  c. Vascular damage

  d. Hypercoagulable state secondary to decrease in antithrombin III due to surgery stress & trauma

6. Diagnosis

  a. Venography

  b. Non-invasive

    i. Doppler Ultrasound

    ii. Plethysmography

    iii. ^{125}I-fibrinogen studies

  c. Differential Diagnoses

    i. Baker's cyst

    ii. Popliteal aneurysm

    iii. Muscle tears

    iv. Deep hematoma

    v. Cellulitis

    vi. Postphlebitic syndrome

vii. Lymphedema
7. Preop Prophylaxis
   a. Mechanical devices
      i. Continuous passive motion is ineffective
      ii. Effective
        (a) Leg elevation
        (b) Elastic compression gradient pressure
        (c) Pneumatic stockings – intermittent
        (d) Electrical stimulation of calf muscles
   b. Pharmacological
      i. Anticoagulation
        (a) Low-dose heparin – risk of DIC
        (b) Warfarin
        (c) Low molecular weight heparin: enoxaparin
      ii. Platelet inhibition (ASA)
      iii. Plasma expander
        (a) Dextran
        (b) Generally not advisable in podiatric surgery
      iv. Co-administer of supplemental antithrombin III & low-dose heparin
8. Anesthesia
   a. General correlates to higher DVT incidence
   b. Regional or local best for podiatric surgery
9. Treatment
   a. Immediate – to prevent PE
   b. Physical
      i. Antiembolic positioning
      ii. Warm, moist heats packs to increase flow around affected area
      iii. Hydrate patient
      iv. Intermittent pneumatic compression for calf thrombis when risk of embolization is low
   c. Pharmacological
      i. Anticoagulation
        (a) Unfractionated Heparin
          (1) Can induce thrombocytopenia
            - In 2-20% of patients receiving hep
            - More common in bovine than porcine
            - Recognized within 2-10 days after start
          (2) Monitor platelet counts
            - If reduced by 30%, then thrombocytopenia is likely
            - D/c heparin
            - Begin antithrombolytic therapy
          (3) Administration, dosage, and monitoring
            - Draw blood for a coagulation profile
            - Administer bolus of Hep IV 5000-10,000 U (or 100-150U/kg)
            - Constant drip infusion of 1000-5000 U/hr
            - Monitor PTT q12h and keep at 2X baseline control
            - Keep PT at 1 1/2 X baseline (although not directly related)
          (4) Reversal achieved with protamine sulfate

          (5) Start adding warfarin for ultimate switching before discharging from hospital

      (b) Warfarin (Coumadin, Coumarin)

          (1) Used to help prevent PE

          (2) Crosses placental blood barrier
- Known to be teratogenic
- Risk of fetal bleeding
- Avoid pregnancy
- If already pregnant, use subQ heparin or LMWH instead

          (3) Lower doses associated with less bleeding complications

          (4) Start upon recognition and diagnosis of DVT simultaneously with heparin (b/c warfarin takes 3-5 days to achieve therapeutic effect in body)

          (5) Dosage and Administration
- Goal is 1.2-1.5 X baseline Patient This is as effective as higher doses with less bleeding problem
- INR = 2-3 (INR monitoring standarizes therapy and improves safety)
- Continue warfarin for 1 yr after DVT episode

      (c) Low Molecular Weight Heparin (LMWH)

          (1) Improved bioavailability
- Longer plasma 1/2 life
- Higher plasma levels after subQ injection

          (2) Less variability in coagulant response to fixed dose

          (3) PTT is not affected and need not be monitored

          (4) Dosage and Administration
- qd or bid yields sustained and stable effect
- Outpatient -1mg/kg subQ q12h
- Inpatient - 1mg/kg subQ q12h or 1.5 mg/kg subQ qd at the same time each day

          (5) Begin warfarin as soon as appropriate, usually within 72 hrs, preferbly shortly after the 1st subQ injection of LMWH

          (6) Continue LMWH for minimum of 4 days and until therapeutic level of warfarin has been achieved, with an INR of 2-3

  ii. Antithrombolytic Therapy – Antithrombin III

      (a) Action: dissolution of thrombus already formed

      (b) Helps prevent veinous incompetency by preserving valvular function

      (c) Usually inadequate for occlusive iliofemoral DVT (although cathetor delivery has relatively good results)

      (d) Fewer postthrombotic symptoms

      (e) Use as supplement to heparin

  iii. Fibrinolysis

      (a) CONTRAINDICATED in postopertive or post-traumatic patients

      (b) Types

          (1) Streptokinase

          (2) Urokinase

          (3) Tissue Plasminogen Activator (TPA)

      (c) Activate the intrinsic plasmin system

      (d) Associated with relatively high incidence of hemorrhagic complication

        (e) No advantage over heparin in treatment of recurrent venous thrombosis or one existing over 72 hours

  d. Surgical

     i. Rarely employed

    ii. Phlegmasia alba or phlegmasia cerulea dolens necessitates performing venous thrombectomy

   iii. Venous ligation to prevent PE

   iv. Vena cava filtration devices to prevent PE

CHAPTER 9
SURGICAL CRITERIA AND COMPLICATIONS

1.   All are risks of general anesthesia in diabetics EXCEPT:

     A.   Increased insulin demands
     B.   Decreased risk of silent MIs
     C.   Greater risk of nausea/vomiting
     D.   Delayed post-op food and oral medication intake

2.   Aspirin should be held pre-operatively for how many days?

     A.   3 days
     B.   5 days
     C.   7 days
     D.   14 days

3.   Immunosuppressive drugs can decrease the risk of infections.

     A.   True
     B.   False

4.   Which of the following are True?

     A.   Atlantoaxial subluxation is present 40% of RA patients.
     B.   Pre-op flexion-extension lateral cervical neck radiographs should be done for all RA patients
     C.   Avoid elective surgery on RA that cannot be protected
     D.   All of the above
     E.   None of the above

5.   Which of the following results in post-op gouty attacks?

     1. local surgery trauma
     2. continuation of uricosuric medications
     3. dehydration

     A.   1 & 2
     B.   2 & 3
     C.   1 & 3
     D.   1, 2, & 3

6.   If a patient has had a MI in less than 6 months, then elective surgeries should be postponed.

     A.   True
     B.   False

7.   Which of the following do not require antibiotic prophylaxis?

     A.   Synthetic valves
     B.   History of Rheumatic fever
     C.   Mitral valve prolapse
     D.   All of the above
     E.   None of the above

8.   Which of the following are true for patients susceptible to malignant hyperthermia?

        A.   Genetic markers (chromosome 19)
        B.   Increased incidence in children with strabismus
        C.   Increase in masseter muscle rigidity
        D.   Patients with repeatedly elevated CPK values
        E.   All of the above

9.   Which of the following are clinical signs of malignant hyperthermia?

        A.   Bradycardia
        B.   Tachycardia
        C.   Respiratory and metabolic acidosis
        D.   A & B
        E.   B & C

10.   Virchow's Triad consists of the following:

        A.   Venous stasis
        B.   Endothelial damage
        C.   Hypercoagulablity
        D.   All of the above
        E.   None of the above

Chapter 10

ANESTHESIA

*by Maria M. Griffiths, updated for 2004 edition
by P.R. Krishna and Annemarie A. Edwards*

CHOICE OF ANESTHESIA

I. Patient considerations

   A. Preoperative evaluation

      1. History and physical examination

         a. Allergies

            i. Medications and reactions to each

               (a) True allergy or unpleasant side effect

               (b) Nausea, emesis, or upset stomach

               (c) Itching, hives, or swelling

               (d) Bronchospasm, hypotension, or cardiac arrest

         b. Smoking, alcohol, and/or recreational drug addiction

            i. Quantity and duration

            ii. Time of most recent ingestion

         c. Medications

            i. Complete list of all medications and dosages

         d. Systems/physical exam

            i. Cardiovascular

               (a) History of myocardial infarction or congestive heart failure

               (b) Angina, orthopnea, paroxysmal nocturnal dyspnea, and/or rheumatic fever and valvular disease

               (c) Distended neck veins

               (d) Shortness of breath

               (e) Hypertension

                   (1) Duration and management

               (f) Pacemaker

                   (1) Type and time of last pacer check

                   (2) AICD implant: Check type and time of implant

               (g) Nitroglycerin paste / pills spray

    ii. Pulmonary
      (a) Asthma, COPD/emphysema, or chronic bronchitis
        (1) Use of inhalers
        (2) Use of steroids
        (3) Shortness of breath/wheezing
        (4) Home oxygen/c-pap machine
   iii. Renal
      (a) History of kidney stones/infections
      (b) History of chronic renal insufficiency
        (1) BUN/creatinine
        (2) History of dialysis
   iv. Endocrine
      (a) Diabetes mellitus
        (1) Duration
          • Likelihood of organ damage
          • Neurological (central and peripheral)
          • Ischemic heart disease, retinopathy
        (2) Renal insufficiency
        (3) Method of control: Diet, oral hypoglycemic, or insulin
        (4) Consider reglan as prophylactic treatment for gastric paresis
      (b) Thyroid
        (1) Hypothyroid: Obese, cold, constipated, decreased heart rate, or arrhythmias
        (2) Hyperthyroid: Thin, tremors, diarrhea, increased heart rate, or arrhythmias
        (3) Neck mass: Difficulty with breathing
      (c) Evaluate the patient for proper steriod use preoperatively for stress dose
    v. Central nervous system
      (a) History of stroke/TIA
        (1) Residual effects
        (2) Carotid artery stenosis
        (3) Anticoagulation status
      (b) History of seizures
        (1) Duration
        (2) Type and frequency
        (3) Medication
   vi. Hematologic
      (a) History of hemophilia
      (b) History of sickle cell disease or trait Thallasimia
        (1) Warm operating room needed
        (2) Avoidance of tourniquet use
        (3) Avoidance of excessive sedation
        (4) Regional pain control helpful
        (5) Presence of sickle cell disease requires hemoglobin electrophoresis
        (6) Transfusion may be needed depending on hematocrit
   vii. Airway
      (a) Teeth: Loose, chipped, capped, missing, or dentures
      (b) Neck
        (1) Degree of extension/flexion

        (2) History of rheumatoid arthritis or Down syndrome: Increased likelihood of subluxation of cervical vertebrae and decreased range of motion of the neck

        (3) History of neck injury or cervical fusion

        (4) Should consider C-spine series radiographs

        (5) Thyromental distance
- Hyoid bone to chin
- Assessment of ability to push soft tissue for intubation

        (6) Malampati score
- Faucil pillars and soft palate visible
- Only soft palate visible
- Soft palate not visible

        (7) Elective or emergency surgery

     viii. Likelihood of increased gastric contents

     ix. Time of last meal in relationship to injury (The standard is usually 6 hours since the last meal)

  e. American Society of Anesthesiologists (ASA) classification

     i. No physiologic or psychiatric disturbance other than reason for surgery

     ii. Mild to moderate systemic disturbance with no functional limitations

     iii. Severe systemic disturbance with definite functional limitation

     iv. Severe systemic disturbance that is a constant threat to life

     v. Moribund patient, who is likely to die within 24 hours with or without surgery

     vi. Any patient requiring an emergency procedure

  f. Previous anesthetics

     i. History of poor or good experience with previous anesthesia: Spinal headache and/or postoperative nausea and vomiting

     ii. History of malignant hyperthermia

       (a) Regional anesthesia when possible

       (b) Avoidance of triggering agents

       (c) Invasive monitoring may be necessary

       (d) Family history or occurrence with previous surgical operation

     iii. Pseudocholinesterase deficiency

       (a) Avoidance of succinylcholine

B. Psychological profile
1. Level of anxiety
2. Pain/discomfort tolerance
3. Restless leg syndrome
4. Comprehension of awareness level
5. Ability to tolerate pressure/pulling sensation
6. Lack of tolerance of local, MAC, or regional anesthesia even with adequate block

C. Patient's choice of anesthesia

II. Surgical considerations

A. Length of procedure
1. Patient's ability to be still for length of procedure without sedation
2. Patient's need for a urinary catheter due to prolonged duration of procedure
3. Duration of block

B. Positioning of patient

      1. Patient's ability to lie comfortably: Arthritis or back pain

      2. Patient's ability to maintain an airway: Obesity, congestive heart failure or orthopnea

C. Type of procedure

      1. Ability to block area with regional or local anesthesia

      2. Requirement of muscle paralysis

      3. Use of a tourniquet

         a. Location

         b. Inflation pressure with associated tourniquet pain

         c. Duration of inflation

         d. Sympathetic mediated pain

D. Recovery time needed

      1. Patient's ability to be admitted for postoperative care

      2. Patient's presence at an ambulatory care center or an office

      3. Patient's history of postoperative nausea and/or vomiting

      4. Anticipation of amount of postoperative pain

E. Ability to provide good working conditions for the surgeon

      1. Adequate area anesthetized

      2. Adequate depth of anesthesia: Sensory block or motor block (if necessary)

      3. Correct positioning of patient

F. Surgeon's preference (general vs regional)

III. Anesthesia considerations

A. Availability of anesthesia

B. Availability of materials

      1. Proper equipment

      2. Proper back-up equipment for failure of primary technique

C. Time constraints: Length of anesthesia in proportion to case and recovery time

D. Availability of personnel

      1. Proper assistance for regional anesthesia

      2. Proper assistance for invasive fine placement

      3. Proper assistance for difficult intubation

E. Anesthetist's preference: Anesthetist's comfort level and familiarity with technique

F. Discuss with patient type of anesthetic and technique to be used and alternative techniques

G. Discuss with patient risks and complications of anesthetic technique

EPINEPHRINE

I. Total Dose Modification

A. Addition of epinephrine to the local anesthetic facilitates slow absorption of the anesthetic and reduces a potential toxic reaction

B. Total dose should not exceed 200-250 mcg

C. Clinical evidence: Near maximal vasoconstriction at 5 mcg/ml (1:200000)

II. Site of injection

A. Absorption of region

1. Increased absorption decreases length of effective block
    a. Greater from highly vascular sites
    b. Intercostal > caudal > epidural > brachial plexus
    c. Slower from sites with large amounts of fatty tissue and infected sites

III. Test Dose: Heart rate increase of > 15 bpm with the addition of 10-15 mcg of epinephrine to a small dose of local anesthetic indicates an inadvertent intravascular block

IV. Drug interaction

  A. Use of epinephrine with general anesthesia
1. Inhaled anesthetics (e.g., Halothane) can sensitize the heart to arrhymias
2. Recent use of cocaine can increase the incidence of coronary vasospasm and ischemia
3. Patients with coronary artery disease may not tolerate increase in blood pressure and heart rate

PROPERTIES OF COMMONLY USED LOCAL ANESTHETICS

I. Onset

  A. pKa
1. Definition: pH at which 50% of the local anesthetic exists in ionic and nonionic states
2. Onset of action related to the concentration of the anesthetic present in the nonionic form
3. Only the nonionic form can penetrate the cell membrane
4. Higher pKa correlates with higher percentage of molecules in ionic form and, therefore, slower onset

  B. Total dose: Greater dose correlates with greater number of nonionic molecules

  C. Tissue diffusion: Greater diffusion correlates with decreased duration of action

  D. Induced vasodilation
1. In general local anesthetics, except cocaine and epinephrine, cause local vasodilatation
2. Allows drug to be removed from the site of action and decreases duration of block

  E. Added vasoconstriction
1. Addition of epinephrine causes decreased uptake of local anesthetic and lower peak blood levels
2. Combined with some agents, this causes prolonged duration of the anesthetic

  F. Alkalization
1. Increased proportion of nonionized drug facilitates diffusion across cell membranes and increases onset
2. Localized tissue acidosis (e.g., infection) increases ionization and, therefore, decreases diffusion, resulting in slow onset or failure of anesthesia

  G. Potency: Increased lipid solubility penetrates cell membranes, which more readily creates molecules intracellularly and results in greater block

II. Differential Onset

  A. Fiber types
1. Myelinated of all subgroups

a. Conduction of motor impulses: Largest diameter fibers and, therefore, most difficult to block
b. Conduction of sensory impulses: Pain, temperature, and cutaneous touch
c. Conduction of temperature and joint proprioception
d. Conduction of pain, heat, cold, and light touch impulses: Responds to pressure; high-threshold receptors

2. Preganglionic sympathetic
    a. Smaller in diameter than "X' fibers
    b. Myelinated
        i. Block needed only at nodes of Ranvier
        ii. Block most easily effected with more rapid onset

3. Conduction of pain, temperature, light touch, and sympathetic postganglionic
    a. Smallest fibers in the body
    b. Unmyelinated
    c. More difficult to block than many other fiber types, which have a larger diameter
    d. Entire nerve (circumference and length) must be blocked
    e. Responds to thermal, chemical, pressure, or mechanic stimulation

III. Progression of clinical anesthesia

A. Peripheral vasodilation and increased skin temperature
B. Loss of pain and temperature sensation
C. Loss of pressure sensation
D. Motor paralysis

IV. Duration

A. Protein binding
1. Agents with greater protein binding have greater attraction for receptor sites
2. Agents with greater protein binding remain with sodium channels for greater periods of time, resulting in longer periods of conduction blockage
3. Local tissue binding may serve as a depot, slowly releasing local anesthetic to the nerve

B. Vasoconstriction
1. Cause of slower uptake of local anesthetic and, therefore, increased duration of block
2. Includes all local anesthetics, except cocaine; bipivicaine and etidocaine bind so tightly to cells secondary to high lipid solubility that uptake is slow and epinephrine will not increase duration
3. Most common are epinephrine

V. Route of metabolism

A. Esters
1. Plasma cholinesterase: Cleaves ester linkage
2. Para-ambiobenzoic acid: A degradation product sometimes associated with hypersensitivity in certain individuals

B. Amides
1. Liver
   a. N-dealkylation of the amide linkage, followed by hydrolysis
   b. Severe abnormalities correlate with decreased metabolism, possibly requiring dosage adjustment

TOXICITY

I. **Systemic**

   A. **Blood levels produce concentration-dependent levels of effects, ranging from sedation to seizures, circulatory collapse, cardiac arrest**

   B. **Free, as opposed to total, concentration determines toxicity**

   C. **Free concentration is determined by the amount of protein binding;** lower protein binding correlates with higher free concentration, therefore resulting in a decreased toxic threshold

   D. **Amount that crosses the blood-brain barrier is determined by the amount in the nonionic form**

   E. **Central nervous system toxicity is increased by the following**

      1. Decreased pH, causing increased ionized form in the brain
      2. Increased PCO_2, causing increased cerebral blood flow and delivery of blood to brain
      3. Increase in the ionized form produced by a decreased pH causes an increase in toxicity, translating into a lower toxic dose

   F. **Barbiturates and benzodiazapines increase seizure threshold and aids in cerebral protection**

   G. **Direct intra-arterial.** Injection can result in central nervous system toxicity at a much lower dose

   H. **Cerebral vascular system**

      1. Low concentrations can be beneficial for prevention and treatment of arrhythmias
      2. High concentrations lead to refractory arrhythmias and arrest

II. **Local**

   A. **Direct intraneural injection**

   B. **Direct trauma from injection needle**

   C. **High volume and concentration in a localized area, producing localized pressure and potential tissue damage or necrosis of skin**

III. **Allergy**

   A. **True allergy to local anesthetics is extremely rare**

   B. **Hydrolysis of aminoesters to PABA sometimes causes an allergic reaction**

   C. **Occasionally to methylparaben preservative**

SPECIFIC AGENTS

I. **Simple mg to percent formulas for dosage limits**

   A. **Basic formula: Percentage of agent multiplied by 10 = mg/cc**

   B. **Examples for common agents/percentages**

      1. Lidocaine 1% = 10 mg/cc
      2. Lidocaine 2% = 20 mg/cc
      3. Bupivicaine .25% = 2.5 mg/cc
      4. Bupivicaine .5% = 5 mg/cc

II. Amino Esters

A. Procaine (Novocaine)

1. Slow onset
2. Short acting: 30-60 minutes, secondary to poor protein binding
3. Low toxicity: Secondary to rapid hydrolysis by plasmacholinesterase
4. Maximum adult single dose: 500 mg
5. Clinical uses
   a. Skin infiltration in limited areas: 0.25-0.5 hours
   b. Spinal anesthesia
6. Metabolite PABA (para-aminobenzoic acid)

B. Chloroprocaine (Nesacaine)

1. Rapid onset
2. Short acting - 30-60 minutes
3. Extremely low toxicity: Secondary to rapid hydrolysis by plasmacholinesterase
4. Maximum adult single dose: 600 mg.; 1000 mg with epinephrine
5. Clinical uses
   a. Epidural anesthesia: 0.5-1 hour
   b. Obstetric anesthesia
      i. Rapid onset
      ii. Limited or no transmission to fetus
   c. Often combined with slow-onset, long-acting agent
6. History of neurologic damage with subarachnoid injection
   a. May be due to preservative bisulfate

C. Tetracaine (Pontocaine)

1. Slow onset
2. Long acting: Secondary to high protein binding
3. Limited toxicity: Secondary to short plasma half life
4. Highly potent and highly lipophilic
5. Maximum adult single dose: 100 mg; 200 mg with epinephrine
6. Clinical uses
   a. Long-duration spinal anesthesia 2-5 hours
   b. Conduction block
      i. Usually in combination with other agents
      ii. Can produce a motor block longer in duration and of greater intensity than a sensory block

D. Cocaine

1. Causes vasoconstriction
2. Slow onset
3. Short duration of action
4. Impairs reuptake of catecholamines; can have adrenergic responses (e.g., hypertension, tachycardia, arrhythmias)

E. Benzocaine

1. Slow onset
2. Short duration of action
3. Limited to topical use
4. Methemoglobinemia
   a. In doses > 8 mg/kg
   b. Treat with methylene blue

III. Amino amides

    A. Lidocaine (Xylocaine)

        1. Rapid onset

        2. Immediate duration of action

        3. Intermediate toxicity

            a. Ion trapping in newborn

        4. Maximum adult single dose: 300 mg, 500 mg with epinephrine

        5. Clinical uses

            a. Topical

                i. Liquid and viscous solutions for mucous membranes

            b. IV regional anesthesia

            c. Spinal anesthesia: 0.75-1.5 hours

            d. Epidural anesthesia: 0.75-1.5 hours

            e. Peripheral conduction blockade: 2-4 hours

    B. Mepivacaine (Carbocaine)

        1. Rapid onset

        2. Intermediate duration of action

        3. Intermediate toxicity

            a. Fetal metabolism limited

            b. Not indicated for use in obstetrics

        4. Maximum adult single dose: 300 mg-, 500 mg with epinephrine

        5. Clinical uses

            a. Skin infiltration 0.5-2 hours

            b. Epidural anesthesia: 1-2 hours

            c. Peripheral conduction block: 3-5 hours

    C. Bupivacaine (Marcaine, Sensorcaine)

        1. Slow onset

        2. Long duration of action: Secondary to high protein binding

        3. Toxicity

            a. Cardiovascular collapse

            b. Narrow range between therapeutic and toxic levels

        4. Maximum adult single dose: 175 mg-, 225 mg with epinephrine

        5. Clinical uses

            a. Skin infiltration: 2-4 hours

            b. Spinal anesthesia: 2-4 hours

            c. Epidural anesthesia: 2-4 hours

            d. Peripheral conduction block: 6-12 hours

    D. Etidocaine (Duranest)

        1. Rapid onset

        2. Long duration of action

        3. Maximum adult single dose: 300 mg-, 400 mg with epinephrine

        4. Clinical uses

            a. Epidural anesthesia: 2-4 hours for 1-2 segment regression

                i. Can have profound motor block with limited sensory block

            b. Peripheral conduction block: 6-12 hours

    E. Prilocaine HCL

        1. Rapid onset

        2. Intermediate duration of action

3. Low toxicity
   a. Metabolite associated with methemoglobinemia
4. Maximum adult single dose: 400 mg
5. Clinical uses
   a. Skin infiltration: 1-2 hours
   b. IV regional anesthesia: 0.75-1 hour
   c. Epidural anesthesia: 1-3 hours
   d. Peripheral conduction block: 1.5-3 hours

F. **Dibucaine**
   1. Intermediate onset
   2. Long duration of action
   3. High toxicity
   4. No clinical use in United States
   5. Laboratory assessment of the activity of cholinesterase in the serum

PEDIATRIC ANESTHESIA

I. **Total Doses**

   A. **Must be calculated on a mg/kg basis**
   B. **Lower concentration may be necessary to obtain adequate volume for infiltration**
   C. **Lidocaine 4 mg/kg, with epinephrine 7 mg/kg**
   D. **Bupivacaine 2.5 mg/kg-, with epinephrine 3.6 mg/kg**
   E. **EMLA cream, a topical anesthetic, for IV placement to decrease pain**

II. **Level of cooperation:** Consider age of patient and ability to cooperate for administration of block

III. **Adjunct to general anesthesia**

   A. **Cooperation not a factor**
   B. **Postoperative pain relief**

THERAPEUTICS

I. **Local sympathectomy**

   A. **Methods**
      1. Spinal
      2. Continuous epidural
      3. Single-shot epidural
      4. Specific nerve block: Stellate ganglion block, lumbar sympathetic block, IV regional blockade
   B. **Indications**
      1. Peripheral vascular disease
      2. Peripheral vascular surgery
      3. Post-herpetic neuralgia
         a. Spontaneous and continuous occurrence of burning pain without stimulation

       b. Exacerbation by light touch and/or temperature change

       c. Most effective block if done within two weeks of onset

  4. Reflex sympathetic dystrophy

       a. Local tissue damage or injury in some form may initiate a reflex response which involves the sympathetic nervous system

       b. Improved or cured with interruption of the sympathetic pathways

       c. Characterized by triad of pain, vasomotor disturbances, and trophic changes

       d. Significantly longer relief than the expected duration of the local anesthetic block

       e. More effective and better chance of cure correlated with blocks performed earlier relative to the onset of symptoms

DIFFERENTIAL NERVE BLOCK

I. Physiological <u>mechanism</u> of pain

  A. Identification of the physiologic mechanism of the patient's pain

    1. Sympathetic

    2. Somatic

    3. Central/psychogenic

II. Physiology of block

  A. Different size nerve fibers blocked by different concentrations of local anesthesia

  B. Varying concentration and dose of local anesthetic allows blockade of individual fiber types

III. Technique

  A. Spinal

    1. Antegrade

       a. Single spinal needle placed

       b. A placebo dose (normal saline) is injected, and pain is assessed

         i. If the pain is relieved by the placebo dose, the patient may have had a placebo reaction, and relief is usually of short duration

        ii. If pain is psychogenic in origin, relief is usually long lasting and/or permanent

       c. A dose of local anesthetic is then given to achieve a sympathetic block; and pain is reassessed; if pain is relieved with sympathetic blockage, it is of sympathetic origin

       d. Additional anesthetic is injected to achieve sensory block, and pain is reassessed; pain relief with sensory blockade indicates a somatic or organic basis

       e. A final dose of anesthetic is injected to achieve motor block, and pain is reassessed; pain relief following motor blockade also indicates a somatic or organic origin, but the patient has an elevated sensory blocking threshold

       f. If complete blockade of all modalities fails to provide relief, pain is felt to be psychogenic

       g. The onset of block modality is correlated with relief of pain

    2. Retrograde

       a. Single spinal needle is placed

       b. Placebo dose, followed by a dose of local anesthetic, is administered to reach block of all modalities (motor, sensory and sympathetic)

     c. As each modality returns, pain is assessed and evaluated using same criteria as antegrade method outlined above

     d. The recovery of various modalities is correlated with return of pain

     e. There is finer differentiation between sympathetic and somatic block

B. Epidural

    1. Can be performed either antegrade or retrograde

    2. May prevent spinal headache with addition of blood patch

    3. Requires longer time for onset and recovery

C. Assessment

    1. Assess by observation of patient and patient's subjective relief

    2. May need to have patient perform movements that normally produce pain

    3. Look for changes in amount, quantity, and duration of pain relief

    4. Assess changes in pulse, blood pressure, and peripheral skin temperature

D. Post-operative considerations

    1. Control nausea and vomiting

       a. Inapsine

       b. Dexamethasone

       c. Zofran

IV. Emergency Drugs

A. Hypotension

    1. Vasopressors

       a. Ephedrine sulfate

       b. Phenylephrine HCL

       c. Epinephrine HCL

       d. Dobutamine HCL

       e. Dopamine HCL

    2. Hypertension

       a. Vasotec

       b. Nitroglycerine

       c. Hydralazine HCL

       d. Esmolol HCL

B. Malignant Hyperthermia

    1. Dantrolene

C. Antiseizure Medications

    1. Phenobarbitol

    2. Diazepam

    3. Barbtiturates

    4. Sodium pentothal

D. Narcotic antagonist

    1. Naloxone HCL (narcan)

BIBLIOGRAPHY

Carpenter RIL, Mackey DC. Local anesthetics. In: Barish PG, ed, Clinical anesthesia, pp. 371-403.J.B. Lippincott Co., Philadelphia, 1989.

Dershwitz M. Local anesthetics. In Firestone LL, ed, Clinical anesthesia procedures of the Massachusetts General Hospital, pp. 195-198. Little, Brown & Co., Boston, 1988.

Eige SA, BeR C. Pediatric pain management. In Bell C, ed, The Pediatric Pain Handbook, pp. 503-528. Moseby Yearbook, St. Louis, 1991.

Murphy TM. Chronic pain. In Millder RD, ed, Anesthesia, pp. 1927-1950. Churchill Livingstone, New York, 1990.

Stoelting RD, Dierdorf SF. Handbook for anesthesia and co-existing disease. Churchill. Livingstone, New York, 1993.

Stoelting W Millder RD. Basics of Anesthesia, pp. 81-89. Churchill Livingstone, New York, 1989.

Strichantz GR, Covino BG. Local Anesthetics. In Miller RD, ed, Anesthesia. Churchill Livingstone, pp. 437-470, New York, 1990.

Winnie AP, Collins NU. The pain clinic. I: Differential neural blockade in pain syndromes of questionable etiology. Med Clin North Am 52:123-129, 1968.

CHAPTER 10
ANESTHESIA

1.   Which of the following local anesthetics, when added with another local anesthetic, slows the absorption and reduces a potential toxic reaction?

      A.   Bupivacaine
      B.   Lidocaine
      C.   Epinephrine
      D.   Prilocaine

2.   A test dose of 10 or 15 mcg of epinephrine, when added to a local anesthetic, may cause a heart increase of greater than 15 bpm and indicate an advertent intravascular block.

      A.   True
      B.   False

3.   The ASA classification of an insulin dependent diabetic with a previous above knee amputation and a severe infection in the contralateral leg would be classified as which of the following ASA level?

      A.   ASA I
      B.   ASA II
      C.   ASA III
      D.   ASA IV
      E.   ASA V

4.   Which of the following is a common postoperative cause of hypertension?

      A.   Pain
      B.   Bladder distention
      C.   Hypoxemia
      D.   Agitation
      E.   Orthopnea

5.   The maximum single adult dose of lidocaine with epinephrine is 500mg/kg.

      A.   True
      B.   False

6.   Which of the following is the treament for malignant hyperthermia?

      A.   Naloxone HCL
      B.   Diazepam
      C.   Dantrolene
      D.   Esmolol HCL

7.   Which of the following may cause neurologic damage when injected into the subarchnoid space?

      A.   Tetraciane
      B.   Chloroprocaine
      C.   Procaine
      D.   Benzocaine

8.   A prolonged motor block may occur with which of the following amino esters?

        A.   Cocaine
        B.   Tetracaine
        C.   Nesacine
        D.   Benzocaine

9.   The site of injection may determine the rate of absorption. Which of the following sites are most likely affected by this?

        A.   Highly vascular
        B.   Fatty tissue
        C.   Infected sites
        D.   All of the above

10.   Which of the following may decrease central nervous system toxicity?

        A.   Decreased pH
        B.   Decreased PCO2
        C.   Benzodiazepines
        D.   Hydrolysis of aminoesters to PABA

Chapter 11

EMERGENCY MEDICINE

*by William J. Martin and Alexandra Grulke,
based on chapter originally written by Steven F.
Boc, Donna Myers and D. Scott Malay*

INTRODUCTION

Life threatening emergencies may occur in any practice of podiatric medicine, whether performing surgical procedures or rendering medical care in your office. This chapter is designed to identify first steps in management of common office emergencies. Most, if not all, emergencies will need the patient further evaluated; however it is important for the practicing podiatric physician to be aware of the protocols to effectively treat emergency situations as they arise in their practice. Additionally the office staff needs to be aware of the signs and symptoms precipitating an emergency event. All medical staff should be trained in regard to their responsibilities in the event of a medical emergency and should have certification in basic life support.

The most important step in management of a medical emergency is to prevent emergencies from occurring whenever possible. The key to this is to know the patient's medical history. In history taking, the practitioner should always review current medications, history of allergies including type of reaction, cardiovascular disease, stroke, diabetes, seizure disorder, history of fainting and any emotional/mental health problems. The staff should be fully informed as to the steps that need to be taken in the event an emergency is encountered, especially if a patient would need to be transported to a hospital. Also the staff should receive regular training on emergency management including signs and symptoms of common emergencies, CPR, Heimlich Maneuver, administration of oxygen, patient positioning and medication location and usage.

There are basic steps in management: proper positioning of the patient, maintenance of an airway, maintenance of breathing and maintenance of circulation. Definitive treatment, including the administration of medications, requires complete knowledge of the medications prior to their administration.

Note: For information relevant to care of the multiple trauma patient, refer to the chapter "Trauma to the Foot and Ankle."

EMERGENCY EQUIPMENT AND MEDICATION

All emergency medications and equipment should be kept in a designated location easily accessible by all staff and should be clearly marked to avoid delay and error in administration of any definitive medications. The medications should be in already preloaded syringes in their appropriate dose. All supplies and medications should be regularly checked to ensure that the expiration date has not gone by. Oxygen tanks should be also checked to be sure that there is an adequate amount of oxygen present in the event it would be needed.

I. **Recommended Emergency Equipment**

   A. **AED** (Automated external defibrillator)
   B. **Glucometer**
   C. **Self inflating resuscitation bag with clear mask in various sizes**
   D. **Oral and nasopharyngeal airways**
   E. **Water based lubricant for airways and tubes**
   F. **Portable oxygen tank, non rebreather mask and nasal cannula**
   G. **Tongue blades**
   H. **Aspiration bulb or suction**
   I. **Flashlight**
   J. **Sphygmometer and stethoscope**
   K. **Paper bag**
   L. **Tourniquet**
   M. **Alcohol swabs**
   N. **Tape**
   O. **Intravenous administration sets and IV solutions** (500 cc NSS)

II. **Recommended Emergency Medications**

   A. **Oxygen**
   B. **Intravenous fluids** (NSS)
   C. **Aromatic spirits of ammonia ampules**
   D. **Epinephrine 1:1000, 3 prefilled syringes**
   E. **Nitroglycerine tablets 0.4 mg**
   F. **Diphenhydramine** (Benadryl) 50 mg injectable and 50 mg oral tablets
   G. **Albuterol aerosol**
   H. **Carbohydrates, such as candy, juice or soda**
   I. **Diazepam** (Valium), injectable
   J. **50% Dextrose solution**
   K. **Atropine 0.5 mg/ml for bradycardia**
   L. **Corticosteroid** (Solu-Cortef) 50 mg per ml **and/or Triamcinalone** (Kenalog) 40mg/cc for allergic reactions
   M. **Analgesic such as Meperidine**
   N. **Methoxiamine for hypotension**

GENERAL RESPONSE AND ASSESSMENT

In any office emergency or unexpected patient reaction, the key steps to all management is as follows:

P   **Position** the patient properly. For most emergencies that would involve placing the patient supine and in some instances, Trendelenburg (i.e., with feet elevated)

A   Maintain the patient's **Airway.** Loosen all clothing and be sure that their airway is not obstructed in any way

B   Monitor **Breathing**

C   **Circulation -** Monitor blood pressure and pulse

D   **Definitive treatment** based on your initial assessment. This might include administration of oxygen through nasal cannula or insertion of a nasopharyngeal airway

Cardiopulmonary Resuscitation

A. If spontaneous breathing does not occur, artificial respirations would need to begin at one breath every 1 to 1.5 seconds. When there is no pulse, external cardiac massage should begin. With only one rescuer, two breaths are given followed by 15 chest compressions, but with two rescuers, one breath is given followed by 5 chest compressions. Consider use of automated external defibrillator (AED).

Heimlich Maneuver

A. Dr. Henry Heimlich first described the abdominal thrust or sub-diaphragmatic abdominal thrust in 1975. It is the recommended procedure for the alleviation of objects causing airway obstruction.

B. Technique

1. Stand behind patient wrap arms around waist. Grasp fist with other hand, place thumb of fist against abdomen above umbilicus and below xiphoid process. Perform repeated inward and upward thrusts until airway is unobstructed or patient loses consciousness. When patient is on the floor, straddle the patient's legs while facing the patient. If the patient is in the treatment chair, place the patient supine with head/neck neutral and perform abdominal thrusts standing slightly to one side. (Figure below)

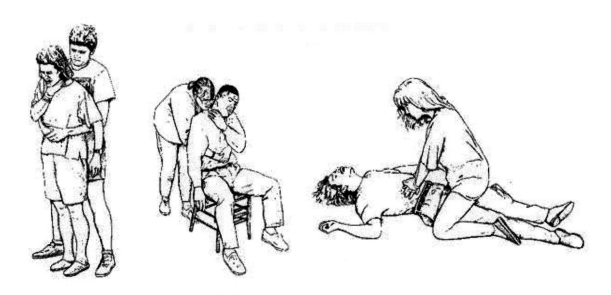

Prevention

In order to avoid airway obstruction in the office, especially if patients will be lying down, it is highly recommended that patients remove all objects from their mouth, such as chewing gum, chewing tobacco, food, lollipops, etc.

SYNCOPE

A patient who suddenly faints during a procedure is usually responding to an external stimulus, which causes a strong emotional response and/or pain. Syncope is caused by bradycardia and peripheral vasodilatation due to activation of a parasympathetic response as a result from over activity in the sympathetic system from the external stimuli. Ordinarily vaso/vagal type reactions are relatively harmless and can account for 50% of all fainting episodes. However, during the process, the patient may fall and strike their head or have an obstruction of their airway leading to hypoxia with further consequences. When syncope is recognized properly and managed properly, few individuals experience complications. To avoid this, patients should be positioned supine or in slight Trendelenburg for all procedures.

I. **Pre-syncope early warning signs:**
    A. **Loss of color / pallor**
    B. **Increased sweating**
    C. **Feeling of warmth**
    D. **Nausea**
    E. **Tachycardia**

II. **Late signs of syncope:**
    A. **Pupillary dilation**
    B. **Loss of consciousness**
    C. **Hypotension**
    D. **Bradycardia**
    E. **Dizziness**
    F. **The recognition of syncope is usually rather easy since most times it occurs in the presence of a physician or medical assistant.** A podiatric physician needs to be aware of the early signs of a syncope episode and by taking the appropriate steps, it might be avoided. Other causes of loss of consciousness are associated with other symptoms and therefore syncope is usually very easy to recognize

III. **Treatment**
    A. **Lay the patient flat or place in Trendelenburg**
    B. **Loosen or remove any tight clothing especially those around the neck to maintain their airway**
    C. **Administer oxygen at 2 to 4 liters per minute**
    D. **Reassure the patient**
    E. **Aromatic spirits of ammonia to the nose**
    F. **Check and record vital signs that include respirations, blood pressure and pulse. If there is persistent bradycardia** (typically a heart rate less than 60 bpm) transport to hospital where the cause will need to be determined, e.g., myocardial infarction, cardiac dysrythmia or

heart block. Atropine 0.5 mg-1mg should only be used in serious cases and in a hospital setting with the patient properly monitored. If atropine is given without close observation, other complications could develop such as worsening of a myocardial infarct or heart block. Atropine may also worsen glaucoma. All of these potential risks need to be considered prior to administration of atropine

IV. **Other causes of Loss of Consciousness or altered Mental State**
  A. **Orthostatic hypotension**
  B. **Seizure disorder**
  C. **CVA/TIA**
  D. **Hypoglycemia**
  E. **Hyperglycemia**
  F. **Myocardial infarct**
  G. **Cardiac dysrhythmia**
  H. **Airway obstruction**
  I. **Allergic reaction**

HYPERSENSITIVITY/ALLERGIC REACTIONS

Hypersensitivity/allergic reactions are IGE antibody responses to an antigen. This causes the release of histamine from mast cells causing severe vasodilatation resulting in urticaria and/or angioedema and/or smooth muscle contraction that may lead to profound bronchospasm and airway constriction. A reaction will usually occur within 1 to 15 minutes, with the patient feeling uneasy, becoming agitated and flushed and leads to palpitations, pruritis and difficulty breathing.

Anaphylactoid reactions mimic IGE mediated anaphylaxis; clinically they are similar in presentation but usually occur after the first exposure and are dose related. This reaction is a toxic-idiosyncratic reaction, not immunologically mediated. Common substances to cause anaphylactoid reactions include aspirin, NSAIDs, contrast media and opoids.

I. **Types of Immediate Hypersensitivity Reactions**
  A. **Generalized systemic anaphylaxis**
  B. **Urticaria and angioedema**
  C. **Asthma attack-Bronchospasm**

II. **Allergic Skin Reactions**
  A. **Urticaria** – pruritus, tingling and warmth, flushing, hives
    1. This can be an early sign of impending anaphylaxis; however, it is usually the mildest form of hypersensitivity. It can occur within seconds of administration of the antigen and if so, is the worst form
  B. **Treatment**
    1. Monitor vital signs, blood pressure, pulse and respirations
    2. Administer Benadryl 50 mg IM
    3. Epinehrine 0.3-0.5 cc subcutaneous (s.c.), if reaction continues or is severe
    4. Consider giving an IM injection of long acting cortisone such as Triamcinolone 60 mg to prevent the reaction from returning. Continue benadryl for 24 hours

5. Finally, if the reaction does not stop, transfer the patient to the hospital for further monitoring

III. Angioedema

A. **Symptoms**
    1. Swelling of the mucous membranes affecting the eyelids, cheeks, lids, pharynx or larynx usually occurs along with urticarial rash
    2. It may lead to lower airway edema that causes hoarseness, wheezing, bronchospasm, and subsequent development of diagnosis

B. **Treatment**
    Same measures as for urticarial rash

IV. Anaphylactic Shock

Rapid progressive onset, life threatening. May cause death within five minutes of the symptoms.

A. **Symptoms**
    Pruritus, urticaria, angioedema, cutaneous flushing, perioral and periorbital edema, laryngospasm, bronchospasm, lightheadedness, weakness, sense of impending doom, hypotension, tachycardia and tachypnea

B. **Treatment**
    1. Place the patient in supine
    2. Establish an airway and administer oxygen
    3. Start IV NSS
    4. Inject Epinephrine 0.3 cc-0.5cc 1:1000 s.c. for a maximum of 3 doses. If reaction is from a local injection in the foot/ankle, a tourniquet can be placed proximal to injection site and 0.2 cc epinephrine injected to prevent further absorption
    5. Diphenhydramine 50 mg IM
    6. Consider hydrocortisone 250 mg IV
    7. Monitor vital signs and transport to hospital

V. Asthmatic Attack

An asthmatic attack would be bronchospasm and edema with wheezing causing difficulty of breathing. It may or may not be part of a hypersensitivity reaction. If the patient has a history of asthma, the patient should be advised to use their own inhaler such as Albuterol, using two puffs every four hours to break the bronchospasm. If the asthmatic attack was brought on by an extrinsic source, Epinephrine 0.3cc 1:1000 every 5 to 10 minutes up to three doses to break the spasm. Oxygen, 2-3 liters/minute nasal cannula. Transport patient to hospital

LOCAL ANESTHETIC TOXICITY AND HYPERSENSITIVITY

I. Types of Local Anesthetics

A. **Esters** — Esters are broken down by pseudocholinesterase in the plasma before being renally excreted.
    1. Examples of esters include Procaine and chloroprocaine

B. **Amides are metabolized in the liver;** therefore, liver function affects its rate of metabolism

and break down.
1. Examples of amides include lidocaine, mepivacaine, bupivacaine

C. **Many local anesthetics contain Epinephrine 1:100,000 or 1:200,000, which is often highlighted in red on the vial.** The addition of the Epinephrine reduces absorption by limiting blood flow by means of vasoconstriction at the injection site.

D. **Toxicity of local anesthetics occurs because of overdosage of the agent, rapid systemic absorption, or inadvertent intravascular injection.** Therefore, it is prudent for the practitioner to know the maximum number of milliliters that can be injected for each various types of solutions. The maximum doses are as follows: Lidocaine 300 mg, (with Epinephrine 500 mg), Bupivacaine 175 mg plain (225 mg with Epinephrine).

E. **Overdose reactions are often characterized by a phase of apprehension and agitation with the following signs and symptoms:**
1. Confusion
2. Apprehension
3. Excitedness
4. Slurred speech
5. Elevated blood pressure
6. Elevated heart rate
7. Elevated respiratory rate

F. **This is followed by:**
1. Lightheadedness
2. Dizziness
3. Ringing in the ears
4. Metallic taste in mouth
5. Flushing
6. Drowsiness
7. Disorientation
8. Loss of consciousness
9. Seizures
10. CNS depression and cardiovascular collapse

II. **Management of Toxic Reaction**

A. **Position the patient so they are lying supine**
B. **Administer oxygen 2-3 liters per minute. Start IV**
C. **Monitor vital signs, blood pressure and pulse**
D. **Diazepam 10 mg IM during excitement phase**
E. **Methoxamine 10 mg IM to correct severe hypotension.** Hypotension may respond to IV fluid
F. **Transport to hospital**

HYPERVENTILATION REACTION

Hyperventilation type reactions occur when a patient has a high level of anxiety. It results in rapid and shallow breathing which leads to loss of CO_2 and alterations of the body's pH with respiratory alkalosis developing.

I. **Symptoms**

- Tachypnea
- Apprehension
- Chest tightness
- Shortness of breath
- Palpitations
- Epigastric distress
- Dizziness
- Paresthesia

II. **Treatment**

A. **Reassurance of the patient**
B. **Encourage regular breathing**
C. **If that has no effect, have the patient breathe into a paper bag** (rebreathing can counteract the respiratory alkalosis)
D. **If this is not effective, administer Diazepam 5-10 mg IM to alleviate anxiety**

SEIZURE

Seizures will usually develop secondary to pre-existing epilepsy or it may also occur in drug toxicity as has been described with an anesthetic overdose.

I. **Treatment**

A. **Protect the patient from injury and allow the seizure to run its course without restraint**
B. **Remove eyeglasses and any tight clothing**
C. **Position the patient in a lateral decubitus position to prevent aspiration of any gastric contents in the event there is vomiting**
D. **Provide oxygen by means of nasal cannula**
E. **In the event the seizure does not stop after a few minutes, or a second seizure begins give Diazepam 10 mg IM**

CEREBRAL VASCULAR EVENT

A cerebral vascular event may present as a transient ischemic attack (TIA) or cerebral vascular attack (CVA). Both are brought on by alterations in cerebral arterial flow.

TIAs are transient, rapid in onset, and last about 5-10 minutes.

I. **Symptoms**

A. **Numbness or weakness of the extremity**
B. **Vision disturbance**

A **cerebral vascular attack** is the result of infarction, embolism or hemorrhage in a cerebral vessel.

I. **Symptoms**

A. **Neurologic symptoms may present for a few hours or over a few days.** These include:
   1. Paralysis on one side of the body
   2. Difficulty in swallowing or breathing

3. Slurred speech
4. Facial dropping
5. Loss of bowel or bladder control
6. Pupils that are unequal in size

B. Headaches, if present, are mild and generally on the side of infarct

C. Vomiting is unusual unless the infarction involves a massive area of the brain or brain stem

HYPOGLYCEMIC SHOCK

Hypoglycemia is the most commonly encountered acute complication of diabetes. In adults, hypoglycemia is equated with a blood glucose value below 50 mg and is characterized by varying degrees of neurologic dysfunction

I. **Symptoms**

A. **Hunger**

B. **Nausea**

C. **Increase in gastric motility**

D. **Hyperactivity**

E. **Sweating**

F. **Tachycardia**

G. **Increased anxiety**

H. **Cold wet skin**

I. **The individual is usually conscious but may begin to exhibit bizarre behavior similar to those that have alcohol or drug intoxification**

J. **As the condition progresses, the hypoglycemic patient will lose consciousness and in fact, seizures may develop**

II. **Treatment**

A. **Immediate step is to do a finger stick blood glucose to determine the blood sugar level**

B. **If the patient is still conscious, give the patient carbohydrates such as candy, juice, soda or Dextrosol glucose tablets**

C. **Additionally, the patient can be given an IM injection of Glucagon 1 mg**

D. **If the blood glucose level does not return to 60 or above, the patient should be transported to the hospital for management**

HYPERGLYCEMIC EVENT

An uncontrolled Diabetic may develop severe hyperglycemia leading to metabolic acidosis (ketoacidosis)

I. **Symptoms**

A. **Ketoacidosis depresses cardiac contractility**

B. **When the blood pH drops below 7.3 Kussmaul respirations begin** (deep respirations slow or rapid); eventually the patient will loose consciousness

    C. **Fruity/sweet breath**

    D. **Low blood pressure**

    E. **Dry/warm skin**

    F. **Altered mental state**

II. Treatment

    A. **This patient needs prompt medical evaluation and blood glucose control with normalization of the pH.** This cannot be done in an office

AIRWAY OBSTRUCTION

Usually occurs from a foreign body in the oropharynx or larynx

I. Symptoms

    A. **Choking**

    B. **Violent respiratory effort**

    C. **Retractions in the supraclavicular, super-sternal and intercostal areas**

    D. **Cyanosis**

II. Treatment

    A. **If the patient is able to cough or speak, allow coughing to continue to alleviate the airway obstruction**

    B. **Should the problem continue, perform the Heimlich maneuver or chest thrust.** Administer oxygen

    C. **Begin the ABCs of cardiopulmonary resuscitation, if the patient loses consciousness**

RESPIRATORY ARREST

Respiratory arrest may occur from airway obstruction, cardiovascular collapse or from drug overdose such as a narcotic or barbiturate use

I. Symptoms

    A. **Cyanosis**

    B. **Absence of breathing**

If drug overdose is suspected, the patient should be ventilated with an Ambu bag and given 0.4 to 2 mg of Naloxone every 2 to 3 minutes up to 10 mg

HYPERTENSIVE CRISIS

Hypertensive crisis occurs when the diastolic blood pressure is above above 140 mm Hg

I. **Symptoms**

   A. In addition, signs and symptoms of **malignant hypertension encephalopathy** such as severe headache, confusion, dizziness, vomiting, visual disturbances, convulsions stupor and coma may occur

      1. The cause is spasm of cerebral vessels and cerebral edema. Hypertensive crisis occurs in less than 1% of hypertensive patients. It is unusual to occur in patients under hypertensive treatment

II. **Treatment**

   A. **Monitor vital signs**
   B. **Take blood pressure in both arms.**

      1. If blood pressure remains diastolic above 140 mm Hg, transport patient to hospital where one of the following will be considered: Nitroprusside (Nitropress), Labetalol (Normodyne), Diazoxide (Hyperstat), Enalaprilat (Vasotec) or Hydralazine (Apresoline). Nifedipine sublingually may also be considered for use but has fallen out of favor since severe hypotension may develop
      2. Note: The patient **must** be monitored extremely close to prevent a hypotensive crisis from developing.

CHEST PAIN

The symptom of chest pain may occur from cardiovascular disease or from a patient who has acutely developed a pulmonary embolus.

Pulmonary embolism would be manifested by a sudden, rapid, onset of chest or back pain, shortness of breath, tachycardia, which may lead to a cardic event. Clinically this may be difficult to differentiate for a myocardial infarct.

I. **Treatment of Pulmonary Embolism**

   A. **Surgical patients should be monitored for signs of DVT and at risk patients should receive Heparin or low molecular weight heparin perioperative**
   B. **In those patients who tolerate aspirin, aspirin can be given 1.3g/day in 2 to 4 divided doses until patients have returned to normal acitivity**
   C. **Patients suspected of having an acute DVT should be evaluated immediately by duplex venous Doppler and/or a D-dimer study**
   D. **Those patients suspected of pulmonary emboli need prompt medical assessment to prevent a cardiac event and /or further embolization**

Angina pectoris occurs secondary to coronary artery disease and is usually a chronic problem for many cardiac patients. Patients with angina often are on Nitroglycerin and it usually is self-limiting being alleviated in three to five minutes if untreated. Angina is commonly brought on by stress or physical activity.

I. **Treatment of Angina**

    A. **Nitroglycerin tablet sublingually**

    B. **Repeat two additional times at 5-minute intervals**

    C. **If the symptoms continue, the patient should be transported to the hospital**

MYOCARDIAL INFARCTION

Myocardial infarct is caused by coronary artery disease and may occur as part of an angina pectoris episode. Symptoms are similar to angina but will last much longer, lasting longer than 5 to 10 minutes and will be described as crushing, burning, pain in the substernal region, feeling as if there is a heavy object or someone sitting on the patient's chest. The pain may radiate to the back, shoulder, arm, or jaw. It will be associated with sweating, nausea, weakness, and perhaps cyanosis of the fingertips or lips. May lead to cardiac arrest

I. **Treatment**

    A. **The patient should be transported to the hospital as soon as possible**

    B. **Oxygen may be administered**

    C. **Nitroglycerine tablet may be administered sublingually and aspirin, 1 tablet, should be given**

    D. **Monitor the patient and transport as soon as possible**

    E. **Morphine may be given to control pain**

    F. **If patient loses consciousness, begin cardiopulmonary resuscitation**

    G. **Consider use of AED if available**

    H. **MONA -** M—morphine

                  O—oxygen

                  N—nitroglycerine

                  A—aspirin

BIBLIOGRAPHY
Berkow, Robert, Editor. The Merck Manual 17th edition, Merck& Co, Rahway, 1998.
Fauci, et al, Harrison's Principles of Internal Medicine, 14th edition, McGraw-Hill, 1998.
Malamed SF, Medical Emergencies in the Dental Office, 5th edition, Mosby Co, 2000.
Malay DS, Editor. The P.I.Manual, The Podiatry Institute, Tucker, 1999.
Taber's Cyclopedic Medical Dictionary, 18th edition, F.A.Davis, Philadelphia, 1997.

CHAPTER 11
EMERGENCY MEDICINE/PODIATRIC EMERGENCIES

1. The proper timing of artificial respirations during cardiopulmonary resuscitation is:

    A. One breath every 10 seconds
    B. One breath every 5 seconds
    C. One breath every 3 seconds
    D. One breath every 1 second

2. Some early signs of syncope include:

    A. Pupillary dilation
    B. Tachycardia
    C. Bradycardia
    D. Loss of consciousness

3. The toxic dose of Lidocain (Xylocaine) without epinephrine is:

    A. 300 mg
    B. 225 mg
    C. 175 mg
    D. 500 mg

4. Symptoms of overdose of a local anesthetic include all of the following EXCEPT:

    A. CNS excitation
    B. Tinnitus
    C. Seizure
    D. Slurred speech

5. A 50-year-old female presents with past medical history significant of diabetes, hypertension and GERD. The patient upon examination is noted to be hyperactive and diaphoretic. Her hands feel cold and wet. The patient's daughter relates that her mother is exhibiting bizarre behavior since entering your office. The most likely diagnosis is:

    A. Post ictal
    B. Myocardial infarction
    C. Hypogylcemia
    D. Asthma

6. Which of the following is true of an **anaphylactoid** reaction:

    A. Hypersensitivity reaction of the IgE antibody response to an antigen
    B. Occurs after the first dose
    C. Toxic-idiosyncratic reaction not immunologically mediated
    D. These reactions are not dose related

7.   The treatment of anaphylaxis include the following EXCEPT:

        A.   Establish airway and administer 02
        B.   Ephineprhine 0.3-0.5 cc of a 1:1000 solution
        C.   Hydrocortisone 250 mg IV
        D.   Inhaled bronchodilator

8.   Characteristics of ester local anesthetics include of all the following EXCEPT:

        A.   Metobolized by the liver
        B.   Broken down by pseudocholinesterases
        C.   Examples include Procaine, chloroprocaine
        D.   Renally excreted

9.   Concerning the treatments of seizures which of the following are true:

        A.   Place the patient in Trendelenberg position
        B.   No oxygen is needed
        C.   Fingers should be placed in a patient's mouth to prevent the swallowing of the tongue
        D.   All tight clothing should be removed

10.   The proper treatment of a hypertensive crisis includes all of the following EXCEPT:

        A.   The blood pressure should be taken in both arms
        B.   A hypertensive crisis occurs when the systolic blood pressure is greater than 140 mmHg
        C.   Consider giving sublingual Nifedipine
        D.   Most concerning complication following treatment of hypertension is hypotension

Chapter 12

Cutaneous Signs in the Diagnosis of Skin Lesions of the Foot

Harvey Lemont, DPM
Joseph Witkowski, MD
Larry R. Goss, DPM

INTRODUCTION

As a practical matter, physicians are often confronted with skin lesions of varying shapes, sizes, arrangements and contents. This can cause confusion with both diagnosis and treatment. We have arranged this chapter in a manner which systematically approaches a variety of common skin lesions. For example, when confronted with blisters exhibiting a cigar or football shape containing clear fluid, think of Hand and Foot disease. When confronted with blisters, which exhibit triangular edges, think of Diabetic bullosis. When you see a patient with blood filled blisters think of Herpes zoster, Epidermolysis bullosa or Gonococcemic skin lesions. We believe that this approach will be helpful also when taking board examinations since oral or written questions often contain a morphologic description of the skin lesion from which you will be expected to form a diagnosis.

CLEAR-TO-SEROUS FILLED BLISTERS OF THE FOOT

   I.   **Acute Tinea Pedis** (Figures 1a and 1b)
       A.   **Tendency to be unilateral** (65%)
       B.   **Blisters on an erythematous base usually seen in crops exhibiting a *"sponge-like"* appearance**
       C.   **On puncture, serous fluid is noted**
       D.   **If significant inflammation is present an ID reaction involving the palms consisting of non-inflammatory vesicles may be noted**

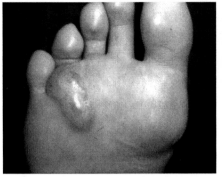
Figure 1a

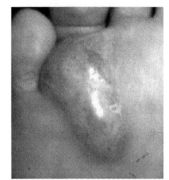
Figure 1b

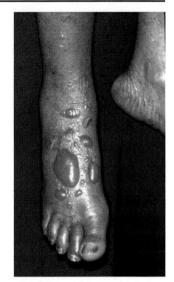
Figure 2a

II. Diabetic Bullosis (Figures 2a and 2b)

A. Think of diabetic bullosis when you see blisters which have a *"triangular shape"* or squared corners

III. Dyshidrotic Eczema (Figure 3)

A. Blisters are small, resembling tapioca
B. Referred to as *"Sago grain"* in appearance
C. Usually bilateral, symmetrical, often non- inflammatory but at times mild inflammation may be present
D. Lesions occur on the arch, sides of toes and fingers, thenar and hypothenar eminencies

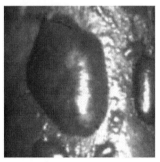
Figure 2b

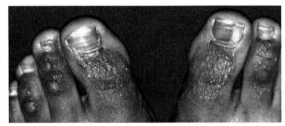
Figure 3

IV. Allergic Eczematous Dermatitis (Figure 4)

A. Known as *"contact dermatitis"*
B. Wet blistering disorder on an erythematous base with sharp demarcation, corresponding to the allergen

V. Hand and Foot Disease (Figures 5a and 5b)

A. Reddish somewhat *"hemorrhagic cigar or football shaped vesicles"*
B. Usually present on the dorsal or lateral surfaces of the hands and feet and on the fingers and toes
C. Lesions are preceded by macules or small papules
D. The disease is caused most frequently by Coxsackie virus A16
E. Most commonly affects young children (six months to 5 years are most susceptible)
F. Presence of concomitant oral mucosa ulcers supports the diagnosis

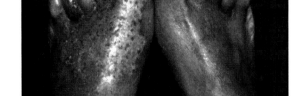
Figure 4

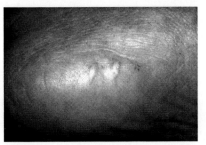

Figure 5a

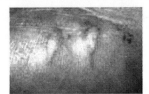

Figure 5b

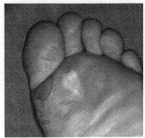

Figure 6b

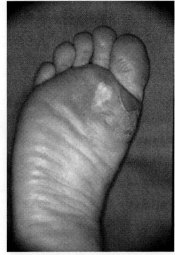

Figure 6a

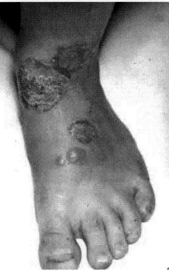

Figure 7

VI. Localized Epidermolysis Bullosa Simplex (Figures 6a and 6b)

    A. Known as *"Weber Cockayne"* disease

    B. Recurrent bullous eruption of the hands and feet

    C. An autosomal dominant disease

    D. Usually appears after prolonged walking or marching

    E. Hyperhidrosis may be an associated finding

VII. Impetigo (Figure 7)

    A. Vesicles or bulla that breaks easily forming an erosion which becomes covered with a *honey-colored crust*

    B. Most commonly caused by *Staph. aureus* and/or Group A beta Hemolytic streptococcus

    C. Think of impetigo when faced with significant crusting and a history of vesicles or bulla appearing in crops and a prior history of puncture wound or abrasion of the skin

PUSTULAR DERMATOSIS OF THE SOLES

    I. Localized Pustular Psoriasis (Barber) (Figures 8a and 8b)

        A. Bilateral pustular eruption on plantar aspect of the feet

        B. Small sterile pustules and lakes of pus on a red glassy base, with brown crusts are characteristic

        C. Pressure bearing areas are involved initially, then the entire plantar surface

        D. The lesions may be painful

        E. Nail changes are common and arthritis is present in thirty percent

        F. The spongioform pustules contain polymorphonuclear leukocytes

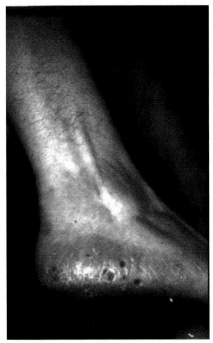

Figure 8a

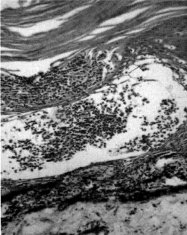

Figure 8b

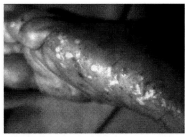

Figure 9

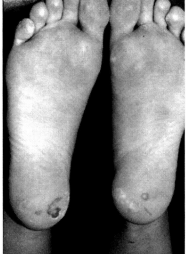

Figure 10a

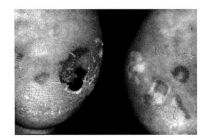

Figure 10b

II. Palmoplantar Pustulosis (Figure 9)

   A. **Can mimic localized pustular psoriasis**

   B. **Requires biopsy to demonstrate lack of psoriasis and the spongiform pustule**

   C. **Mononuclear cells and polys are present histologically**

   D. **In this condition, deep seated vesicles become pustules and then brown crusts**

   E. **It most frequently involves middle-aged women who are smokers**

   F. **The condition begins on non-pressure bearing parts of the soles but may be more extensive**

   G. **It is often pruritic**

   H. **Sternocostoclavicular hyperostosis and hyperthyroidism may be present**

BLOOD-FILLED BLISTERS

I. Dystrophic Form of Epidermolysis Bullosa (Figures 10a and 10b)

   A. **Epidermolysis bullosa (EB) is a group of inherited mechano-bullous diseases**

   B. **Often termed "*friction blisters*"**

   C. **It is classified as simplex, junctional, or dystrophic based on histology (level of the vesicle)**

   D. **The dystrophic variety is characterized by the appearance of bullae which are frequently blood-filled**

   E. **Lesions are induced by minor trauma and are located on pressure points of the foot**

   F. **Nails are often absent, lesions are present on other parts of the skin and the mucous membranes**

II. Herpes Zoster (Figures 11a and 11b)

  A. **Blood-filled vesicles or bulla appearing in crops following a dermatomal pattern**

  B. **It is often associated with or preceded by pain**

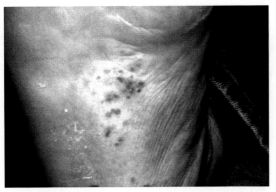

Figure 11a   Figure 11b

III. Gonococcal Skin Infection (Chronic Gonococcemia) (Figure 12)

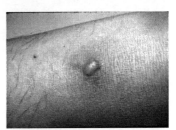

  A. **Pustules and hemorrhagic pustules characteristically occur over bony prominences**

  B. **The lesions tend to be painful**

  C. **Recurrent arthritis and tendonitis are often present**

  D. **Smear and culture of the lesion often shows gonococci**

Figure 12

RED PAPULES/NODULES

I. Eccrine Poroma (Figures 13a and 13b)

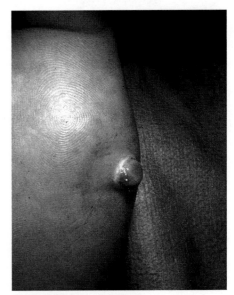

  A. **Small reddish papule that resembles granulation tissue or pyogenic granuloma**

  B. **There may be a groove surrounding the lesion and separating it from the adjacent skin** (called a "*moat*")

  C. **This is a tumor of the eccrine sweat duct origin**

  D. **It should not to be confused with porokeratosis plantaris discreta (plugged duct cyst)**

  E. **Think of eccrine poroma when faced with an *isolated granulating lesion of the sole***

  F. **Lesions may resemble granulation tissue or paronychia associated with ingrown toenail**

  G. **Misdiagnosis is common and may result in legal action against the treating physician**

Figure 13a

  H. **It is for this reason that routine submission of granulation tissue for pathologic evaluation is judicious to rule out amelanotic melanoma**

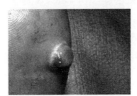

II. Bacillary Angiomatosis

  A. **Small cherry colored papules seen in HIV-**

Figure 13b

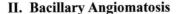

positive individuals caused by *Bartonella henselae*

B. **A history of a cat scratch may be elicited**

C. **Cats appear to serve as a reservoir for the transmittal of the disease**

D. **Bartonella henselae is also responsible for cat scratch fever in immunocompromised persons**

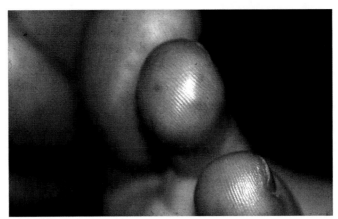

Figure 14

III. **Oslers' Nodes** (Figure 14)

   A. **Small tender pea-sized papules seen at the tips of the toes**

   B. **Tend to last a few days representing infective emboli containing the offending organism** associated with bacterial endocarditis, infected arterial catheters, gonococcemia, and typhoid fever

IV. **Kaposi Sarcoma** (Figure 15)

   A. **The lesions often appear as isolated firm smooth surfaced papules red to eggplant in color**

   B. **No histologic differences are noted in AIDS related Kaposi sarcoma versus European forms**

   C. **Recent evidence suggests that it may be due to Type 8 herpes simplex virus**

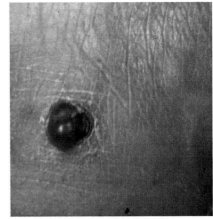

Figure 15

V. **Pyogenic Granuloma** (Figure 16)

   A. **Red loosely formed capillary proliferation commonly seen in association with ingrown** toenail

   B. **The lesions bleed easily**

   C. **Chronic lesions tend to lose the red color due to fibrous replacement of its vascular** stroma and epithelial re-surfacing

   D. **While most commonly seen in association with ingrown toe nails, these lesions frequently** occur as isolated lesions on the plantar aspect of the foot

   E. **Must rule out an amelanotic melanoma by biopsy**

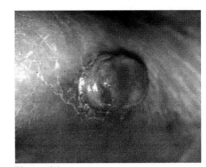

Figure 16

VI. Erythema Nodosum (Figures 17a and 17b)

  A. Tender nodules in crops located on the anterior aspect of the leg
  B. Associated with collagen vascular disease, infection, and oral contraceptives

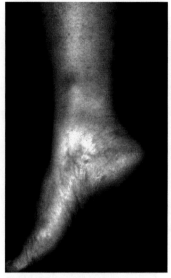

Figure 17a

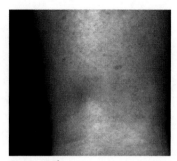

Figure 17b

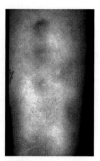

Figure 18

VII. Sporotrichosis (Figure 18)

  A. *Sporothrix schenckki* is a dimorphic fungi that invades the lymphatics through a puncture wound
  B. Starts as an ulcerative nodule which spreads to lymphatic system

VIII. Frostbite (Figure 19)

  A. Tips of the toes are involved
  B. Lesions tend to be erythematous purplish swelling with areas of pallor noted within some lesions
  C. Blistering in severe cases
  D. Lesions are tender, itch and burn
  E. Most occur repeatedly in the cold weather when they become more clinically obvious
  F. Lesions tend to be associated with tingling and numbness

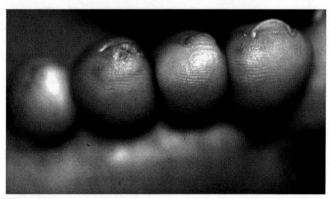

Figure 19

BLUE NODULES OF THE FOOT

I. Thrombosed Vein (Figure 20)

    A. Blue superficial tender to painful bluish nodule of recent onset

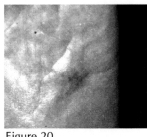

Figure 20

II. Glomus Tumor (Figure 21)

    A. Small blue papule few millimeters in size most commonly seen beneath the nail plate within the dermis of the nail unit

    B. Severe pain is the hallmark of this lesion

    C. The lesion is a tumor of the Suquet-Hoyer canal (connection between the arteriole and venule in the pads of the digits and is responsible for thermoregulation)

III. Blue Nevus (Figure 22)

    A. Commonly seen as an isolated blue-black lesion slightly raised to nodular papule which may be confused with a melanoma

    B. The blue color results from melanocytes limited to the mid-dermis

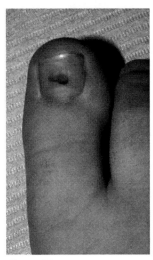

Figure 21

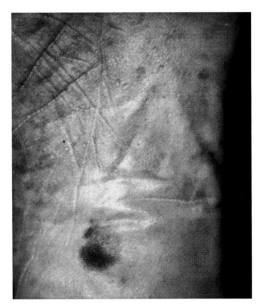

Figure 22

IV. Tattoo Reaction

    A. Implantation of lead from a pencil, metallic particle or detritus into the skin presents itself as a blue to black lesion mimicking a blue nevus

    B. A history of stepping on "something" is often elicited

    C. Sometimes pressure causes pain

V. Venous Lake

    A. A small blue to black lesion resulting from a dilated venule

    B. The lesion can be differentiated from a melanoma which it often is confused with by the ability to push blood out of the lesion by manual compression and its soft consistency

VI. Angiokeratoma of Mibelli

    A. Small blue to black lesions a few millimeters in size composed of small-dilated venules capped by a scaly, keratinous or verrucous surface seen on dorsum of the toes and fingers

BLACK LESIONS

I. Angiitis (Figure 23)

    A. Appears as small multiple discrete purpuric papules commonly seen in association with collagen-vascular disease

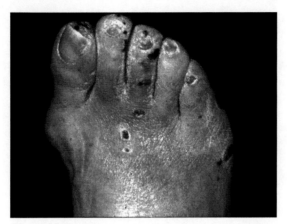

Figure 23

    B. *Bywaters lesion* is a small black lesion located on the pulp of the toe resulting from leukocytoclastic angiitis associated with rheumatoid arthritis

    C. The hallmark of the condition is a *purpuric papule*

II. Talon Noir (Figure 24)

    A. Focal areas of coagulated blood following a history of injury or trauma

    B. Commonly seen in athletes on the sides of the heels

    C. The lesion can be removed by sharp debridement

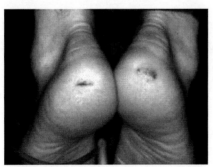

Figure 24

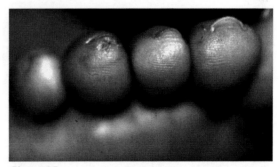

Figure 25

III. Frostbite (Figure 25)

    A. Appears as areas of dried blood with ruborous, purple swollen toes

    B. Tingling and burning are common symptoms

    C. There is erythema edema, vesicles, bullae, superficial and deep gangrene

IV. Tinea Nigra Plantaris

    A. Tinea nigra is a superficial fungal infection caused by a class of fungus called dematiaceous fungi

   B. The causative organism is *Exophiala Wernicke* (Phaeoanellomyces werneckii)
   C. As the name suggests, patients present with an asymptomatic, well demarcated, slow growing pigmented macule on the palms or soles may be mistaken for a melanoma

NEVUS

I. **Junctional Nevus** (Figure 26)
   A. Lesion flat uniform pigmentation common on soles less than 6 mm
   B. Histology consists of melanocytes limited to the dermo-epidermal junction

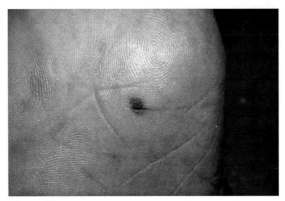

Figure 26

II. **Compound Nevus** (Figure 27)
   A. Elevated lesion usually plaque shaped or domed in appearance
   B. Histology: Melanocytes found in both the dermo-epidermal junction and the dermis the epidermis and dermis

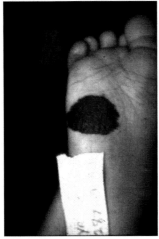   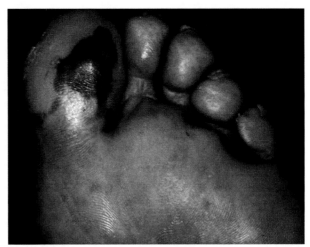

Figure 27   Figure 28

III. **Intradermal Nevus**
   A. Dome shaped soft flabby lesion common around the toes
   B. Histology: Melanocytes found mostly in dermis only

MELANOMA

I. **Acral Lentiginous Melanoma** (Figure 28)

   A. **Frequently affects the soles, palms and toes, especially the nail unit**

   B. **Appearance:** Flat, hyperpigmented (black or brown) lesion sometimes described as a spill, or spreading stain, on the skin of the palm or sole

   C. **Its black/blue appearance is not raised, although its invasiveness under the surface is often underestimated and may be extensive**

   D. **May present as an extensive surface lesion which may occupy as much as 12.0 cm**

   E. **Grows much more slowly than other melanomas**

   F. **Subungual lesions appear as a macular, irregular, laterally growing area of pigmentation in the nail** (melanonychia) and surrounding tissues

   G. **Leakage of pigment proximally away from the nail fold is called the *"Hutchinson sign"* and should be considered diagnostic**

   H. **Location:** Great toe are the most frequently involved sites

   I. **Treatment:** Amputation if present in the digit

   J. **Prognosis:** Poor prognosis because often diagnosed in later stages however, extremely rare recurrence if amputation performed

II. **Nodular Melanoma** (Figure 29)

   A. **Incidence:** Second most common melanoma; typically more common in males (2:1); occurs most often in the fifth or sixth decade

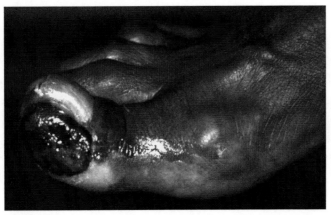

Figure 29

   B. **A very fast-growing nodular event that occurs in a period of 3 months to 2 years**

   C. **Patient reports the sudden appearance of a "bump" that started to grow recently**

   D. **Appearance:** An elevated, dark blue, brown, or black nodule that is 1.0 to 3.0 cm or larger if untreated, is almost spherical, and generally smooth; the appearance may be distorted in individuals that have bumped or rubbed the area

   E. **Does not have a horizontal growth phase, starts vertically from the beginning**

   F. **Treatment:** Best possible method of biopsy: total excision of the lesion

   G. **Must be biopsied to rule out all other diagnoses (e.g., hemangioma)**

   H. **May be confused with a pyogenic granuloma**

   I. **Prognosis:** Most malignant of any melanoma because depth tends to be deeper

III. Lentigo Mailgna Melanoma (Figure 30)

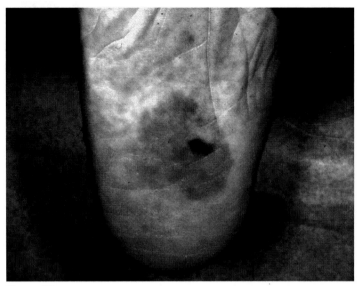

Figure 30

How wide should the margins be when removing a melanoma?

Thin   1mm or less = 1cm border
Intermediate   1mm-4 mm = 2 cm
Thick   > 4 mm = 2 cm border

Sentinel node biopsy and lymphatic mapping
   A. **A technique for tracing the flow of lymph from a melanoma site to the nearest lymph node that first receives lymph drainage is termed the** *"sentinel node"*
   B. **Tracers using PCR techniques are used to increase sensitivity**
   C. **Biopsy of this node then takes place**
   D. **If the sentinel node biopsy is negative node, no other lymph nodes are biopsied and the patient is spared the morbidity and complications associated with more extensive lymph node biopsies**
   E. **Most clinicians agree that sentinel lymph node biopsy is not indicated for tumors less than 0.76 mm in thickness, since the yield is zero in most large series**
   F. **Only patients with high-risk lesions of 0.76-0.99 mm should be considered for sentinel lymph node biopsy if their melanomas are at Clark level IV or V or if the tumors are ulcerated**
   G. **Sentinels node biopsies are indicated for intermediate thickness melanomas which measure between 1mm and 4 mm**

Clark Classification System	5 year survival rate
Level I - Tumor in situ	100% - 98%
Level II - Papillary dermis	96% - 72%
Level III - Tumor cells are found throughout the papillary dermis with impingement on the reticular dermis	90% - 46%
Level IV - Tumor cells are clearly in reticular dermis	67% - 31%
Level V - Tumor cells show invasion of the subcutaneous fat.	48% - 12%

Breslow Classification System	5 year survival rate
0.00 - 0.76 mm	98% - 99%
0.76 - 1.49 mm	85%
1.50 - 2.49 mm	84%
4.00 mm	44%

VII. **"ABCD Rule" for Detection of Melanomas**
   A. **NIH Publication No. 99-1563 modified 12/12/2000**
   B. **Melanomas can vary greatly in the ways they appear**
   C. **Many show all of the ABCD features**
   D. **However, some may show changes or abnormalities in only one or two of the ABCD features**
   E. **None of the ABCD features are present in amelanotic melanoma**

   F. **Asymmetry** (Figure 31)
      1. The shape of one half does not match the other
      2. The edges are often ragged, notched, blurred, or irregular in outline; the pigment may spread   into the surrounding skin

   G. **Border Irregularity** (Figure 32)

   H. **Color** (Figure 33)
      1. The color is uneven
      2. Shades of black, brown, and tan may be present
      3. Areas of white, grey, red, pink, or blue also may be seen

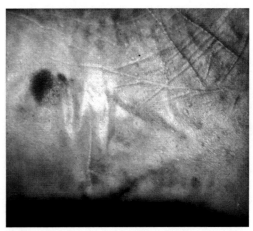

Figure 31

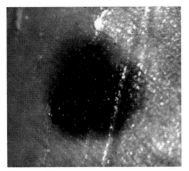

Figure 32

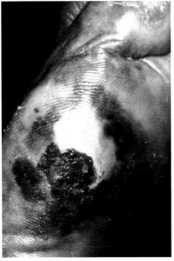

Figure 33

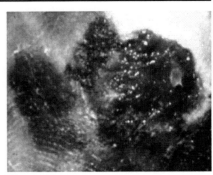

Figure 34

I. **Diameter** (Figure 34)
   1. There is a change in size, usually an increase
   2. Melanomas are usually larger than the eraser of a pencil (5 mm or 1/4 inch)

J. **Melanoma of Nail Bed** (Figure 35)
   *   Pigmentation of the nail plate in Caucasians usually represents melanoma whereas pigmentation of the nail plate in African Americans is benign and represents simply pigmentation of the basal layer (ephelides)

ABCDEF of Nail Melanoma (Figure 36)

A ge 50-70 years

A frican-Americans > Native Americans >Asians

B and – brown – black > or equal to 3 mm in. width, irregular border or blurred border

C olor change (rapid)

D igits: thumb > hallux > index finger >multiple; usually the dominant hand

E xtension of pigment to periungual skin

F amilial or personal history of melanoma or dysplastic nevus syndrome

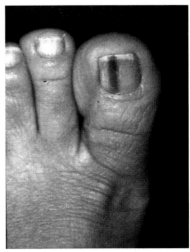

Figure 35

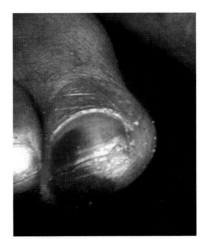

Figure 36

NODULES (MISCELLANEOUS)

I.   **Pretibial Myxedema** (Figure 37a and 37b)

   A.   **Raised nodular yellowish, skin colored or waxy plaques on the anterior surfaces of the legs and occasionally on the dorsum of the feet**

   B.   **The lesions often show dilated hair follicles and feel cooler than normal skin**

   C.   **It may be associated with exopthalamos and acropachy**

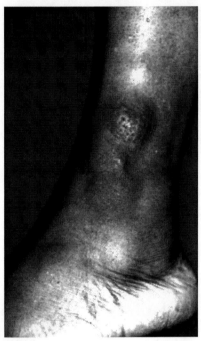

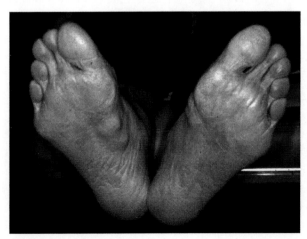

Figure 37b

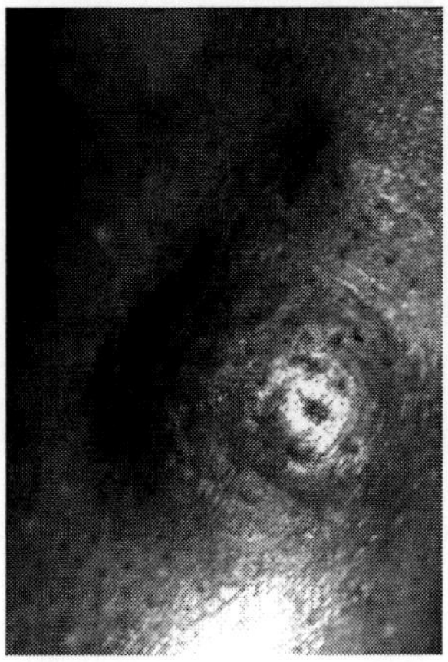

Figure 37a

II.   **Fibromatosis** (Figure 38)

   A.   **Bilateral symmetric nodules composed of fibrous tissue involving the plantar fascia medially**

   B.   **May be associated with diabetes, epilepsy and alcoholism**

Figure 38

III. Ganglion Cyst (Figure 39)

    A. Cystic fibrous lesion most often lined by fibrous tissue not synovium

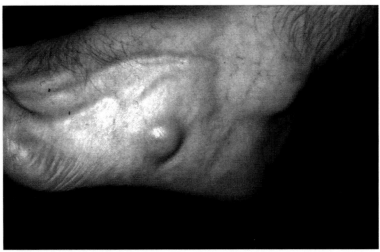

Figure 39

ULCERATIVE NODULES OF THE FOOT AND LEG

    I. Basal Cell Carcinoma (Figures 40a and 40b)

        A. While basal cell carcinoma is rarely reported on the foot the lesion does with some frequency develop on the foot usually its plantar aspect

        B. The lesion may present itself as a foot ulcer that does not heal or a nodule with central ulceration and a raised pearly border

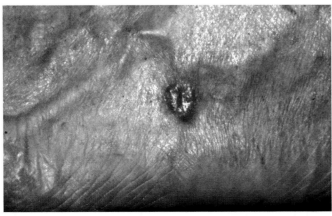

Figure 40b

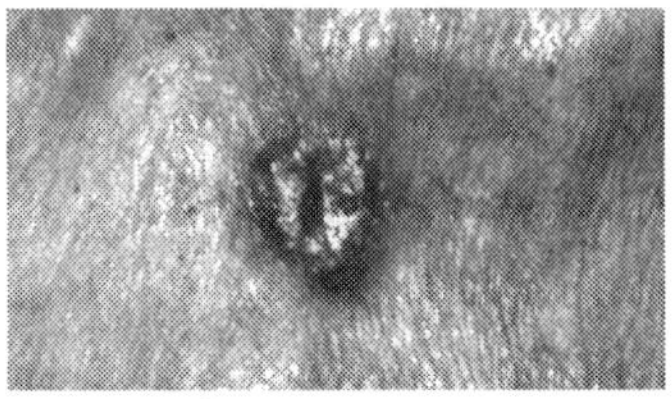

Figure 40a

    II. Keratoacanthoma (Figure 41)

        A. A dome shaped lesion with central ulceration filled with keratin

        B. Occurs beneath the nail plates causing erosion of the tip of the distal phalanx as well as occurring as a isolated lesion on the top of the foot

        C. The lesion has been associated with various viral serotypes, is self limiting and spontaneously regresses

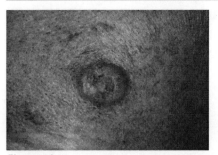

Figure 41

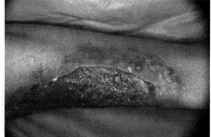

Figure 42a

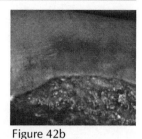

Figure 42b

    D. Because of its histologic similarity to squamous cell carcinoma biopsy material must be large enough for proper interpretation

III. **Erythema Induratum** (Bazin's Disease)
    A. Ulcerative nodules involving the calf due to mycobacterium tuberculosis
    B. Products, demonstrated by PCR
    C. Lesions are more common in women
    D. Recurrences occur in the winter
    E. PPD is positive

IV. **Pyoderma Gangrenosum** (Figures 42a and 42b)
    A. The ulcers tend to be found most commonly on the lower extremity
    B. It exhibits a ragged border with a blue-red overhanging edge
    C. A history of trauma at the site is often elicited (pathergy)
    D. The ulcers may be preceded by small pustules at the site or nodules, which breakdown
    E. The borders tend to be dusky red
    F. An association between ulcerative colitis has been established
    G. Biopsy findings are non-diagnostic

V. **Squamous Cell Carcinoma**
    A. Should be suspected in an ulcer that has not healed and neuropathy and vascular disease has been ruled out
    B. Skin changes are not clinically diagnostic and biopsy is required to establish the diagnosis

VI. **Ecthyma** (Figure 43)
    A. The lesions caused by group A beta hemolytic streptococcus
    B. Lesions are deep seated and ulcerative in nature
    C. Adherent hemorrhagic crusts are present like ice bergs above the level of the skin
    D. The lesions tend to affect the legs more than the feet and are painful

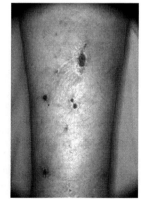

Figure 43

VII. **Venous Stasis** (Figures 44a and 44b)
    A. Ulcers with an irregular sloping border with red granulating base and are as a rule not painful

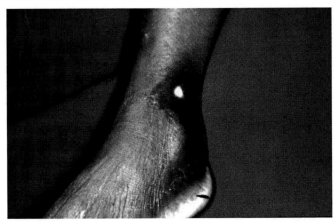

Figure 45a

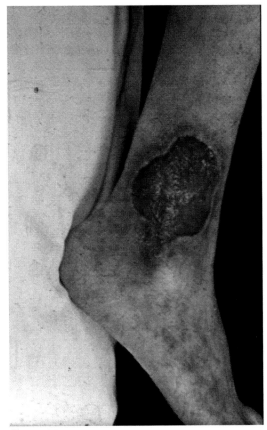

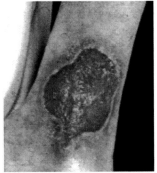

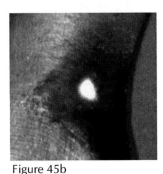

Figure 45b

Figure 44a   Figure 44b

    B.   Medial ankle above the malleolus is a common location due to incompetent communication veins between deep and superficial systems at that site

VIII. Sickle Cell Ulceration (Figures 45a and 45b)

    A.   Sickle cell ulcers usually begin as small, punched out painful ulcers on the lower third of the leg, above the ankle and over and around the medial or lateral malleolus

    B.   Surrounding zone of hyperpigmentation is common

    C.   Accompanying cellulitis and regional inguinal adenitis may be present

    D.   Ulceration is common in patients with SS hemoglobinopathy

IX. Sporotrichosis Ulceration

    A.   Ulcerative nodule due to sporotrichosis schenckii exhibiting a trail of dermal and subdermal nodules involving the lymphatics

X. Hypertensive Ulceration (Figure 46)

    A.   Common lateral lower leg

    B.   Ulcer is punched out and has sharply demarcated border

    C.   Base is necrotic and the lesion is extremely painful

    D.   Etiology usually to cutaneous small vessel arterial ischemia usually resulting from compression of surrounding tissue, as opposed to large vessel disease of ASO causing toe ulcers

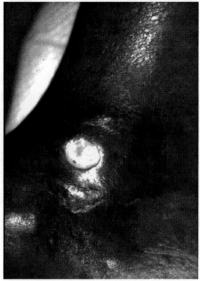

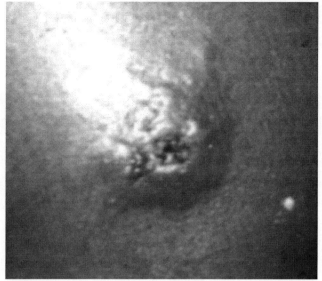

Figure 46   Figure 47

XI. Anthrax Ulceration (Figure 47)

    A. Anthrax begins as a painless papule, resembling an insect bite

    B. As the papule enlarges as vesicle or bulla within the lesion may be noted

    C. Beneath the lesion induration is present

    D. As the lesion progresses, it may become necrotic forming a black eschar

XII. Antiphospholipid Syndrome

    A. These patients commonly present to podiatrists with skin ulcers and/or recurrent deep venous thrombosis

    B. The diagnosis is established by detecting the presence of anti cardiolipin antibodies and lupus anticoagulant

    C. Coagulation studies may be helpful

    D. Patients often show reddish or purplish mottling of the skin ("*livido reticularis*")

XIII. Klinefellter Syndrome

    A. A chromosomal disease affecting the 48XXYY chromosome, hypogonadism, resulting in small genitalia, slipped femoral epiphysis, breast enlargement and foot and leg ulcers

ANNULAR / SERPIGINOUS / CIRCULAR LESIONS

I. Erythema Chronicum Migrans (Figure 48)

    A. Rapidly expanding erythematous flat lesions with clear center usually greater than 5 cm in diameter

    B. Can expand to 50 cm

    C. The center is usually clear but at times the early lesion can be entirely red lacking a clear center

    D. No scale is present

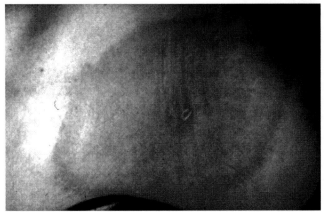

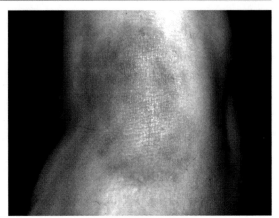

Figure 48   Figure 49

II. Granuloma Annulare (Figure 49)

   A. Annular or ring shaped lesions occurring on the dorsum of the feet and hands in young adults, usually female

   B. The border is composed of papules

   C. No scale is present and the lesion does not itch

   D. Biopsy is diagnostic demonstrating complete and incomplete zones of collagen

III. Cutaneous Larva Migrans ("*Creeping Eruption*") (Figure 50)

   A. Initially linear then serpiginous in shape the larvae of parasites found in dogs and cattle are deposited in sand and soil and penetrate and travel within human skin

   B. The lesion lacks a scale seen in tinea circinata and is extremely itchy and travels over days within the skin which helps differentiate the disorder

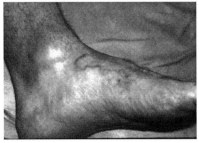

Figure 50

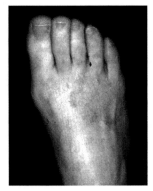

Figure 51

IV. Tinea Circinata (Figure 51)

   A. Circinate lesion composed of peripheral papules covered by a scale

   B. The lesion gradually clears centrally as the lesion develops

V. Sarcoidosis

   A. Lesions tend to be circinate but lesions frequently coalesce forming reddish brown plaques

   B. Associated with high uric acid levels and an arthritis that responds to colchicine

   C. Biopsy helpful

    D. **A test for angio converting enzyme may be helpful**

VI. **Pityriasis Rosea**

    A. **While usually affecting the trunk, on occasion the lesions of Pityriasis rosea may affect the feet**

    B. **These lesions are oval occurring along Langer's lines of cleavage**

    C. **The herald or mother patch is usually larger appearing before the onset of the other lesions**

VII. **Triangular shape lesions**

VIII. **Atrophie Blanche** (Figure 52a and 52b)

    A. **White atrophic plaques exhibiting triangular edges seen in venous disease**

    B. **May have an immununologic etiology**

IX. **Neurotic Excoriations** (Figure 53)

    A. **Triangular gauges in the skin within scratch marks**

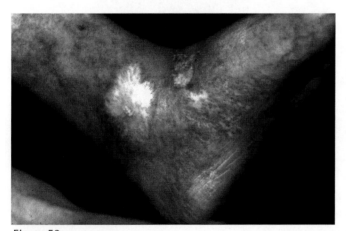

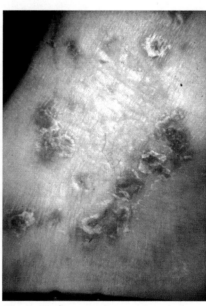

Figure 52a

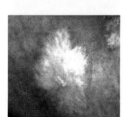

Figure 52b

Figure 53

X. **Lichen Planus** (Figure 54)

    A. **Think of Lichen planus when confronted with a violaceous papule(s) that are polygonal or triangular in shape**

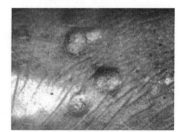

XI. **Diabetic Bullosis**

    A. **Characterized by triangular edges to bulla**

Figure 54

XII. Painful Lesions

XIII. GC Pustule (Gonoccemia) (See Figure 12)

   A. Painful hemorrhagic pustule seen on palms and soles resulting from dissemination of gonnococcal infection
   B. Associated with tenosynovitis and septic joints
   C. Present over bony prominences

XIV. Oslers' Nodes (Figure 55)

   A. Erythematous papules located on tips of toes representing infective emboli
   B. Associated with acute and subacute infective endocarditis
   C. Janeway's nodes non-painful lesions palms & soles small vessel vasculitis no organisms

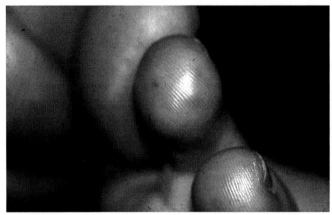

Figure 55

XV. Leiomyoma

   A. Small movable flesh colored intradermal of subcutaneous lesions usually arising from tunica media of veins (arrector pili muscles elsewhere)
   B. Common located in the rearfoot region
   C. Pain and tenderness are present in most but not all lesions

XVI. Glomus Tumor

   A. Bluish lesion usually located subungually, representing a tumor of the Suquet-Hoyer canal

XVII. Erythema Nodosum

   A. Small red warm tender to painful nodules affecting the anterior leg due to inflammation of the fibrous septa between fat lobules
   B. May be associated with systemic disease
   C. Differential diagnosis is cellulitis

XVIII. Hypertensive Ischemic Ulcer

   A. Painful punched-out circumscribed ulcer exhibiting a grey necrotic base and a cyanotic edge
   B. Seen most commonly on side of lower leg and ankle due to small vessel arterial disease

XIX. **Arterial Ulcer**

    A. **Painful ulcer associated with systemic disease (see ulcers section)**

    B. **Found on foot and toes secondary to large artery occlusion**

XX. **Calciphylaxis**

    A. **Chronic renal disease produces high phosphorous and low calcium levels**

    B. **The parathyroid gland compensates by producing parathormone causing osteoclastic leaching of calcium from bone to skin and soft tissue causing skin calcification**

    C. **Painful skin breakdowns and ulcers can also develop due medial and intimal calcifications of small vessels**

    D. **Painful patchy livedo reticularis that becomes superficially gangrenous star shaped eschars is an early sign**

XXI. **Zoster Blisters**

    A. **Painful bulla may be blood filled, arranged in crops located along a dermatome**

    B. **Severe pain may precede lesions**

XXII. **Frostbite**

    A. **Small rounded mildly elevated painful papules involving the toes**

    B. **Toes may appear red-purple but warm**

    C. **Can be confused with Oslers nodes**

    D. **A history of cold exposure, areas of necrotic skin change and reddish toe color are helpful diagnostic features**

VERRUCOUS LESIONS OF THE FOOT

I. **Tuberculosis of Skin** (Figure 56)

    A. **Known as "*tuberculosis verrucosis cutis*"**

    B. **Begins as a flat soft papule enlarging into verrucous plaques which are easily compressible**

    C. **Commonly seen in immunosuppressed individuals**

    D. **PPD is positive**

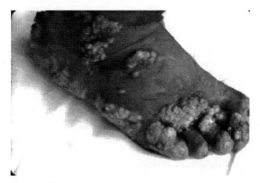

Figure 56

II. Verrucous Carcinoma (Figures 57a and 57b)

    A. **Most commonly on the soles simulating as a large mosaic wart with channels or fissures extending to the deep dermis where foul smelling keratinous material may be extruded to the skin's surface**

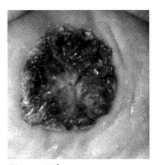

Figure 57b

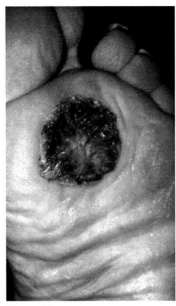

Figure 57a

III. Warts

    A. **While usually seen on the plantar surface of feet may take on a cauliflower appearance on non-weight bearing surfaces such as the dorsum of the foot**

IV. Stucco Keratosis (Figure 58)

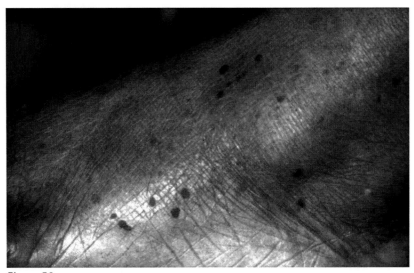

Figure 58

    A. **Small grey to black papules located on the dorsum of the feet and ankle**
    B. **Lesions may also be seen on the face**
    C. **These lesions represent a form of seborrheic keratosis and are genetically inherited**

V. **Acrokeratosis Verruciformis** (Hopf) (Figures 59a and 59b)

    A. **Multiple tiny white or light flat topped minute papules on the dorsum of the hands and feet with a predilection to fingers and toes**

    B. **Stucco keratosis and warts are larger lesions**

    C. **Flat warts and Lichen planus like lesions can cause difficulty in diagnosis but can be differentiated by their histology**

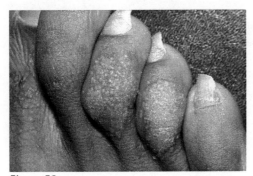

Figure 59a

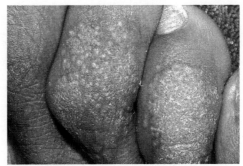

Figure 59b

VI. **Epidermodysplasia Verruciformis** (Lewandowsky & Lutz)

    A. **Epidermodysplasia verruciformis a rare familial disorder characterized by flat warts on the dorsum of the feet and hands with facial, check and back lesions noted**

    B. **HPV may be associated**

    C. **Lesions may lead to squamous cell carcinoma**

VII. **Verrucous Skin Change Associated with Lymphedema**

    A. **Small spiny lesions in plaques are commonly seen on the toes, ankles and lower legs in lymphedema**

VII. **Round Plaques of Dermatitis**

IX. **Bowens Disease** (Figure 60)

    A. **Bowens disease is a squamous cell carcinoma in situ and should be considered when confronted with an isolated patch of dermatitis that looks like Psoriasis in an elderly patient**

    B. **Often responds temporarily to topical therapy**

X. **Lichen Simplex Chronicus** (Figure 61)

    A. **Looks like psoriasis and is often misdiagnosed as psoriasis**

    B. **Usually lacks the sharp border of psoriasis and exhibits increased depth of the skin lines *"ichenification"***

    C. **It is characteristically associated with itching**

XI. **Psoriasis** (Figure 62)

    A. **Sharply outlined erythematous patches with overlying white silvery scale**

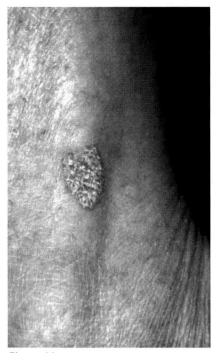

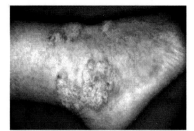

Figure 61

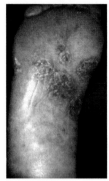

Figure 62

Figure 60

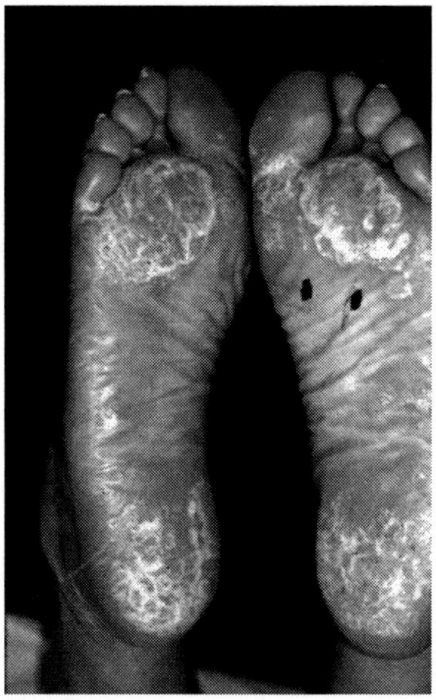

Figure 63

B. No increase in skin lines and usually not itchy

C. Tend to be bilateral and symmetric mistaken for fungal infection but no clearing center

XII. **Nummular Eczema** (Figure 63)

  A. Rounded plaques of dermatosis looking like psoriasis but not as defined

  B. Lesions also tend to be bilateral and symmetric and extensor surfaces like psoriasis

  C. Key to diagnosis is looking for the primary lesion which is small vesicles

  D. Absence of a clearing center helps to differentiate from a fungal infection

  E. Presence of exudation helps to differentiate from psoriasis

XIII. **Necrobiosis Lipoidica Diabeticorum** (Figure 64)

TOE LESIONS

  I. **Synovial Cyst** (Figure 65)

  A. Known as a "*myxoid cyst*"

  B. Small fluctuant cystic lesions containing mucin

  C. Identical histologically to a ganglionic skin cyst with the exception that it is located within the dermis

  D. It is found exclusively at the DIP joint of the toes and in the proximal nail fold

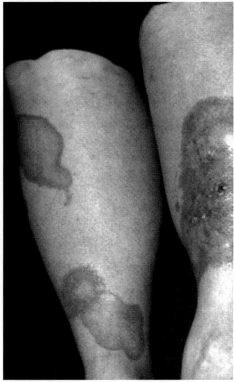

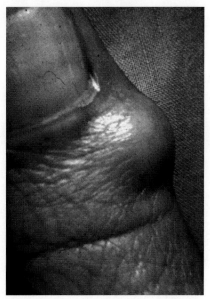

Figure 65

Figure 64

II. Angiofibroma (Koenen)

    A. Flesh colored lesion around or under the nail plate seen either idiopathically or in association with Tuberous sclerosis

III. Giant Cell Tumor of Tendon Sheath (Figure 66)

    A. Small firm lesion representing a reactive fibroproliferative response commonly seen on the toes

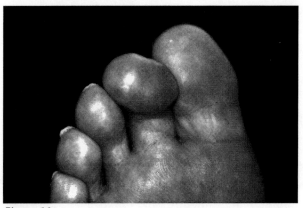

Figure 66

    B. Giant cells are admixed with spindled fibroblasts

TOENAIL PATHOLOGY/ONYCHOMYCOSIS

I. Pterygium (Figures 67a and 67b)

    A. Adhesion of the posterior nail fold to its underlying nail matrix and bed results in permanent central loss of nail plate production

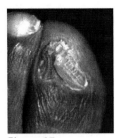

Figure 67a

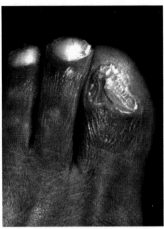

Figure 67b

II. Mee's Lines (Figure 68)

    A. Mee's lines, or *"transverse striate leukonychia"*, are classically associated with arsenic poisoning, but have been described in other cases of acute or chronic illness and other poisons

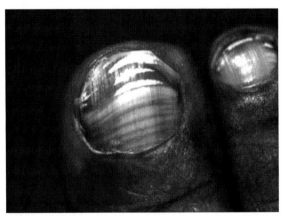

Figure 68

III. Advanced Psoriasis of the Nail Unit (Figure 69)

    A. Note sharp outline of skin which helps differentiate this from fungal infection

    B. Pitting and oil spots usually lacking in advanced psoriasis of the nail unit

IV. Pitting of Nails in Psoriasis (Figure 70)

    A. Small pits arranged haphazardly in the nail plate is diagnostic of psoriasis

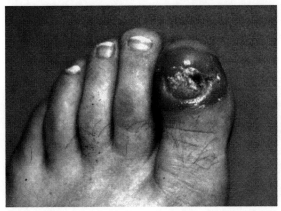
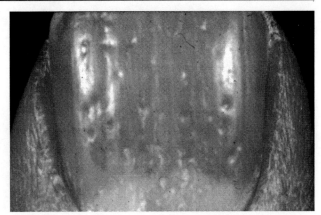

Figure 69   Figure 70

    B. **Few pits in a nail are considered normal**

    C. **"*Oil spot sign*" represents brownish spots under the nail plate and possibly the most specific nail sign of psoriasis**

V. **Pincer Nail**

    A. **Represents a nail that is laterally convex causing constriction of the underlying tissue**

    B. **Sometimes painful condition**

    C. **May be related to a subungual exostosis**

VI. **Yellow Nail Syndrome**

    A. **The nail is excessively curved from side to side and has a yellow or greenish color**

    B. **The nail is usually onycholytic and has stopped growing**

    C. **Usually associated with lympthedema of the ankles, bronchitis, bronchiectasis and pleural effusions**

    D. **May be associated with malignant neoplasms**

ONYCHOMYCOSIS

I. **Zaias Classification**

    A. **Distal subungual onychomycosis (*T. Rubrum*)**

    B. **Proximal subungual onychomycosis (*T. Rubrum can be associated with AIDS*)**

    C. **Superfical white onychomycosis (*T. Mentagrophytes*)**

    D. **Posterior nail fold onychomycosis (*Candida albicans*)**

II. **Proximal Subungual Onychomycosis** (Figure 71)

III. **Dematiaceous Fungus of Nail** (Figure 72)

    A. **Exophiala jeanselmei is a dematiaceous fungus that may cause invasive diseases, particularly among immunocompromised hosts**

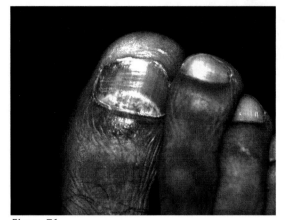

Figure 71

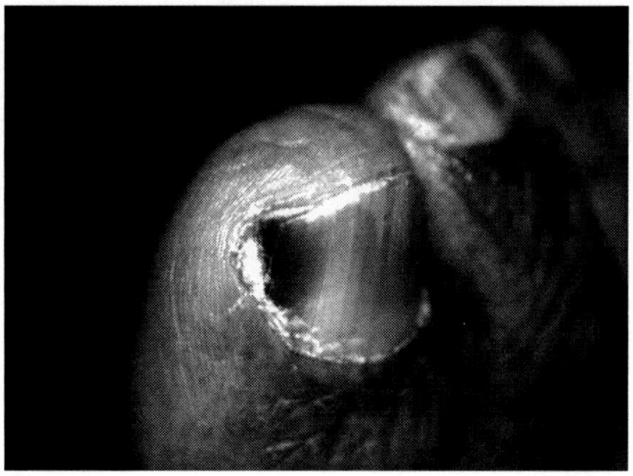

Figure 72

IV. Treatment of Nail Fungus

A. Lamisil (Terbinafine)

1. Mycologic cure of 70% of toenail, fungicidal
   a. Clinical cure
   b. Complete cure (mycologic + clinical cure)
2. Adverse events are GI (nausea, diarrhea) and skin rash, pruritis (mild, transient, reversible)
3. Adverse events less common: perversion of taste; happens more in women
4. No evidence of drug-drug interactions
5. Just one week of therapy and it is at the nail bed
6. 250 mg (1 tablet) PO x 3 months by mouth
7. Diabetic patient? Yes, you can use it
8. No hypoglycemic episode in diabetics on Lamisil (Br J Derm Farkas 2002) in NIDDM and IDDM
9. Liver? <1% have risk of acute liver injury
10. 3% develop elevated liver enzymes
11. Risk increases with prior history of PO use
12. Pre-existing liver disease a RELATIVE contraindication
13. Liver function tests (AST & ALT) prior to prescription. Also, CBC

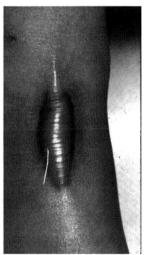

Figure 73

B. Sporonox (Itraconazole)

1. Pulse dosing is not FDA approved for toenails
2. Fungistatic
3. Mycologic cure is 67%
4. After two weeks therapy, it is at nail bed
5. Drug interactions: lovastatin, simvastitin, triazolam, midazolam
6. Hepatitis more likely to occur - in continuous therapy especially
7. Do not give to patients with pre-existing cardiac dysfunction
8. 200 mg bid for one week per month x 3 months (pulse dosing)
9. Liver function tests (AST & ALT) prior to dosing. Also, CBC.

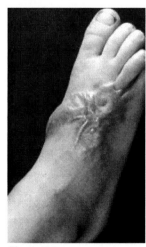

Figure 74

C. **Relapse Rate with oral antifungals**
1. Tosti et al (1998) showed 22% relapse with no significant difference between drugs
2. Consider the following factors if patient relapses:
   a. Presence of untreated or chronic tinea
   b. Age
   c. Hyperhidrosis
   d. Immunosuppression
   e. Hereditary

D. **Diflucan** (Fluconazole)
1. 300 mg weekly x 6-12 months or 50-100 mg every other day until nail fungus grows out
2. Not FDA approved for toenail onychomycosis

E. **Penlac** (Ciclopirox 8%)
1. Broad spectrum (antifungal and antibacterial) lacquer
2. If it is at the lunula, it won't be effective; but is effective for superficial white onychomycosis
3. Mycologic cure 7-36%
4. 6.6 mL bottle
5. Need to use for 52 weeks or more with monthly debridement
6. Adverse reactions: skin rash. Otherwise, no drug interactions
7. Getting it covered: when patient refuses oral treatment, patient is diabetic, patient has liver disease and cannot take orals, there is nothing else out on the market FDA approved to treat topically

F. **Keralac Gel** (Urea 50%)
1. Topical debriding agent that can be used to soften the nail before Penlac therapy
2. Some antifungal properties

V. **Treatment of Tinea Pedis**

A. **Oral Antifungals** - In general, topicals are the first line of defense but
1. Ultra-microsized Griseofulvin (Gris-Peg) 375-750 mg/day in an adult for 4-8 weeks
   a. No effect on bacteria or candida
2. Terbinafine (Lamisil) 250 mg qd x 2-4 weeks
3. Itraconazole (Sporonox) 400 mg/day x 7 days or 100 mg x 2 weeks
4. Fluconazole (Diflucan) 150 mg weekly x 2 weeks
5. Only Gris-Peg is FDA approved for tinea pedis
6. Use these when patient compliance is an issue or a moccassin version that doesn't respond to topicals

B. **Topical Antifungals**
1. Castellani's paint
   a. Modified Clear does not have coloring additive
2. Gentian Violet
3. Whitfield's ointment (benzoic acid)
4. Undecylenic Acid
5. Miconazole: Micantin (OTC) powder or cream
6. Dermatophytes, candida, mild anti-bacterial
7. Tolnaftate: Tinactin (OTC) powder or cream
   a. Covers Dermatophytes, no Candida or bacteria
8. Butenafine: (Lotrimin Ultra OTC) also as Mentax Rx, fungicidal, apply qd x 1 month
9. Terbinafine: (Lamisil AF OTC cream) fungicidal, bid x 1 month

10. Clotrimazole: (Lotrimin AF OTC cream) bid x 1 month
   a. Covers dermatophytes, gram +, mild to Candida
11. Econazole: (Specatzole cream)
12. Ketoconazole: (Nizoral cream)
13. Oxiconazole (Oxistat cream)
14. Ciclopirox (Loprox TS, gel)
15. Naftitine (Naftin cream)

C. Antifungal/Steroid combos:
1. Vytone cream is iodoquinol and hydrocortisone 1%
2. Mycolog II is nystatin and triamcinolone
3. Lotrisone is clotrimazole and betamethasone
4. You run the risk of suppressing the fungus temporarily when you use these
5. These meds are for CANDIDIASIS ONLY!!!!
6. Most antifungal topicals have a NATURAL anti-inflammatory property

D. Anti-inflammatory Antifungals
1. The best in order of most effective
   a. Ciclopirox
   b. Naftitine
   c. Terbinafine
   d. Ketoconazole
   e. Oxiconazole
2. Can also combine keratolytic moisturizers
   a. Namely, urea or lactic acid preparations
   b. Best to use separately in order to de-scale the foot
   c. Not enough research on combining the antifungal and keratolytic at the same time

E. Hyperhidrosis Therapies
1. Use Zeasorb or Zeasorb AF powder
2. Drysol (Al Cl 20%) use for 3 days at night
3. LazerFormalyde solution (Formaldehyde 10%) use at night for 3 days

CHAPTER 12
DERMATOLOGY

1.   Which of the following disorders are associated with cigar shaped blisters?

    A.   Acute Tinea Pedis
    B.   Dyshidrotic Exzema
    C.   Diabetic Bullosis
    D.   Allergic Eczematoid dermatitis
    E.   Hand & Foot Disease

2.   All of the following lesions may be blood filled except:

    A.   Herpes Zoster
    B.   Dystrophic form of ED
    C.   Friction blisters
    D.   Gonococcal skin infection
    E.   Osler's nodes

3.   All of the following lesions are red in color except:

    A.   Bacillary Angiomatosis
    B.   Amelanotic Melanoma
    C.   Kaposi sarcoma
    D.   Eccrine poroma
    E.   Glomus tumor

4.   All of the following lesions are characterized by ulceration except:

    A.   Basal cell carcinoma
    B.   Keratoacanthoma
    C.   Erythema induratum (Bazins Disease)
    D.   Antiphospholipid syndrome
    E.   Erythema nodosum

5.   All of the following lesions are black in color except:

    A.   Frostbite
    B.   Cuntaneous angiitis
    C.   Talon noir
    D.   Tinea Nigra plantaris
    E.   Amelanotic melanoma

6.   Which of the following nevi are located within the epidermis of skin?

    A.   Junctional nevus
    B.   Compound nevus
    C.   Intradermal nevus
    D.   Blue nevus

7.   All of the following lesions are serpiginous or circular except:

        A.   Erythema Chronicum Migrans
        B.   Granuloma Annulare
        C.   Cutaneous Larva Migrans (Creeping eruption)
        D.   Tinea corporis
        E.   Lichen planus

8.   Aids have been associated with which of the following types of Onychomycosis?

        A.   Distal subungual onychomycosis
        B.   Proximal subungual onychomycosis
        C.   Superfical white onychomycosis
        D.   Posterior nail fold onychomycosis

9.   How wide should the margins be when removing a melanoma?

        A.   1mm or less = .5cm border
        B.   1mm or less = 1cm border
        C.   1mm - 4mm = 3cm border
        D.   4mm or >   = 5cm border

10.   Sentinel node biopsy and lymphatic mapping should be performed on melanomas measuring:

        A.   .5mm or less
        B.   1mm or less
        C.   1mm – 4mm
        D.   > 4mm

Chapter 13

RHEUMATOLOGY

Robert S. Marcus
Ralph E. Marcus
Roger W. Marcus

RHEUMATOID ARTHRITIS

I. Epidemology

    A. Etiology

        1. Unknown, but postulated to be triggered by infectious agent or trauma in genetically susceptible individual

        2. Heritable factors include HLA-DR4 and DR1 molecules

    B. Rheumatoid factor

        1. An IgM antibody directed against IgG

        2. Produced in the synovium

        3. Present in the serum of 70% of patients with rheumatoid arthritis

        4. High titers generally associated with more severe disease

    C. Pathogenesis

        1. Putative antigen presented to helper T-lymphocytes which proliferate with macrophages in synovium. B-cells secrete immunoglobulins, including rheumatoid factor

        2. Angiogenesis and fibroblast proliferation causing villous synovitis, pannus

        3. Liberation of a number of pro-inflammatory cytokines including TNF-alpha, IL-1, and IL-6 which modulate T-cell proliferation and activate collagenase

        4. Articular cartilage collagen degradation and subchondral erosions occur by action of proteases in synovial fluid and pannus

II. Presentation

    A. Articular manifestations

        1. Symmetric small joint involvement especially involving MCP and PIP joints of hands, wrists, MTP joints, subtalar and ankle joints

        2. Marked morning stiffness with painful, swollen joints

   3. Joint effusions, most prominent in large joints
   4. Gradual progression of joint subluxation, deformities with loss of hyaline cartilage and
       subchondral bone erosions

B. Extra-articular manifestations

   1. Skin: Rheumatoid nodules, particularly over the elbows as well as the fingers and
       Achilles tendons
   2. Ocular
       a. Keratoconjunctivitis sicca, most common
       b. Episcleritis, scleromalacia
   3. Pulmonary
       a. Interstitial lung disease
       b. Infrequent pleural effusions
       c. Rheumatoid nodules, uncommon in lung, can mimic malignancy
   4. Cardiac
       a. Pericarditis, rarely of clinical significance
       b. Myocarditis, conduction abnormalities, rare
   5. Gastrointestinal
       a. Effects of NSAIDs causing ulceration, bleeding, perforation, dyspepsia, gastritis
       b. Less common with use of COX-2 drugs and with concurrent misoprostol or
           lansoprazole
   6. Renal
       a. Effects of anti-inflammatory drugs
       b. Amyloidosis in long-standing severe disease
   7. Neurologic
       a. Entrapment syndromes: carpal tunnel and tarsal tunnel
       b. Severe myelopathy can occur with cervical subluxation, especially C1-C2
       c. Neuropathies due to rheumatoid vasculitis

C. Hematologic

   1. Anemia of chronic disease
   2. Leukopenia, which is seen in Felty's syndrome
       a. Platelet counts, which act as acute phase reactants, generally elevated

III. Diagnosis:

   A. Based on clinical findings and typical history
   **B. Supported, but not necessarily confirmed, by the presence of rheumatoid factor and
         elevated sedimentation rate**

IV. Treatment: Recent findings of increased morbidity and mortality and early radiographic joint
damage has led to more aggressive therapy

   **A. Non-steroidal anti-inflammatory drugs (NSAIDs) generally used initially or COX-2
         drugs in patients at higher risk of GI bleeding**
   **B. Prednisone in low doses, generally 10 mg. or less, to improve patient function and act as
         bridge until DMARDs take effect. Can also have disease-modifying effects including
         slowing joint damage**
   **C. Disease-modifying anti-rheumatic drugs (DMARDs) used within first few months of
         disease onset to prevent disease progression and disability. Frequently used in
         combinations. Careful monitoring for side effects necessary**

1. Methotrexate, weekly oral or subcutaneous dose of 7.5-20 mg
2. Sulfasalazine
3. Hydroxychloroquine
4. Leflunomide
5. Intramuscular gold
6. Cyclosporine

D. Biologic agents that target specific cytokines. Used for patients who continue to have active synovitis, joint destruction after treatment with DMARDs. These slow or arrest radiographic progression of disease. Expensive

1. Anti-TNF drugs
   a. Entanercept
   b. Infliximab
   c. Adalimumab
2. Anti-IL-1 drug
   a. Anakinra

V. Complications

A. Rheumatoid nodules can cause both cosmetic and functional problems on elbows and hands. May be exacerbated with use of methotrexate

B. Ruptured popliteal cyst, diagnosed by ultrasound, may mimic thrombophlebitis

C. Vasculitis with digital gangrene, leg ulcers, neuropathy in severe disease

D. Felty's syndrome with weight loss, Sjogren's syndrome, lymphadenopathy, neutropenia

E. Rheumatoid lung disease may lead to pulmonary fibrosis

F. Nerve entrapment syndromes

G. Paraplegia due to cervical myelopathy

H. Osteoporosis

I. Lymphoma, increased risk

SJÖGREN'S SYNDROME

I. Overview

Autoimmune disease with lymphocytic infiltration of lacrimal and salivary glands. The disease is "primary" if it occurs alone and termed "secondary" if occurs in association with other autoimmune disease such as rheumatoid arthritis, scleroderma

II. Manifestations

A. Dry eyes (xerophthalmia) and dry mouth (xerostomia)

B. Parotid gland enlargement

C. Arthralgias, fatigue

D. CNS involvement rare

E. Dysphagia, atrophic gastritis

F. Primary Sjögren's syndrome associated with lymphoma (5%) and pseudolymphoma

III. Diagnosis

A. Positive rheumatoid factor, ANA, SS-A and SS-B antibodies in 50-80%

B. Lip biopsy confirmatory showing lymphocytic infiltration in salivary glands

IV. Treatment

A. Eye lubricants, oral pilocarpine, and cevimeline helpful symptomatically for sicca syndrome

B. Hydroxychloroquine, methotrexate, corticosteroids may be of benefit in systemic disease

JUVENILE CHRONIC ARTHRITIS

I. **Overview**

Characterized by synovial inflammation in childhood. Sub-types are polyarticular, pauciarticular, and systemic. No diagnostic laboratory test with diagnosis based on American College of Rheumatology criteria

A. **Systemic** (Still's disease)
   1. 10% of patients with JCA
   2. Equal incidence in males, females
   3. Spiking fevers, evanescent salmon pink rash usually in early evening
   4. Diffuse lymphadenopathy, hepatosplenomagaly
   5. Fatigue
   6. Leukocytosis and anemia are common
   7. Rheumatoid factor and ANA are usually negative

B. **Polyarticular**
   1. 40%
   2. Girls more than boys
   3. Five or more joints involved, insidious onset, fatigue, weight loss, low grade fever, mild hepatosplenomegaly, mild lymphadenopathy, anemia, and growth retardation
   4. Rheumatoid factor positive in 20% of patients
   5. ANA in 60% of patients
   6. Destructive arthritis occurs in patients with positive rheumatoid factor more frequently than those with negative rheumatoid factor

C. **Pauciarticular**
   1. 50% of patients
   2. Fewer than four joints affected within the first 6 months
   3. Females more often affected than males
   4. Usually have positive ANA but negative rheumatoid factor
   5. No systemic features
   6. Frequent ocular manifestations
   7. Uveitis major cause of morbidity

II. **Treatment**

A. **Aspirin or non-steroidal anti-inflammatory drugs** (ibuprofen, tolmetin, naproxen) **or COX-2 drugs are initial treatment**

B. **Disease-modifying anti-rheumatic drugs for patients with polyarticular or pauciarticular disease with inadequate response to anti-inflammatory drugs**

    1. Methotrexate
    2. Intramuscular gold
    3. Hydroxychloroquine
    4. Sulfasalazine
C. **Biologic agents**
    1. Etanercept (anti-TNF)
D. **Low dose prednisone** (can cause growth retardation). **High doses for life-threatening complications or severe iridocyclitis**
E. **Physical therapy to increase muscle strength and maintain range of motion**
F. **Serial casting or splinting to prevent soft-tissue contractures**

JUVENILE SPONDYLOARTHROPATHIES

I. **Overview:** Ankylosing spondylitis, reactive arthritis, psoriatic arthritis, and spondyloarthropathies associated with regional enteritis present a diagnostic dilemma in children. There is usually little radiologic evidence of spine involvement in the first few years of onset. A symmetric lower-extremity involvement largely appears in children with a positive family history. Other features include involvement of the first MPJ and heel spur syndrome. In addition, it is important to search for early signs of psoriasis. Reiter's syndrome usually is associated with shigella-, salmonella-, or yersinia-associated diarrhea. Of children with Reiter's syndrome, 90% have positive HLA B-27. Among cases of juvenile psoriatic: arthritis, 40% are familial. Incidence in girls exceeds that in boys by 2 to 1. Management includes education; physical therapy; NSAIDs, sulfasalazine, etanercept, or methotrexate, according to the patient's age. Corticosteroids are reserved for severe inflammatory bowel disease or aggressive iridocyclitis

PEDIATRIC VASCULOPATHIES

I. **Henoch-Schöenlein purpura**
    A. **One of the most common forms of vasculitis in childhood**
    B. **Consists of rash, arthritis, gastrointestinal pain, and renal pathology**
    C. **Skin changes consist of palpable purpura on the buttocks and lower extremities, especially around the sock line; the rash will progress from red to purple to brown**
    D. **Some of these patients have arthritis or arthralgias in the large joints**

II. **SLE:** In children younger than 6, girls predominate, with symptoms and signs similar to those in adults

III. **Dermatomyositis**
    A. **Characterized by vasculitis in the skin, the muscle; calcinosis; and lack of association with malignancy**
    B. **Diagnosis requires the typical rash and elevated muscle enzymes, symmetrical weakness, evidence of vasculitis, and EMG confirming inflammatory myopathy**

IV. **PSS**
   A. **In children, localized forms are more common than either limited or diffuse sclerosis, and severe growth abnormalities occur**
   B. **Prognosis is usually good, with the exception of morbidity from growth retardation**
   C. **Progression from localized scleroderma. to diffuse systemic sclerosis is very rare**

SYSTEMIC LUPUS ERYTHEMATOSUS

I. **Overview**
   A. **Definition:** Autoimmune disease with multisystemic manifestations characterized by a variety of autoantibodies, including antinuclear antibodies and, frequently, anti- double-stranded DNA antibodies
   B. **Incidence:** Approximately 2.5 per 100,000 in white females and 3 times higher in black females; 90% of patients are female
   C. **Genetic factors:** Many loci found on BI.A genes, which correlate with specific clinical manifestations; increased incidence in monozygotic twins: Some increased risk of disease with HLA-B8, DR2, and DR3 alleles.
   D. **Environmental factors**
      1. Many drugs can induce lupus, including procainamide and hydralazine
      2. Other environmental factors are speculative

II. **Clinical Presentation**
   A. **Constitutional signs and symptoms:** Fatigue, fever, arthralgias or arthritis, and weight loss
   B. **Dermatologic manifestations**
      1. Butterfly malar rashes and photosensitivity are most common
      2. Occasional nasal septum perforation and oral ulcers
      3. Alopecia
      4. Other rashes, such as urticaria, are common
   C. **Vascular/vasculitis**
      1. May occur with typical cutaneous lesions or digital gangrene
      2. Raynaud phenomenon and livedo reticularis frequently seen but are nonspecific

III. **Fifteen preliminary American College of Rheumatology criteria for classification of SLE, used for epidemiology purposes only**
   A. **Musculoskeletal**
      1. Arthralgias more common than arthritis
      2. Arthritis is non erosive in general and in small joints symmetric, can resemble rheumatoid arthritis, and deformities, but not erosions
      3. Weakness may result from muscle atrophy or myositis
      4. Aseptic necrosis may be a consequence of lupus itself or of treatment with corticosteroids
   B. **Neurologic**
      1. Dementia
      2. Seizures
      3. Peripheral neuropathy is uncommon
      4. Transverse myelitis occurs infrequently but may have disastrous consequences
      5. CVAs associated with lupus anticoagulant or antiphospholipid antibody syndrome

C. **Other manifestations:**
1. Renal involvement is common and may lead to nephrotic syndrome or kidney failure
2. Vasculitis and digital gangrene, myocardial infarction secondary to coronary arteritis (rare) or in association with antiphospholipid antibody syndrome
3. Gastrointestinal manifestations occur in 50% of patients with nonspecific dysphagia of dyspepsia; abdominal pain may be manifestation of serositis; and pancreatitis may develop in up to 8% of patients; mesenteric vasculitis is uncommon; hepatosplenornegaly
4. Ocular: Sjögren's syndrome; retinal vasculitis is uncommon but can cause blindness
5. Pregnancy increases morbidity with low birth weight babies common and markedly increased risk of miscarriage, still birth, or prematurity, particularly in association with anti-phospholipid antibodies; when renal disease is present or other severe manifestations are present, pregnancy is hazardous

IV. **Laboratory findings**

A. **ANA positive in 98% of patients**
B. **Anti-double-stranded DNA antibodies are more specific but occur in less than 30% of patients**
C. **Anti-Sm antibodies are present in 25% of patients and are also very specific; C3, C4, and total complement levels are frequently low in active disease, particularly in renal disease**

V. **Differential diagnosis:** Mixed connective tissue disease, overlap with polymyositis, rheumatoid arthritis, and systemic vasculitis

VI. **Management**

A. **Oral corticosteroids: The mainstay treatment, with dosage varying for the severity of organ involvement**
B. **Immunosuppressant drugs such as azathioprine and cyclophosphamide used for central nervous system, renal, and vascular complications**
C. **Steroids can also be used in high-dose pulses, as can cyclophosphamide. Hydroxycholoroquine is used to treat the skin and joint disease and serositis**

PROGRESSIVE SYSTEMIC SCLEROSIS (SCLERODERMA)

I. **Clinical manifestations**

A. **Skin**
1. Bound down and thickened
2. Superficial ulcers can occur at the PIP and DIP joints of the hands, elbows
3. May be limited oral aperture and frequently there is flattening of the normal creases in the face
4. Involvement of the fingers is termed "sclerodactyly"
5. Frequent involvement in the feet
6. Raynaud's phenomenon is almost always present
7. Calcinosis, particularly in patients with crest syndrome; a form of the illness limited to

skin involvement at the fingers and face, Raynaud's phenomenon and esophageal disease

    8. Frequently dilated capillaries in the nail folds, which is characteristic of scleroderma

B. Bones and joints

    1. Initially edematous changes in the hands and wrists, which progressively decreases range of motion in involved joints as a result of fibrosis of joint capsule

    2. Joint pain frequent

    3. Frequent marked crepitus over the tendons (poor prognostic sign)

C. Skeletal muscle

    1. May be progressive fibrosis of skeletal muscle and weakness

    2. Inflammatory changes in patients with overlap syndrome (lupus/scleroderma)

D. Organs

    1. Esophagus and gastrointestinal tract

        a. Dysphagia caused by dysmotility is common

        b. Fibrosis of smooth muscle in the distal esophagus can lead to marked reflux and stricture formation

        c. Small bowel involvement includes symptoms of abdominal cramps, bloating, chronic diarrhea, and sometimes malabsorption

        d. Bacterial overgrowth occurs frequently and may be the cause of diarrhea

        e. Colonic involvement may produce symptoms suggestive of obstruction

        f. Characteristic wide mouth diverticula sometimes seen

        g. Patients occasionally develop primary biliary cirrhosis

    2. Lungs

        a. Primary cause of long-term mortality

        b. Progressive, restrictive lung disease and decreased diffusion capacity due to pulmonary fibrosis

        c. Progressive pulmonary hypertension and respiratory failure

    3. Heart

        a. Myocardial fibrosis common

        b. Patients may develop arrhythmias or pericardial inflammation

        c. Conduction disturbances may occur

    4. Kidney

        a. Sudden onset of malignant hypertension and rapidly progressive renal failure usually associated with proteinuria ("renal crisis")

        b. If detected early, can be treated successfully with ACE inhibitors

    5. Nerves: Occasionally carpal tunnel syndrome, trigeminal neuralgia, and facial palsies

E. Limited systemic sclerosis, also known as CREST (<u>C</u>alcinosis, <u>R</u>aynaud phenomenon, <u>E</u>sophageal involvement, <u>S</u>clerodactyly, and <u>T</u>elangiectasias) syndrome: Generally heralds a more benign course but is associated with pulmonary hypertension, digital gangrene, biliary cirrhosis

F. Serology

    1. Anticentromere antibody characteristic of CREST syndrome

    2. Anti-Scl antibody is seen in 30% of patients with diffuse disease

    3. Rheumatoid factor: Present in 30% of patients

    4. ANA: Present in more than 90% of patients

G. Localized scleroderma

    1. Morphea: Characterized by small, discrete, sparse, or large patches of indurated skin; over a period of months or years, these target appearing lesions may gradually expand with an erythematous border and central clearing

    2. Linear scleroderma

         a. Very uncommon
         b. Characterized by a band of sclerotic induration and hyperpigmentation that occurs only in one extremity or on the face
         c. Usually seen in children and young adults, with women affected three times more than men
         d. Coup de sabre is facial involvement in children

     3. Eosinophilic fasciitis
         a. Skin disease is similar to scleroderma but with deposition of eosinophils, lymphocytes, and plasma cells that infiltrate the deep fascia
         b. Patients generally do not have Raynaud's phenomenon
         c. Generally occurs after marked physical exertion or trauma, with usual rapid onset of pain and swelling of the extremities followed by progressive induration of skin
         d. Frequently a peripheral eosinophilia is seen in the early stage of the disease

VASCULITIS

I. **Polyarteritis nodosa: A multisystem vasculitis affecting small and medium arteries**

   A. **Pathology:** Necrotizing vasculitis
     1. Necrotizing inflammatory changes involve entire arterial wall, particularly at bifurcations
     2. Thromboses with ischemia and aneurysms frequently occur

   B. **Clinical signs**
     1. Dermal: Palpable purpura, digital, ischemia, or gangrene involving the fingers and/or toes, cutaneous ulcers, and livedo reticularis
     2. Musculoskeletal: Myalgias, intermittent claudication with vascular involvement to muscles; asymmetric recurrent polyarthritis particularly involving large joints in lower extremities occurs in 20% of cases
     3. Mononeuritis multiplex or multiple mononeuropathy or symmetric polyneuropathy involving both sensory and motor function
     4. Segmental necrotizing glomerulonephritis
     5. Intestinal, myocardial and cerebral infarction

   C. **Laboratory**
     Hepatitis B and Hepatitis C infection common

   D. **Treatment**
     1. Steroids frequently given by intravenous pulses for 3 days, followed by a high dose of oral corticosteroids
     2. Intravenous or oral cyclophosphamide given for severe or resistant cases

II. **Churg-Strauss syndrome:** Associated with asthma, vasculitis, granulomata, and eosinophilia

   A. **Pathology:** a necrotizing granulomatous vasculitis involving arterioles and venules
   B. **Clinical signs**
     1. Patient may present with asthma or pneumonia
     2. Eventually will develop fever, weight loss, and other systemic manifestations, including nodular infiltrates of the lung and diffuse interstitial lung disease
     3. Otherwise similar to polyarteritis nodosa

III. **Wegener's granulomatosis:**

A. **Overview**
1. Necrotizing granulomas commonly involving the respiratory tract, kidneys, and other organs
2. Classic triad: Upper respiratory tract involvement, such as chronic sinusitis or nasal ulceration; respiratory tract involvement, including hemoptysis, benign infiltrates, or cavitation; and renal involvement with manifestations of glomerulonephritis
3. Skin involvement, arthralgias, and eye involvement common
B. **C-ANCA a specific test for condition is present in 90% of cases.** Antineutrophil cytoplasmic antibodies (AntiP-ANCA) positive in other forms systemic vasculitis, including polyarteritis nodosa
C. **Treatment:** Generally with corticosteroids, cyclophosphamide, and, in some cases, methotrexate

IV. **Leukocytoclastic vasculitis**

A. **Cutaneous vasculitis generally caused by a drug allergy**
B. **Skin lesions appear as petechia, which progress to papules or palpable purpura and are focally seen on the forearms and the hands as well as on the lower extremities or the back**
C. **Can be associated with rheumatoid arthritis, SLE, or Sjogren's syndrome, in addition to drug hypersensitivity**

V. **Henoch-Schönlein purpura**

A. **Generally occurs in children and teenagers**
B. **Frequently occurs after upper respiratory infection**
C. **Classic triad in 80% of patients:** Palpable purpura, arthritis, and abdominal pain
D. **Vascular lesions are prominent in the lower extremities;** arthritis is usually transient; gastrointestinal lesions are characterized by abdominal pain, cramps, hemorrhage and, rarely, perforation. Intussusception is an important complication in children
E. **Mild renal involvement occurs in up to 50% of patients**
F. **Diseases generally last 2-4 months**

VI. **Essential mixed cryoglobulinemia**

A. **Syndrome consists of purpura, arthralgias, weakness.** Mixed cryoglobulins are detected in warmed blood that has been allowed to clot in centrifuge; under refrigeration, there is a cryoprecipitate jelly containing IgG and IgM
B. **Mononeuritis multiplex can occur**
C. **Hepatitis B surface antigen or Hepatitis C antibody can be present in cryoglobulin or even in serum**
D. **Rheumatoid factor may be present in the cryoprecipitant**
E. **Treatment:** Generally with prednisone, cyclophosphamide, and, occasionally, plasmapheresis

POLYMYALGIA RHEUMATICA

I. **Clinical presentation:** Abrupt or insidious onset of profound stiffness and achiness, specifically in the shoulder girdle, low thigh, and buttocks; there also may be a low-grade synovitis of the hands and wrists and, occasionally carpal tunnel syndrome; patients have profound disability

II. Treatment

    A. Prednisone 10-15 mg. daily, which is then gradually tapered over a 12 to 18 month period

    B. There is a dramatic response within the first several days of treatment

    C. Patients have characteristically very high sedimentation rates; although a subset of patients, particularly males, may have only slightly elevated or even normal sedimentation rates

III. Associated with giant cell arteritis: Up to 30% of patients will have an associated giant cell arteritis with characteristic symptoms, such as temporal headaches, diplopia, jaw claudication, or scalp sensitivity; rule of thumb is that patients with symptoms above the neck should have bilateral temporal artery biopsies to help confirm this diagnosis

POLYMYOSITIS AND DERMATOMYOSITIS

I. Polymyositis

    A. A progressive, predominantly proximal muscle weakness, often with very little or no pain

    B. Classifications

        1. Polymyositis (Type I): Generally occurs in middle-age females, who are twice as commonly affected as males; primarily, symptoms are those of proximal muscle weakness, which progresses over several months

        2. Dermatomyositis (Type II): Same as Type I, except that patients have skin involvement, particularly with involvement of the eyelids, cheeks, and bridge of the nose; Gottron's papules, which are flat plaques, can be seen at the PIP joints; involvement of airways; and heliotrope rash

        3. Malignancy associated myositis (Type III): Same as Type I, except that in 5%-8% of patients with dermatomyositis and polymyositis there is an underlying malignancy, which is generally found in the first 2 years of diagnosis; the incidence is much greater in dermatomyositis than in polymyositis, particularly in patients over the age of 40 years

        4. Pediatric dermatomyositis (Type IV): polymyositis; clinical features are the same as those of adult dermatomyositis. Calcinosis and vasculitis are important complications

        5. MCTD (Type V): Overlap of scleroderma, polymyositis and lupus characterized by very high titers of anti-RNP antibodies; there are six new cases per million population per year (i.e., rare)

    C. Clinical presentation

        1. Dermatologic: Manifestations as described above

        2. Arthritis: Joint pain is common, particularly in patients with dermatomyositis and malignancy; true synovial disease is uncommon

        3. Muscular: Profound weakness in proximal muscle groups; when the upper esophagus is involved, dysphagia occurs with nasopharyngeal aspiration

        4. Respiratory distress with involvement of diaphragm or respiratory muscles

        5. Arrythmias, heart failure with myocarditis

    D. Laboratory findings

        1. Characteristic EMG findings: Numerous fibrillation potentials, positive sharp waves at rest, and increased exertional activity of the muscle

2. Characteristic myopathic changes in motor unit action potentials
3. Muscle enzymes are usually markedly elevated but may be slightly elevated
4. Muscle biopsy is usually indicated

E. **Treatment**
1. High-dose corticosteroids; after a few months, patients may be switched to alternate day steroids
2. Addition of inummosuppressive drugs, including azathioprine or methotrexate, may be necessary in resistant cases or with life threatening disease

II. **Prognosis:** Generally respond incompletely to treatment; muscle weakness may persist for many years, and relapses are common

MIXED CONNECTIVE-TISSUE DISEASE

I. **Serology:** High levels of anti-RNP antibodies

II. **Description, presentation and course**
A. **Symptoms:** Features scleroderma, polymyositis, and lupus with Raynaud's phenomenon, arthritis, myositis, muscle weakness, diarrhea, and pulmonary disease
1. Raynaud's phenomenon commonly seen
2. Arthritis: Seen in 60% of patients similar to changes seen in rheumatoid arthritis; puffiness in the hands and hand deformities can occur without joint erosions
3. Skin involvement: Occasional nasal septal perforation and oral ulcerations
4. Sclerodactyly
5. Myalgias common, as is inflammatory myopathy
6. Organ involvement
    a. Heart: Pericarditis is the most common form of involvement; occasional involvement of myocardium, arrhythmias, and conduction abnormalities are sometimes seen
    b. Lungs: Pleurisy commonly seen, as in lupus; may be associated with significant pleural effusion
    c. Esophagus: Involvement similar to that in scleroderma, including dysphagia, involvement of the lower esophagus, acid reflux, and development of strictures
    d. Kidney: Development of glomerulonephritis and renal failure or a renovascular hypertension crisis, as seen in scleroderma; patients generally respond to oral corticosteroids

III. **Treatment:** Patients generally respond to oral corticosteroids in addition to Imuran

ANKYLOSING SPONDYLITIS

I. **Introduction:** The seronegative spondyloarthropathies (negative rheumatoid factor, inflammatory disorders of the spine and peripheral joints) comprise ankylosing spondylitis, Reiter syndrome and reactive arthritis, and the arthritides of inflammatory bowel disease; in addition to being "seronegative spondyloarthropathies" these disorders have the following features in common:

A. **Incidence of HLAB-27**
   1. Caucasian American population   8%
   2. African American population   2%-4%
   3. Ankylosing spondylitis   90%
   4. Reiter's syndrome and reactive arthritis   80%
   5. Psoriatic arthritis w/spondylitis   65%
   6. Ankylosing spondylitis associated with inflammatory bowel disease   50%
B. **Sacroiliitis**
C. **Heel involvement**
   1. Achilles tendonitis
   2. Plantar fasciitis
   3. Achilles tendon and plantar aspect calcaneal erosions and periostitis Dactylitis (sausage digit with involvement of the MITP, PIP, and DIP joints often with associated periostitis)

II. Clinical manifestations

A. **Spinal pain**
   1. Daily chronic pain
   2. Morning stiffness with nocturnal pain. Pain improves with motion and exercise. The persistent daily pain with morning stiffness and nocturnal pain is distinctive from episodic mechanical back pain of lumbar disc disease and lumbar spondylosis
   3. Limitation of lumbar spine motion
   4. Marked limitation of chest expansion (less than 2.5 cm)
   5. Radiographic sacroiliitis necessary for definitive diagnosis; ankylosing spondylitis can be clinically defined as symptomatic sacroiliitis

B. **Skeletal complications:**
   1. Tarsal tunnel syndrome
   2. Arachnoiditis
   3. Cl-C2 subluxation
   4. Spinal fracture, either overt or occult, with eventual diskitis, which are actually spinal pseudoarthroses
   5. Carpal tunnel syndrome

C. **Extraskeletal complications**
   1. Acute anterior uveitis
      a. Incidence is 20%-30%
      b. Must be recognized and treated promptly to avoid anterior chamber scarring and glaucoma
   2. Ascending aortic aneurysm and aortic insufficiency
   3. Cavitary upper lobe pulmonary lesions (very rare)
   4. IgA nephropathy (rare)

D. **Differential Diagnosis**
   1. Sacroiliitis must be differentiated from osteitis condenthans ileum, which is a non erosive sclerotic lesion limited to the iliac side of the SI joint
   2. Syndesmophytes must be differentiated from osteophytes and from the flowing spinal calcification of dissemination (idiopathic skeletal hyperostosis)

III. Radiographic features

A. **Sacroiliitis** (subchondral erosion, subchondral sclerosis, and eventual effusion)

B. **Vertebral squaring**

C. **Syndesmophyte formation** (syndesmophytes are thin, vertically based growth of new bone along the annulus fibrosis that bridge the vertebral body and give the "bamboo spine appearance"; vertically oriented syndesmophytes differ from thick, pointed, laterally directed osteophytes)

D. **Apophyseal joint fusion**

E. **Achilles tendon and plantar calcaneal erosions and periostitis**

F. **Concentric glenohumeral and hip joint space narrowing**

IV. **Management**

    A. **Indomethacin and other NSAIDs**

    B. **Sulfasalazine**

    C. **Methotrexate**

    D. **Physical therapy and postural exercise**

    E. **Avoidance of corticosteroids**

    F. **Avoidance of bedrest**

REITER'S SYNDROME AND REACTIVE ARTHRITIS

I. **Epidemiology:** A post infectious reactive disorder after genitourinary tract infections with chlamydia and after gastrointestinal infections with Shigella, Salmonella, and Yersinia organisms

II. **Manifestations:** Classical Reiter's syndrome is the tetrad of a characteristic lower extremity, large joint polyarthritis; characteristic mucocutaneous lesions; and urethritis and conjunctivitis

    A. **Musculoskeletal features**
        1. Large joint, lower extremity predominant polyarthritis
        2. Achilles tendonitis
        3. Plantar fasciitis
        4. Sacroiliitis
        5. Dactylitis (sausage-like distal swelling)

    B. **Mucocutaneous features**
        1. Onycholysis
        2. Keratoderma blennorrhagica (hyperkeratotic pustules of psoriatic-like lesions on the soles of the feet)
        3. Circinate balanitis (shallow ulcer or psoriatic lesions on the glans penis)
        4. Shallow painless oral ulcerations

    C. **Radiographic features**
        1. Heel erosions and/or periostitis
        2. Digital periostitis
        3. Sacroiliitis

    D. **Laboratory features**
        1. Elevated sedimentation rate
        2. Leukocytosis
        3. Normal synovial fluid glucose and normal or elevated synovial fluid complement

III. **Treatment**

A. **Tetracyclines may be effective for some patients with post Chlamydia Reiter's syndrome**
B. **NSAIDs**
C. **Intra-articular steroids**
D. **Sulfasalazine**

IV. **Prognosis:** Can be a single-episode illness, a polycyclic illness, or a severe chronic destructive disease

PSORIATIC ARTHRITIS

I. **Incidence:** Five percent of patients with psoriasis

II. **Manifestations:**
   A. **Several patterns of joint distribution**
      1. Asymmetric oligoarticular arthritis
      2. Predominant distal interphalangeal joint disease
      3. Polyarticular: Usually very asymmetric
      4. **Clinical Pearl: Inflammatory arthritis involving three joints of a single digit; more commonly represents psoriatic arthritis than any other disorder, although similar dactylitis can be seen in Reiter's syndrome**
      5. Sacroiliitis and spondylitis
      6. Arthritis mutilans: Digital osteolysis with telescoping digits
   B. **Skin disease**
      1. Psoriasis precedes the arthritis in 4 of 5 patients
      2. Skin disease need not be extensive
      3. Nail changes (often but not necessarily associated with contiguous DIP joint inflammation)
         a. Hyperkeratosis
         b. Onycholysis
         c. Nail ridging
         d. Nail pitting

III. **Radiographic findings**
   A. **Pencil-in-cup deformity** (distal osteolysis) **with widening of the articulating proximal bone**
   B. **Periostitis**
   C. **Lack of peri-articular osteoporosis**
   D. **Sclerosed erosions**
   E. **Spondylitis similar to ankylosing spondylitis but with larger, more asymmetrical syndesmophytes**

IV. **Treatment**
   A. **NSAIDs**
   B. **Intra-articular injection**
   C. **Sulfasalazine, hydroxychloroquine, methotrexate, gold, and PUVA**

ENTEROPATHIC ARTHRITIS

I. **Diagnosis**

    A. **Considered in presence of inflammatory joint disease and gastrointestinal symptoms;** there are many inflammatory rheumatic diseases that may have gastrointestinal manifestations but that are not classified as enteropathic arthritides

    B. **Diagnosis of enteropathic arthritis is made when there is a direct causative relationship between the intestines and the joints;** these include arthritis associated with inflammatory bowel disease, ulcerative colitis and Crohn's disease, reactive arthritis triggered by bacteria, undifferentiated spondyloarthropathies, and Whipple's disease

II. **Manifestations**

    A. **Extra-articular manifestations:** Diarrhea, intestinal blood loss, abdominal pain, weight loss, fever, erythema nodosum, pyoderma gangrenosum, and thrombophlebitis

    B. **Articular manifestations:** Two patterns
        1. Twenty percent of patients have joint manifestations (pauciarticular, asymmetric transient, and migratory); large and small joints of the lower extremities are usually involved and nondestructive; usually subsides within 2 months
        2. Ankylosing spondylitis often with achilles tendonitis, heel spur syndrome, plantar fasciitis, sausage fingers and toes, and occasional periostitis

III. **Therapy**

    A. **Intra-articular corticosteroid injections may be beneficial**

    B. **Sulfasalazine in conjunction with corticosteroids may be employed**

IV. **Undifferentiated spondyloarthropathies:** Same as above

V. **Reactive arthritis post infectious enteritis:** Refers to sterile synovitis with evidence of antecedent infection; characterized by asymmetric oligoarthritis in the knees, ankles, and MPJs may have mucocutaneous features of Reiter's syndrome

    A. **Treatment**
        1. Indomethacin
        2. Sulfasalazine when NSAIDs response is inadequate
        3. Tetracycline may shorten the course of post Chlamydia-reactive arthritis

OSTEOARTHRITIS

I. **Pathogenesis**

    A. **Loss of proteoglycans and decrease in proteoglycan aggregation**

    B. **Damage to restraining collagen fibers**

    C. **Increased water content**

    D. **Increased proteoglycans synthesis by chondrocytes**

    E. **Impact-loading stress can initiate or accelerate the process**
        1. Probable increased incidence of osteoarthritis of the knees in competitive runners

2. Increased incidence of osteoarthritis of the shoulders and the elbows in baseball pitchers

II. Pathology

A. **Longitudinal tears in the superficial cartilage layers parallel to the superficial collagen fibers**

B. **Deeper vertical tears**

C. **Eventual irregular loss of the cartilage surface, with ulcerative lesions in the cartilage**

D. **New bone formation**
1. Eburnation (production of ivory like, polished, dense bone)
2. Osteophyte formation

E. **Subchondral pseudocyst formation**

III. Signs and symptoms

A. **Pain on weight bearing or motion of the affected joint, pain is least severe in the mornings and worsens with activity**

B. **Nocturnal pain unusual except in end-stage disease**

C. **Hallmark physical signs:** Crepitus and bone enlargement

D. **Joint effusion**

E. **Joint instability**

F. **Osteophytes** ("spurs" produce symptoms only when there is neural impingement or an associated bursitis or tendonitis)

IV. Radiographic findings

A. **Irregular joint space narrowing**

B. **Subchondral sclerosis**

C. **Subchondral pseudocyst formation**

D. **Osteophyte formation**

V. Laboratory findings

A. **Synovial fluid with high viscosity**

B. **Few white blood cells, normal glucose, and good mucin clotting**

VI. Differential diagnosis: Unusual patterns of osteoarthritis seen in hemochromatosis, Wilson disease, ochronosis, and chondrocalcinosis

VII. Treatment

A. **For most patients, analgesics are as effective as anti-inflammatory drugs and are far safer**

B. **Occasionally patients respond with the intermittent use of NSAIDs**

C. **No drugs positively modify the course of osteoarthritis, and there is concern that anti-inflammatory drugs may have a negative effect on cartilage**

D. **Joint injections** (corticosteroids)

E. **Physiotherapy**

F. **Joint replacement surgery**

NEUROPATHIC ARTHROPATHY

I.   **Overview:** A severe destructive arthropathy resulting from impaired joint position sensation

II. **Pathogenesis**
    A. Definition
        1. Joint damage secondary to repetitive trauma of an insensitive joint
        2. Alterations in sympathetic nerve system, leading to increased blood flow, which causes active hyperemia and bone absorption
    B. Clinical manifestations
        1. Swelling, warmth, dry feet, bounding pulses, edema
        2. Pain may or may not be present
        3. Spontaneous fractures, dislocation, and infection are common complications
        4. Can lead to progressive joint destruction
    C. Radiographic findings
        1. Extensive bone resorbtion without evidence of bone repair and sharp transitional zone between resorbed bone and remaining bone with bone around resorbed area normally mineralized
        2. Early changes may mimic osteoarthritis
        3. Other changes include large osteophytes, bony fragments, bony dislocation and/or subluxation, and "bag of bones" appearance
    D. Associated conditions
        1. Diabetes
        2. Tabes Dorsalis
        3. Syringomyelia
        4. Spinal cord injury
        5. Peripheral nerve damage
        6. Leprosy
        7. Amyloidosis
        8. Multiple sclerosis
        9. Tumor
       10. Charcot-Marie-Tooth disease
       11. Riley-Day syndrome

III. **Arthrocentesis**
    A. Definition: Non-inflammatory fluids and hemorrhagic effusions frequently described; severe cases can mimic septic joint
    B. Management
        1. Attack the etiology
        2. Use casting orthotics and/or prosthetics
        3. Immobilize and elevate part, cast, implement surgical revision, and replace joint

OSTEOCHONDRITIS

I.   **True osteonecrosis**

    A. **Legg-Calvé-Perthes disease**

    B. **Freiberg's disease**

II. **Non-necrotic abnormalities**

    A. **Osgood-Schlatter's disease**

    B. **Blount's disease**

    C. **Severs' disease**

    D. **Köhler's disease** (may be true osteonecrosis on occasion)

    E. **Treves' disease**

    F. **Diaz's disease**

    G. **Islins' disease**

    H. **Osteochondritis dissecans**

III. **Osteonecrosis as a marker for disease**

    A. **Cortico-steroid therapy**

    B. **Alcohol abuse**

    C. **SLE**

    D. **Gaucher's disease**

    E. **Decompression related illness**

SEPTIC ARTHRITIS

I. **Presentation**

    A. **Children**

       1. Sources of infection:

          a. Direct inocculation

          b. Hematogenous spread: Otitis media; mouth and nose catheters; central lines; femoral venous punctures

          c. Spread from adjacent osteomyelitis

       2. Gram stain and blood cultures are positive in 30% of cases

       3. Type of organism is age dependent

       4. Antibiotics

          a. Selection adjusted when culture results are available

          b. IV antibiotics

          c. Repeated needle drainage of the synovial pus. If ineffective or organism relatively resistant

          d. Residual abnormality seen in approximately 15%-25% of the cases (staph, gram negative bacilli) open debridement and drainage is indicated

    B. **Elderly**

       1. Seventy-five percent have had history of prior arthritis such as RA or prosthetic joints; majority have pre-existing diseases, such as diabetes, malignancy, renal failure, SLE, COPD, ETOH, IV drug abuse

       2. An extra-articular source of infection is evident in 75% of cases; permanent joint damage tends to be substantial

    C. **Sexually active adults:** Gonococcal arthritis

II. Pathogenesis

A. Organisms
1. Childhood: Beta strep, Strep Pneumonia, Staphylococus
2. Health Adults: Gonococcus, Staph, Strep
3. Immunocompromised Adults: Gram negative bacilli in addition to the above

B. Diagnostic approach
1. Synovial fluid analysis is the most important test in acute septic arthritis. Aspiration must be performed as an emergency procedure
2. Positive gram stain and positive synovial culture are fundamental for diagnosis
3. The white blood cell count is usually greater than 55,000 and can be greater than 100,000
4. Neutrophils are usually greater than 85%-90%
5. Synovial glucose is often less than 25% of serum glucose; increased synovial levels of lactic acid can be seen
6. After 2 weeks, destructive changes of the joint space, including narrowing, erosions, or foci of subchondral osteomyelitis, become evident
7. Rarely gas formation is seen in cases of E. coli and anaerobes

C. Therapeutic approach
1. Empiric antibiotics directed at the age, history, extra-articular foci, and synovial fluid gram stain findings; this is modified once the causative organism is identified and its sensitivities known
2. IV administration of antibiotics for several weeks, followed by oral administration
3. Synovial fluid should be aspirated frequently to drain intra-articular pus
4. For relatively resistant organisms or if the joint cannot be fully aspirated, surgical arthrotomy may be necessary

D. Outcome is dependent on time it takes to make the diagnosis and get clinical response

LYME DISEASE

I. **Overview:** A complex, multi-system, tick-borne (deer tick) illness caused by *Borrelia* Bargdorferia occurring in stages with remissions and exacerbations

II. Clinical findings and manifestations

A. Skin: Erythema migrans
1. A red macule or papule that expands slowly to form a large annular lesion with bright red outer border and central clearing
2. Appear 1-2 weeks after disease transmission
3. May have central necrosis
4. Additional signs include neck stiffness, fever, chills, myalgias, fatigue, and arthralgias
5. Occur in 80-90% of all cases

B. Neurologic
1. Meningitis, Lyme encephalopathy, and cranial neuritis, including bilateral Bell's palsy and sensory neuropathy, and mononeuritis multiplex
2. Lesions with severe and encephalopathy may resemble those of Alzheimer disease
3. Possible lymphocytic meningradiaelitis (Bannwarth's Syndrome)

C. Cardiac involvement

    1. First-degree block very common
    2. Some patients have diffuse cardiac involvement, including electrocardiogram changes consistent with acute myopericarditis

D. Arthritis

    1. Early symptoms include migratory joint pains, tendonitis, and bursitis
    2. Several months later, approximately half of untreated patients develop arthritis
    3. Typical patterns:
       a. Short attacks involving one or two joints, usually the knees and ankles
       b. Resistant monoarticular or oligoarticular synovitis

III. Laboratory findings

A. The best way of making a diagnosis is by finding the positive antibody test determined by ELISA and confirmed by Western Blot

B. The organism may also be detected in synovial fluid

IV. Radiographic findings: Cartilage loss can occur

V. Treatment

A. Early Lyme disease: Doxycycline 100 b.i.d., which should not be administered to children or pregnant women. Amoxicillin is an alternative drug

B. Late Lyme disease: Ceftriaxone 1 gm IV b.i.d.

C. Patients with infection localized to the skin, 10 days seems to be sufficient, but 14-28 days is not unreasonable

D. In patient with disseminated disease, 20-30 days is necessary

E. Patients with neurologic pathology need Ceftriaxone 2 gm per day for 30 days

F. Patients with arthritis: Doxycycline 100 mg. b.i.d. for 30 days is usually successful, but response is usually slow

VI. Prevention

A. Avoid tick-infested areas

B. Wear protective clothing

C. Apply insect repellents (DEET or Permethrin)

SARCOIDOSIS

I. Rheumatic manifestations:

A. Ten to fifteen percent of cases

B. Lofgren's syndrome - Associated with acute arthritis, erythema nodosum, and bilateral hilar adenopathy

C. Other

    1. Late arthritic changes associated with chronic cutaneous sarcoidosis and not with erythema nodosum
    2. Radiographs include cystic lytic lesions in the middle of the phalanges; honey-comb appearance in trabecular patterns

3. Other manifestations: Pulmonary disease, cutaneous lesions, Bell's palsy changes similar to Sjogren's syndrome

II. Diagnosis: Based on clinical picture and histologic evidence of noncaseating granulomas

III. Treatment: NSAIDs; corticosteroids and methotrexate are utilized in severe cases

RHEUMATIC FEVER

I. **Clinical aspects**
    A. **An acute condition following Beta-hemolytic Streptococcus infections involving the joints, skin, heart, central nervous system, and subcutaneous tissue**
    B. **Most important manifestations:** polyarthritis, carditis, chorea, erythema marginatum and subcutaneous nodules

II. **Clinical manifestations**
    A. **Acute migratory polyarthritis in the knees, the ankles, the elbows, and the shoulders**
    B. **Subcutaneous nodules, erythema marginatum, Sydenham's chorea, and heart pathology**

III. **Laboratory findings:** ASO titers are positive in 80%-85% of patients, especially if changes between the acute and the convalescent times are reviewed

IV. **Treatment**
    A. **For people with arthritis, salicylates and other NSAIDs for 3-4 weeks;** if abandoned too soon, symptoms may recur
    B. **Eradication and prevention of streptococcal infection**

GOUT

I. **Epidemiology**
    A. **Overall prevalence:** 2-2.6:1,000 population base; some cases are familial; 95% of patients are men; and it occurs only infrequently before the age of 20 in men and 50 in women
    B. **Classification of hyperuricemia**
        1. Ninety-five percent of hyperuricemia patients never develop gout and generally require no treatment
        2. Due to a decrease in renal excretion of uric acid and/or an excessive rate of uric acid production
        3. Overproduction occurs (10% of gout patients) as a result of increased rate of purine synthesis denovo or increased turnover of nucleic acids; the latter is seen in such disorders as myeloproliferative and lymphoproliferative disorders, multiple myeloma, certain hemoglobinopathies, hemolytic anemias, and certain carcinomas
        4. The largest proportion of patients with gout have underexcretion of uric acid in the urine; diuretic therapy causes enhanced tubular reabsorption of uric add and decreased uric acid

filtration, which increases serum levels; other agents that decrease renal excretion include low-dose aspirin and alcohol

5. Measurement of 24-hour urine uric acid levels differentiate over producers from under excretors

C. Pathogenesis of gouty inflammation

1. Hyperuricemia leads to the deposition of monosodiumurate crystals in cartilage and synovium in association with proteoglycans; there are periodic episodes of inflammation secondary to crystals in the synovial fluid

2. The crystals are phagocytosized by leukocytes and activate the complement and kallikrein system with the disruption of lysosomes within the leukocytes that lead to the destruction of the white blood cells and release of the proteolytic enzymes into the synovial fluid

D. Acute gouty arthritis

1. Most common manifestation: Acute monoarticular arthritis

2. Exquisite pain, tenderness, erythema, and swelling of the affected joint, most commonly the first MTP joint (podagra); other commonly involved joints include the ankles, the midtarsal joints, the knees, and less frequently, joints in the distal upper extremities

3. Even slight pressure on involved joints causes exquisite pain

4. Frequently patients have low-grade fevers and may present with a fever of an unknown origin

5. Frequently precipitated by dehydration, dietary excess, surgery, serious medical illness or trauma

E. Chronic tophaceous gout

1. Large accumulations of monosodium urate crystals at various locations, including the olecranon bursas and the elbows, the Achilles tendons, the first CMPJs, the PIP and DIP joints of the hands and feet, and the helix or antihelix of the ears, causes marked structure changes in the involved joints and crippling

2. Chronic tophii can lead to draining sinuses and secondary infection

II. Complications

A. Urate nephrolithiasis (resulting from increased excretion of uric acid, especially over 1,100 mg per day)

B. Urate nephropathy results from the deposition of MSU crystals in the kidneys or from obstructive uropathy

III. Radiographic findings

A. Acute attack demonstrates soft-tissue swelling

B. Chronic disease is characterized by sharp, marginated erosions with overhanging edges; the erosions are usually round or oval, with a sclerotic border and punched-out appearance

IV. Laboratory findings

A. Normal serum uric acid levels occur in many patients with acute gout, but low normal values occur only rarely

B. A definitive diagnosis of gout can only be made where needle-shaped MSU crystals, which are negatively birefringent are demonstrated with compensated polarized light microscopy-, the crystals can be seen in the synovial fluid, both in the acute attack and intercritical periods between gouty attacks

V. Treatments

A. Acute

1. In the medical community, peripheral nerve blocks are rarely used, except in patients resistant to all other modalities; however, it is very effective and commonly utilized in the podiatric community

2. NSAIDs: Indomethacin is most commonly used, generally 150-200 mg in divided doses with food for the first 3-5 days; almost all NSAIDs with rapid onset of action can be used to treat acute gout, if maximal doses are used

3. Steroids: Patients with polyarticular gout with or without tophi may require a brief course of prednisone

4. Colchicine use for acute gout has fallen out of favor because of suboptimal efficacy, the common occurence of diarrhea with oral use and the fear of leukopenia with IV administration

5. Allopurinol or probenicide have no role in controlling gout inflammation

B. Prophylactic treatment

1. Urate-lowering drugs
   a. Probenicid in slowly increasing doses is used primarily in patients who are under excretors < 1200 mg/24 hrs of uric acid
   b. If patients are over producers, or have a history of urate renal stones, allopurinol should be used starting at 200-300 mg daily. Allopurinol has potentially fatal toxicity and should be used properly
   c. The goal must be to lower serum uric to a level at which attacks cease to occur and tophii resorb. This usually requires level at < 6.5

2. Colchicine 0.6 mg BID can be used temporarily in patient with frequent attacks until the disease is controlled with probenicid or allopurinol

CALCIUM PYROPHOSPHATE CRYSTAL DEPOSITION DISEASE

I. Classification

A. Hereditary
B. Associated with metabolic diseases
C. Idiopathic

II. Pathogenesis

A. Occurs in association with hyperparathyroidism, hemochromatosis, hypomagnesemia, hypophosphatasia, hypothyroidism, Wilson disease, and gout

B. Crystals of calcium pyrophosphate are found in cartilage and are shed into the synovial fluid; this may occur after trauma or after degradation of the cartilage by proteolytic enzymes

C. Acute arthritis occurs where the crystals are phagocytosed by leukocytes and release lysosomal enzymes. This mimics acute gout, hence "pseudogout"

D. The synovium is infiltrated by polys, and a chronic synovitis can occur

III. Clinical features

A. Pseudogout (25% of patients)

B. **Pseudorheumatoid disease** (polyarthritis with recurrent attacks)

C. **Chondrocalcinosis characterized by progressive degenerative changes in the involved joints, frequently with intermittent attacks of pseudogout**

IV. **Radiographic features**

  A. **Abnormal calcifications seen in articular hyaline cartilage or in fibrocartilage**

  B. **Calcifications most commonly occur in the wrist, the knee, the elbow, and the hip**

  C. **Calcification parallels the subchondral bony plates and may also be calcification of the menisci of the knee, the triangular ligaments of the wrists, or the labra of the glenoid or symphysis pubis**

  D. **There may also be amorphous calcifications in the synovium or the bursas**

  E. **There is joint space narrowing, bony sclerosis, and subchondral cysts**

V. **Laboratory findings**

  A. **Crystals should be identified in fresh synovial fluid samples; they are usually rhomboidal weakly birefringent, usually intracellular, and can be difficult to see**

  B. **Synovial fluid and white blood cell counts are generally less than 50,000**

  C. **Serum calcium, phosphorus, alkaline phosphatase, iron, and magnesium levels should be obtained to exclude hypoparathyroidism, hemochromatosis, hypomagnesemia, and hypophosphatasia**

  D. **Tests for hypothyroidism, diabetes, and gout should also be obtained**

VI. **Arthrocentesis: Gold standard for diagnosis**

VII. **Treatment**

  A. **A short course of high dose corticosteroids can effectively treat pseudogout**

  B. **NSAIDs in high doses**

  C. **IV or oral colchicine is also somewhat effective but rarely necessary**

  D. **Acutely inflamed joints may be injected with corticosteroids**

STORAGE AND DEPOSITION DISEASES

I. **Hemochromatosis**

  A. **Rheumatic manifestations**

    1. A common hereditary disorder characterized by excessive body iron stores and hemosiderin deposits causing tissue damage and organ dysfunction

    2. Characterized by chronic arthritis of the peripheral joints, mostly of the upper extremities and spine; there is a higher association with chondrocalcinosis and pseudogout

    3. Joint symptoms: controlled by NSAIDs

    4. Agents requiring liver metabolism should be avoided

    5. Phlebotomies are utilized frequently to decrease iron stores and prevent liver and cardiac damage

II. **Alcaptonuria**

A. **A rare, inherited disorder from a deficiency of homogentisic acid oxidase**

B. **There are pigmented areas in the cartilage, skin, and sclera.** This darkening is referred to as ochronosis

C. **Causes severe spondylosis with disc calcification, and osteoarthritis often with chondrocalcinosis**

D. **Diagnosis is suspected when patient has history of passing dark urine or when fresh urine turns black on standing**

E. **Synovial aspiration reveals debris resembling ground pepper**

III. **Wilson disease**

A. **Abnormal deposition of copper, leading to central nervous system, hepatic, and renal dysfunction**

B. **Copper accumulation leads to Kayser-Fleischer rings in the eyes and basal ganglia, resulting in lenticular damage and movement disorders;** kidney deposition results in tubular damage

C. **Arthropathy is characterized by premature osteoarthritis of the knees, the wrists, and the spine**

D. **Of patients with Wilson disease, 50% develop osteoporosis**

E. **Treatment:** Copper chelation with penicillamine and dietary copper restriction

IV. **Gaucher disease**

A. **Lysosomal, glycolipid storage disease with accumulations of glucose cerebroside in the reticular endothelial cells of the spleen, the liver, and the bone marrow**

B. **Rheumatic manifestations:** Spontaneous fracture, aseptic necrosis of the hip and the proximal tibia

C. **Treatment:** Enzyme replacement

HEMATOLOGIC ARTHROPATHIES

I. **Hemophilic arthropathy**

A. **Rheumatic manifestations:** Recurrent and chronic hemarthrosis with cartilage breakdown secondary to hemosiderin deposits

B. **Treatment for the acute bleeding replacement of Factor VIII**

II. **Sickle cell disease**

A. **Diffuse swelling and tenderness of the fingers and toes, hand/foot syndrome:** Occurs in approximately one third of patients

B. **Radiographic signs:** Widening of the medullary cavities, thinning of the cortices, abnormal trabeculae, and sclerosis of the phalanges

III. **Multiple myeloma**

A. **Signs and symptoms:** Two thirds of patients with multiple myeloma present with bone pain

B. **Radiographic findings:** well-circumscribed lytic lesions or moth-eaten appearance of the vertebrae, ribs, sternum, skull, pelvis, and proximal long bones

C. **Laboratory findings:** Monoclonal immunoglobulin on serum or urine immunoelectrophoresis

IV. Leukemia: Can present with joint pain and swelling, especially in children. Ten to fifteen percent of patients develop Leukemic infiltrate in the synovium and bone

V. Lymphoma: Primary lymphoma of bone constitutes 10% of all extranodal lymphomas joint infiltrations are occasionally reported

OSTEOPOROSIS

I. Definition: Low bone mass and micro architectural changes in bone, resulting in increased bone fragility and increased incidence of fracture

II. Epidemiology
   A. **> 50-year-old women:** 40% will eventually have an osteoporotic fracture
   B. **> 50-year-old women:** 17% will eventually have a hip fracture
   C. **Osteoporotic fractures in 1994 cost 10 billion dollars**
   D. **Causes of osteoporosis**
      1. Hereditary
      2. Sex-hormone deficiency
         a. Menopause
         b. Prolonged premenopausal estrogen deficiency (i.e., anorexia nervosa)
         c. Male hypogonadism
      3. Low calcium intake
      4. Corticosteroid treatment

III. Diagnosis
   A. **Vertebral compression, hip, wrist and proximal humeral fractures are the classical osteoporotic fractures, all fractures are increased in incidence in patients with low bone density;** the presence of any fracture in a mature adult in the absence of serious trauma should lead to a suspicion that osteoporosis is present
   B. **X-ray:** Thirty percent of bone must be lost in order for osteoporosis to be detected by X-ray; detection of osteoporosis is also a highly subjective diagnosis, with inaccuracies produced by many variables inherent in X-ray technique
   C. **Bone-density measurement:** The cornerstone of diagnosis of osteoporosis; dual X-ray of soft geometry (DEXA) is the prevailing and preferred technique
   D. **Treatment**
      1. Establish normal calcium intake of 1,500 mg/day taken in divided doses with food
      2. Insure intake of vitamin D of at least 400 RJ/day
      3. Medications that slow bone loss (anti-result of ages):
         a. Estrogens
         b. Calcitonin
         c. Bisphosphenates

FIBROMYALGIA

I. **Clinical manifestations**
    A. **Diffuse pain generally in all four body quadrants in women much more frequently than in men**
    B. **Associated symptoms frequently include insomnia, non refreshing sleep, and fatigue;** many of the classic 18 tender points (at specific locations); spastic colon, chronic headaches, chest pain, mitral valve prolapse, and depression

II. **Differential diagnosis:**
    A. **Diffuse disabling symptoms may be confused with rheumatoid arthritis, which also may be seen secondary to other rheumatic disease, such as lupus, rheumatoid arthritis, Sjögren's syndrome, Lyme disease**
    B. **Malingering should also be ruled out, but this is sometimes difficult**

III. **Treatment**
    A. **Low-dose tricyclate antidepressants at nighttime** (e.g., Cyclobenzaprine, or other SSRI antidepressants)
    B. **NSAIDs may have synergistic effects**
    C. **Low-impact aerobic exercises are frequently effective**
    D. **Biofeedback may be useful as well as support groups**

BIBLIOGRAPHY

Bennett C, Plum F. (ed.) Cecil textbook of medicine/Textbook of medicine. Saunders, Philadelphia, 1996.
Harrison RJ. Textbook of medicine: with relevant physiology and anatomy. Wiley, New York, 1977.
Kelley WN, et al. Textbook of rheumatology/Rheumatology. W.B. Saunders, Philadelphia, 1997.
McCarty DJ. Arthritis and allied conditions: a textbook of rheumatology. Lea & Febiger, Philadelphia, 1993.
Schumacher HR Jr. et al. Primer on the rheumatic diseases. Arthritis Foundation, Atlanta, GA, 1988.

CHAPTER 13
RHEUMATOLOGY

1.   Which of the following is normally a true osteonecrosis (a septic necrosis):

        A.   Kohler's disease
        B.   Blount's disease
        C.   Treves disease
        D.   Osgood Schlatter's disease
        E.   Frieberg's disease

2.   Which of the following is most commonly associated with true osteonecroses?

        A.   Systemic lupus erythematosis
        B.   Brown tumors
        C.   Acromegaly
        D.   Marfan's disease
        E.   Osteoporosis

3.   What is the most appropriate drug to treat Lyme arthritis?

        A.   Cefadyl – IV
        B.   Doxycycline – PO
        C.   Roecephin – IV
        D.   Biaxin – PO
        E.   Cipro – PO

4.   A patient presents with pain in the digits. X-ray findings are consistent with sarcoidosis. What is the best
        test result to confirm your findings?

        A.   + Chest x-ray
        B.   - Kviem test
        C.   + VDRL with + Rheumatoid Factor
        D.   + ANA, - RPR, Increase in IgG
        E.   + Tzank smear, + ANA, Leukopenia

5.   Erythema marginatum is most commonly seen in:

        A.   Steven-Johnson syndrome
        B.   Rheumatic fever
        C.   Pediatric dermatomyositis
        D.   Penicillin allergy

6.   Which of the following has the highest incidence of (causing) secondary gouty arthritis?

        A.   Non-Hodgkin Lymphoma
        B.   Lesch-Nyhan disease
        C.   Diabetes
        D.   Marfan's disease
        E.   Pseudo-pseudo hypoparathyroidism

7.   Which of the following storage diseases causing ankle arthritis will best respond to chelation therapy?

      A.   Fabry's disease
      B.   Gaucher's disease
      C.   von Gierke's disease
      D.   Wilson's disease
      E.   Acute Weber's syndrome

8.   Which of the following endocrine disorders will result in brachymetatarsia?

      A.   Hyperparathyroidism
      B.   Pseudopseudohypoparathyroidism
      C.   Hypoparathyroidism
      D.   Thyroid acrapachy
      E.   Hashimoto's thyroiditis

9.   Of the following, what is the best drug utilized for the management of fibromyalgia?

      A.   Elavil
      B.   Darvon
      C.   Haldol
      D.   Percocet
      E.   Tylenol #3 with Codeine

10.   Which of the following describes a potentially fatal complication of rheumatoid arthritis?

      A.   Rheumatoid lung
      B.   Rheumatoid liver
      C.   Felty's syndrome
      D.   Baker's cyst
      E.   Disseminated rheumatoid nodules

11.   Which of the following diseases will show the most profound decrease in sedimentation rate with 5mg of
      Prednisone?

      A.   Dermatomyositis
      B.   Juvenile rheumatoid arthritis
      C.   Polymyalgia rheumatica
      D.   Juvenile lupus
      E.   Rheumatic fever

12.   Which of the following is most associated with Sjogren's syndrome in a 30-year-old black male presenting
      with joint stiffness in MPJs 2-5 bilaterally?

      A.   HIV
      B.   Male breast cancer
      C.   Acute tropical spastic paraparesis
      D.   Hepatitis B
      E.   Cytomegalovirus

13.   Which of the following is most associated with Reynaud's phenomenon?

    A.   Systemic lupus erythematosis
    B.   Rheumatoid arthritis
    C.   Polyarteritis nodosa
    D.   Progressive systemic sclerosis
    E.   Giant cell arteritis

14.   Which of the following will most likely cause effusion of both the DJPJs and PIPJs at the same time?

    A.   Psoriatic arthritis
    B.   Reactive arthritis
    C.   Reiters' syndrome
    D.   Juvenile ankylosing spondylitis
    E.   Ulcerative colitis

15.   Paralysis of the lower extremities will most likely occur from cauda equina syndrome. This is a complication of which disease?

    A.   Reiters' syndrome
    B.   Ulcerative colitis
    C.   Psoriatic arthritis
    D.   Primary radiculopathy
    E.   Ankylosing spondylitis

16.   Which of the following findings in Reiter's syndrome occur least frequently?

    A.   Urethritis
    B.   Conjunctivitis
    C.   Ankle arthritis
    D.   Sacroiliitis
    E.   Fluffy periostitis

17.   Which disease has the highest incidence of association with HLA B-27?

    A.   Ankylosing spondylitis
    B.   Reiters' syndrome
    C.   Psoriatic arthritis
    D.   Reative arthritis
    E.   Crohn's disease

18.   Which joint is most associated with diabetic neuroarthropathy?

    A.   Choparts
    B.   Ankle
    C.   Knee
    D.   Lisfranc
    E.   Talo-calcaneal

19. Rheumatoid arthritis usually:

    A.   is bilateral, symmentrical and highly associated with HLA B-8
    B.   is bilateral and asymmetrical
    C.   is unilateral and asymmetrical
    D.   does not affect the sacroiliac joint
    E.   affects the hips in over 75 % of cases

Peripheral Vascular Disease

Jeffrey C. Page
Brad Newswander
Chad Thompson

ARTERIAL DISORDERS AFFECTING THE LOWER EXTREMITIES

I. **Anatomy of arteries and hemodynamics**

 A. **Anatomy of lower extremity arteries**

 B. **Arterial anatomy:** intima, media and adventitia

 C. **Artherosclerotic lesions**

 D. **Pathophysiology**

   1. Occlusive disease

   2. Aneurysmal disease

   3. Vasospastic disease

II. **Patient history**

 A. **Present complaints**

   1. Pain, numbness, coldness, tenderness, burning, fullness and pallor

   2. Questions to rule out: neuropathy, arthritis, anemia, trauma and musculoskeletal abnormalities

 B. **Intermittent claudication**

   1. Changes with fast versus slow walking

   2. Changes with walking up or down hills

   3. Distance walked before pain occurs

   4. Correlation with pain and location of occlusion

 C. **Rest pain**

 D. **Past vascular history**

   1. Risk factors for atherosclerosis

2. Conditions associated with embolic phenomena
3. Other relevant history, including presence of angina, impotence, syncope, intra-vascular clotting, ischemic ulcers and previous vascular surgery
4. History of previously diagnosed peripheral arterial occlusive disease, inflammatory or connective tissue disease, vasculitis, or vasospastic disease
5. Conditions in which blood flow is adequate but healing might be impaired, including anemia, alcohol use, connective tissue disease, polycythemia, poor nutrition, neuropathy, aged tissue, high dose prednisone use, anti-neoplastic drug use or hemodialysis

III. Physical exam
A. General
1. Heart rate and rhythm
2. Blood pressure
B. Inspection
1. Skin appearance
2. Temperature
3. Hair growth
4. Condition of nails
5. Color
6. Pallor on elevation, rubor with dependency
C. Palpation of pulses
1. Common femoral
2. Popliteal
3. Dorsalis pedis
4. Posterior tibial
5. Perforating peroneal
D. Clinical testing
1. Capillary refill time
2. Elevation-dependency test
3. Five minute reactive hyperemia test:
   a. Color return
   b. Intensity
   c. Time for maximum erythema return

IV. Noninvasive arterial testing
A. Doppler
1. Quality of arterial waveforms
   a. Femoral
   b. Popliteal
   c. Dorsalis pedis
   d. Posterior tibial
   e. Perforating peroneal
2. Segmental pressures, including ABI
   a. Vessels/segment pressure measured
      i. Posterior tibial
      ii. Dorsalis pedis
      iii. Perforating peroneal
      iv. Below knee

       v. Above knee

      vi. High thigh

    b. Interpretation of data

       i. Correlation of sound with ABI

      ii. Interpretation of ABI

      iii. Identification of falsely elevated ABI

      iv. Interpretation of meaning of segmental pressure difference

        (a) 20mmHg difference as pressure progresses distally and when compared to same level on contralateral limb

  3. Stress test

    a. One minute exercise test in a supine position with leg elevated (Carter's test) note changes in pressure of pedal arteries

    b. Five minute reactive hyperemia test, note change in digital artery sound

B. Photoplethysmography

  1. Waveforms of high thigh, above knee, below knee, ankle, mid-foot and toe

  2. Correlation with doppler and photophlethysmography

C. Volume plethysmography

D. Duplex scanning

E. Transcutaneous oximetry

F. Laser doppler

G. Interpretation of above tests to determine whether blood flow compatible with:

  1. Contemplated surgery

  2. Maintenance of tissue nutrition

  3. Healing of ulcer

V. Invasive arterial testing

A. Arteriography

B. Digital subtraction arteriography

C. Magnetic resonance imaging (MRA)

D. 3D CT re-construction

VI. Arterial diseases and/or syndrome

A. Chronic occlusive arterial disease (peripheral arterial occlusive disease)

  1. Risk factors

    a. With ASO

       i. Hyperlipidemia

      ii. Cholesterol

    b. Major risk factors

       i. Smoking

      ii. Diabetes

      iii. Hypertension

      iv. Family history

    c. Minor risk factors

       i. Hyperlipidemia

      ii. Obesity

      iii. Stress

      iv. Sedative life style

  2. Patterns of disease

     a. Aortoiliac disease (type 1)

     b. Combined aortoiliac and femoropopliteal disease (type 2)

     c. Isolated femoropopliteal disease (type 3) good femoral pulses

3. Arterial pathology

     a. Gradual stenosis

     b. Embolic phenomena

     c. Utilization of collateral vessels

4. Symptoms

     a. Intermittent claudication

     b. Rest (pre-trophic) pain

     c. Ulceration and gangrene

     d. Ischemic neuropathy

5. Physical findings

     a. Diminished pulses

     b. Bruits

     c. Color changes

     d. Temperature changes

     e. Trophic changes

6. Laboratory findings

     a. Doppler

     b. Photoplethysmography

     c. Volume plethysmography

     d. Trancutaneous oximetry

     e. Laser doppler

     f. Arteriography

     g. Oscillometer

7. Differential diagnosis

     a. Arterial embolism

     b. Mönckeberg's sclerosis

     c. Thromboangiitis obliterans (Buerger's disease)

     d. Vasculitis

     e. Infection overlying presence of peripheral arterial occlusive disease (PAOD)

8. Medical treatment

     a. Treatment

         i. Increase in physical activity

        ii. Control of risk factors

       iii. Increase care of skin

       iv. Precautions against bacterial infection, fungi, heat and cold

        v. Drug therapy:

          (a) Aspirin

          (b) NSAID's

          (c) Pentoxifylline

          (d) Cilostazol

          (e) Clopidogrel

          (f) Prostaglandins

          (g) Nitroglycerine ointment/patch

          (h) Therapeutic blocks

     b. Head of bed elevation dependency of affected limb

     c. Surgical intervention:

          i. Bypass
          ii. Stent
          iii. Angioplasty

B. Arterial embolism and acute arterial thrombosis
1. Etiology
   a. Atherosclerosis
   b. Atheromatous detachment
   c. Atrial fibrillation
   d. Myocardial infarction
   e. Cardiac valve pathology or prosthesis
   f. Aneurysm
   g. Endocarditis
   h. Trauma
2. Symptoms: Same as for PAOD, but with sudden onset
3. Signs: Same as for PAOD, but with sudden onset
4. Treatment
   a. Local care
   b. Anti-coagulants
      i. Heparin
      ii. Low molecular weight heparin
      iii. Warfarin
   c. Referral to PCP/Internist for work up to find source

C. Aneurysms
1. Etiology
   a. Atherosclerosis
   b. Syphilis
   c. Peri-arteritis
   d. Trauma
2. Location
   a. Abdominal aorta
   b. Iliac
   c. Popliteal
3. Diagnosis
   a. Palpation
   b. Auscultation
   c. Non-invasive testing
   d. Invasive testing
4. Treatment
   a. Vascular surgeon

D. Thromboangiitis obliterans (Buerger's disease)
1. Non atherosclerotic segmental inflammatory disease that most commonly affects the small and medium sized vessels of upper and lower extremities
2. Etiology unknown, associated with cigarette smoking
3. Clinical findings
   a. Rest pain
   b. Foot or arch claudication progressing to digital ulceration
4. Treatment
   a. Complete cessation of all tobacco use
   b. Local care

E. Vasculitis
  1. Systemic lupus erythematous
    a. Pathology: autoimmune disease that leads to deposits of damaging biologic substances in tissue
    b. Signs
        i. Livedo reticularis
        ii. Painful ulcerations
        iii. Recurrent arterial and venous thromboses
        iv. Digital gangrene
        v. Vasospasm
    c. Treatment
        i. Local
        ii. Heparin/Warfarin
        iii. Referral to other health care specialist
  2. Rheumatoid arthritis
    a. Vascular pathology
    b. Signs
        i. Ulceration
        ii. Vasospasm
        iii. Digital gangrene
    c. Laboratory findings consistent with RA
    d. Treatment
        i. Local
        ii. Referral to health care specialist for systemic care
  3. Erythema nodosum
    a. Signs
        i. Subcutaneous and cutaneous nodules, extremely painful
    b. Etiology
        i. Streptococcal infection
        ii. Ingestion of certain compounds
    c. Treatment
        i. Local
        ii. Referral to health care specialist
  4. Erythema induratum
    a. Signs
        i. Reddish, deep seated nodules most commonly in posterior aspects of skin and the subcutaneous tissue of calves and legs
    b. Almost always associated with active tuberculosis
    c. Treatment
        i. Local
        ii. Referral to health care specialist for systemic treatment
  5. Polyarteritis nodosa (necrotizing arteritis)
    a. Necrotizing vasculitis of small and medium sized muscular arteries
    b. Signs and symptoms
        i. Fever
        ii. Decline in overall health
        iii. Involvement of several organ systems
        iv. Ischemic ulcers of skin
    c. Treatment

     i. Local

     ii. Oral steroid use

     iii. Referral to other health care specialist

   6. Miscellaneous vasculitic disease that can have lower extremity manifestations

    a. Systemic giant cell arteritis (temporal arteritis)

    b. Idiopathic medial arthropathy (Takayasus' disease)

    c. Dermatomyositis

F. Vasoplastic conditions/disease

   1. Raynaud's phenomenon (primary)

    a. Episodic digital ischemia

     i. Patient experiences digital blanching, cyanosis followed by rubor

     ii. Phenomena occur after cold exposure and during subsequent re-warming

    b. Treatment aimed at alleviation of symptoms

   2. Raynaud's phenomenon (secondary)

    a. Progressive systemic sclerosis (scleroderma) and CREST

    b. Other disease/conditions associated with Raynaud's phenomenon

     i. Systemic lupus erythematosis

     ii. Dermatomyositis

     iii. Rheumatoid arthritis

     iv. Sjogren's syndrome

     v. Mixed connective tissue disease

     vi. Cryoglobulinemia

     vii. Complex regional pain syndrome

     viii. Ergot poisoning

     ix. Post traumatic disorders

    c. Diagnosis

     i. History and physical

     ii. Non-invasive tests

     iii. Invasive tests

    d. Treatment

     i. Local

     ii. Keeping warm

     iii. Medications

     iv. Referral to other health care specialist

   3. Acrocyanosis

    a. Characterized by coldness and bluish discoloration of fingers and hands for many years

    b. Arterial vasoconstrictions secondary to dilation of the capillaries and venules

    c. Benign condition

    d. Different from Raynaud's in that it is constant

   4. Livedo Reticularis

    a. Characterized by blotchy, mottled pattern

    b. Primary livedo

    c. Secondary livedo

     i. Associated with conditions related to secondary Raynaud's, infections, drug side effects and endocrine disorders

G. Temperature related

   1. Cold induced

    a. Chilblains

           i. Vasculitic disorder associated with exposure to cold
           ii. Acute and chronic
           iii. Raised erythematous lesions on extremities
           iv. Treatment
               (a) Avoid cold temperatures
      b. Trench foot (immersion foot)
           i. Prolonged exposure to subfreezing temperature
           ii. With re-warming:
               (a) Rapid swelling
               (b) Cyanosis
               (c) Ecchymosis
               (d) Vasodilatation
               (e) Nerve damage
               (f) Tissue necrosis
           iii. Treatment:
               (a) Debride nonviable tissue
               (b) Local wound care
      c. Frost bite
           i. Tissue damage due to cold temperature and vasodilatation
           ii. Re-warming of affected tissue
           iii. Local care
      d. Cryoglobulinemia
           i. Digital ulcerations
           ii. Associated with lymphoma and myeloma
  2. Erythermalgia, heat-related
      a. Burning, pain and erythema to the extremities
      b. Primary erythermalgia
           i. Genetic
           ii. Females more than males
      c. Secondary erythermalgia
           i. Myeloproliferative disorders
           ii. Hypertension
           iii. Venous insufficiency
           iv. Diabetes
           v. Systemic lupus erythematous
           vi. Rheumatoid arthritis
      d. Treatment
           i. Cooler temperatures
           ii. Elevation of affected extremity

H. Arteriovenous fistulae
  1. Traumatic and Congenital
      a. Characteristic
           i. Thrill
           ii. Bruit
           iii. Venous insufficiency
           iv. Gangrene
  2. Diagnosis
           i. Compression of large AV fistula may result in reflex slowing of heart rate
           ii. Arteriography

3. Treatment
   a. Surgery

I. Infection overlying pre-existing PVD
1. Treat infection
2. Local care

J. Popliteal artery entrapment (Popliteal entrapment syndrome)
1. Developing head of gastrocnemius, as it crosses from lateral to medial during development, traps popliteal artery and vein against medial condyle of femur
2. Diagnosis:
   a. H&P
   b. Physical
   c. Imaging modalities, CT, Ultrasound and angiographies
3. Treatment:
   a. Resection of muscle
   b. Reconstruction of occluded segment of artery

K. Blue toe syndrome
1. Etiology
   a. Peripheral arterial occlusive disease
   b. Emboli
   c. Thrombosis
   d. Infection with PVD
   e. Vasculitis
   f. Vasospastic disease
2. Treatment
   a. Local
   b. Treatment of cause

VII. Methods of treating peripheral vascular disease

A. Oral medications
1. Aspirin, NSAID's
2. Prostaglandins
3. Platel, Plavix, Trental
4. Heparin, low molecular weight heparin, warfarin
5. L-carnitine, L-arginine

B. Local anesthetic blocks

C. Use of nitroglycerine ointment/patch

D. Increase in exercise, appropriate patient selected needed

E. Head of bed elevation, dependency of affected limb

F. Heart assist device or circulator boot

G. Surgical treatment
1. Vascular surgeon
   a. Bypass
   b. Stent
   c. Angioplasty

H. Future
1. Gene therapy

VENOUS DISEASES AFFECTING THE LOWER EXTREMITIES

I. **Clinical assessment**

    A. **Anatomy of veins and hemodynamics**
    B. **Venous history**
        1. Relevant family history, including episodes of superficial and deep thrombophlebitis and primary varicosities
        2. Past history
            a. Repeated attacks of superficial or deep thrombophlebitis
            b. Spontaneous ulcers or bleeding ulcerations
            c. Spontaneous pitting or nonpitting edema of lower extremities
            d. Systemic conditions associated with venous manifestations in the lower limbs, including heart disease, pregnancy, and hypercoagulability
            e. Trauma, fractures, and bed rest
            f. Previous treatment, including venous stripping and injection therapy
        3. Habits and medication
            a. Tobacco use
            b. Use of birth control pill
            c. Anticoagulants
            d. Use of support hose
        4. Presenting complaints
            a. Fatigue and heaviness in the feet and legs
            b. Nocturnal cramps
            c. Responsiveness of unilateral swelling to sitting, standing, and lying down with the lower limbs elevated
            d. Presence of stasis dermatitis, ulceration, or edema
    C. **Physical examination**
        1. Inspection
            a. Varicosities, superficial thrombophlebitis, and dilated prominent veins that remain full on elevation of the limb
            b. Swelling (location, pitting, and nonpitting)
            c. Pigmentation, induration, brawniness, stasis dermatitis, or ulceration
        2. Palpation
            a. Determination of superficial thrombophlebitis
            b. Determination of presence of masses in the femoral triangle and muscles
            c. Determination of quality of the edema
        3. Clinical testing
            a. Tourniquet (Trendelenburg and Perthe's)
            b. Homan's
        4. Laboratory testing
            a. Doppler
            b. Photoplethysmography
            c. Volume plethysmography
            d. Duplex scanning
            e. Radioactive fibrinogen
            f. Contrast venography
            g. Radionucleotide venography
            h. Equilibrium RBC Phleboscintigraphy

      i. GD-Enhanced subtraction MR venography

II. Specific venous diseases

A. Varicose veins
1. Clinical presentation
2. Medical treatment
   a. Avoidance of prolonged sitting and standing, obesity, and constrictive garments
   b. Use of support hose
   c. Improvement of musculovenous pump through exercise or physical therapy
3. Sclerotherapy
4. Surgical treatment

B. Venous thromboembolism
1. Prevention of venous stasis by exercise and support
2. Prevention of hypercoagulability
3. Diagnosis
   a. Characteristics of superficial thrombophlebitis
   b. Characteristics of deep thrombophlebitis
   c. Pulmonary embolism
4. Treatment
   a. Superficial thrombophlebitis with elastic support, heart and anti-inflammatory medications, and anticoagulants
   b. Deep thrombophlebitis with anticoagulant therapy, bed rest, elevation, local heat, analgesics, support hose, and thrombolytic therapy (high pressure, rapid-inflation compression)
   c. Pulmonary embolism

C. Postphlebitic syndrome (chronic venous insufficiency)
1. Prevention through use of elastic supports, foot elevation, and skin care
2. Venous ulcerations
   a. Location and characteristics
   b. Treatment, including use of topical dressings and unna boot
   c. Multilayer compression
   d. Circaid boot

LYMPHATIC DISEASES AFFECTING THE LOWER EXTREMITIES

I. Anatomy and physiology

II. Primary lymphedema (idiopathic)

A. Congenital
1. Hereditary or familial (e.g., Milroy's disease, Meige's disease, Turner's syndrome)
2. Simple

B. Lymphedema precox - manifests usually in females between 10 to 25 years of age

C. Lymphedema tarda - occurs after 35 years of age

III. Secondary lymphedema

A. **Traumatic**
   1. Direct impacting
   2. Surgical disruption
   3. Pressure
B. **Malignant occlusion (angiosarcoma, kaposi sarcoma)**
C. **Inflammatory**
   1. Secondary to recurrent lymphangitis and cellulitis
   2. Complicating venous insufficiency
   3. Filariasis
   4. Local tissue injury
D. **Neuroplegic**
E. **Vasospastic disorders**
F. **Infection**

IV. **Diagnosis**

   A. **ACI edema tester**
   B. **MR imaging**
   C. **CT**
   D. **Lymphoscintigraphy**
   E. **Ultrasonography**

V. **Differential diagnosis**

   A. **Myxedema**
   B. **Myocardial failure**
   C. **Nephrosis**
   D. **Nephritis**
   E. **Deficient Proteinemia**
   F. **Sarcoma**
   G. **Lipoma**
   H. **Bone neoplasms**
   F. **A-V fistulas**

V. **Medical treatment**

   A. **Diuretic therapy**
   B. **Elastic support**
   C. **Massage, exercise, and elevation**
   D. **Gene therapy**
   E. **Benzopyrones (Coumadin)**

BIBLIOGRAPHY

Abramson DI. Circulatory Problems in Podiatry. Karger, New York, 1985.

Kempczinski RF. The Ischemic Leg. Mosby Year Book, Chicago, 1985.

Levin J, Zier BG, Hoffman AF. Peripheral vascular disease. In: Zier BG, ed., Essentials of Internal Medicine in Clinical Podiatry. W.B. Saunders Co., Philadelphia, 1990.

Robbins. M. Peripheral vascular disease in the lower extremity. Clin Podiatric Med & Surg 9:1,1992.

REFERENCES:

Anthony SF, etal: "Fever and Rash" in *Harrison's Principles of Internal Medicine*. Vol I, ed SF Anthony, etal, p 97, McGraw-Hill, San Francisco, 1998.

Anthony SF, etal: "Vascular Disease of the Extremities" in *Harrison's Principles of Internal Medicine*. Vol I, ed SF Anthony, etal, p1401-3, McGraw-Hill, San Francisco, 1998.

Anthony SF, etal: "The Vasculitis Syndromes" in *Harrison's Principles of Internal Medicine*. Vol II ed SF Anthony, etal, p1912-3, McGraw-Hill, San Francisco, 1998.

Astrom KG, Abdsaleh S, Brenning GC, Ahlstrom KH: MR imaging of primary, secondary, and mixed forms of lymphedema. Acta Radiologica. 42(4) 409-16, 2001 Jul.

Cardia G, Cianci V, Iusco, Nacchiero M. Ultrasound duplex as a sole exam for surgical purposes in lower limb arterial obstructive disease. Minerva Cardioangiol, 49: 349-55, 2001.

Cesarone MR, Belcaro G, Nicolaides AN, Arkans E, Laurora G, De Sanctis MT, Incandela L: The edema tester in the evaluation of swollen limbs in venous and lymphatic disease. Panminerva Medica. 41(1): 10-4, 1999 Mar.

Clude D, etal. Exercise rehabilitation improves functional outcomes and peripheral circulation in patients with intermittent claudication: a randomized controlled trial. J Am Geriatr Soc, 49: 755-62, 2001.

Department of Medicine, Temple University Medical Center, Philadelphia, Carnitine and its role in cardiovascular disease. Heart Dis, 1: 108-13, 1999.

Einfeldt H: Lymph drainage with secondary lymphedema caused by Kaposi sarcoma. Zeitschrift fur Lymphologie – Journal of Lymphology. 16(1):10-3, 1992 Dec.

Gianetti J, etal. Intravenous prostaglandin E1 reduces soluble vascular cell adhesion molecule-1 in peripheral arterial obstructive disease. Am Heart J, 142: 733-9, 2001.

Giordano A, Calcagni ML, Rulli F, Muzi M, Martino G, D'Andrea G, Galli M, Zanella E: Correlation of Tc-99m-red blood cell phleboscintigraphy with clinical severity of chronic venous disease. Vascular Surgery. 35(4):273-83, 2001 Jul-Aug.

Hooi JD, etal. Peripheral arterial occlusive disease: prognostic value of signs, symptoms and the ankle-brachial pressure index. Med Decis Making, 22: 99-107, 2002.

Hoshi T, Hachiya T, Kanauchi T, Hando Y, Homma T: Gd-enhanced subtraction MR venography. Nippon Igaku Hoshasen Gakkai Zasshi – Nippon Acta Radiologica, 59(12):674-8, 1999 Oct.

Irwin MS, etal. Neuropathy in non-freezing cold injury (trench foot). J R Soc Med, 90: 433-8, 1997.

Irwin MS. Nature and mechanism of peripheral nerve damage in an experimental model of non-freezing cold injury. Ann R Coll Surg Engl, 78: 372-9, 1996.

Jahnke T, etal. Endovascular placement of self-expanding nitinol coil stents for treatment of femoropopliteal obstructive disease. Vasc Interv Radiol, 13: 257-66, 2002.

Jahss MH: "Chemical, Environmental and Foreign-Body Injuries to the Foot and Ankle" in *Disorders of the Foot & Ankle*, Vol III ed by MH Jahss, p 2576-7, W.B. Saunders Company, Philadelphia, 1991.

Karkkainen MJ, Saaristo A, Jussila L, Karila KA, Lawrence EC, Pajusola K, Bueler H, Eichmann A, Kauppinen R, Kettunen MI, Yla-Herttuala S, Finegold DN, Ferrell RE, Alitalo K: A model for gene therapy of human hereditary lymphedema. Proceedings of the National Academy of Sciences of the United States of America. 98(22):12677-82, 2001 Oct 23.

Karmazanovski GG, Savchenko TV: Computed tomographic symptomatology of lymphedema of the lower extremities. Vestnik Rentgenologii I Radiologii.

Kidawa AS: Vasospastic disorders. Clinics in Podiatric Medicine & Surgery. 9(1):139-50, 1992 Jan.

Labropoulos N, etal. Acute Effects of Intermittent Pneumatic Compression on Popliteal Artery Blood Flow. Arch Surg, 133: 1072-1075, 1998.

Lammer J, etal. Peripheral arterial obstruction: prospective study of treatment with transluminally placed self-expanding stent graft. International Trial Study Group. Radiology, 217: 95-104, 2000.

Malone MD, Cisek PL, Comerota AJ Jr, Holland B, Eid IG, Comerota AJ: High-pressure, rapid-inflation pneumatic compression improves venous hemodynamics in healthy volunteers and patients who are post-thrombotic. Journal of Vascular Surgery. 29(4):593-9, 1999 Apr.

Mandell GA, Alexander MA, Harcke HT: A multiscintigraphic approach to imaging of lymphedema and other causes of the congenitally enlarged extremity. Seminars in Nuclear Medicine. 23(4):334-46, 1993 Oct.

Pecking A: Medical treatment of lymphedema with benzopyrones. Experimental basis and applications. Journal des Maladies Vasculaires. 15(2):157-8, 1990.

Radonic V, etal. Popliteal artery entrapment syndrome: diagnosis and management, with report of three cases. Tex Heart Inst J, 27: 3-13, 2000.

Rissanen TT, Vajanto I, Yla-Herttuala S. Gene therapy for therapeutic angiogenesis in critically ischeamic lower limb – on the way to the clinic. Eur J Clin Invest, 31: 651-66, 2001.

Rutherford RB: "Initial Patient Evaluation: The Vascular Consultation" in *Vascular Surgery*, Vol I, ed RB Rutherford, p3-9, W.B Saunders Company, Philadelphia, 2000.

Rutherford RB: " Anatomy of Commonly Exposed Arteries" in *Vascular Surgery*, Vol I, ed RB Rutherford, p56-60, W.B Saunders Company, Philadelphia, 2000.

Rutherford RB: " The Vascular Laboratory" in *Vascular Surgery*, Vol I, ed RB Rutherford, p130-8, W.B Saunders Company, Philadelphia, 2000.

Rutherford RB: "Magnetic Resonance and Angiography" in *Vascular Surgery*, Vol I, ed RB Rutherford, p274-7, W.B Saunders Company, Philadelphia, 2000.

Rutherford RB: "Principles of Arteriography" in *Vascular Surgery*, Vol I, ed RB Rutherford, p286-302, W.B Saunders Company, Philadelphia, 2000.

Rutherford RB: "Uncommon Arteriopathies" in *Vascular Surgery*, Vol I, ed RB Rutherford, p423, W.B Saunders Company, Philadelphia, 2000.

Rutherford RB: "Antithrombotic Therapy" in *Vascular Surgery*, Vol I, ed RB Rutherford, p435-54, W.B Saunders Company, Philadelphia, 2000.

Schmitz-Rixen T, Horsch S. Arnold G, Peters PE: Angiosarcoma in primary lymphedema of the lower extremity—Stewart-Treves Syndrome. Vasa. 13(3):262-6, 1984.

Sepa G, etal. Popliteal artery entrapment syndrome. Magy Seb, 53: 17-20, 2000.

Strandness DE Jr, etal. Effect of cilostazol in patients with intermittent claudication: a randomized, double-blind, placebo-controlled study. Vasc Endovascular Surg, 36: 83-91, 2002.

Textbook: The Merck Manual of Diagnosis and Therapy. 2000.

Tsyb AF, Mukhamedzhanov Ikh, Bardychev MS, Guseva LI: Ultrasonic examination in secondary lymphedema of the lower extremities. Khirurgiia. (11):61-7, 1990 Nov.

Turpie AG, Mason JA. Review of enoxaparin and its clinical applications in venous and arterial thromboembolism. Expert Opin Pharmacother, 3: 575-98, 2002.

Vowden KR, Goulding V, Vowden P. Hand-held Doppler assessment for peripheral arterial disease. J Wound Care, 5: 125-8, 1996.

Weissleder H, Weissleder R: Lymphedema: evaluation of qualitative and quantitative lymphoscintigraphy in 238 patients. Radiology. 167(3):729-35, 1988 Jun.

CHAPTER 14
PERIPHERAL VASCULAR DISEASE

1.   Each of the following is always a sign or symptom of clinically significant arterial disease EXCEPT:

        A.   pain or fatigue in the calf after walking two blocks
        B.   transient ischemic attacks
        C.   absence of hair on the toes
        D.   A & B
        E.   A & C

2.   Which of the following is an invasive vascular study?

        A.   Laser Doppler
        B.   Arteriography
        C.   Oscillometry
        D.   Volume Plethysmography
        E.   Magnetic Resonance Angiography

3.   Which of the following is the most effective method of treatment for thromboangiitis obliterans?

        A.   Exercise
        B.   High dose prednisone
        C.   Aspirin
        D.   Cessation of all tobacco use
        E.   Oral hemorrheologic agents

4.   Acrocyanosis differs from Raynaud's Disease in that it:

        A.   involves females more than males
        B.   is intermittent
        C.   is constant
        D.   manifests with cyanosis of the digits
        E.   only affects the elderly

5.   All of the following are used to increase arterial blood flow to the extremities EXCEPT:

        A.   popliteal/dorsalis pedis bypass
        B.   aspirin
        C.   nitroglycerin patches
        D.   capsaicin
        E.   exercise

6. A 43-year-old female presents to your office with an increase in erythema, edema and tenderness to her right leg. She claims that four days ago while riding a bike she jammed her leg into the ground. She smokes one and a half packs of cigarettes a day and is taking oral contraceptives. She denies fevers, chills or nausea and claims that her pain has decreased in the past 24 hours. She took two aspirin yesterday, which helped to resolve the pain. Homan's and Pratt's tests are negative. What is the best course of treatment for this patient?

    A. Have the patient rest, use warm compresses, take 650 mg aspirin qd and return to your clinic in four days or sooner if symptoms worsen
    B. Admit the patient immediately, order coagulation studies, chem 7, CBC, radiographs of the foot and leg, and begin heparin therapy
    C. Obtain a D-dimer test, radiographs and venous duplex studies. Start the patient on low molecular weight heparin and send her home with instructions to rest and return to see you in one week
    D. Obtain D-dimer, radiographs and venous duplex studies. Admit patient to hospital, initiate heparin and coumadin therapy

7. All of the following are risk factors for venous thromboembolism EXCEPT:

    A. Age over 60
    B. Paraplegia
    C. Past history of prostate cancer
    D. Absence of anticardiolipin antibodies
    E. Birth control pills

8. Which of the following is NOT an etiological factor associated with varicose veins?

    A. Primary idiopathic dilation of vein walls
    B. Valvular incompetence
    C. High-pressure flow in perforator veins during muscular contraction
    D. Prolonged standing
    E. Pregnancy

9. Which of the following clinical findings are consistent with Turner's syndrome?

    A. Brachymetatarsia of the 4th, short stature, webbing of the neck and lymphedema of the feet
    B. Lymphedema of the hands and feet, brachymetatarsia of the 2nd and low hair line on the back of the neck
    C. Lymphedema of the hands and feet, brachymetatarsia of the 2nd, and hypoplasia of the nails
    D. Lymphedema of the feet, broad chest, long feet, brachymetatarsia of the 1st

10. Which of the following would be LEAST likely to be a cause of lymphedema?

    A. Ewings sarcoma of the tibia
    B. Hypothyroidism
    C. Multiple shrapnel wounds to the lower extremities
    D. Hyperthyroidism
    E. Adenocarcinoma of the breast

Infectious Disease and Wound Care of the Lower Extremity

By Gregg K. Young, updated for the 2004 edition by Gregg K. Young, Marianne Misiewicz, and Cindy Bullock

DIAGNOSTIC TECHNIQUES (SEE ALGORITHM 1 & 2)

I. **Evaluation of infection** - a problem-directed history and physical should be obtained in every patient. While additional history and physical based information may be desirable for some patients, the following represents the minimum information that should normally be obtained

   A. **History of the chief complaint**
      1. Wound/infection site history
         a. Appearance of area prior to development of the infection or wound
         b. Onset and duration
         c. Drainage, swelling, color changes around ulcer - always determine normal level of edema based on uninvolved limb. The effect of elevation and dependency on swelling and color changes should be determined
         d. Pain and/or numbness - the reported onset and duration of a wound or infection should be considered unreliable in a patient with neuropathy
      2. Previous/present treatment - home remedies should be specifically queried
      3. Previous ulcerations/infections - at present site or any other site
      4. Trauma (including surgeries) at or near the wound/infection site should be reviewed. The setting in which the trauma occurred may assist in the selection of empiric antibiotics (i.e, puncture wounds through athletic shoes have a higher incidence of pseudomonas infection). Antibiotic prophylaxis at the time of surgery with a subsequent infection may represent an organism that is resistant to the drug used for prophylaxis
      5. Constitutional symptoms - nausea, malaise, fatigue, vomiting, fever, chills, etc. If these are present sepsis must be considered

B. Past medical history

1. Potential causes of immunocompromise should be determined
   a. Diabetes - the most common associated disease for lower extremity infections
   b. Rheumatoid arthritis, connective tissue diseases (SLE, etc.)
2. Neurological - neurologic diseases resulting in neuropathies or fixed deformities will complicate treatment and in the case of neuropathy patient compliance
3. Vascular disease - patients with significant arterial disease are unlikely to heal an infection and should be identified as soon as possible (see algorithm 1)
   a. Arterial
      i. Intermittent claudication - limitation of walking distance is consistent over repeated episodes and normally requires less than 5 minutes of recovery time
      ii. Rest pain - pain on elevation of legs relieved by dangling legs. Patients often must sleep sitting up
   b. Venous - venous stasis disease can mimic cellulitis; venous ulcers are rarely infected
      i. Deep venous thrombosis (DVT) acute event can mimic an infection. Imaging studies should be used for diagnosis since clinical impression is unreliable
4. Dermatological diseases such as bullous diseases and carcinomas can appear to be infections/ulcerations. These should be considered if the presentation is atypical or if wounds are located in non-classical sites (i.e, the dorsum or arch of the foot)
5. Atypical infection - these infections all require interventions that are beyond the scope of this chapter. However, identification of these causes when present is essential for patient care
   a. Syphilis - history of multiple sexual partners, unsafe sex, urogenital symptoms
   b. Hansen's disease - history of patchy plaque-like areas of numbness; history of foreign travel; recent immigrants
   c. Other mycobacterium - mycobacterium ulcerans - history of travel to tropical areas; mycobacterium tuberculosis - history of nodule formation, slow indolent course, pulmonary symptoms (chronic cough)
   d. Parasitic - history of travel to tropical areas; injuries associated with swimming or diving

C. Medications: may either interfere with planned treatments or indicate that standard treatments are likely to be ineffective

1. Antibiotics - chronic use of antibiotics can develop resistant organisms; failure of an antibiotic course can relate to selecting a drug with poor or intermediate activity against the suspected organism or because of poor penetration into the infected site (i.e, cephalosporins have poor penetration into skin structures)
2. Anticoagulants - many lower extremity infections require surgical drainage for resolution; anticoagulants present a relative contraindication to surgery. Excess anticoagulation may lead to hematomas that can become secondarily infected. Warfarin effects the bioavailability of many antibiotics
3. Antidiabetic - control of blood sugars is necessary to optimize the immune response of diabetic patients. Diabetics on oral medications often must be switched to insulin to control their glucose levels when they are infected
4. Prednisone and anti-neoplastic drugs are immunosuppressive and should be stopped or reduced when possible in infected patients. These drugs may suppress many of the signs and symptoms of an infection. Antibiotics should be considered in wound management even in the absence of clinical and laboratory evidence of infection if wound fails to respond to therapy

D. Allergies to both antibiotics and topical wound treatments should be ruled out.
Cephalosporin and thienamycin (imipenem) antibiotics have a cross-allergic reaction with penicillin only in patients with a history of anaphylaxis. The cross reactivity is probably less than 10%. The type of reaction should always be determined since patients often relate cases of gastrointestinal distress as an allergic reaction. Reactions such as gastrointestinal distress are not contraindications to using an antibiotic

E. Previous surgeries should be reviewed to determine if the patient has had an unusually high incidence of infection or a history of slow healing. Patients with these problems may require more intensive therapy

II. Physical exam

A. Vital signs - pulse and respirations are often increased in patients with infections. Hypotension is a sign of septic shock and requires immediate intervention

1. Temperature elevation is seen in individuals with normal immune response. The elevation usually correlates well to the severity of the infection (i.e, higher temperature equals more severe infection). However, diabetics and immunosuppressed patients may have normal temperatures even with severe infections

B. Vascular/Lymphatic

1. Pulses should be evaluated from distal to proximal until a normal pulse is reached
2. Capillary filling time of less than 5 seconds with the foot elevated above the heart indicates satisfactory blood flow
3. Elevation pallor is the most reliable clinical indicator of significant vascular disease
4. Dependent rubor is a hyperemic response in a patient with arterial disease of a magnitude great enough to cause partial deoxygenation of the blood by the vascular tree prior to reaching the capillary beds. Dependent rubor differs clinically from cellulitis in that the limb is generally cool and the color disappears completely with elevation

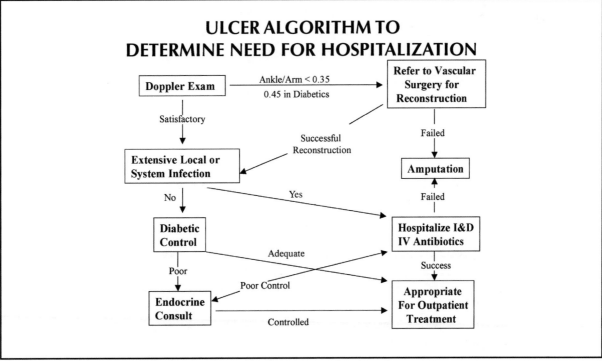

Figure 1.   Initial steps in evaluating a patient with a lower extremity ulceration.

5. Cyanosis is the result of deoxygenated blood most commonly associated with venous insufficiency. It can be the result of pulmonary disease. However it does not correlate with arterial disease

6. Skin temperature will be increased in infection except with severe vascular disease. The temperature should be assessed relative to the other limb and to the more proximal areas of the affected limb. Limbs should be symmetrical and show a mild temperature gradient (cool distally to warm proximally)

7. Edema is a nonspecific finding. When seen in association with an infection it is normally unilateral and is more severe surrounding a wound if present and in areas of cellulitis. If it is diffuse or symmetrical the present level of edema should be viewed in light of the average amount of edema the patient reports

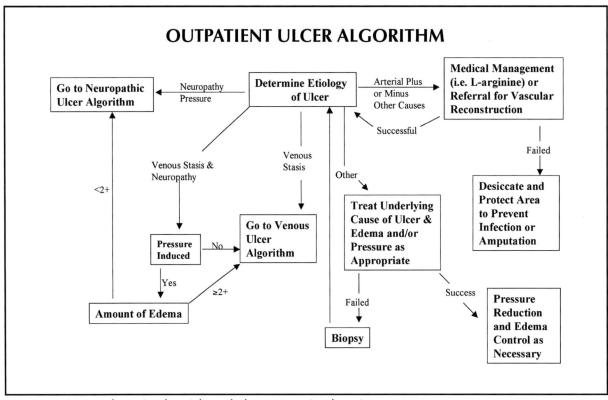

Figure 2. Steps to determine the etiology of a lower extremity ulceration.

8. Hemosiderin pigment associated with venous stasis is easily confused with cellulitis particularly when it is inflammatory. If the problem is chronic with varicosities, venous stasis disease is favored. Unfortunately, venous stasis can also mask cellulitis. In these cases the use of sequential compression boot therapy followed by re-evaluation is helpful. Venous stasis appears to improve while cellulitis does not. Laboratory tests (CBC with differential) may be necessary in differentiating the two

9. Deep venous thrombosis may mimic infection and should always be considered in cellulitic-appearing limbs where no portal of entry can be identified or where the cellulitis is not contiguous with the potential site of entry (i.e, leg cellulitis with a digital ulcer and no foot cellulitis)

10. Lymph nodes should be evaluated if infection is suspected. Popliteal nodes are difficult to feel, particularly if marked swelling is present. However, tenderness should be assessed relative to the normal limb. Femoral nodes should be checked also and are much easier to palpate

C. Neurological - Patients with neuropathy tend to be less likely to stay off their feet than other individuals and are less likely to be conscientious about wound care. Patient education is extremely important in the care of these individuals

1. Monofilament testing (5.07) divides patients into two groups, one with significant risk for ulceration on the basis of neuropathy (can't feel the 5.07 monofilament) and the other group that has enough sensation to alert them to possible injuries

D. Wound/infected site - For wound management to be effective the progress of wounds must be tracked in an objective manner. If measurable improvement hasn't occurred within 2-3 weeks modification of therapy should be considered. Remember that it is not unusual for wounds to enlarge initially as callous and necrotic tissue are removed

1. Location including the relationship of the wound to any potential pressure points
2. Size: width, length, and depth should be determined at each visit and used as the basis for determining progress
   a. Area may be tracked periodically to determine healing rate
3. Drainage/odor - wounds with significant amounts of either of these should be worked up for infection. Occlusive dressings tend to hold drainage and may be malodorous. The significance of these findings should be correlated with the appearance of the wound following cleansing and the frequency with which the dressing must be changed to prevent it from leaking. If the cleansed wound appears uninfected and the dressing can be left at least 3 days, the likelihood of these findings indicating an infection is low
4. Fibrin in base/amount of granulation - the appearance of the base of the wound is a good indicator of whether the wound environment has been sufficiently optimized to promote healing. Wounds with marked amounts of fibrous debris and/or a lack of granulation tissue generally indicate one of three things: 1) severe arterial insufficiency; 2) poor systemic nutrition; 3) the use of tissue toxic treatments such as iodine

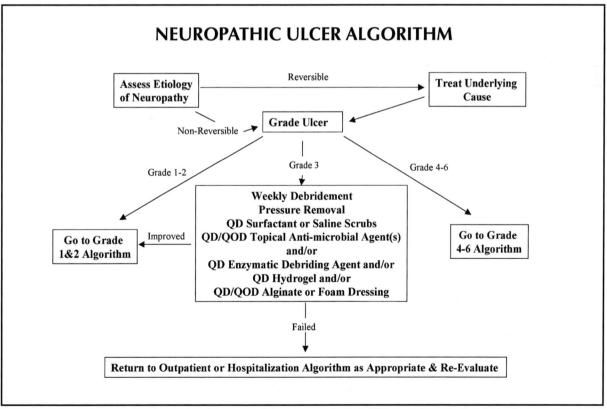

Figure 3.   It is important to determine the cause of the neuropathy in addition to the severity of the ulcer.

5. Erythema/edema - when these are restricted to the immediate area of the wound they are usually indicative of infection. However, if they are more generalized other possibilities should be considered (see above under Vascular section)

6. Probe for sinus tract or exposed bone or tendon - tendon sheaths are a common route for the spread of infection. If bone is exposed it is assumed that there is osteomyelitis until proven otherwise

7. Foreign bodies including nail borders - explore all wounds for possible foreign bodies. Foreign bodies provide a nidus for infection and should be considered in infections that respond to antibiotic therapy only to flare up after the antibiotics have been discontinued

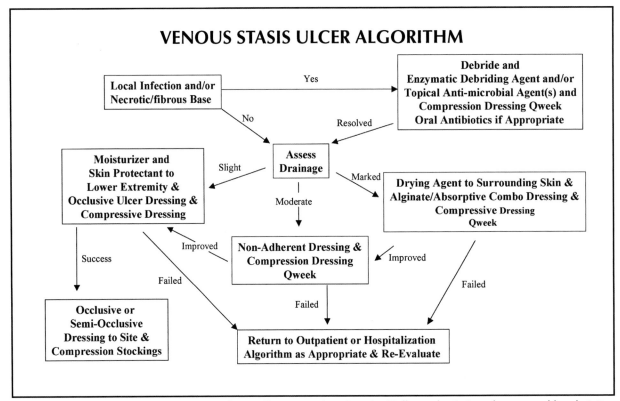

Figure 4. Diagrammatic representation of monofilament testing sites. 1—Hallux pulp; 2-6—submetatarsal heads 1-5; 7—plantar heel.

E. Orthopedic deformities and biomechanical faults are often secondary causes of ulcerations in neuropathic patients. These deformities should be identified early and treatment should include addressing them both on an immediate and a long-term basis

1. Bony deformities causing ulceration are usually the result of direct pressure and often require surgical intervention

2. Gait abnormalities causing ulceration are usually the result of shearing forces and require modification of shoes and either orthotics or shear dispersing inserts

III. Additional studies are often helpful in determining if a wound or suspicious closed lesion is infected. These studies are also useful in determining the underlying etiologies and the likelihood of healing

A. Initially for most wounds - minor wounds in healthy individuals (i.e., an ingrown toenail of two days duration in a young patient with no medical problems) usually don't require any additional studies. However, any wound where infection is suspected, chronic wounds, and wounds in compromised individuals should have additional workups. The timing of these studies should be determined by the clinical severity of the presentation. In wounds where the index of suspicion for infection is low, the studies can often be deferred to the second visit and canceled if the area has resolved

1. Radiographs to rule out osteomyelitis and/or gas in the tissues *(See chapter on Imaging)*
2. CBC with differential should be obtained to determine if an infection is present and its severity. In compromised individuals the values obtained should be compared to their previous studies. They often do not mount a significant immune response and an increase from their baseline should be considered a positive test even if the values are normal or only slightly elevated
3. Random/Fasting glucose - glucose levels should be obtained in all diabetics or suspected diabetics. A markedly elevated glucose may be their only sign of infection. The significance of a given value should be considered in comparison to their usual level of control. While fasting glucose is preferable, do not wait. Obtain a random glucose in individuals where the index of suspicion for infection is high

B. **Arterial disease should be evaluated with appropriate non-invasive studies**

C. **Clinical evidence of infection** - Wounds without evidence of infection should not be cultured. Cultures are a test to determine the organisms that are causing the infection, not a test to determine if there is an infection. Remember, if you have cultured the wound you have declared it infected and must treat the infection
1. Culture and sensitivity (aerobic) - deep tissue should be sent; swabs are not reliable. Needle aspirate can be considered in closed infections. Tissue obtained at the time of an incision and drainage is the most reliable. If osteomyelitis is suspected bone cultures are best but the value of the information obtained must be balanced against the possibility of contaminating non-infected bone
2. Anaerobic cultures, fungal cultures, and/or acid fast bacterial cultures should be considered in compromised individuals, atypical presentations, or infection refractory to treatment

D. **Patient with venous disease**
1. Studies should be obtained if DVT is suspected because clinical judgment regarding DVT is false positive approximately 50% of the time and false negative approximately the same amount

E. **Patients with suspected nutritional deficiencies** (chronically out of control diabetes, low socioeconomic status, homeless, substance abuse)
1. Healing potential is nutritionally compromised if total lymphocyte count is less than 1500 or albumin is less than 3

F. **Advanced imaging** *(see Osteomyelitis in Imaging chapter)*

MICROBIOLOGY

I. **Gram positive cocci** (aerobic)

A. **Most common organisms in lower extremity infections** *(see table of organisms)*

B. **Community acquired use narrow spectrum antibiotic** *(see antibiotic tables)*

C. **Methicillin resistant or in life-threatening infection use IV vancomycin**
1. Vancomycin-resistant strains particularly of enterococcus but also S. aureus have

developed. Vancomycin should be reserved for the two situations above

   2. Alternatives: TMP/SMX (test susceptibility first), doxycycline, minocycline (some strains), linezolid, quinupristin/dalfopristin, rifampin, and fluoroquinolones may be active but must be used in combination regimens to prevent in vivo emergence of resistance
   3. Enterococcus is seen more frequently as a pathogen in many areas and may be resistant; consider ampicillin and/or vancomycin
   4. If vancomycin resistant, therapeutic options include linezolid, quinpristin/ dalfopristin, teicoplanin (compassionate use may be available)

II. Gram positive cocci (anaerobic)

   A. **Usually susceptible to narrow spectrum antibiotics** (see Tables 1 and 2)
   B. **Rarely a major problem**

III. Anaerobic bacteria (other)

   A. **Generally susceptible to clindamycin or metronidazole** (see Tables 1 and 2 for other possibilities)
   B. **More common in compromised patients such as diabetics**

IV. Gram negative rods

   A. **See Tables 1 and 2 for common organisms**
   B. **Levofloxacin and penicillin beta-lactam combinations are effective against many of these**
      4. If resistant use imipenem, meropenem, or antipseudomonal penicillins. Many strains susceptible to aztreonam, third and fourth generation cephalosporins (increasing concerns regarding resistance)
      5. Check susceptibilities

ANTIBIOTIC THERAPY

I. Empiric therapy

   A. **Always use narrow spectrum antibiotics except in compromised host or limb/life threatening infection** (see Tables 1 and 2)
   B. **Very resistant organisms** (Pseudomonas, Enterococcus, etc.) should not be taken into consideration when choosing empiric therapy. They occur infrequently and develop resistance quickly. Their treatment is more effective when based on culture and sensitivity information. In life-threatening infections where resistant organisms are suspected, a combination of vancomycin or linezolid and imipenem, meropenem, levofloxacin or piperacillin/tazobactam with or without gentamicin should be considered
   C. **Fluoroquinolone antibiotics in general should not be used as first line therapy for lower extremity infections except possibly in PCN/cephalosporin allergic patients with significant infections.** Most in this group have poor gram positive activity. The indiscriminate use can lead to development of new resistant organisms. Levaquin may have some empiric indications (see above)
   D. **Imipenem and the beta-lactam antibiotics** (see Tables 1 and 2) should only be used empirically in compromised patients or life-threatening infections
   E. **Bone infections** – Generally cannot be resolved in small foot bones with antibiotics alone.

Use amoxicillin/clavulanate for less serious infections. More severe infections use carbapenems or penicillin beta-lactam combo with or without vancomycin/linezolid
1. Hematogenous – nafcillin
2. Puncture wounds – consider antipseudomonal therapy (see Tables)

II. Culture-proven infections

A. Organisms grown in cultures may be contaminates

B. Do not change antibiotic if they are working

C. Remember sensitivities are in vitro not in vivo

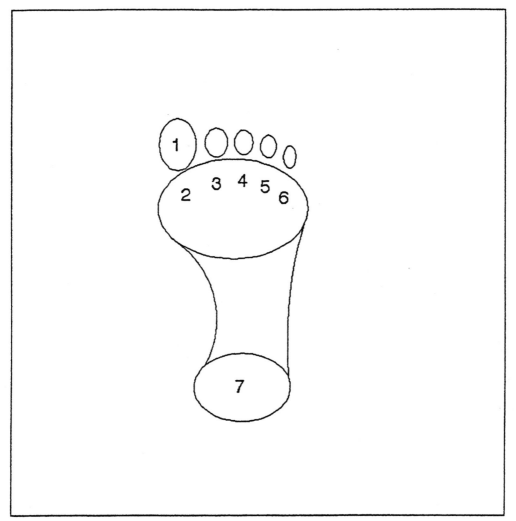

Figure 5.   In patients with systemic causes for their edema (i.e., congestive heart failure) compressive therapy should be used with caution to avoid decompensation of their underlying disease.

III. Hospitalization and consultation (see Algorithm 1)

Table 1: Bacteria Seen in Lower Extremity Infections

Bacteria	Antibiotic Therapy	Resistance	Comments
Gram-Positive			

Staphylococcus aureus	1°-Semisynthetic penicillins/1st generation cephalosporins 2°-Clindamycin, TMP/SMZ, vancomycin (only in PCN-allergic) 3°-Tetracycline, imipenem, b-lactam/ b-lactamase inhibitor, fluoroquinolones, erythromycin, clarithromycin, azithromycin	90%+ of isolates are resistant to Pen G. 30-40% of nosocomial isolates are resistant to methicillin (MRSA); this varies by area of the country	Most common organism found in lower extremity infections. Empiric therapy for any foot infection must include coverage for PCN-resistant non-MRSA
	MRSA 1°-Vancomycin 2°- Linezolid TMP/SMX, quinu/dalfo	A small number of isolates are resistant to vancomycin; this group is extremely difficult to treat. >60% ciprofloxacin resistant in US	
Staphylococcus epidermidis	1°-Vancomycin ± rifampin 2°-Rifampin + TMP/SMX or fluoroquinolone	As many as 50-80% of isolates are methicillin resistant with marked variation between centers	Most common organism in late post operative infections involving implants. Superficial cultures may grow this as a contaminate; consider quality of culture before initiating therapy.
Streptococci Group A & B	1°-Penicillins 2°-All b-lactams, erythromycin, azithromycin, dirithromycin, clarithromycin	No significant resistance	Very common in lower extremity infections
Enterococci (Streptococci Group D)	1°-Ampicillin with or without gentamicin 2°-Vancomycin with or without gentamicin 3°-Quinupristin/Dalfopristin, Linezolid	Many resistant strains, including vancomycin (VRE). Nosocomial rate as high as 25%. Some strains resistant to nearly all antibiotics including gentamicin (30-60%)	Majority are *E. faecium*. While these organisms may occasion be contaminates; they should be aggressively treated, particularly in compromised hosts

Gram-Negative

Gonococci (N. gonorrhoeae)	For septic arthritis 1°-Ceftriaxone, cefotaxime, N. gonorrhoeae cefpodoxime 2°-Ofloxacin, ciprofloxacin. levofloxacin, spectinomycin 3°-Switch to orals after improvement, i.e., cefixime	Quinolone-resistant 0.2% res in USA. Hawaii ~ 14%, increasing in California.	Lower extremity infections are primarily septic arthritis.
Enterobacter Citrobacter Morganella Serratia	1°-Imipenem, meropenem, 3rd gen ceph (Mor, Ser) 2°-Tic/Clav, Pip/Taz, quinolones 3°-Cefipime, (Citro, Mor), aztreonam (Mor, Ser), gentamicin (Ser)	Up to 40% strains from ICUs may be resistant to ceftazadime. May see resistance develop during therapy as the result of inducible b-lactamase.	Mostly seen in nosocomial infections.
Klebsiella Proteus mirabilis	1°-3rd/4th generation cephalosporin, levofloxacin, ampicillin (Pro) 2°- Parental b-lactam combo, aminoglycosides, TMP/SMX (Pro) 3°-Anti-pseudomonal penicillin, imipenem, meropenem, aztreonam	K. pneumoniae most likely to show resistance; ceftazadime reported up to 10%.	P. mirabilis is most common gram-negative organism isolated from lower extremity infections (normal foot flora). Klebsiella is rare in lower extremity infections and is usually nosocomial.
Providencia Proteus vulgaris	1°- Amikacin, 3rd/4th gen cephalosporin, quinolones, 2°-TMP/SMX (Prv), aminoglycoside (Prt), 3°-Anti-pseudomonal penicillin + amikacin, imipenem, aztreonam	Resistant to 1st generation cephalosporins	Primarily seen in nosocomial infections, not common in lower extremity infections.
E. coli	Most drugs with activity against gram-negative organisms. b-lactam/b-lactamase inhibitors, cephalosporins, fluoroquinolones, TMP/SMX, aminoglycosides	Some nosocomial infections show resistance to ceftaz or ciprofloxacin	Second most common gram negative organism seen in lower extremity infections

Pseudomonas aeruginosa	1°-Anti-pseudomonal penicillin, anti-pseudomona 3rd gen cephalosporin, imipenem, meropenem tobramycin, ciprofloxacin (priority with bone)	Resistance patterns vary greatly between facilities. Resistance shown ~10-20% ceftaz, aminoglycosides, carbapenems. Resistance to b-lactams may emerge during treatment. Therapy should be guided by sensitivities.	Many individuals recommend using two agents for all pseudomonal infections. Pseudomonas should not be targeted with empiric therapy.
Eikenella corrodens	1°-Penicillin G, ampicillin, 2°-TMP/SMX, fluoroquinolone 3°-cefoxitin, cefotaxime, imipenem	Clindamycin, cephalexin, erythromycin and metronidazole	Primarily seen in bite wounds.
Pasteurella multocida	1°-Penicillin G, ampicillin, amoxicillin 2°- Doxycycline, AM/CL, cephalosporin 2nd gen, TMP/SMX 3°-Ceftriaxone, cefpodoxime		Primarily seen in bite wounds.
Anaerobic Bacteria	b-lactamase inhibitor combinations, clindamycin, metronidazole are effective against most anaerobes		b-lactamase inhibitor combinations should be reserved for severe infections with mixed flora.
Bacteroides	1°-Metronidazole 2°-Clindamycin 3°-Cefoxitin, imipenem, meropenem, b-lactamase, inhibitor combos, cefotetan	Penicillin and many cephalosporins are ineffective particularly against B. fragilis.	Common in mixed diabetic foot infections.
Clostridium perfringens	1º - Penicillin ± clindamycin 2°-Doxycycline 3°-Erythromycin, chloramphenicol, cefazolin, cefoxitin, anti-pseudomonal PCN, imipenem	Rare	
Clostridium tetani	1°-Metronidazole or Penicillin G 2°-Doxycycline 3°-Imipenem		C. tetani produces a neurotoxin (see table on Immunization)

Table 2: Antibiotics for Possible Use in Lower Extremity Infections

Drug/Drug Group	Spectrum	Dosage/Admin.	Comments
Penicillin G/V	Streptococci Gonococci	Procaine penicillin 1.2 mil units q12-24h IM Benzathine penicillin 1.2 mil units once IM Pen V 250-500mg qid	Most organisms in LE infections are resistant. Probenicid 1-2 g/day markedly increases serum levels.
Ampicillin	Streptococci (better Group D than Pen	250-500mg qid PO 150-200mg/kg/d IV	Bacteriostatic against Strep Grp D
Amoxicillin	G), P. mirablis. ±Community-acquired E. coli, H. influenza, Salmonella, Shigella	500mg q8h PO or 875mg q12h PO	(consider using with aminoglycosides). Of limited use in LE infections.
Semisynthetic Penicillins (penicillinase resistant)	Staph, strep except methicillin-resistant	Nafcillin 1-2g q4h IV/IM Cloxa 250-500mg q6h PO Dicloxa 125-500mg q6h PO	Cloxacillin and dicloxacillin are drug of choice for mild to moderate Staph infections. Nafcillin's frequent administration increases its cost.
Anti-pseudomonal Penicillins	P. aeruginosa, Proteus, Morganella, and the Enterobacteriaceae	Ticarcillin 3g q4-6h IV Piperacillin 3-4g q4-6h IV or 200-300mg/kg/d up to 500mg/kg/d Mezlocillin 3g q4h IV	Ticarcillin has decreased activity and increased K+ load relative to other two. Resistance via lactamase induction can develop when used as single agents. Combine with aminoglycosides or quinolones for gram negative infections. Add anti-staph drug in combination for severe mixed infections.

Penicillin b-lactam inhibitor combinations	Staph except methicillin resistant. Strep and gram negative activity same as parent drug. Gram negative organisms that produce plasmid-mediated b-lactamase are more sensitive than to parent drug. AMP/SUL, AMO/CLAV not effective vs Pseudomonas	Ticarcillin/ Clavulanate 3.1g q4-6h IV Piperacillin/ Tazobactam 3.375g q6h IV Ampicillin/ Sulbactam 150-300mg q6h IV Amoxicillin/ Clavulanate 875/125mg bid PO or 500/125mg tid PO	These antibiotics should not be used for mono-microbial infections except when resistance to narrow spectrum antibiotics has been documented. Empiric therapy should be limited to compromised hosts (i.e. diabetics), mixed infections (i.e. bites), or severe life-threatening infections.
Cephalosporins 1st Generation	Staph except methicillin resistant, Strep except group D, P. mirablis, E. coli Shigella, Salmonella, anaerobes except Bacteroides	Cefazolin 0.5g-1.5g q6-8h IV/IM Cephalexin/ Cephradine 250-500mg q6h PO Cefadroxil 0.5-1.0g q12h PO	For Staph infections particularly of skin structures, oral semisynthetic penicillins are generally superior to oral cephalosporins. Cefazolin is empiric drug of choice for non-limb-/life-threatening community-acquired infections. It is also an excellent agent for prophylaxis during foot and ankle surgery.
Cephalosporins 2nd Generation	Less active against Staph than 1st generation. Otherwise same as 1st generation plus H. influenzae, Proteus, Morganella, Klebsiella, and some Bacteroides	Cefoxitin 1g q8h-2g q4h IV/IM Cefotetan 1-3g q12h IV, IM Cefuroxime 750-1500mg q8h IV/IM Cefaclor 250-500mg q8h PO Cefuroxime axetil 125-500mg q12h PO (500mg rarely needed) Loracarbef 400mg q12h PO	2nd generation cephalosporins have no significant advantages over 1st generation cephalosporins for treatment of lower extremity infections and should be limited to cases where they are more cost effective or as dictated by sensitivities.

Cephalosporins 3rd Generation	Decreased Staph coverage, increased gram negative coverage relative to 1st and 2nd generations. Gonococci.	Parenteral: Cefotaxime 1g q8-12h- 2g q6-8h IV Ceftizoxime 1g q8-12h-4g q8h IV Ceftriaxone 1-2g qd IV Ceftazidime l-2g q8-12h IV/IM (amt depends on soft tissue vs bone and joint) Cefaperazone 2g q12h- 4g q6h IV(max 8g qd, must use q6h for anti- pseudomonas) Oral: Cefixime 0.2-0.4g q12-24h Ceftibuten 0.4g qd Cefpodoxime 0.1-0.2g q12h Cefdinir 0.3g q12h	Cefotaxime/ Ceftizoxime in combination with clindamycin are excellent for diabetic foot infections. Ceftriaxone is the drug of choice for gonococcal septic arthritis. Ceftazidime is the most active against pseudomonas; can be used as a single agent or in combination with aminoglycosides or aztreonam. Increasing resistance occurring, use should be limited.
Cephalosporins 4th Generation	Increased Staph, Strep, Enterobacteriaceae, and N. gonorrheae coverage relative to 3rd generation. Pseudomonas resistance up to 50%.	Cefepime 1-2g ql2h IV	Cefepime should be reserved for infection where older agents are ineffective.
Imipenem/Cilastatin	Staph including inhibition of many strains of MRSA (MRSA activity is not dependable). Strep except for some strains of enterococcus. Gram negatives except for P. cepacia, Y. Maltophilia and Legionella. Anaerobes except C. difficile Cross-reactivity in 50% of pts with PCN anaphylaxis.	500 mg q6h IV	Drug of choice in life-/limb-threatening infections particularly in diabetics. Known to cause seizures in patients with history of seizures. Caution in renal failure and elderly. Treatment for multiple drug resistant organisms. Resistance of P. aeruginosa reported.
Meropenem	Aerobic gram neg increased over imipenem, staph/strep slightly decreased, anaerobes.	0.5-1.0g q8h IV	Known to cause seizures in patients with history of seizures. Caution in renal failure and elderly.
Ertapenem	MSSA, Strep, E. coli, H. influenzae, Klebsiella, Bacteroides (incl. B. frag)	1g qd IV, IM	Skin and skin structure. infections. MRSA and enterococcus are resistant.

Aztreonam	Gram negatives except P. cepacia, X. maltophilia, Legionella, and Acinetobacter. No gram positive or anaerobic activity.	1g q8h-2g q6h IV	In combination with clindamycin for diabetic foot infections in patients with penicillin or cephalosporin allergies. Severe gram negative infections.
Fluoroquinolones	Gram negatives except P. cepacia, X. maltophilia. Gram positive coverage is inconsistent. Poor activity against anaerobes.	Ciprofloxacin 500-750mg bid PO 200-400mg q12h IV Ofloxacin 200-400mg bid PO/IV Levofloxacin 250-500mg qd PO/IV Trovafloxacin 200mg qd PO/IV	May be useful against MRSA when used in combination with rifampin. Oral treatment for gram negative osteomyelitis including Pseudomonas. Use in combination with clindamycin for diabetic foot infections in PCN/ Ceph allergic patients. These antibiotics should not be used in empiric therapy except for life- or limb-threatening infections. Levofloxacin enhanced vs gram positive cocci Trovaflacin may worsen glycemic control
Metronidazole	Anaerobic bacteria	7.5mg/kg (~500mg) q6h (not to exceed 4g qd) IV. If life-threatening infection loading dose 15mg/kg IV 500 mg qid PO.	For lower extremity infections must be used with other agents because of narrow spectrum. Drug of choice for pseudomembranous colitis.
Clindamycin	Gram positive except enterococcus and MRSA. Anaerobes except C. difficile	600-900mg q8h IV or 150-450mg q6h PO	PO for mild infection (including diabetic wounds) in PCN/Ceph-allergic patients. IV - Excellent for staph osteomyelitis; use in combination with anti-gram negative drug in moderate to severe diabetic foot infections.

Vancomycin	Gram positive including MRSA, enterococcus. Resistant strains of enterococcus have become more common and some resistant strains of staph have developed.	15mg/kg q12h IV administered slowly. 125mg q6h PO for C. difficile only	Drug of choice for MRSA/MRSE. Nephrotoxicity can occur with elevated serum levels. Use with aminoglycoside for resistant strains of enterococcus (VRE). Monitor renal function closely when using this combination.
Rifampin	Staphylococcus. Mycobacteria in combination with other agents.	300mg bid PO	Combination therapy with quinolones, vancomycin, or trimethoprim/ sulfamethoxazole for MRSA/MRSE. Turns all body fluids red.
Trimethoprim/ sulfamethoxazole (TMP/SMX)	Bacteriostatic; Staph including some MRSA. Poor against Strep. Gram negative except P. aeruginosa and some Serratia.	TMP 160mg/SMX 800mg bid PO	Drug of choice for P. cepacia and X. maltophilia. Consider combining it with rifampin for MRSA.
Macrolides	Staph not MRSA/ MRSE Strep not enterococcus Some common gram negative	Erythromycin 250-500mg q6h PO or 15-20mg/kg IV(up to 4g/day) over 30 min. Azthromycin 500mg day 1, 250mg days 2-5 PO, 500g/day IV	Third line drugs for gram positive infections.
Linezolid	Staph (MRSA, VRSA), Enterococcus (VRE), Strep A, B, pneum	600mg q12h PO or IV 400mg q12h for skin inf that are uncomplicated	Reserved for serious infections with no alternate therapy, i.e. sepsis, skin and skin structure infections. Not approved for osteomyelitis treatment. Myelosuppression reported so must get weekly CBC.
Quinupristin/ Dalfopristin	Enterococcus faecium (VRE), MSSA, S. pyogenes. No activity	7.5mg/kg q8-12h IV for 21-72 days. Ratio Q:D (30:70)	Reserved for serious or life-threatening infection associated with VRE. Inhibits cyt against E. faecalis. P450 3A4 so may interfere with metabolism of other drug products associated with this.

| Tetracycline | Staph/strep except enterococcus; some gram negative and anaerobes Borrelia burgdorferi (Lyme disease), actinomyces, rickettsial diseases. | Tetracycline 250-500mg q6h PO 500-1000mg q12h IV Minocycline/doxycycline 100mg q12h PO | Third line drugs for gram positive infections. Useful for unusual infections of the lower extremity. |
| Aminoglycosides | Gram negative except for P. cepacia, X maltophilia, and Acinetobacter. Useful as synergistic agent with ampicillin for enterococcus. No anaerobic activity. | Loading doses: Gentamycin/ tobramycin 2mg/kg Maintenance doses: Gent 1mg/kg q8h Tobr 3-5mg/kg/d div q8h Amikacin 7.5mg/kg q12h Spectinomycin 2g q12-24h | Renal and ototoxic; must monitor peak and trough levels and adjust dose or dosing intervals accordingly. Because of toxicity these drugs should be used only for infection where no other agents are effective or where synergy against organisms that rapidly develop resistance is needed. |

A. All limb- or life-threatening infections should be hospitalized
   1. Medicine consult - all (may be a medical subspeciality, i.e, Diabetology)
   2. Infectious disease consult (may include physician with significant experience with lower extremity infections) if available in the community. If not available transfer to a tertiary care center should be considered
   3. Surgical consult - as indicated by the type and location of infection. (Diabetics tolerate surgery well—they do not tolerate undrained pus)
   4. Individuals with little or no experience in managing major infection should refer these patients

B. Immunocompromised patients should be considered for hospitalization if they are systemically ill, nutritionally compromised, or in the case of diabetics in poor control
   1. The patient's primary physician should be consulted in all these patients
   2. If the patient has no primary physician a medicine consult is indicated
   3. Individuals with little or no experience in managing infections in compromised hosts should refer these patients

IV. Antibiotic dosing

A. Patients with renal and hepatic disease often need dosage modifications

B. Patients on dialysis do not clear antibiotics; consider vancomycin and aminoglycosides and adjust doses based on blood levels at the time of dialysis

C. Antibiotics can interact with other medications

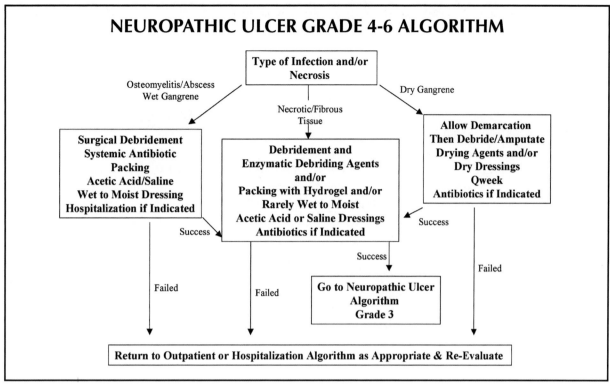

NEUROPATHIC ULCER GRADE 4-6 ALGORITHM

Figure 6.   Many patients presenting with grade 4-6 ulcerations will require hospitalization for initial therapy.

LOCAL WOUND CARE AND ADJUNCTIVE CARE

I.   **Wound care** (see Algorithms)
  A. **Goal-reduction microbial load in wound**
    1. Topical antibiotics are useful in reducing the bacteria counts in wounds. Some topical antibiotics may be as effective as oral antibiotics for mild localized infections in wounds
      a. The following comprises a list of five types of vehicles in order of occlusiveness from most to least: ointment > cream > emollient > liquid > powder. The amount of moisture in and around a wound affects the rate of healing. Ideally, wounds should be moist without causing maceration
      b. Silver: Broad spectrum inactivating almost all known bacteria. Different vehicles available for repeated applications or silver-coated dressings
      c. Cadexomer iodine: Slow, sustained release of iodine. Minimal tissue toxicity
    2. Antifungals - superinfection with fungi occur in compromised hosts and chronic broad-spectrum antibiotic use. A very small percentage of wounds are primarily fungal
      a. Systemic antifungals should be reserved for culture-proven infections
      b. Topical antifungals may be used empirically in wounds not responding to care
    3. Antiseptics are all toxic and should not be used in wounds
    4. Soaks are not recommended because of their potential to macerate, spread infections, and cause burns in neuropathic patients
    5. Potential complications to topical antimicrobial therapy include allergic reactions and delayed healing secondary to toxicity to tissue
  B. **Goal - remove necrotic tissue including hyperkeratosis**
    1. Surgical debridement is often necessary initially; excessive destruction of healthy tissue should be avoided

      a.   Laser has no advantage over conventional means and should be avoided because of cost

   2. Chemical debridement with silver nitrate, phenol, salicylic acid, for example, should be avoided except in cases where excessive granulation tissue is present. Care should be taken to limit their use to the areas where tissue reduction is required

   3. Topical enzymes can be useful to remove small amounts of fibrin or necrotic tissue. Collagenase and papain-urea are the only enzymes that have been demonstrated to be effective in this respect

      a.   Collagenase digests only collagen in necrotic tissue to prepare wound base for granulation tissue and epithelialization. It is neutralized by silver

      b.   Papain-urea. Enzyme derived from papaya with urea as reducing agent. Inactive against collagen. May complex with chlorophyllin and copper to promote collagen matrix structural integrity. This adds healing action to the debriding action of the papain-urea

   4. Mechanical debridement using scrubs can be effective. Non-toxic scrubs should be used, surfactant cleansers can be helpful in removing debris

      a.   Wet to dry dressings tend to cause tissue impairment through desiccation, cooling, and mechanical removal of granulation tissue and should be used cautiously

C. Goal - optimum temperature and humidity for cell function

   1. Occlusive membranes are effective in maintaining a moist warm environment. The major problem is maceration of the surrounding tissue that can be controlled with drying agents (i.e., gentian violet). Wounds treated with occlusive dressings should be cleansed prior to wound assessment to avoid confusing the breakdown products of the dressing with an infection

      a.   Absorptive dressings

          i.   Hydrogel. Keeps moist wound environment while absorbing up to five times its own weight (for moderately exudating wounds)

         ii.   Hydrocolloid. Maintains moist environment of wound while aiding in healing and exudate removal

       iii.   Alginate. For highly exudative wounds. Turns to stable gel with absorption of exudates

       iv.   Foams. Highly absorbent dressing generally made from hydrophilic polyurethane foam. For heavy exudate wounds, deep cavity wounds, packing to prevent premature closure to absorb exudate while maintaining a moist environment. May leave on for several days, comfortable

        v.   Absorbent combination dressings. Highly absorbent, nonadherent dressing. May be used wet, dry, or with a variety of topical agents

           (a) Hyaluronic acid - Reepithelialization agent

           (b) Collagen sponge

      b.   Silver-impregnated absorptive dressings

D. Goal - optimize nutrition of wound tissue

   1. Extrinsic/topical

      a.   Irritants that may promote granulation

          i.   Silver

      b.   Platelet healing factors

          i.   Platelet-derived growth factor

            (a) Fibroblast mitogen and chemoattractant

         ii.   Platelet-derived angiogenesis factor

            (a) Capillary formation

        iii. Platelet-derived epidermal growth factor
            (a) Mitogenic peptide involved in skin cell synthesis
        iv. Platelet factor 4
            (a) Neutrophil chemoattractant

    c. One or more of the platelet factors can be obtained through the following mechanisms: extraction from the patient's own blood, gel-based products, bioengineered tissues

2. Intrinsic

    a. Hyperbaric oxygen therapy (systemic) is probably helpful in a small group of patients with marginal blood flow. Local hyperbaric therapy is probably contraindicated since high surface oxygen can be toxic to tissue and since it tends to halt granulation tissue growth by reversing the oxygen tension gradient

    b. Revascularization
        i. Surgery
        ii. tPA
        iii. Clopidogrel, L-arginine

    c. Reversal of vasospasm
        i. Vasodilators

    d. Venous disease
        i. Compression is the cornerstone of treatment for venous ulcerations. Without surgical intervention and sometimes even with it, surgery patients will require compressive therapy for life to prevent recurrent ulcerations. Protect bony prominences—this may require extra padding. Instruct patient on correct usage.
            (a) Unna boots
            (b) Elastic wraps
            (c) Multilayer compression systems
            (d) Stockings
            (e) Compression boots
        ii. Surgical intervention to eliminate any incompetent venous perforators may be the best long-term solution for patients with recurrent or intractable ulcers

E. Goal – Re-epithelialization

1. Grafts can be useful particularly in non-weight bearing areas. They should be used as a last resort in weight-bearing areas

    a. Porcine
    b. Amnionic membrane
    c. Skin
        i. Split thickness
        ii. Full thickness
        iii. Flaps
        Can result in new nonhealing wound at donor site
    d. Cadaver skin
    e. Living skin substitutes-May close ulcerations faster than conventional therapy alone (compression, saline dressings, off-loading)
        i. Graftskin-epidermis and dermis
        ii. Human fibroblast-derived dermal substitute- dermis only

F. Goal - Pressure removal

1. Padding such as a felted foam post-op type shoe can be effective if the patient limits his or her activity and wears it all the time. Modified insoles in athletic shoes and felt pads adhered directly to the patient's foot can also be effective

   2. Cast boots and/or healing shoes with a removal plug system in the sole are useful
       provided that care is taken to identify the appropriate sites for pressure relief
   3. Casts should be used with care particularly in neuropathic patients due to the risk of
       creating new ulcerations. Cast should be avoided in patients with marked edema until the
       edema can be controlled
       a. Total contact casts are best. Only individuals with experience should apply them.
           Poorly applied casts can cause additional ulcers
   4. Non-weight bearing is the ideal way to treat ulcers. However it is almost never practical
       in practice. The following adjunctive methods should be encouraged to promote non-
       weight bearing
       a. Complete bed rest
       b. Crutches, walker, wheelchair

II. **Adjunctive therapies**
   A. **Goal - Optimize patient's health status**
      1. Appropriate nutrition is very important particularly in patients from a low socioeconomic
          background. Appropriate nutrition including diabetes control is as important as pressure
          removal in the treatment of ulcers. Vitamin and mineral supplementation should be
          considered in all patients. Protein supplementation in patients with renal disease should
          be approached with caution
      2. Systemic disease
          a. Optimize management
              i. L-arginine may be useful to improve blood flow (nitric oxide pathway)
              ii. Anodyne therapy using MIRE (monochromatic infrared energy) to close wounds,
                  increase circulation, decrease neuropathy (nitric oxide pathway)
          b. Eliminate imunosuppressing drugs where possible
      3. Patient compliance
          a. Patient education is the key to success
   B. **Tetanus prophylaxis**
      1. Recommendation by CDC for the following persons to be vaccinated:
          a. People traveling to a country where the risk for diphtheria is high (tetanus and
              diphtheria vaccines are usually given together)
          b. Persons requiring tetanus vaccine for prophylaxis in wound management
              (see Table 3)
          c. People who have not received at least three doses of tetanus vaccine in the past
          d. Pregnant women who have not received tetanus vaccine within the past ten years

III. **Evidence-based approach** - Essential for maximizing healing and minimizing complications.
     Improvement in healing rates and prevention while reducing costs of care can come from
     incorporating staff training, validated patient and wound assessment tools, and evidence-based
     treatment with a formulary of modern wound and skin care products

Table 3: Tetanus prophylaxis in wound management, adapted from MMWR 1991;40:1-28

History of adsorbed tetanus toxoid (doses)	Minor Clean Wounds		All Other Wounds[*]	
	TD[+]	TIG	TD[+]	TIG
Uncertain through 3[&]	No[@]	No	No[**]	No[**]

TD = Tetanus and diphtheria toxoids.

TIG = Tetanus immune globulin.

[*]Such as, but not limited to, wounds contaminated with dirt, feces, soil, and saliva; puncture wounds, avulsions, and wounds resulting from missiles, crushing, burns, and frostbite.

[+]For children <7 years old; DTP (DT if pertussis vaccine is contraindicated) is preferred to tetanus toxoid alone. For persons greater than or equal to seven years of age, TD is preferred to tetanus toxoid alone.

[&]If only three doses of fluid toxoid have been received, then a fourth dose of toxoid, preferably an adsorbed toxoid, should be given.

[@]Yes, if greater than ten years since last dose.

[**]Yes, if greater than five years since last dose. (More frequent boosters are not needed and can accentuate side effects.)

PREVENTION AND PRECAUTIONS

I. **Prevention**
   A. **Orthotics should be utilized for all patients in an attempt to redistribute the forces that caused the original ulcer.** Functional orthotics should be utilized where the causative factor appears to be dynamic forces. Accommodative orthotics should be used where direct pressure is the primary cause. Combination therapy (i.e., a functional orthotic and a metatarsal bar) is often necessary
   B. **Padding can prove useful in many cases such as digital ulcerations**
   C. **Shoes are a very important part of the equation.** Patients should never wear worn out shoes
      1. Running/walking shoes normally have soft uppers, good supportive soles, and ample toe room. Patients should be educated on shoe fitting. The most common misfit is a shoe that is too short and wide. If the shoe is too wide a narrower width, not a smaller size, is in order
      2. Extra-depth or molded shoes should be utilized whenever marked deformities or recurrent ulcers are present
   D. **Surgery should be considered for severe deformities, refractory ulcers, or recurrent ulcers**

II. **Universal precautions:** All patients are treated as if infected

OSTEOMYELITIS AND SEPTIC ARTHRITIS

I. **Classification**
   A. **Hematogenous**
   B. **Contiguous or direct extension from an existing wound**

  C. **Acute (initial)**
  D. **Chronic (recurrent)**

II. **Patient risk patterns**

   A. **Hematogenous osteomyelitis is much more common in children because of the anatomy of the vasculature surrounding open epiphyses**
      1. Elderly
      2. Septic arthritis - gonococcal in young adults
   B. **Contiguous osteomyelitis is more commonly seen in patients with the following:**
      1. Diabetes (most common cause in the foot)
      2. PVD
      3. Rheumatic disease
      4. Neoplastic disease
      5. Drug abuse
         a. Corticosteroids
         b. Antimetabolics
      6. Surgery
         a. Nail and bone at the same time (20.8% of infections)
         b. Implants (polymethylmethacrylate decreases PMN function)
      7. Open fractures

III. **Signs and symptoms**

   A. **Hematogenous**
      1. Abrupt onset pain, tenderness, and inflammation
      2. Elevated ESR, PMNs, and CRP
   B. **Contiguous**
      1. Pain, tenderness, and inflammation
      2. Sinus tract formation usually probes to bone with marked drainage

IV. **Radiology** (see Imaging chapter for additional information)

   A. **Plain radiographs**
      1. Lag 10 to 18 days
      2. Serial radiographs may be helpful in questionable cases
      3. Periosteal lifting, resorption of bone sequestrum, involucrum
      4. Joint effusion followed by destruction in septic arthritis
   B. **Scintigraphy**
      1. Tc^{99}
         a. Specific for bone
         b. Label WBCs
   C. **CT scan**
   D. **MRI with contrast is best**
   E. **Magnification views**

V. **Bacteriology**

   A. **Must culture bone/joint directly**
      1. Needle aspiration is more useful in septic arthritis
      2. Bone biopsy is the gold standard. Ideally bone should be sent for both culture/sensitivity

(aerobic, anaerobic, acid fast, and fungal) and pathology to confirm both that osteomyelitis is present and the organism. However, identifying the organism is the most important aspect of the biopsy

B. **Most common organisms**
1. Staphylococcus aureus, epidermidis, and streptococci
   a. 70-80% of cases
   b. S. epidermidis after implant (delayed)
2. Gram negative or mixed
   a. Compromised host (diabetic)
   b. After prophylaxis
3. Pseudomonas aeruginosa, < 10% of all cases
   a. Puncture wounds
   b. DM, PVD
4. Bacteroides
   a. DM, PVD

VI. **Treatment**

A. **Hematogenous**
1. IV antibiotics 4-6 wks followed by 2 months oral antibiotics
2. Surgical debridement sometimes necessary

B. **Contiguous**
1. Surgical debridement is cornerstone of treatment
2. Antibiotics as above unless entire infected bone is removed, in which case antibiotics can be discontinued as soon as soft tissue infection is resolved
3. Implanted material should be removed particularly if it is loose
4. Wound closure should be delayed or drains should be placed if wound is closed
   a. Polymethylmethacrylate impregnated with an aminoglycoside has been used in cases of osteomyelitis. However there is no documented advantage to this technique over systemic antibiotics with drains, ingress/egress systems, or open packing

BIBLIOGRAPHY

Boxer AM et al. Debridement of dermal ulcers and decubiti with collagenase. Geriatrics 24, 75-86, 1969.
Carek PJ. Diagnosis and management of osteomyelitis. Am Fam Phys 63, 2001.
Centers for Disease Control. Diphtheria, tetanus, and pertussis. Recommendations for vaccine use and other preventative measures: recommendations of the Immunization Practices Advisory Committee. MMWR 1991:40 (No. RR-10).
Centers for Disease Control. Sexually transmitted diseases treatment guidelines 2002. MMWR 2002:51 (No. RR-6).
Falanga V. Leg and Foot Ulcers: A Clinician's Guide. C.V. Mosby Co., St. Louis, 1995.
Falanga V. Classifications for wound bed preparation and stimulation of chronic wounds. Wound Rep Reg 8, 347-352, 2000.
Frykberg P. (Ed.) The High Risk Foot in Diabetes Mellitus. Churchill Livingstone, New York, 1991.
Gentzkow GD, et al. Improved healing of diabetic foot ulcers after grafting with a living human dermal replacement. Wounds 11, 77-84, 1999.
Gilbert DN, Moellering RC Jr, Sande MA. The Sanford Guide to Antimicrobial Therapy 2002. 32nd edition. Antimicrobial Therapy, Inc. Hyde Park, Vermont. 2002.
Joseph W. Handbook of Lower Extremity Infections. Churchill Livingstone, New York, 2002.
Joseph WS. Treatment of lower extremity infections in diabetics. Drugs 42:984-996, 1991.

Marcinko D. Infections of the Foot, Diagnosis and Management. C.V. Mosby Co., St. Louis, 1994.

Owens RC and Ambrose PG. Antibiotic therapy. Clinic use of the fluoroquinolones. Med Clin of NA 84, 2002.

Wright JB, Lam K, and Burrell RE. Wound management in an era of increasing bacterial antibiotic resistance. A
    role for topical silver treatment. Am J Infect Control 26, 572-577, 1998.

www.fda.gov.

Young G, Johnson, JD. An algorithmic approach to the diagnosis and management of lower extremity ulcerations.
    Lower Extremity 1:29-36, 1993.

Special thanks to Pippin, Max, Cheeky, Mara, and Bellaluna for their vast assistance in this project.

CHAPTER 15
INFECTIOUS DISEASE AND WOUND CARE OF THE LOWER EXTREMITY

1.   The most commonly seen organism(s) in diabetic foot infections is (are) as follows:

   A.   Gram positive cocci
   B.   Gram negative rods
   C.   Anaerobes
   D.   A & C
   E.   A, B, & C

2.   Drainage, swelling, color changes, AND pain are all clinical signs of:

   A.   ulceration
   B.   neuropathy
   C.   vasculitis
   D.   infection
   E.   none of the above

3.   Prednisone and other anti-neoplastic drugs should be discontinued or reduced when possible in infected patients because they are agents that:

   A.   increase the bioavailability of other antibiotics
   B.   suppress and mask infection
   C.   promote development of resistance to antibiotics
   D.   all of the above

4.   A patient with a non-infected, fibrotic, partial thickness venous stasis ulceration would BEST benefit from which of the following treatments:

   A.   Panafil, Duoderm and Unna's boot
   B.   Accuzyme and 4X4's
   C.   Unna's boot alone
   D.   Wet-to-dry dressings

5.   Of the following, which are classified as a bilayered living skin substitute:

   A.   Dermagraft
   B.   Apligraf
   C.   Allograft
   D.   Xenograft

6.   Goals in wound care include the following principles:

   A.   reducing the microbial load
   B.   removal of necrotic tissue, including hyperkeratosis and macerated tissue
   C.   maintaining optimum temperature, humidity and nutrition to maximize cell function
   D.   reepithelialization with off-loading of pressure
   E.   all of the above

7.   When considering empiric therapy for antibiotic coverage, the following principle does NOT apply:

      A.   use narrow spectrum antibiotics except in a limb or life threatening infection
      B.   a quinolone would be a good choice for a healthy patient with a simple foot infection
      C.   Imipenam and beta-lactamase antibiotics should be used in a compromised patient or a patient
            with limb or life threatening infection
      D.   very resistant organisms should not be considered when choosing empiric therapy unless the
            suspicion for these organisms is high

8.   The most common organism found in Osteomyelitis is:

      A.   Staphylococcus aureus
      B.   Pseudomonas aeruginosa
      C.   Bacterioides fragilis
      D.   All of the above
      E.   None of the above

9.   A penicillin-allergic, diabetic patient presents to your office having sustained a puncture wound on a rusty
      nail on the plantar aspect of his foot. Appropriate treatment(s) would include the following:

      A.   Assess tetanus status and treat with appropriate prophylaxis if necessary
      B.   Take radiographs to determine if foreign body is present
      C.   Begin antibiosis with Clindamycin + Levoquin
      D.   A & B
      E.   A, B, & C

10.   The patient above develops pseudomembranous colitis subsequent to antibiotic use. The drug of
      choice is:

      A.   Cefipime
      B.   Loperamide
      C.   Metronidazole
      D.   Imipenan
      E.   None of the above

SOFT TISSUE TUMORS AND SKIN NEOPLASMS

Larry R. Goss
John H. Walter

I. **Introduction to Soft Tissue Tumors**
   A. **Soft tissue tumor involvement of the foot and ankle region is a relatively common event when compared to their osseous counterparts**
   B. **Soft tissue tumors of the foot and ankle are much more likely to be benign than malignant (soft tissue sarcomas) (100:1) However, many times sarcomas are overlooked or mistaken as "simple lesions" when they do occur**
      1. For example, ganglion cysts occur so frequently in the foot and ankle that it has all too often led to the careless assumption that every asymptomatic, soft, movable mass represents a benign lesion
      2. Unfortunately, this lackadaisical confidence can lead to misdiagnosis and disaster in certain situations
      3. Although rare, some "simple lesions" may actually represent a malignant process that goes undiagnosed until skeletal metastasis occurs or amputation is required
      4. This undesirable tragedy could potentially propagate malpractice litigation against the treating physician for negligent care
      5. Therefore, proper identification and differentiation is required for appropriate treatment management
   C. **Evaluation of any foot and ankle soft tissue tumor should include a comprehensive patient history, systematic physical examination, essential laboratory studies and appropriate diagnostic studies**
   D. **Adherence to early treatment and management principles diminishes complications and optimizes clinical results**
   E. **If a lesion turns out to be malignant, serious consideration should be given for an oncology consultation**
   F. **Chapter is divided into four sections:**
      1. **Part I**: *Soft Tissue Tumors (benign and malignant)*
      2. **Part II**: *Epidermal (skin) Neoplasms (benign and malignant)*

3. **Part III**: *Metastatic Tumors*
4. **Part IV**: *Systemic Carcinoma*

II. **Soft Tissue Tumor Terminology**

   A. **Soft tissue tumor**: Enzinger and Weiss defined them as a swelling or tumefaction of non-epithelial extraskeletal tissue of the body exclusive of the reticuloendothelial system, glia, and supporting tissue of various mesenchymal (mesoderm) organs; more than 20 varieties are known to affect the foot and ankle areas; most common clinical presentation is soft-tissue swelling

   B. **Sarcoma**: A connective soft tissue neoplasm; usually malignant; formed by proliferation of mesodermal cells

   C. **Carcinoma**: Any of the various types of malignant neoplasms derived from epithelial tissue; occurs more frequently in the skin, glands, ducts and internal organs; identified histologically on the basis of invasiveness and the changes that indicate anaplasia

   D. **Carcinosarcoma**: A malignant neoplasm that contains elements of a carcinoma and sarcoma so extensively intermixed as to indicate neoplasia of epithelial and mesenchymal tissue

   E. **Neoplasm**: A term that refers to any new growth; an abnormal tissue that grows by cellular proliferation more rapidly than normal; continues to grow after the stimuli that initiated the new growth cease; usually a distinct mass of tissue which may be either benign or malignant; it may refer to relatively commonplace and generally harmless verrucae to devastating forms of cancerous tumors

   F. **Lesion**: Represents a pathological change of a neoplasm

   G. **Benign**: Denoting non-malignant characteristics of a neoplasm

   H. **Malignant**: A lesion that invades surrounding tissues; usually capable of producing metastases; may recur after attempted removal; may cause death of the patient unless adequately treated

   I. **Cancer**: General term frequently used to indicate any of the various types of malignant neoplasms; most invade surrounding tissues; potential to metastasize to various sites

   J. **Neoplasia**: Pathologic process that results in the formation and growth of a neoplasm

   K. **Anaplasia**: Loss of cell differentiation (e.g., the cells of the parenchymal tissue involved no longer resemble the original tissue from which they arose); a benign tumor may be well differentiated and, therefore, look almost exactly like the normal cells of origin; cellular function may also be considered in determination of differentiation

   L. **Metaplasia**: Adaptive response in which there is a change in the type of mature cells of a tissue that is not normal for that tissue but may not be abnormal in the strictest sense of the word; may occur in tissue repeatedly disturbed or irritated

   M. **Hyperplasia**: Represents an increase in the number of cells occurring in tissue during normal physiological processes as well as in abnormal responses to various hormonal stimuli; a normal response would be as in the menstrual cycle, when the lining of the uterus becomes enlarged

   N. **Hypertrophy**: An enlargement of a group of cells in response to stimuli (e.g., physical activity; hormonal cues, as in pregnancy); the size of the individual cells increases

   O. **Dysplasia**: A condition very closely related to hyperplasia that occurs when cells are found to be very different in shape, size, or character; often used to connote a change in the cells found in an area that is characteristic or implied to characterize a tendency toward malignancy; usually regarded as a reversible finding (e.g., the cells involved may return to a more normal appearance and functional state)

   P. **Metastasis**: Spread of cancerous cells distant to the primary site of a malignancy; the cells are not in contact with the primary site and the spread may occur through the lymphatics, hematogenously, or by direct implantation to a body cavity or surface; the hallmark of malignancy

III. Systematic Approach to Soft Tissue Tumors
A. Comprehensive history
1. NLDOCAT
   a. Nature
   b. Location
   c. Duration
   d. Onset
   e. Course
   f. Aggrevating factors
   g. Treatment
2. Past medical history
3. Family history
   a. Any family history of cancer
   b. Any family history of death caused by cancers
4. Social history
   a. Cigarette smoking
   b. Drug use
5. Review of systems
B. History of the lesion
1. When presented with a soft tissue tumor, the first step is to determine whether the lesion is benign or malignant
   a. Usually the initial presentation is a "bump" on the foot with some report of pain in shoegear or a limp during ambulation
2. Most soft tissue neoplasms involving the foot and ankle present earlier in their course than those with tumors at other sites in the body because of the relative thin soft tissues covering these areas
   a. Most small masses are usually easily palpable in the foot and ankle regions
   b. Dorsal neoplasms often produce symptoms because of pressure from shoegear, while plantar lesions are typically aggravated by weightbearing and ambulation forces
3. Documentation to determine duration of symptoms, rate of growth, and any associated pain is essential
4. Common clinical symptoms, such as pain, discomfort, tenderness and localized swelling may be secondary to mechanical obstruction of tightly bound gliding mechanisms of muscles, tendons and ligaments that encompass the foot and ankle areas
5. However, not all soft tissue neoplasms are painful or small
   a. Statements such as "benign lesions are painless" and "malignant lesions are painful" are grossly inaccurate
   b. Likewise, size is not a predictor of malignancy; a large tumor had to start out as a small lesion at one point
C. Exam of the lesion
1. Visual inspection of skin: observe for the ABCD's signs of melanoma
   a. Asymmetric lesion
   b. Irregular border: Cut out or scallop edge
   c. Variegated color: Various shades of brown, black, or other colors

       d.   Diameter greater than 5.0 mm
       e.   Elevated: Note whether nodular or raised lesion
       f.   Document rate of growth of the lesion

2. Palpation of soft tissue lesions
    a.   Is lesion fixed or mobile?
    b.   Document any attachment of skin, tendons, ligaments, fascia, or bone
    c.   Note consistency of lesion
    d.   Any pulsations within the lesion?
    e.   Any bogginess present?
    f.   Any pain or tenderness with palpation or ROM?
    g.   However, diagnosis based on palpation alone is notoriously unreliable
       i.   For example, the physical examination of a ganglion cyst may be soft, firm, or hard

3. Transillumination and auscultation can provide valuable information in the initial evaluation of fluid-containing and vascular lesions, respectively
4. A positive Tinel's sign may be present in association with peripheral nerve tumors
5. Diascopy of skin lesions is beneficial in certain circumstances
    a.   Involves the application of or pressing of a flat transparent glass on the skin to blanch away redness
    b.   Allows true color evaluation, as well as, helping to differentiate between purpura and vessel inflammation

PART I: SOFT TISSUE TUMORS

I. **Classification of Soft Tissue Tumors**

   A. **Current histological classification of soft-tissue tumors is based on the apparent differentiation of the tumor cell** (Table 1)

   B. **This table is based largely on the classification of soft tissue tumors by the World Health Organization, with subsequent modification as described by Enzinger and Weiss**

   C. **Lesions may arise from any of the mesenchymal tissues** (embryonic mesoderm) and are categorized according to their differentiated or adult histology

   D. **Tissue types include fibrous, vascular, neural, adipose, synovial, and muscular components**

   E. **However, this classification of soft tissue tumors does not imply that the histologic appearance of the tumor is related to the tissue of origin**

   F. **Most tumors arise from an undifferentiated precursor cell and acquire phenotypic traits of various normal cells during neoplastic transformation**

   G. **It is this appearance by which the tumors are classified rather than by the tissue of origin**

   H. **Tumors are classified as benign or malignant based on their perceived capability of metastasis**

   I. **Malignant tumors are subcategorized as low-grade or high-grade based on their histologic characteristics including tumor necrosis, cellular anaplasia, and the number of mitotic figures**

Table 1. Classification of Soft Tissue Tumors

Tissue Type	Benign	Malignant
Fibrous	Fibroma Plantar fibroma (Ledderhose's syndrome) Fibromatosis (desmoid) Xanthoma	Fibrosarcoma Malignant fibrous histiocytoma
Vascular	Glomus tumor Hemangioendothelioma Hemangioma	Angiosarcoma Malignant hemangioendothelioma Hemangiopericytoma
Neural	Neurilemoma (schwannoma) Neurofibroma Neurofibromatosis (von Recklinghausen's disease)	Neurosarcoma
Adipose	Lipoma Angiolipoma	Liposarcoma
Synovial	Ganglion cyst Synovial cyst Giant cell tumor of tendon sheath Pigmented villonodular synovitis Synovial chondromatosis	Synovial sarcoma
Muscle	Leiomyoma	Leiomyosarcoma Rhabdomyosarcoma
Miscellaneous	Tumoral calcinosis Myositis ossificans	Kaposi's sarcoma
Pseudotumors	Neuroma Hematoma formation Phleboliths Pyogenic granuloma Epidermal inclusion cyst Keloid	

II. Diagnostic Modalities

A. Standard Radiographs:

1. Are an extremely useful imaging modality for osseous neoplasms; however they are much less informative when dealing with soft tissue lesions
2. In spite of this fact, they should be the first imaging modality performed
3. An increased soft tissue density and volume may be appreciated
4. Presence of soft tissue calcification is an important diagnostic consideration in certain soft tissue lesions
5. Plain radiographs allow for visualization of concomitant osseous involvement, such as bony destruction, erosion, periosteal reaction or remodeling
   a. For example, pigmented villonodular synovitis frequently causes bony juxta-cortical bony erosions that are easily appreciated on plain films
6. Chest films are indicated for suspected metastasis

B. Ultrasonography:

1. Extremely helpful in differentiation of solid versus cystic (fluid-filled) lesions

    2. Fluid-filled lesions present as an anechoic mass or homogeneously black on ultrasound, while solid lesions typically appear as hypoechoic mass and purely cystic masses are not likely to be malignant

    3. It also can help determine the size and depth of the neoplasm

    4. Color Doppler ultrasonography has proven useful in demonstrating the vascular supply of certain vascular tumors, thereby eliminating certain lesions from a differential diagnosis

    5. Additionally, it can be used to constantly visualize the location of a percutaneous needle biopsy if neurovascular structures are in proximity

    6. Despite its value as a rapid and inexpensive diagnostic medium, ultrasound remains an underutilized modality in soft tissue tumor evaluation

C. Radionuclide Scans:

    1. Provides information regarding the intensity of uptake in a specific lesion

    2. Soft tissue lesions that show increased uptake may be benign or malignant; however, lesions that show no uptake on scanning are invariably benign

    3. Standard practice if skeletal metastasis is strongly suspected is a technetium 99m (^{99m}Tc) bone scan

D. Angiography:

    1. May provide information regarding proximity of lesions to neurovascular bundles; however, its role has been limited in soft tissue tumors by the advent of computed tomography (CT) and magnetic resonance imaging (MRI)

E. Computed Tomography (CT):

    1. CT can provide valuable information regarding calcification or ossification within the lesion and penetration into osseous structures of soft tissue lesions if present

F. Magnetic Imaging Resonance (MRI):

    1. For the vast majority of soft tissue tumors, MRI has become the imaging method of choice

    2. MRI provides superior soft tissue contrast, multiplanar images, eliminates ionizing radiation and defines marrow involvement if osseous extension is evident

G. New Technology:

    1. Recently, two new imaging techniques have evolved to show promise with soft tissue tumor identification

    2. One is called dynamic contrast-enhanced MRI and uses contrast material (gadolinium or gadopenteate dimeglumine) to provide excellent evaluation of anatomic localization in pre-operative surgical planning of soft tissue tumors

    3. The other is called positron emission tomography (PET), which uses 2-fluoro-2-deoxy-D-glucose molecule to enter tumor cells using glucose transporters

    4. These sophisticated scanning tests are primarily used to determine the stage of the tumor, response to therapy and monitor recurrence in difficult cases

H. Laboratory Screening:

    1. Standard screening with CBC and differential

    2. SMA panel or Chemistry 21 panel

    3. Carcinoma Embryonic Antigen

    4. Serum protein electrophoresis

    5. Immunologic studies

I. One must remember that despite the continuing advances in these diagnostic imaging studies, sometimes these techniques do not adequately distinguish between benign and malignant disease processes

J. Establishing a benign versus malignant diagnosis should definitively be made with histology examination of the tumor

K. Biopsy is the critical step in determining the nature of the tumor

L. It is recommended that all imaging and laboratory studies be performed prior to biopsy

III. Biopsy of Soft Tissue Tumors (non-epithelial lesions)

A. Introduction to Biopsy of Soft Tissue Tumors

1. Although a biopsy is considered simple practice, its significance should not be taken too lightly, and should be considered as an important surgical procedure
2. Biopsy is often used as a diagnostic tool, but in malignant lesions it is also used as part of the staging sequence
3. Biopsy is not technically demanding, however the planning for it is
4. Additionally, a "simple biopsy" is not without inherent risks and may result in tumor implantation and/or extension if the lesion turns out to be malignant
   a. For that reason, all biopsies carry the potential risk to a patient's limb or life
   b. Lesions at greatest risk are those in which a malignant diagnosis was not considered in the initial differential diagnosis
5. A physician must rely on clinical judgment, appropriate imaging techniques, laboratory studies, combined with patient history and physical findings to determine when to biopsy

B. Considerations for a Soft Tissue Biopsy

1. One must choose between closed biopsy (*needle aspiration or a percutaneous core needle*) versus an open biopsy (*excisional, incisional, or wide excision*) method
2. Technique is crucial and serious complications may result from an improperly or poorly executed biopsy
3. Consequently, all biopsies must be carefully planned and well-executed to minimize complications from poor incision placement, sampling error, inadequate tissue resection, and soft tissue implantation
4. It is essential to consider the surgical margins that may be needed for definitive treatment before the biopsy so that the incisions may be placed in a position to be completely excised as part of the specimen at final resection
5. Poorly planned or executed biopsies can result in misdiagnosis and a delay in treatment or overly aggressive treatment
6. Planning for a biopsy relies on the knowledge of the origin of soft tissue tumors and the ability to develop a differential diagnosis
7. A differential diagnosis guides the relative indication for a biopsy and the various possible definitive treatments of the tumors being considered
8. One must always consider the possibility a lesion is malignant so that the needle tracts or skin incisions from the biopsy do not interfere with possible future reconstruction

C. Closed Biopsy Techniques for Soft Tissue Tumors

1. Needle aspiration
   a. Is a beneficial diagnostic tool often used to differentiate fluid-filled (cystic) from solid lesions
   b. This requires a large-bore needle (18-guage) and lesions that do not yield fluid should be treated as potentially malignant in nature until proven otherwise
   c. Aspiration causes no morbidity if the lesion proves to be a ganglion cyst, and if the lesion is found to be solid, it may be treated as a needle tract site which can later be removed during biopsy
   d. Cautious aspiration of a suspected ganglion is an easy and acceptable method of verifying a supposed diagnosis, but if typical ganglion fluid is not obtained serious consideration should be given to the possibility of the lesion being a solid tumor

2. Percutaneous core needle biopsy
    a. Is commonly used for large soft tissue masses; however they are not routinely employed in the foot and ankle areas
    b. Most core needle biopsies are reserved for lesions with an obvious diagnosis from the staging studies
    c. Disadvantages of core needle biopsy techniques include the quantity of specimens obtained may not be sufficient for adequate diagnosis, inadvertent extension of the lesion by the depth of needle penetration or subsequent hematoma formation

D. Open Biopsy Techniques for Soft Tissue Neoplasms
1. For the vast majority of soft tissue tumors in the foot and ankle, open biopsy is the preferred method
2. However, each technique carries its own potential advantages and disadvantages
3. Excisional biopsy
    a. A technique of removing the entire lesion at the time of biopsy
    b. It should be performed for lesions that are assumed benign or small enough that they can be removed in toto with a small surrounding section of normal tissue
    c. In the foot and ankle, it is generally reserved for lesions less than 3.0 cm
    d. Advantages of excisional biopsy include: removes the entire lesion, avoiding potential seeding, and increases diagnostic accuracy because of the larger sample size
    e. It serves as adequate treatment for small benign or low-grade malignant lesions
4. Incisional biopsy
    a. Involves directly cutting into the lesion to remove a sample without excising the entire lesion
    b. It is preferred for larger lesions (greater than 3.0 cm) or possibly malignant lesions that would require undue sacrifice of normal tissue to achieve a wide margin with the biopsy
    c. A disadvantage is potential implantation of tumor cells
5. Wide excision biopsy
    a. Involves removal of the entire lesion while excise a large portion of normal, healthy tissue
    b. Surrounding rim of the tumor is attached and left undisturbed with the resection
    c. This technique is used only when malignancy is highly suspected and when the risk of contaminating major neurovascular structures is great
    d. Disadvantages of this of biopsy technique often include major functional and cosmetic defects
    e. This is the most aggressive biopsy technique and should be used with caution in light of the fact the patient may be better served with a functional amputation and fitted prosthesis
6. A multidisciplinary approach involving primary care physician, surgeon, pathologist, internist, oncologist, and plastic surgeon is essential in difficult cases

E. Important Technical Points for a Successful Biopsy of Soft Tissue Neoplasms
1. It is recommended that biopsies be performed under tourniquet control but without exsanguination and should be deflated prior to wound closure
2. Biopsy incisions should be made longitudinal where possible
3. One should avoid unnecessary dissection to prevent potential implantation
4. Do not violate anatomic compartments other than those containing the tumor
5. Do not expose or contaminate important vascular or neural structures
6. Hemostasis should be obtained prior to closure and a drain be used if necessary
7. If used, the drain site should be positioned so that it may be excised at definitive surgical

resection

8. Do not use widespread infiltration of local anesthetic around the lesion or place sutures at a distance from the wound

9. Major vascular bundles and tendon sheaths should be avoided because of the potential for spread

10. Frozen-section histologic confirmation should be obtained from all lesions suspected of malignancy at their biopsy

IV. **Staging of Benign Soft Tissue Lesions** (non-epithelial neoplasms)

    A. **Pre-operative staging of lesions provides a basis for definitive surgical treatment and long-term prognosis**

    B. **Staging combines radiographic, histologic, and clinical data to categorize tumors**

    C. **Enneking has devised both benign (*Table 2*) and malignant staging systems**

    D. **Benign soft tissue tumors are classified into three stages based on latent, active and local aggressive growth, respectively**

Table 2. Enneking Classification for Benign Soft Tissue Tumors

STAGE	ACTIVITY LEVEL	EXAMPLES
Stage 1	Lesions are latent or inactive (static) and usually have no clinical symptoms.	Lipoma, Ganglionic cyst, Fibroma
Stage 2	Lesions are active growing and are associated with clinical symptoms.	Xanthoma, Glomus tumor, Neurilemoma, Neurofibroma
Stage 3	Lesions are locally aggressive, histologically immature and show progressive growth that is not limited by normal anatomic boundaries.	Hemangioma, Plantar Fibromatosis, PVNS

V. **Staging of Malignant Sarcomas**

    A. **Staging and grading of sarcomas is performed to act as standard for physicians all across the United States**

    B. **It serves as a basis for determining prognosis and treatment protocols**

    C. **The most commonly used prognostic variables for extremity soft tissue sarcoma are histologic grade, tumor size, tumor depth, compartment status and the presence or absence of metastases**

    D. **Different groupings of these characteristics define the most commonly used staging systems for soft tissue sarcomas**

    E. **The Enneking Surgical Staging System (SSS) is the most commonly used (*Table 3*)**

        1. Soft tissue sarcomas (malignant) are graded into low-grade (Stage I) and high-grade (Stage II) tumors

            a. **G1** = low grade

            b. **G2** = high grade

        2. They are based on histologic appearance coupled with diagnostic imaging characteristic and anatomical location

            a. **T1** = intracompartmental

            b. **T2** = extracompartmental

        3. Sarcomas with the presence of distant metastasis are considered Stage III

            a. **M0** = no distant metastasis

            b. **M1** = any regional or systemic metastasis

    F. **Sarcomas unlike carcinomas disseminate almost exclusively through the blood**

    G. **If a malignant sarcoma is suspected, a consultation or referral with a musculoskeletal oncologist is highly recommended**

Table 3. Enneking Surgical Staging System for Malignant Soft Tissue Sarcomas

STAGE	STAGE DESCRIPTION	GRADE	ANATOMICAL SITE	METASTASIS
IA	G1, T1, M0	Low	Intracompartmental	None
IB	G1, T2, M0	Low	Extracompartmental	None
IIA	G2, T1, M0	High	Intracompartmental	None
IIB	G2, T2, M0	High	Extracompartmental	None
III	Any G, any T, M1	Either	Either	Present

  V. Additional Staging Classifications of Sarcomas

    A. **There are three other commonly employed staging systems for sarcomas**

    B. **Each classification and staging system is not perfect, as various tumor types are more difficult than others to stage and grade**

    C. **Additionally, the less differentiated the cells, the more difficult it becomes to classify**

    D. **First is called *The Union Internationale Contre Cancer* and uses a TNM system**

      1. **Cancers are graded as T for tumor, N for lymph nodes, or M for metastasis**

    E. **Second is the *American Joint Committee on Cancer Staging Manual (AJCC)* considers in each stage the size of the primary tumor as well as nodal and metastatic spread (Table 4)**

      1. This staging of cancers is considered to be based on a system that looks at the size of a tumor

        a. **T1** = small size (< 5 cm); T1a is superficial to fascia; T1b is deep to fascia

        b. **T2** = large size (> 5 cm); T2a is superficial to fascia; T2b is deep to fascia

      2. Lesions are staged according to there histologic grade

        a. **G1** = well differentiated

        b. **G2** = moderately differentiated

        c. **G3** = poorly differentiated

        d. **G4** = undifferentiated

      3. Determine whether there is any lymph node involvement

        a. **N0** = no regional lymph node spread

        b. **N1** = regional lymph node metastasis

      4. Presence of metastasis

        a. **M0** = no systemic metastasis

        b. **M1** = systemic metastasis

Table 4. American Joint Committee on Cancer Staging

STAGE OF TUMOR	STAGE DESCRIPTION	TUMOR DESCRIPTION
IA	G1-2, T1a-1b, N0, M0	Low grade, small, superficial or deep tumor
IB	G1-2, T2a, N0, M0	Low grade, large, superficial tumor
IIA	G1-2, T2b, N0, M0	Low grade, large, deep tumor
IIB	G3-4, T1a-1b, N0, M0	High grade, small, superficial or deep tumor
IIC	G3-4, T2a, N0, M0	High grade, large, superficial tumor
III	G3-4, T2b, N0, M0	High grade, large, deep tumor
IV	Any G, ant T, N1 or M1	Any metastasis

A. Memorial Sloan-Kettering Cancer (MSK) Center System

1. Simplest staging classification (Table 5)
2. Assigns stage based on accumulated number of favorable or adverse prognostic factors
3. Favorable factors include:
   a. Low grade
   b. Small size (< 5 cm)
   c. Superficial location of tumor (above fascia)
   d. No lymph node involvement
   e. No metastasis
4. Adverse factors include:
   a. High grade tumor
   b. Large size (> 5 cm)
   c. Deep location (below fascia)
   d. Presence of lymph node involvement
   e. Presence of metastasis

Table 5. Memorial Sloan-Kettering (MSK) Cancer System

STAGE	DESCRIPTION OF TUMOR
0	No adverse factors
1	One adverse factor
2	Two adverse factors
3	Three adverse factors
4	Any metastasis

VII. Definitive Management of Soft Tissue Lesions

A. Definitive treatment for both benign and malignant soft tissue tumors is surgical resection

B. Clinical success rates are directly related to the adequacy of the surgical margins (Table 6)

C. Extent of surgical margin is determined by the type and stage of the lesion

D. Surgical resection is also determined by the anatomic location and the estimated disability from the resection

E. Most benign stages 1 and 2 soft tissue lesions are generally treated by marginal excision if this can be achieved without sacrifice of vital structures

F. Benign stage 3 and malignant stage I (low-grade sarcoma) soft tissue lesions typically require wide margins for definitive treatment

G. If there is involvement of adjacent tendons, neurovascular structures, and bone, wide excision may sacrifice too much tissue to leave a functional foot and ankle

H. Because of the disability that would result from achieving an appropriate surgical margin, an amputation will not only achieve the desired margin but also offer the best method of reconstruction and rehabilitation

I. Most malignant stage II (high-grade sarcoma) lesions and all malignant stage III lesions require margins that require radical resection or amputation as definitive treatment

J. Occasionally, malignant sarcomas may benefit from adjunct radiation or chemotherapy. For this reason, a referral to a musculoskeletal oncologist is highly suggested

Table 6. Surgical Margins

Surgical Technique	Surgical Pathology	Recommended Stage
Intralesional	Removal of the lesion from within the reactive pseudocapsule	Rarely utilized
Marginal	Removal of the lesion by dissection around the outside of the pseudocapsule (may leave microscopic disease)	Stage 1 and 2 lesions
Wide	Removal of the lesion (and biopsy tract site) with a modest amount of normal tissue so that the reactive pseudocapsule is not exposed	Stage 3 lesions Low-grade malignant
Radical	Removal the entire anatomic compartment(s) containing the lesion (may include amputation)	High-grade malignant

BENIGN SOFT TISSUE TUMORS

I. Soft Tissue Lesions

A. Mesenchymal (mesoderm origin) (see Table 7)
1. More than 20 varieties known to affect the foot and ankle areas
2. Most common clinical presentation is soft-tissue swelling
3. Many are asymptomatic and painless
4. See Table 7 for the summary of the most common to affect the foot and ankle

MALIGNANT SARCOMAS

I. Types

A. Malignant fibrous histicytoma (MFH)
1. MFH is the most common soft tissue sarcoma
2. Basic cellular elements of MFH includes fibroblasts and histiocyte-like cells
3. Lesions are either solitary or multinodular and can be mistaken for a hematoma especially where there are areas of hemorrhage superficial to the tumor

B. Epithelioid sarcoma
1. This is a small tumor of uncertain histiognesis that tends to occur in the hand and forearm regions of adolescents and young adults
2. This lesion has a high propensity for lymph node involvement
3. Tumor usually arises in the deep soft tissues and presents as a firm nodular mass

C. Fibrosarcomas
1. Extremely rare tissue sarcoma
2. Usually arises from fascial or aponeurotic structures of the deep soft tissues
3. Classified by level of differentiation
4. Higher potential for metastasis
5. Usually larger than plantar fibromatosis
6. Generally painless until late in the course
7. Seventy percent found in extremities with the majority in the lower extremity
8. Rarely affects the foot and ankle
9. Incidence may be greater in area of irritation
10. Microscopic view demonstrates reticular fibers increasingly pleomorphic and possibly mixed with malignant spindle cells
11. Treatment is amputation

Table 7. Summary of Common Benign Soft Tissue Tumors in the Lower Extremities

Type of Tumor	Clinical Description and Common Characteristics	Imaging Features	Treatment Options	Recurrence Rates
Lipomas	Lipomas may occur in the soft tissue, muscle, tendon sheaths or bone. The mass is soft, non-tender, mobile, and usually asymptomatic unless it compresses neural structures. Most lipomas of the foot are slow growing, located in the subcutaneous tissue and are usually solitary. They frequently occur in obese, post-menopausal women along the anterolateral aspect of the ankle, but may occur anywhere in the foot and ankle. Commonly they occur with patients with hypercholesterolemia.	Radiographs may reveal a well-marginated, fat-like density with possible calcification secondary to fat necrosis. MRI is diagnostic and shows a well-defined lesion with the same density as normal fat.	Treatment consists of observation or marginal excision if symptomatic.	Low with extremely little chance for local recurrence (less than 5%).
Angiolipoma	These tumors are composed of mature fat with multiple vascular channels. They are usually subcutaneous, well encapsulated, movable, less than 2.0 cm in size, and exquisitely tender to palpation. Rarely do they occur before puberty.	An angiogram or MRI image may show the tortuous blood vessels as seen in hemangiomas.	Because of its infiltrative nature, marginal excision is more difficult to treat than simple lipomas.	Associated with a higher recurrence rate than with simple lipomas (30%).
Hemangiomas	Benign vascular tumors believed to represent hamartomatous malformations of normal vascular tissues or benign neoplasms. Most are soft, compressible and subcutaneous in location. Tumors can be of the cavernous, capillary, or mixed type, with the port-wine capillary hemangiomas being most common in the foot. Hemangiomas generally arise in childhood and adolescence. When these tumors are superficial, a noticeable bluish discoloration is observed, associated with a soft, doughy mass. More extensive lesions may have associated localized gigantism of adjacent bone and soft tissue. Hemangiomas may be seen in conjunction with dyschondroplasia, also known as *Maffucci's syndrome*.	Plain radiographs characteristically show multiple small calcified phleboliths. Other imaging studies, such as MRI, CT, angiography can further identify the hemangioma's anatomic extent.	Best treated based on symptomatology. NSAIDs have been found useful, as have compression stockings, which in some early presentations have led to partial involution. Surgical resection should be reserved for those cases that cause significant functional disability.	Because of these lesions' infiltrative nature and lack of a pseudocapsule, marginal excision is associated with a high local recurrence rate.
Glomus Tumor	Glomus tumors arise from the hemangiopericyte, a cell type seen at the periphery of the capillary vascular network. They are extremely painful benign vascular tumors that have their peak incidence in the 20 to 40 year-old age range. They represent less than 2% of soft tissue tumors. If glomus tumors are subungual in location, they are associated with a female predominance of 3:1. These tumors typically present with a bright-red to bluish discoloration and are associated with intense, lancing pain that worsens with cold exposure or direct pressure. They are usually less than 1.0 cm in diameter and commonly found beneath the nail bed.	Radiographs may show a well-marginated bony erosion over the dorsal surface of the distal phalanx in long standing cases (20%).	Treatment involves marginal excision for this benign lesion. In any lesion found under the nail, the possibility of malignant melanoma should always be considered in the pre-operative differential diagnosis.	Pain relief is dramatic after primary marginal excision. Recurrence is low (less than 10%).
Fibroma	Fibroma is a soft tissue lesion composed of dense mature fibrocytes. It usually occurs around fibrous structures and fascial planes, may be noticed at any age, and is usually asymptomatic. This entity has a much different prognosis and should be distinguished from plantar fibroma and fibromatosis (desmoid).	Ultrasound is diagnostic and reveals a hypoechoic mass.	If symptomatic, marginal extra-capsular excision is easily accomplished.	Has an extremely low recurrence rate.
Plantar Fibromatosis (Ledderhose's syndrome)	Usually presents as a solitary lesion or multiple nodules, occurring most often along the medial and central band of the plantar fascia. It occurs more often in adolescents and young adults. Males are twice as likely to develop these lesions. Lesions are typically unilateral (75%) which are firm and fixed to the plantar fascia. They may produce discomfort with weightbearing because of the irregular contour of the plantar surface in the arch of the foot, however most lesions are asymptomatic. Growth is usually slow and stops once the lesion reaches a size of approximately 3.0 cm. Local adherence to the overlying skin is a common characteristic. Nodules consist of a hyperplasia of fibroblasts embedded within the plantar aponeurosis. Older patients may have associated palmer (*Dupuytren's disease*) contracture of the hands or penile (*Peyronie's disease*) fibromatosis. Although no specific staging study helps to separate this benign disease from its malignant counterparts, the location along the medial and central border of the plantar fascia makes the diagnosis clinically quite evident. Certain systemic conditions are associated with a higher incidence: epilepsy, alcoholism, hypothyroidism and DM.	MRI images reveal that the lesion is not encapsulated but well circumscribed. MRI reveals that the tumor is typically of low signal on both T1- and T2-weighted images because of the large collagen content. Fat saturation images are helpful in distinguishing more aggressive lesions.	Asymptomatic individuals require observation and no treatment. Symptomatic patients should be given a persistent trial of non-surgical therapy, including padding, shoegear modification and non-steroidal anti-inflammatory drugs. Attempted surgical resection is reserved for problematical cases. If excision is to be undertaken, a radical resection with a significant amount of normal appearing plantar fascia is recommended.	Because the lesion may extend into the dermis and skin as well as the underlying fascia, it may be difficult to obtain satisfactory surgical margins. Accordingly, the recurrence rate after marginal excision is quite high and sometimes rapid. However, metastasize is unlikely.
Fibromatosis (desmoid)	Fibromatosis (**desmoid**) is distinguished from plantar fibroma by its different anatomic site, more aggressive clinical course, more aggressive pathologic characteristics, and different response to treatment. It is more frequently encountered in and around the large muscles of the proximal portions of the extremities and the trunk. It may be present in the foot as a soft tissue mass deep in the plantar arch and not superficial as is a plantar fibroma. Fibromatosis grows actively and occasionally rapidly, producing a mass of considerable size.	MRI reveals that the tumor is typically of low signal on both T1- and T2-weighted images because of the large collagen content.	Radical excision is the treatment of choice. Adjunct treatment in the form of radiation therapy is often considered. Estrogen blockade or chemotherapy may be considered in selected circumstances.	Intermediate recurrence (20%). Amputation may be required after multiple recurrences. Radiation has decreased recurrence rates.
Ganglion Cyst	Most patients are between 20-40 years old and present with a lesion of varying size that is usually painless. Females are 3 times more likely to develop them. Aspiration with a large-bore needle (18-guage) is diagnostic. Fluid is clear yellow and viscous. Ganglionic fluid is the product of mucoid degeneration in an area of the joint capsule or tendon sheath. Ganglia may remain stationary, increase in size, or spontaneously rupture and disappear. Ganglion cysts may occur at any location in the foot and ankle, but most commonly arise from the dorsal surface. They are the most common soft tissue tumor in the foot and ankle. They often occur is close apposition to tendons or joints.	Plain radiographs are usually of little benefit unless underlying arthritic changes are seen in the joint adjacent to the lesion. CT and MRI can identify the well-defined reactive pseudocapsule with decreased density within the lesion.	Treatment is usually reserved for symptomatic cases that produce mechanical pain or irritation of neural structures. Marginal excision is usually curative if the entire cyst wall with surrounding degenerative capsular or tendon sheath is removed.	Although aspiration is an excellent diagnostic tool for verification, a 70%-80% rate of recurrence is common. Recurrence rates with local excision is less than 10%.
Neurilemoma (schwannoma)	Neurilemoma (**schwannoma**) is a benign tumor of nerve sheath origin (Schwann cell) with a peak incidence in the fourth and fifth decades of life. No predilection toward either gender is shown. The tumor is usually solitary, less than 2.0 cm, well encapsulated, and on the surface of a peripheral nerve. Patients present with a painful nodule associated with a positive Tinel's sign in the distribution of the nerve affected.	MRI scan often shows that this tumor is of very bright signal on T2-weighted images and is usually homogeneous. These are usually stage 2 benign lesions.	Marginal excision is usually curative. The tumor is shelled out of the nerve sheath without damage to the nerve fibers themselves.	Recurrence is rare, and little malignant potential exists.
Neurofibroma	Neurofibromas are slow growing spindle cell tumors of peripheral nerves that may be solitary or multiple. Ninety percent are solitary and usually located in the dermis or subcutaneous tissue. Ten percent	Diagnosis is usually based on history and physical examination. However, it is	Marginal resection usually is required and removal of affected portions of the	Recurrence may occur and 10% of patients with Recklinghausen's

Table 7 – continued

	of cases are associated with von Recklinghausen's disease and present with multiple lesions that may be associated with scoliosis, localized gigantism, or tibial pseudoarthroses. Neurofibromas are the most common tumor of neurogenic origin. They are stage 2 benign lesions and diffusely invasive, permeating between nerve fibers with no clear plane of dissection.	often difficult to distinguish from a neurilemoma.	nerve as well. Must choose between the disability caused by the lesion and that which will result from resection.	disease may develop into neurosarcomas.
Pigmented villonodular synovitis	PVNS is defined as a benign inflammatory condition of unknown etiology. PVNS may occur as two forms, either localized (nodular) or diffuse. Localized form consists of a discrete mass that usually arises from tendon sheath, also known as *giant cell tumor of tendon sheath*. The more devastating is the diffuse form that often occurs around joints but may also occur around the sheath of tendons and bursae linings. PVNS presents as an intermittent monoarticular swelling, with minimal discomfort, and without a history of antecedent trauma. Joint aspiration reveals bloody or brownish fluid and does not appreciably reduce the swelling because of the residual capsular thickening. PVNS rarely involves the foot and ankle (less than 3%). Histological examination reveals synovial hyperplasia, increased number of histiocytes, giant cells, fibroblasts and lipid-laden macrophages (foam cells) within a fibrous stroma.	Radiographic findings are variable, and longstanding involvement may show bone juxta-cortical erosions, lack of hypertrophic callus formation, absence of calcification and degenerative changes within the affected joint. MRI demonstrates the heterogeneity of the lesion. Angiography typically reveals increased vascularity to the lesion.	When the lesion is symptomatic or has radiographic evidence of progressive joint destruction, synovectomy is the treatment of choice. Synovectomy can be performed arthroscopically or open depending on the location and extent of involvement. En bloc resection is an alternative in severe cases with bone loss.	Risk of recurrence vary with the lesion's stage but is extremely common (40%) and often disabling. Radiation therapy has been used as an adjuvant for recurrences and when surgical intervention is contra-indicated.
Synovial chondromatosis	Results from chondral metaplasia within the synovial tissue. This tumor has a peak incidence in 3rd decade of adult life with a male predominance. This tumor may cause numerous cartilaginous bodies within a joint, bursa, or tendon sheath, or it may be solitary. On gross examination, multiple cartilaginous and osteocartilaginous nodules are embedded in the synovium, often with additional free loose bodies in the joint. Microscopically these nodules are composed of cartilage with varying degrees of calcification or ossification and may have atypical cytology that should not be misinterpreted as low-grade chondrosarcoma. Greater than 50% of cases occur around the knee, but synovial chondromatosis may also occur in and around the ankle.	Radiographs may show variable amounts of speckled calcifications depending on the maturity of the lesions, and often more disease is present than radiographs indicate because of numerous uncalcified nodules. Persistent, longstanding synovial chondromatosis leads to severe degenerative arthritis.	Treatment consists of synovectomy and removal of the extruded, loose cartilaginous bodies from the joint. Arthroscopic excision is often difficult.	Recurrence after marginal excision and synovectomy is common. Various isolated case reports of sarcomatous transformation exist.
Leiomyoma	Benign soft tissue tumor originating in smooth muscle. They present as a well localized, slow growing mass, causing paroxysmal pain. In long standing conditions, they may calcify. Most lesions are located on the dorsum of the foot. Men and women are equally affected and the majority of patients are in their 4th decade at diagnosis.	Radiographs may reveal a calcific lesion if present. MRI reveals a homogenous mass with the same consistency as muscle.	Treatment consists of wide excision.	Recurrence or malignant transformation is rare.
Xanthoma	Xanthomatous deposits may develop in tendons as an expression of essential familiar hypercholesterolemia. A common site is the Achilles tendon. Clinically it presents as a painful fusiform swelling, which may suggest an inflammatory synovitis. The slowly enlarging swelling is firm and moves with the tendon.	MRI reveals fusiform enlargement, increased intra-tendinous signal represented by linear strand-like heterogeneity with well-defined margins of lesion.	Treatment should be symptomatic. Debulking of the tendon has been reported to reduce pain but is technically difficult.	Intermediate recurrence (less than 15%).

D. Liposarcoma

1. Origin: Fat tissue
2. Found in deep planes
3. Not considered a malignant degeneration
4. Pseudoencapsulated
5. Lobulated like fat
6. Predisposed to lung metastasis
7. Common in lower extremities
8. Treatment by wide excision

E. Rhabdomyosarcoma

1. This is a common myogenic tumor (Striated muscle tumor)
2. It is usually found in the thigh, shoulder, and upper area of adult patients.
3. Various types:
   a. Adult form
   b. Young adult form
   c. Child form
4. The most common malognant sarcoma in children less than 15
5. Disorganized myoblasts and myofibrils
6. May rapidly invade locally
7. High potential for metastasis
8. Predisposed to lung metastasis
9. High percentage of lower-extremity lesions

10. Diagnosis is often late
11. Alveolar form in young adults: Very aggressive, with rapid mitotic alveolar appearance
12. Treatment is by amputation
13. Entire treatment team, including prosthetist, psychologist, and radiologist

F. Leiomyosarcoma
1. Origin: smooth muscle, usually in stomach or uterus
2. Solid tumor
3. Sharp-edged appearance, "cleaved"
4. Blunted nuclei
5. Anaplastic
6. Cellular material: Bizarre and interwoven
7. Frequently found in extremities
8. Very aggressive with lung metastasis

G. Clear cell sarcoma
1. This is a small and rare neoplasm arising from tendons or aponeuroses
2. Clear Cell Sarcomas occur most frequently (50%) around the foot and ankle in persons between 20 and 40 years of age
3. About half of these lesions contain melanin
4. Lymphatic as well as hemotogenous spread occurs (so regional lymph nodes must carefully be examined for any enlargement)

H. Hemangioendothelioma
1. Malignant endothelium
2. Usually in deep tissue structures
3. Rarely occurs in the lower extremity
4. Very aggressive with intimate access to bloodstream

I. Hemangiopericytoma
1. Pericytes
2. Normal endothelial lining
3. Painless compared to glomus tumor
4. Generally a local malignancy

J. Lymphangiosarcoma
1. Primarily in the upper extremity
2. Rarely in the lower extremity
3. May be associated with post-mastectomy

K. Neurofibrosarcoma (NFS)
1. These are malignant tumors of peripheral nerves
2. They account for about 10% of all sarcoma
3. Fifty percent of these are associated with von Recklinghausen's Disease
4. Unlike other sarcomas, NFS presents with neurological symptoms, such as, pain and paresthesia

L. Synovial sarcoma
1. Synovial sacromas are deep seated, well-circumscribed, multinodular, firm tenosynovial tumors that occur predominantly in the flexor aspect of the extremities close to joints
2. Although these tumors are of a synovial origin, they do not arise from joints
3. They occur in younger age groups than other sarcomas, with a propensity for the distal portions of the lower extremity (25% occur in the foot and ankle)
4. Radiographs often show small calcifications with a soft tissue mass; this is diagnostic finding

5. All synovial sarcomas are considered to be high grade

M. Kaposi sarcoma

1. Current evidence suggests that Kaposi's sarcoma is a viral-associated, if not viral-induced, tumor (may be associated with a retrovirus)
2. It has a predilection for the skin of the hands and feet, particularly the great toe
3. The lesions present as flat, pink patches that slowly enlarge, becoming blue-violet and papular in appearance
4. Violaceous nodule(s) that begin to merge may grow rapidly and become tuberous
5. Associated with HIV-positive status
6. They are often associated with edema secondary to lymphatic obstruction
7. Often presents initially on lower extremity
8. The microscopic findings are variable
9. Early lesions may show a proliferation of miniature vessels that are so bland that they resemble normal capillary or lymphatic endothelium
10. The more advanced stages demonstrate a characteristic spindle cell component but are typically devoid of pleomorphism and significant miotic activity
11. As for treatment, surgery is no longer indicated except for tissue diagnosis
12. Radiation and chemotherapy are the preferred therapies
13. Staging of Kaposi's sarcoma provides a means of comparing treatment protocols

PART II: SKIN NEOPLASMS

I. Biopsy for Epidermal Lesions

A. Which Lesions to Biospy?

1. Lesions which are not well defined
2. Established efficacy of a therapeutic procedure
3. To establish a diagnosis of benign versus malignant

B. Types of Skin Biopsy Methods

1. Punch: preferred size is 2-6 mm in diameter
2. Shave (scissor): is reserved for elevated lesions or those in which a more complex technique is not warranted
3. Curettage
4. Incisional
5. Excisional

C. Important Technical Points for Biopsy of Skin Lesions

1. Tourniquet control is not usually used for purely epidermal lesions
2. Do not use widespread infiltration of local anesthetic directly around the lesion or place sutures at a distance from the wound
3. A working differential is extremely important as the kind, type and depth of appropriate biopsy will change
4. For a punch biopsy, the skin should be stretched taut perpendicular to relaxed skin tension lines before the punch is made
5. A punch biopsy is inadequate for pathological processes of fat such as morphea, erythema nodosum, and scleoderma
6. A punch biopsy of less than 4.0 mm is inadequate for inflammatory conditions
7. Excisional biopsy when possible is always preferred for small lesions
8. Incisional biopsy for large lesions is acceptable

9. Processes in the deep to lower dermis require scalpel incisional biopsy
10. Shave or curettage biopsies are never appropriate for suspected malignant lesions
11. Areas of excoriation, rubbing and the application of medications should be avoided
12. Biopsies are typically placed in 10% neutral buffered aqueous formalin for transportation to a laboratory

BENIGN SKIN LESIONS

I. **Benign Vascular Lesions**
   A. **Hemangiorna** (vascular nevus)
      1. Congenital, localized vascular lesions of the skin and subcutaneous tissue that generally involute or disappear with time
   B. **Nevus flammeus** (port wine stain)
      1. Flat, pink, red, or purple as a result of vascular ectasia
      2. Often facial and will not disappear
      3. May indicate Sturge-Weber syndrome
   C. **Capillary hemangioma** (strawberry mark)
      1. Bright red
      2. Appears after birth
      3. Involutes in a few years
      4. Generally best to leave untreated, as treatment causes scarring
   D. **Raised cavernous hemangioma**
      1. Red or purple lesion
      2. Large vascular bed
      3. Will have venous or arterial shunts
      4. Will not disappear
      5. Treatment: Specific to site
   E. **Venous stasis**
      1. In differential for various lesions
      2. Chronic hyperpigmented areas around ankle and lowerleg's frequent site of ulceration; ulcers most often seen on the medial ankle
      3. Treated with elevation and compression
   F. **AV malformations:** (AV fistula)
      1. Any abnormal communication between an artery and vein
      2. Can be a large warm mass under on the skin if it is superficial
      3. May also result from a wound or from an aneurysm
      4. Can be very serious causing ischemia

II. **Differential Diagnosis for Benign Skin Neoplasms**
   A. **Moles, pigmented nevus** (nevi)
      1. Flesh color, brown, wart-like, or hairy, and black on a stalk: very common; almost everyone has one or more
      2. Must be observed for change
   B. **Skin tags**
      1. Usually on neck, axilla and groin
      2. Pigmented or unpigmented stalks of skin

3. Not painful unless irritated
4. Best treated with freezing or excision

C. Seborrheic keratoses
1. Stuck-on lesions
2. Found in middle-age and older people
3. Usually appear flat
4. Brown, black, or flesh color
5. Size varies
6. On trunk or temple area of face

D. Dermatofibroma (histiocytoma)
1. Firm, red or sometimes brown papule
2. Found on the lower leg
3. Generally present as small, stalked or nodular, asymptomatic solitary lesions
4. Composed of fibroblastic tissue

MALIGNANT SKIN LESIONS

I. **Describing Pigmented Lesions of the Skin**

A. **ABCD's of melanomas:** Asymmetry, border irregularity, color variation, and diameter change
   1. Asymmetrical lesion
      a. Determine whether shape is symmetric
      b. Determine whether elevation from surrounding tissue is present or whether the underlying tissue is nodular or distorted
   2. Border irregularity
      a. Determine whether border is irregular or there is scalloping of edges
      b. Describe the shape (e.g., oval, round, stellate)
   3. Color variation or variegation
      a. Determine whether color is consistent throughout lesion
      b. Determine whether color has changed recently
      c. Determine whether there is more than one color
      d. Determine whether there is increased or decreased pigmentation
      e. Determine whether pigment appears to be leaking at edges
   4. Diameter enlargement
      a. Size: Measure exact diameter in mm
      b. Any lesion greater than 5 mm should be biopsied

II. **Common Features of Melanomas**

A. **Usually greater than 6.0 mm in greatest diameter before clinically evident as a melanoma**

B. **Lesions are all asymmetrical; you can not bisect the lesion anywhere to make two mirror images**

C. **Varying degree of pigmentation throughout the lesion with varying shades of tan to brown to black in early lesions;** red, white and blue in later lesions

D. **Border irregularity**

E. **Elevation or enlargement is usually present**

F. Each has the ability to metastasize to any organ system, including the brain and heart

G. Metastasis occurs through the lymphatic vessels to regional lymph nodes and through blood vessels

H. Incidence is higher in patients with fair complexion, red hair, blue eyes, feckles and poor tanning ability who live in areas where solar exposure is high

III. Malignant Melanoma

A. Many types of melanoma exist

B. Increases in the incidence of melanoma in the United States are anticipated owing to various factors

C. Socially, the U.S. population glorifies a "tan" appearance, which may be aesthetically pleasing but is a major factor in development of melanoma

D. Melanoma is a skin disease that can be fatal; although it is easily detected and is preventable, it has become endemic to the United States and, therefore, requires adherence to strict surveillance methods

E. There are five types of malignant melanomas, however only four types that frequently present in the lower extremity

1. Superficial spreading melanoma (SSM)
   a. Incidence: Most common form of melanoma in "fair" skinned people typically seen in the late fourth or early fifth decade of life
   b. Etiology: Predisposing or pre-existing nevus (or nevi), relative number of "sunburns" in early adolescence and pre-adolescence, or inability to tan
   c. Appearance: Usually a slow growing, flat papule or plaque that generally is variegated in color, ranges from 0.5 to 25 mm in size, frequently is asymmetric, and generally presents as only one lesion
   d. Location: Look at legs, trunk, and back as well as total body in surveillance of all skin surfaces
   e. Prognosis: Best of any of the melanomas (5 year survival rate of 95% if diagnosed early)

2. Nodular melanoma
   a. Incidence: Second most common melanoma; typically more common in males (2:1); occurs most often in the fifth or sixth decade
   b. A very fast-growing nodular event that occurs in a period of 3 months to 2 years
   c. Patient reports the sudden appearance of a "bump" that started to grow recently
   d. Appearance: An elevated, dark blue, brown, or black nodule that is 1.0 to 3.0 cm or larger if untreated, is almost spherical, and generally smooth; the appearance may be distorted in individuals that have bumped or rubbed the area
   e. Does not have a horizontal growth phase, starts vertically from the beginning
   f. Treatment: Best possible method of biopsy: total excision of the lesion
   g. Must be biopsied to rule out all other diagnoses (e.g., hemangioma)
   h. May be confused with a pyogenic granuloma
   i. Prognosis: Most malignant of any melanoma because depth tends to be deeper

3. Acral lentiginous melanoma
   a. Incidence: Rare, but may be seen during an initial examination as an incidental finding
   b. Etiology: Most commonly affects Japanese and African-American descent; one of the most common melanomas in people with darker skin tones; rarely found in fair-skinned individuals

    c.   Location: Frequently affects the soles, palms and toes, especially the nail unit
    d.   Appearance: Flat, hyperpigmented (black or brown) lesion sometimes described as a spill, or spreading stain, on the skin of the palm or sole
         i.   Its black/blue appearance is not raised, although its invasiveness under the surface is often underestimated and may be extensive
        ii.   May present as an extensive surface lesion which may occupy as much as 12.0 cm
      iii.   Grows much more slowly than other melanomas
      iv.   Subungual lesions appear as a macular, irregular, laterally growing area of pigmentation in the nail (melanonychia) and surrounding tissues
       v.   Leakage of pigment proximally away from the nail fold is called the *"Hutchinson sign"* and should be considered diagnostic
    e.   Location: Great toe are the most frequently involved sites
    f.   Treatment: Amputation if present in the digit
    g.   Prognosis: Poor prognosis because often diagnosed in later stages however, extremely rare recurrence if amputation performed

4.   Amelamotic melanoma
    a.   Incidence: Rare form of melanoma found in people 30-80 years of age; somewhat more common in women
    b.   Etiology: Sun exposure may be the primary cause
    c.   The lesion may have been present for years and is, therefore, mistaken for other non-malignant lesions (e.g., histiocytoma, dermatofibroma)
    d.   Appears as either a macular or a nodular lesion that may or may not be pigmented, sometimes looks blue or blue-gray; usually is solitary and found in an area of tanning

5.   Lentigo melanoma
    a.   Incidence: Least frequent type of melanoma in the lower extremity
    b.   Etiology: Develops from lentigo maligna, the in-situ form
    c.   Location: Not very common in the foot and ankle, most commonly affects the face and upper extremity; sun-exposed parts of the body

IV. General Principles Regarding Management of Malignant Melanomas

A. Excisional biopsy when possible is preferred
B. Incisional biopsy for large lesions is acceptable
C. Shave or curettage biopsies are never appropriate
D. Ulcerated or vegetative lesions have a much poorer prognosis
E. For biopsy surgery, only small margin of normal skin is required
F. For definitive surgery, margin size is determined by lesion depth
G. Excision surgery should be oriented parallel to direction of lymphatic drainage
H. Pigmented bands in nails must be biopsied at the matrix level
I. In general, start with 3.0 cm margin, adding 1.0 cm more for each millimeter of depth

V. Classification of Melanomas

A. Classification of epidermal lesions by level of invasion (*Clark's classification*), or tumor thickness (*Breslow's classification*) are used to set criteria for treatment and prognosis
B. Clark's classification system has become widely accepted and is based on level of invasion
   1.   Level 1: Lesion is confined to the epidermis (< 0.6 mm invasion)
   2.   Level 2: Lesion extends beyond the epidermis and 1 mm into the papillary dermis (up to

0.6 mm)
3. Level 3: Lesion extends to the junction of the papillary and reticular dermis (up to 1.7 mm)
4. Level 4: Lesion invades the reticular dermis (deep as 3.3 mm)
5. Level 5: Lesion invades into the subcutaneous fat layer, (depth of up to 7 mm)
C. **Breslow's classification: based on tumor thickness (depth)**
1. Method of prognosticating based on actual depth in millimeters of extension into the skin
2. Thought to be more reliable and reproducible than Clark's levels

VI. Basal Cell Carcinoma

A. **Most common form of skin cancer, including morpheaform ulcerative with cerutive, nodular, and pigmented lesion forms**
B. **Generally seen in white-skinned individuals with poor ability to tan**
C. **Lesion may be a papular or a nodular translucent area**
D. **There is a pigmented form that may be confused with a nodular melanoma; the lesion is a firm, round to oval area about 2-3 cm in size**
E. **There are cicatrizing and superficial, multicentric forms**
F. **Treatment: Excision**

VII. Squamous Cell Carcinoma

A. **A lesion epithelial keratinocytes, therefore, can be found in skin or mucous membranes**
B. **Etiologies: Several suspected, but sun exposure may be the most important**
C. **Predisposing factors: White skin and a poor ability to tan; exposure to carcinogens**
D. **Many types of lesions classified for in situ squamous cell carcinoma:** Solar, ionizing radiation-induced, arsenical, Bowen's, erythroplasia of Queyrat, and several other forms; these lesions may develop as indurated plaques or as nodules

VIII. Bowen's Disease

A. **In situ squamous cell carcinoma that presents at the junction of skin a mucocutaneous region**
B. **Appears as a longstanding, sometimes crusted, nodular plaque; on debridement, a dull red and moist surface is noted;** may be seen alone or in a group; the dermis is invaded, but the basement membrane is not involved
C. **Noted for its ability to become highly aggressive**

PART III: METASTATIC TUMORS

I. Definition

A. **Lesions that are discontinuous from the primary site, which is a proof of malignancy, benign lesions do not metastasize, although they can locally invade adjacent structures**
B. **Spread of cancerous cells distant to the primary site of a malignancy**
C. **The spread may occur through the lymphatics, hematogenously, or by direct implantation to a body cavity or surface; the hallmark of malignancy**

II. Routes of Metastasis

A. **Direct extension**
   1. Tissue invades other structures immediately adjacent to it
B. **Lymphatic**
   1. Spread to sites of regional lymphatic drainage
C. **Hematogenous dissemination**
   1. Arterial
   2. Venous
   3. Vascular tumors, which increase likelihood of metastasis through a blood-borne route
   4. Local invasion into vasculature permits dissemination
D. **Some types of malignant lesions exhibit specific patterns for sites of metastasis**

III. Primary Tissue Sources of Metastatic Lesions

A. **Connective tissue lesions**
   1. Chondrosarcoma
   2. Fibrosarcoma
   3. Liposarcoma
   4. Myxosarcoma
   5. Osteosarcoma
B. **Blood vessels**
   1. Angiosarcoma
C. **Lymphatic**
   1. Lymphangiosarcoma
D. **Synovial**
   1. Synovial sacroma
E. **Lining of body cavities**
   1. Mesothelioma
F. **Blood cells**
   1. Various tissue; myelogenous leukemia, malignant lymphoma and Hodgkin's disease
G. **Muscle cells**
   1. Smooth muscle; leiomyosarcoma, rhabdomyosarcoma
H. **Squamanous cells**
   1. Simple carcinoma
I. **Basal cells**
   1. Basal dermal layer
J. **Glands and ducts**
   1. Adrenocarcinoma
K. **Liver**
   1. Hepatoma
L. **More than one cell type neoplasm**
   1. Wilms tumor (renal)
M. **More than one cell type from more than one germ layer**
   1. Immature teratoma

PART IV: SYSTEMIC CARCINOMA

I. **Introduction**

A. **Although metastatic carcinoma is the most common malignant tumor of bone, it is seldom found distal to the knee**

B. **There are few common, or directly related, symptoms of systemic carcinoma in the foot**

C. **There are, however, some instances in which the foot and lower extremity may reflect the manifestations of end-organ damage and concomitant processes**

D. **Some of these entities may demonstrate themselves as an obstruction of vascular supply, as changes in bone composition or density, or as changes in the appearance of the skin**

E. **Of the five carcinomas most likely to metastasize to bone** (lung, breast, prostate, kidney, thyroid), *bronchogenic carcinoma* of the lung is most common to occur below the knee

F. **If another primary lesion is found in a metastatic location distal to the knee, the primary carcinoma often has already metastasized to the lung**

G. **Treatment to prevent pathologic fracture or for palliation is indicated to maintain quality of life**

II. **Vascular Changes Associated with Cancer**

A. **Obstruction of arterial flow**
   1. Pain, paresthesia, pallor, pulselessness, and paralysis (5 P's, as in compartment syndrome)
   2. Enlarging abdominal organ blocks the artery
   3. Disseminated intravascular coagulation (DIC) associated with cancer of the prostate, lung, or stomach
      a. Occurs by inappropriate activation and resultant exhaustion of most available clotting components
      b. Emboli form uses up platelets and fibrin
      c. Fibrin-destroying mechanisms exacerbate problem

B. **Obstruction of venous flow**
   1. Also obstructed by tumor mass
   2. Trousseau's syndrome of migrating thrombophlebitis, associated cancer of the pancreas, or lung thrombosis repeatedly recurs in extremities
   3. May be due to hypercoaguable state from substances released by tumor

C. **Obstruction of lymphatic flow**
   1. Obstruction often owing to tumor growth
   2. Obstruction resulting from metastasis along nodes
   3. Must differentiate among infection; Milroy's disease, which is present from birth; and lymphedema praecox, which is associated with females age 10-25 years who have progressing edema in the foot

D. **Vascular tumors**
   1. Benign
      a. Hemangioma
      b. Granuloma pyogenicum
      c. Vascular ectasias
      d. Glomus tumor
   2. Malignant
      a. Angiosarcoma
      b. Kaposi's sarcoma
      c. Hemangiopericytoma
   3. Other neoplasms that are not strictly malignant but affect vessels directly (e.g., hemangioendothelioma, epithelioid hemangioendothelioma) may also be considered

E. Carcinoma of the pancreas
  1. Unusual polyarthritis in the lower extremity that develops in some individuals who have pancreatic cancer
  2. Often mimics erytherma nodorsum in that it will cause subcutaneous nodules and fat necrosis
  3. Early on, the disease will not respond to non-steroid anti-inflammatory drug therapy as will other forms of arthritis

F. Metastatic cancers of the liver
  1. Obstruction of the major ducts and deterioration of liver function manifest themselves with yellow jaundice pruritus over the body, including the lower extremity
  2. Edema resulting from large shifts in proteins may also occur

G. Gardner's syndrome
  1. Age 20-30 years
  2. Rectal bleeding and diarrhea
  3. Tetrad of anomalies: Polyposis of the colon, osteomas, fibromas, and subcutaneous skin lesions
  4. Most common site: Mandibular bone and skull
  5. In feet, involves the tubular bones, dense lobulated and with a thick periosteal reaction

H. Prostatic cancer
  1. Induced postrenal disease
  2. Changes in serum creatinine, BUN, and potassium levels may induce coarse muscular twitching
  3. May cause neuropathic disease or cause cramps in the lower extremity
  4. In worsening renal disease, there may be a uremic frost where crystals have deposited on the skin
  5. Pruritus may be intense

REFERENCES

Akerman M, Rydholm A, Persson BM. Aspiration cytology and soft tissue tumors. The 10-year experience at an orthopaedic oncology center. Acta Orthop Scand 56:407, 1985.

Allard, MM, Thomas RL, Nicholas RW: Myositis ossificans: an unusual presentation in the foot, Foot Ankle Int 18:39, 1997.

Aluisio FV, Mair SD, Hall RL: Plantar fibromatosis: treatment of primary and recurrent lesions and factors associated with recurrence, Foot Ankle Int 17:672, 1996.

American Joint Committee on Cancer - Soft Tissues. In: Fleming ID, Cooper JS, Hensen DE, et al., eds. American Joint Committee on Cancer (AJCC) Cancer Staging Manual, 5th ed. Philadelphia: Lippincott-Raven, 149, 1997.

Ballo M, Zajars G, Pollack A, et al. Desmoid tumor: prognostic factors and outcome after surgery, radiation therapy, or combined surgery and radiation therapy. J Clin Oncol 17:158, 1999.

Barbella R, Fox IM: Recurring desmoid tumor of the foot: a case study, Foot Ankle Int 17:221, 1996.

Begin LR, Guy P, Mitmaker B: Intramural leiomyosarcoma of the dorsal pedal vein: a clinical mimicry of ganglion, Foot Ankle 15:48, 1994.

Berlin S, Binder D, Emiley T, et al.: Leiomyoma of the foot: A review of the literature and report of cases. JAPA 66:450, 1976.

Bernstein KE, Lattes R. Nodular (pseudosarcomatous) faciitis, a non-recurrent lesion: clinicopathologic study of 134 cases. Cancer 49:1668, 1992.

Cohn DL, Judson FN: Absence of Kaposi's sarcoma in hemophiliacs with the acquired immunodeficiency syndrome, Ann Intern Med 101:401, 1984.

Crist W, Gehan E, Rajeb A, et al. The third intergroup rhabdomyosarcoma Study. J Clin Oncol 13:610, 1995.

Curtin JW: Fibromatosis of the plantar fascia: surgical technique and design of skin incision. J Bone Joint Surg 47A:1605, 1965.

Davis JL, Russell RD, Giacopelli JA: Calcific leiomyoma: A unique case report. JAPMA 85(2):96, 1995.

Eary JF, Conrad, EU, Brucker JD, et al: Quantitative [F-18] fluorodeoxyglucose positron emission tomography in pre-treatment and grading of sarcoma. Clin Canc Res 4: 1215-1220, 1998.

Enneking WF, Spanier SS, Goodman MA. A system for the surgical staging of musculoskeletal sarcomas. Clin Orthop 153:106, 1980.

Enneking WF. Musculoskeletal Tumor Surgery. New York: Churchill Livingstone, 1983.

Enzinger FM, Weiss SW: Soft Tissue Tumors. St. Louis: Mosby, 1995.

Fornage BD: Soft tissue masses: The underutilization of sonography. Semin Musculoskel Radiol 3:115-133, 1999.

Fortin PT, et al: Malignant melanoma of the foot and ankle, J Bone Joint Surg 77A:1396, 1995.

Friedman RJ, et al: Malignant melanoma in the 1990's: the continued importance of early detection and the role of physician examination and self-examination of the skin, J Am Cancer Soc 41(4):201, 1991.

Geschickter CF: Tumors of the peripheral nerves. Am J Cancer 25:377-410, 1935.

Gibbs CP, Peabody TD, Mundt AS, et al.: Oncologic outcomes of operative treatment of subcutaneous soft-tissue sarcomas of the extremities. J Bone Joint Surg 79A:888, 1991.

Gibbs CP, Peabody TD, Simon MA: Mini-symposium: Soft tissue tumors of the musculoskeletal system: classification, clinical features, preoperative assessment, and staging of soft tissue tumors, Current Orthopaedics 11:75, 1997.

Giraldo G, Beth E, Buonaqurao FM: Kaposi's sarcoma: a natural model of interrelationship between viruses, immunologic responses, genetics, and oncogenesis, Antibiot Chemother 32:1, 1984.

Giulano AE, Eilber FR: The rationale for planned reoperation after unplanned total excision of soft tissue sarcomas. J Clin Oncol 3:1344, 1985.

Hajdu S: Peripheral nerve sheath tumors. Cancer 72:3549, 1993.

Harrelson JM: Tumors of the foot. In Jahss MH, editor: Disorders of the foot and ankle, ed 2, Philadelphia, WB Saunders, 1991.

Harwood A: Kaposi's sarcoma in renal transplant patients. In AIDS: the epidemic of Kaposi's sarcoma and opportunistic infections, New York, 1984.

Hruban R, Shiu M, Senie R, Woodruff J: Malignant peripheral nerve sheath tumors of the buttock and lower extremity. A study of 43 cases. Cancer 66:1253, 1990.

Johnson MR. Epidemiology of soft-tissue and bone tumors of the foot. Clin Pod Med Surg 10(4):581, 1993.

Johnston JO: Tumors and metabolic disease of the foot. In Mann RA, editor: Surgery of the foot and ankle, ed 6, St Louis, Mosby, 1992.

Jones FR, Soule EH, Coventry MD: Fibrous xanthoma of synovium, J Bone Joint Surg 51A:76, 1969.

Kaufman SL, Stout AP: Histocytic tumors (fibrous xanthoma and histiocytoma) in children, Cancer 14:469, 1961.

Kransdorf MJ, Jelinek, JS, Moser RP: Imaging of soft tissue tumors. Radiol Clin North Am 31:359-372, 1993.

Laredo JD: Percutaneous biopsy of primary soft tissue tumors. Semin Musculoskel Radiol 3:139-144, 1999.

Leeson MCF, Smith MJ: Ewing's sarcoma of the foot, Foot Ankle 10:147, 1989.

Levey DS, Park YH, Sartoris DJ, Resnick D: Imaging methods for assessment of pedal soft-tissue neoplasms. Clin Pod Med Surg 10(4):617, 1993.

Mankin HJ, Mankin CJ, Simon MA: The hazards of biopsy, revisited: Members of the Musculoskeletal Tumor Society. J Bone Joint Surg Am 78:656-663, 1996.

Math KR, et al: Spindle cell lipoma of the foot: a case report and literature review, Foot Ankle Int 16:220, 1995.

Mathews RS, Hart JL: Benign synovioma (pigmented villonodular synovitis), Surg Forum 26:513, 1975.

McNeill TW, Ray RD: Hemangioma of the extremities: a review of 35 cases, Clin Orthop 101:154, 1974.

Mullins F, Beard CW, Eisenberg SH: Chondrosarcoma following synovial chondromatosis, Cancer 18:1180, 1965.

Mykre-Jenson O: A consecutive 7-year series of 1,331 benign soft-tissue tumors: clinicopathologic data and comparison with sarcomas. Acta Orthop Scand 52:287, 1981.

Nishiyama Y, Yamamoto Y, Toyama Y, Satoh K, Ohkawa M, Tanabe M: Diagnostic value of T1-201 and three-phase bone scintigraphy for bone and soft tissue tumors. Clin Nucl Med 25:200-205, 2000.

Peabody TD, Gibbs CP, Simon MA: Evaluation and staging of musculoskeletal neoplasms. J Bone Joint Surg 80A:1204, 1998.

Peabody TD, Monson D, Montag A, et al.: A comparison of the prognosis for deep and subcutaneous sarcomas of the extremities. J Bone Joint Surg 76A:1167, 1994.

Pearlston D, Pisters P, Bold R, et al. Patterns of recurrence in extremity liposarcoma. Cancer 85:85, 1999.

Pontious J, Good J, Maxiam SH: Ganglions of the foot and ankle: A retrospective analysis of 63 procedures. JAPMA 89(4):163, 1999.

Potter GK. Evaluation of a patient with a pedal neoplasm. Clin Pod Med Surg 10(4):609, 1993.

Rao V, Weiss S: Angiomatosis of soft-tissue: an analysis of the histologic featues and clinical outcome in 51 cases. Am J Pathol 16:764, 1992.

Rydholm A, Berg NO: Size, site, and clinical incidence of lipoma: factors in the differential diagnosis of lipoma and sarcoma. Acta Orthop Scand 54:333, 1983.

Rydholm A, Gustafson P, Rooser B, et al.: Subcutaneous sarcoma: A population-based study of 129 patients. J Bone Joint Surg 73B:662, 1991.

Sanders SM, Mandracchia VJ, Kimball DA, Rissman LJ. Pigmented villonodular synovitis: A literature review and usually case report. Clin Pod Med Surg 19:4, 541, 2002.

Schwartz H, Unni K, Pritchard D: Pigmented villonodular synovitis: A retrospective review of affected large joints. Clin Orthop 247:243, 1989.

Schwarzbach MH, Dimitrakopoulou-Strauss A, Willeke F, et al: Clinical value of [18-F] fluorodeoxyglucose positron emission tomography imaging in soft tissue sarcomas 231:380-386, 2000.

Seale KS, et al: Soft tissue tumors of the foot and ankle, Foot Ankle 9:19, 1988.

Shapeero LG, Vanel D, Verstragte KL, et al: Dynamic contrast-enhanced MR imaging for soft tissue sarcomas. Semin Musculoskel Radiol 3:101-113, 1999.

Singer S, Baldini E, Demetri G, et al. Synovial sarcoma: prognostic significance of tumor Size, margin of resection and mitotic activity for survival. J Clin Oncol 14:1201, 1996.

Skrzynski MC, Biermann JS, Montag A, Simon MA. Diagnostic accuracy and charge-savings of outpatient core needle biopsy compared with open biopsy of musculoskeletal tumors. J Bone Joint Surg 78A:644, 1996.

Smith M: Glomus-cell tumor in the lower extremity: report of two cases, J Bone Joint Surg 53A:157, 1971.

Sober AJ: Cutaneous melanoma: opportunity for cure, J Am Cancer Soc 41(4):197, 1991.

Springer KR. Synovial chondromatosis. J Foot Surg 30(5):446, 1991.

Tighe C, Lynn JA: Angiolipoma of the foot: A review of the literature and case report. JAPMA 84(2):85, 1994.

Walling AK, Gasser SI: Soft-tissue and bone tumors about the foot and ankle, Clin Sports Med 13:909, 1994.

Walter JH, Galitz J, Robertson DW: Pigmented villonodular synovitis pedal manifestations. JAPMA 84:574, 1994.

Wapner KL, et al: Fibromatosis: a review of primary and recurrent surgical treatment, Foot Ankle Int 16:548, 1995.

Wu KK: Ganglions of the foot. J Foot Surg 32(3):343, 1993.

Yu GV, Sellers CS: Extensive lipoma of the foot: A case report. JAPMA 85(9):488, 1995.

CHAPTER 16
SOFT TISSUE TUMORS AND SKIN NEOPLASMS

1.   What is the ratio in the foot and ankle of benign soft tissue tumor compared to malignant ones?

    A.   10:1
    B.   50:1
    C.   100:1
    D.   1000:1

2.   What is the general term for any new growth of a lesion that may represent either benign or malignant forms?

    A.   Lesion
    B.   Neoplasm
    C.   Hypertrophy
    D.   Metaplasia

3.   What is the term that represents the hallmark of malignancy?

    A.   Metastasis
    B.   Dysplasia
    C.   Hyperplasia
    D.   Anaplasia

4.   A diagnosis of a soft tissue lesion can usually be made on palpation alone.

    A.   True
    B.   False

5.   Ultrasonography is helpful in differentiating solid versus cystic lesions.

    A.   True
    B.   False

6.   Which biopsy technique removes the entire lesion?

    A.   Excisional
    B.   Incisional
    C.   Wide resection
    D.   Both A and C

7.   Clinical examination of a soft tissue tumor that is located in the anterolateral aspect of the ankle in a post-menopausal female reveals that the mass is soft, non-tender, and mobile. An MRI was taken and revealed a well-defined lesion with the same density as the surround normal fat. What is the correct diagnosis of the neoplasm?

    A.   Lipoma
    B.   Ganglion cyst
    C.   Fibroma
    D.   Neurilemoma

8.   A 35 year-old female presented with a lesion that was located in the subungual area of her great toe. She
        related intense, lancing type pain that is worse with cold exposure. The lesion measured 0.5 mm and had a
        bluish discoloration. Radiographs showed a well-marginated erosion of the distal phalanx. What is the
        most likely diagnosis base on the information given?

        A.   Hemangioma
        B.   Pigmented villonodular synovitis
        C.   Neurilemoma
        D.   Glomus tumor

9.   Which of the following does **NOT** represent an Enneking Stage I (latent) benign soft tissue lesion?

        A.   Ganglion cyst
        B.   Lipoma
        C.   Glomus tumor
        D.   Fibroma

10.   Using the Enneking Surgical Staging System for malignant soft tissue sarcomas, which of the following
        would correspond to a Stage IB (low-grade, extracompartmental lesion without metastasis) tumor?

        A.   G1, T1, M0
        B.   G1, T2, M0
        C.   G2, T2, M0
        D.   G1, T1, M1

11.   Which of the following statements if **FALSE** concerning biopsy of epidermal lesions?

        A.   Shave biopsy is not appropriate for malignant lesions.
        B.   For a punch biopsy, the skin should be stretched taut perpendicular to relaxed skin tension lines
                before the punch is made.
        C.   A punch biopsy is adequate for pathological processes of fat such as morphea, erythema nodosum,
                and scleoderma.
        D.   Excisional biopsy when possible is always preferred for small lesions.

12.   Which of the following is **NOT** a common clinical feature of melanomas?

        A.   Usually greater than 5.0 mm in greatest diameter before clinically evident as a melanoma.
        B.   Lesions are all symmetrical; you can bisect the lesion anywhere to make two mirror images.
        C.   All have border irregularity.
        D.   Incidence is higher in patients with fair complexion, red hair, blue eyes, freckles and poor tanning
                ability who live in areas where solar exposure is high.

13.   What is the most common type of malignant melamona?

        A.   Superficial spreading
        B.   Nodular
        C.   Amelanotic
        D.   Acral lentiginous

14.   Which of the following types of malignant melanomas is the least frequent in the lower extremity?

    A.   Superficial spreading
    B.   Nodular
    C.   Lentigo
    D.   Amelanotic

15.   Which of the following type of malignant melanoma is frequently found in the subungual location?

    A.   Nodular
    B.   Superficial spreading
    C.   Amelanotic
    D.   Acral lentiginous

Chapter 17

OSSEOUS NEOPLASMS

John H. Walter, Jr.
Larry R. Goss
Craig Haueisen

I. **Introduction**
   A. **Bone tumors represent less than 1% of all tumors diagnosed in the United States**
   B. **Only 1% to 2% of these tumors arise in the foot**
   C. **The World Health Organization has identified over 50 types of osseous tumors**
   D. **Only about half of these have been documented to affect the foot and ankle areas**
   E. **Benign neoplasms outnumber malignant neoplasms by approximately 4:1**
   F. **In general, males are more commonly affected than females (2:1)**
   G. **Calcaneus and the metatarsals are the most commonly involved in both benign and malignant lesions**
   H. **With benign lesions, the phalanges and the talus are the next most common sites**
   I. **Represent either a *dysplastic* or *anaplastic* response of the various cellular elements present in bones**

II. **Etiology of Osseous Tumors**
   A. **Cartilaginous elements:**
      1. Chondroblastoma
      2. Chondrosarcomas
      3. Chondromyxoid Fibroma
      4. Osteochondroma
      5. Enchondroma
   B. **Fibroblastic elements:**
      1. Fibrosacroma
      2. Fibrous dysplasia
      3. Non-ossifying fibroma
      4. Desmoplastic fibroma
      5. Malignant fibrous histiocytoma
   C. **Osteoblastic elements:**
      1. Osteosarcoma
      2. Osteoid osteoma

       3. Osteoblastoma
- **D. Hematopoietic elements:**
  1. Myeloma
  2. Leukemia
- **E. Tumors of uncertain origin:**
  1. Ewing's sarcoma
  2. Giant cell tumor
  3. Aneurysmal bone cyst (ABC)

III. Differential Diagnosis of Solitary Radiolucent Bone Neoplasms

- A. Use the Mnemonic "**FOGMACHINES**"

  F - Fibrous dysplasia

  O - Osteoblastoma, Osteochondroma, Osteoid osteoma, Osteosarcoma

  G - Giant Cell Tumor

  M - Metastasis, Myeloma

  A - Aneurysmal bone cyst, Angioma

  C - Condroblastoma, Chondromyxoid fibroma

  H - Hemangioma, Hyperparathyroidism (Brown tumors)

  I - Infection (Brodie's abscess)

  N - Non-ossifying fibroma

  E - Enchondroma, Eosinophilic granuloma

  S - Solitary Bone Cyst (Unicameral)

IV. Osseous Tumors

- **A. Primary bone tumors may be either benign or malignant**
- **B. Metastatic bone tumors are malignant tumors that present in the skeleton secondary to spread from a primary carcinoma**
- **C. Mnemonic: "_BLT_ with _K_etchup & _P_ickle"**
  1. Breast, Lung, Thyroid, Kidney, Prostate
- **D. Breast and prostate carcinomas most commonly metastasize to bone** (*see section on Metastatic Carcinoma*)
- **E. Lung, kidney, and thyroid carcinomas also metastasize but less frequently**
- **F. Bone tumors can frequently be diagnosed from an initial radiographic study**

V. Radiographic Parameters

- **A. Location of lesion:**
  1. Is the lesion located in the epiphyseal, metaphyseal, or diaphyseal area?
  2. Is the lesion limited to the cortex or within the medullary canal?
  3. Specific location of an identifiable lesion will often be suggestive of a specific tumor
- **B. Pattern of destruction:**
  1. The pattern of bone destruction is helpful in determining the specific kind of tumor involved
  2. **Geographic lesions**: usually are well-defined and has sclerotic margins
     a. Unicameral bone cyst
     b. Enchondroma

   3. **Moth-eaten lesion**: this pattern of cortical destruction is suggestive of an aggressive tumor and possible malignancy
      a. Giant cell tumor
      b. Eosinophilic granuloma
   4. **Permeative lesions**: a lesion that permeates through bone with minimal destruction is more aggressive than those that resorb bone in their path and is highly suggestive of malignancy
      a. Ewing's sarcoma

C. **Osseous reaction:**
   1. Well-defined reactive sclerosis suggests a slower growing lesion
   2. An intact periosteal response is evidence of an aggressive lesion
   3. Periosteal reaction that cannot keep up with tumor is termed "***Codman's Triangle***" and is suggestive of an extremely rapid growing malignant lesion

D. **Radiographic characteristics:**
   1. Calcification is diagnostic of a cartilage lesion
   2. Bone production is diagnostic of an osteogenic tumor
   3. A ground glass appearance is diagnostic of fibrous dysplasia

VI. Biologic Behavior of Tumors

A. **Latent Tumor**
   1. No growth of neoplasm and no osseous reaction of host bone
   2. No symptoms or physical findings on examination
   3. No intervention of any kind may be necessary

B. **Active Tumor**
   1. These are lesions with a natural history of progressive growth
   2. Mild or moderate reaction to the tumor by host bone
   3. Progressive pain and dysfunction
   4. Excision of the tumor usually leaves a reactive zone with a possibility of local recurrence
   5. Treatment: Careful diagnosis, biopsy, and surgical removal

C. **Aggressive Tumor**
   1. Progressive growth and may grow rapidly
   2. Host bone shows marked reaction to the tumor
   3. Mass or pathological fracture may occur
   4. Treatment: Complete cancer staging work-up, biopsy, chemotherapy, radiation, and surgery intervention is required

VII. Tumor Mimicking Disorders (Pseudotumors):

A. **Myositis ossifications: known as "*heterotrophic ossification*"**
B. **Accessory ossicles**
C. **Stress fracture**
D. **Osteochondrosis**
   1. Kohler's disease: Navicular
   2. Freiberg's disease: metatarsal head
   3. Islin's disease: 5th metatarsal base
   4. Sever's disease: calcaneus
E. **Subungual exostosis**
F. **Brodie's abscess**
G. **Garre's osteomyelitis**

    H. Seronegative arthritis
    I. Tuberculosis
    J. Madura foot
    K. Coccidioidomycosis
    L. Gaucher's disease
    M. Paget's disease
    N. Gout
    O. Hyperparathyroidism
    P. Brown tumor

VIII. Benign Versus Malignant Bone Tumors

A. Plain radiographs are the primary imaging modalities to establishing a benign versus malignant diagnosis (Table 1)
B. Determine what the tumor is doing to bone
    1. Benign tumors generally are confined by a natural barrier
    2. Benign tumors do not usually destroy the cortex
C. Determine how the bone is reacting to the tumor
    1. Benign tumors usually are slow growing
D. Determine if there is any soft tissue invasion
    1. This is an ominous sign and suggests an aggressive lesion or malignancy
E. Determine the response of the periosteum
F. Determine if there is any matrix mineralization within the tumor
G. Determine the margin between the tumor and the host bone

Table 1. General Radiographic Parameters for Benign and Malignant Tumors

BENIGN VERSUS MALIGNANT	
BENIGN	**MALIGNANT**
Slow growing	Aggressive growth

Walled off (well-defined margins)
   a. sclerotic margins
   b. geographic
	Various patterns of destruction
	   a. moth-eaten
	   b. permeative

Usually no cortical disruption	Cortical disruption

No periosteal reaction
   a. buttress pattern
	Periosteal reactions
	   a. onion-skin
	   b. sun-burst effect

IX. Classification of Benign Bone Tumors

A. Enneking Classification: primary classification for both benign (Table 2) and malignant (Table 3) osseous neoplasms

Table 2. Enneking Classification for Benign Osseous Neoplasms

Stage	Type	Description	Examples
I	*Latent*	A lesion that does not progress and may spontaneous heal	Enchondroma Simple bone cyst Non-ossifying fibroma Osteochondroma Osteoid osteoma Fibrous dysplasia
II	*Active*	A lesion that can expand and even deform bone but is fully contained by the host bone	Giant cell tumor Chondromyoxid fibroma Small aneurysmal bone cyst (ABC) Unicameral bone cyst Eosinophilic granuloma
III	*Aggressive*	A lesion that invades and destroys the bone and may extend into the soft tissues	Osteoblastoma Chondroblastoma Large ABC Epithelioid Hemangioendothelioma

Table 3. Enneking Classification of Malignant Osseous Neoplasms

Stage	Clinical Description	Examples
Low-Grade Malignant	These lesions have a low potential to metastasize. There is no true capsule, but there is a pseudocapsule. Tumor nodules, if they exist, will exist only in the reactive zone. Local control requires removal of the entire tumor, reactive zone, and a margin of normal tissue. Systemic therapy is not required	**Chondrosarcoma**
High-Grade Malignant	These lesions grow rapidly and metastasize early on. Tumor nodules are found beyond the reactive zone at some distance to the tumor. Surgery is necessary for local control and systemic therapy is necessary to prevent metastasis	**Osteosarcoma** **Ewing's sarcoma** **Synovial sarcoma** **Malignant fibrous histiocytoma** **Fibrosarcoma**

X. Differential Diagnosis for Osseous Neoplasms

A. A practical and logical approach should utilize information such as the patient's age, clinical course, growth characteristics of the lesion, and significant objective information to develop an accurate differential diagnosis

B. Age and skeletal location are two of the most important characteristics for developing a differential diagnosis

1. The patient's age is an important piece of information since certain osseous tumors are found more commonly within certain age groups (Tables 4 and 5)

2. Location of a bone tumor is an important characteristic because certain tumors are only found at a specific site or area

C. Location of the questionable lesion should be determined in both the axial and longitudinal directions (Tables 6 and 7)

1. Axial direction

   a. Central

   b. Eccentric

   c. Cortical

   d. Parosteal (juxtacortical)

    2. Longitudinal direction
        a. Epiphyseal
        b. Metaphyseal
        c. Diaphyseal

Table 4. Occurrence of Osseous Neoplasms in Young Patients

YOUNG POPULATION (0-20 years)	
BENIGN	**MALIGNANT**
Aneurysmal bone cyst (90%)	Ewing's sarcoma (100%)
Enchondroma (incidental finding)	Osteosarcoma (95%)
Osteoid osteoma (95%)	
Osteoblastoma (90%)	
Chondroblastoma	
Non-ossifying fibroma	
Simple bone cyst	
Fibrous dysplasia	

Table 5. Occurrence of Osseous Neoplasms in Middle Age Patients

MIDDLE AGE POPULATION (20-50)	
BENIGN	**MALIGNANT**
Chondromyxoid fibroma (90%)	Chondrosarcoma
Giant cell tumor (80%)	Fibrosarcoma
Enchondroma (when pain starts)	Hemangioendothelioma

Table 6. Location of Osseous Neoplasms

EPIPHYSEAL	METAPHYSEAL	DIAPHYSEAL
Chondroblastoma	Chondromyxoid fibroma	Aneurysmal bone cyst
Osteoid osteoma	Giant cell tumor	Enchondroma
Ossifying lipoma	Non-ossifying fibroma	Fibrous dysplasia
Ewing's sarcoma	Osteochondroma	Unicameral bone cyst
All sarcomas:	Osteoblastoma	

Table 7. Location of Osseous Neoplasms

CENTRAL	ECCENTRIC
Enchondroma	Chondromyxoid fibroma
Simple bone cyst	Giant cell tumor
Chondroblastoma	All sarcomas

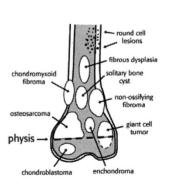

XI. **General Facts Concerning Osseous Neoplasms**
   A. **When there is an identifiable neoplasm in otherwise normal bone, the above four criteria can be used to determine the specific type of lesion**
   B. **Small radiolucent lesions surrounded by a rim of sclerotic bone without periosteal reaction are inactive and usually benign bone tumors**
   C. **Lesions that erode the cortex but are contained within a well-defined periosteal reaction are usually either active benign, low-grade malignant or metastatic lesions**
   D. **Large lesions that destroy the cortex and are not contained by the periosteum are aggressive high-grade malignant lesions**
   E. **Some benign bone tumors are difficult to differentiate from malignant ones, have a significant rate of local recurrence, and may undergo malignant transformation**
   F. **Treatment must be individualized based upon the natural history of the specific tumor**
   G. **Some neoplasms can be treated by simple curettage while others require extensive resection and even possible amputation**
   H. **Aggressive bone tumors require a complete and prompt work-up that includes:**
       1. Plain radiographs
       2. Bone scan
       3. MRI
       4. CT chest/abdomen
       5. Laboratory studies: CBC, electrolytes, LFT's, alkaline phosphatase, and LDH
       6. Consultation with a musculoskeletal oncologist

BENIGN OSSEOUS NEOPLASMS

I. **Osteochondroma**
   A. **These are benign cartilaginous bone tumors with a predilection for the lower metaphysis of the femur and the upper metaphysis of the tibia in the adolescent**
   B. **Most common benign bone tumors in the body accounting for approximately 50% of osseous neoplasms and 10-15% of all tumors in the foot**
   C. **Osteochondromas are aberrant developmental anomalies that arise from the periphery of the cartilaginous growth plates**
   D. **Most often occur around the rapidly growing, long tubular bones (metatarsals) and rarely in the small tarsal bones of the foot**
   E. **They are composed of bone and cartilage, and their cartilage cap has all the features of a physeal growth plate**
   F. **Because of this, osteochondromas continue to enlarge throughout growth**
   G. **Lesion increases in size and moves away from the physeal plate with age**
   H. **Enlargement stops with the cessation of growth and closure of the physeal plates, and the lesion remains inactive**
   I. **They may be sessile (flat) or pedunculated (stalk-like)**
   J. **Radiographs are usually diagnostic and no further tests are required**
   K. **Lesion generally presents as a mass on a stalk with a cauliflower appearance**
   L. **They are covered with a thick cartilaginous cap with the marrow cavity of the osteochondroma contiguous with the marrow of normal bone**
   M. **Rarely, sarcomatous transformation can occur in the cartilage cap, giving rise to a secondary chondrosarcoma**

N. Between 1-2% of osteochondromas may undergo malignant transformation into low-grade chondrosacromas

O. Malignant transformation is much more common in conjunction with multiple hereditary osteochondromas than with the solitary form

P. In general, surgical removal is recommended for symptomatic or for those that arise along the axial skeleton

Q. Osteochondromas may be distinguished from surface osteosarcomas, which do not have a cancellous bridge, and radiographically may demonstrate a *"string sign"*

R. Treatment of osteochondromas usually consists of simple excision by osteotomy through the base of the stalk

1. Excision does not need to remove every vestige of the stalk or base of the tumor to achieve complete resolution of the symptoms
2. Surgical treatment should be deferred until the patient is at or near skeletal maturity, if possible
3. The lesions are less likely to recur and are better defined so that complete removal can be easily accomplished and damage to the growth plate as well as recurrence can be avoided

II. **Bizarre Parosteal Osteochondromatosis Proliferation (BPOP)**

A. Known as *"Nora's lesion"*

B. Rare lesion that is sometimes found in the feet

C. Males and females are equally affected

D. There is a history of a mildly painful mass that seems to increase in size over many weeks or a few months

E. There is usually no history of trauma

F. It most commonly occurs on the proximal and middle phalanges

G. Radiographic features include:

1. Bony mass with well defined margins is seen to be applied to the surface of the bone
2. It may project into the soft tissues, but lacks the characteristic orientation away from the nearby physis that is seen in osteochondromas
3. BPOP usually appears as a mushroom (pedunculated) on plain radiographs

H. Lesion grows rapidly and has aggressive features on imaging studies as well as confusion findings on histopathology, leading to many errors in diagnosis and potentially inappropriate treatments

I. May resemble a subungual exostosis, except for the location

J. Gross pathology features include:

1. Lesion has a nodular surface covered with glistening cartilage
2. The bone in the lesion is said to have a distinct blue tint

K. Complete excision with the best possible margin is the treatment of choice

L. Lesion is benign but may recur locally in as many as 50% of cases

M. Lesion does not metastasize

III. **Osteoblastoma**

A. Benign bone producing tumor which may be found in any bone, but mostly involves the spine (posterior process) and skull

B. Osteoblastoma must be differentiated from osteosarcoma and osteoid osteoma

C. Radiographically, they may present with sclerotic margins and a bulging of the underlying bone

D. Osteoblastoma is arbitrarily designated by its larger size (greater than 2.0 cm) compared with osteoid osteoma

E. However, the histologic picture truly distinguishes one from the other

F. Radiographically, osteoblastoma is more of a radiolucent lesion without the characteristic reactive bone seen with osteoid osteoma

G. Osteoblastoma vs. osteoid osteoma
   1. Inconsistent pain
   2. Irregular tissue pattern
   3. Greater than 2.0 cm

H. Whereas osteoid osteoma is non-progressive and may spontaneously heal, osteoblastoma is progressive and can exhibit both local aggressiveness and malignant transformation

I. Treatment consists of extended intralesional curettage and grafting

J. Recurrences require more aggressive treatment and are at higher risk for more malignant behavior

K. Neoplasms may metastasize following several recurrences

IV. Osteoid Osteoma

A. Represents a small benign painful osteoblastic bone tumor with a strong predilection for the proximal femur (32%) and tibia (24%) of adolescent and young adults (rare <5 and >40)

B. Incidence is 10% to 14% of primary foot tumors and affects males 2:1

C. Osteoid osteomas are *extremely painful* (equivalent to a toothache)

D. Pain is well localized to the area of abnormality and is *worse at night*

E. Although narcotics are not helpful, the *pain is often relieved by NSAIDs or salicylates* (one or two of regular aspirins produces dramatic pain relief)
   1. One of only a few conditions that will cause a teenager to take medicine on a regular basis without prompting

F. In adults, symptoms are exacerbated by alcohol

G. Common sites in the foot are the neck of talus and calcaneus

H. Common radiographs findings include:
   1. Most common site of tumor is intracortical
   2. A "*radiolucent nidus*" surrounded by a zone of sclerosis
   3. Nidus is often obscured by dense reactive bone stimulated in response to the tumor
   4. Nidus is only 3 to 5 mm in diameter
   5. Entire lesion is almost always less than 2.0 cm in diameter
   6. Has a "*bulls-eye*" configuration on plain radiographs
   7. Usually has a zone of sclerosis that surrounds the lesion
   8. When the lesion is intramedullary there is less sclerotic response and detection is more difficult

I. Bone scans are helpful since the lesions will show an intense, highly focal increased radionuclide uptake in the region of the nidus, which is a unique feature of the tumor

J. CT scans and linear tomography are also helpful in demonstrating the nidus

K. Treatment options include:
   1. Surgical removal of the nidus (intralesional excision or en bloc excision is recommended) is often required because of the pain
   2. Simple curettage is not recommended because the risk of leaving a portion of the nidus results in clinical recurrence (20% to 50%)
   3. Sclerotic rim does not need to be removed to obtain healing

4. Tetracycline localization:
   a. Utilizes tetracycline at a dosage of 4 mg/kg, four times daily, 2 days pre-operatively, the nidus will have a golden yellow fluorescence
5. Percutaneous radiofrequency coagulation
   a. Represents a relatively new surgical technique that involves inserting a thermal probe under CT guidance called RTA

L. Pain always resolves upon excision of the nidus

M. However, many lesions undergo spontaneous healing with time
1. Average time is 33 months

N. Rarely undergoes malignant transformation

V. Enchondroma

A. These are benign cartilaginous tumors which may present either as solitary or multiple lesions

B. This is a benign cartilaginous tumor with a predilection for the epiphyseal region of long tubular bones of adolescent males (less than 20)

C. Solitary enchondroma is one of the most common benign tumors in the foot (10% to 15% of bone tumors in the foot)

D. Most common tumor of the phalanges in the foot
1. **Most frequently the proximal phalanx (70%) and middle phalanx (20%)**

E. Rare in the rearfoot

F. 95% present as a solitary lesion that is diagnosed as an incidental finding on a plain radiograph

G. Rarely, multiple lesions may be present
1. Ollier's disease = multiple enchondromas
   a. Known as "*enchondromatosis*"
   b. Characterized by the presence of polyostotic involvement of enchondromas
   c. Osseous involvement is often asymmetric and tends to affect one side of the body more than the other
   d. Malignant degeneration of Ollier's disease is 25% to 50%
2. Maffucci syndrome = multiple enchondromas with hemangiomas
   a. Represents a non-hereditary skeletal mesodermal dysplasia
   b. Characterized by the presence of polyostotic enchondromas in an association with multiple soft tissue hemangiomas
   c. Osseous involvement is often asymmetric, like Ollier's disease, and tends to affect one side of the body more than the other
   d. Chondrosarcomatous transformation with Maffucci's syndrome is greater than 50%

H. They may be difficult to diagnose radiographically, however the lesions are usually expansile and lytic, with a variable amount of matrix mineralization
1. On radiograph, the classic finding is "*popcorn*", "*stippled*", or "*snowflake*" appearance
2. Matrix consists of nodules of cartilage which tend to calcify at the periphery

I. Enchondromas are usually asymptomatic, unless a pathologic fracture exists

J. Extreme pain and pathologic fracture is a sign of local aggressiveness and possible malignancy

K. There is a tendency for malignant transformation especially when they occur in the axial and proximal apendicular skeleton

L. However, they very rarely undergo malignant transformation

M. Can be mistaken as giant cell tumor because both lesions occur in the foot in similar locations

N. Curettage of enchondromas with bone grafting is the treatment of choice

O. Highly expansile lesions in the phalanges with pathological fracture may require amputation of the involved portion of the toe, since the function and cosmetic results are not likely to be acceptable following attempted curettage

P. Rarely do they recur

VI. Chondroblastoma (CB)

A. Chondroblastomas are always *epiphyseal* in location, present as radiolucent lesions, and occur before skeletal maturity

B. Peak incidence is less than 20 years (75% of patients are between 10 and 20 years old)

C. Rare tumor in the foot and ankle regions (< 1% of all primary bone tumors)

D. Patient often complains of a mass near a joint with severe pain

E. Pathological fracture is rare

F. In foot, the primary lesion affects the *talocalcaneal articulation*

G. Radiologically, the tumor is almost exclusively located in the epiphysis
   1. Cortex may be scalloped or expanded
   2. Lesion has a chondroid matrix and "*stippled calcification*" may be seen on plain radiographs

H. CT is useful for defining the relationship of the tumor to the joint, integrity of the cortex, and intralesional calcifications

I. Treatment is biopsy and curettage with possible use of adjuvant liquid nitrogen or phenol or mechanical burr

J. They are aggressive benign lesions with a high recurrence rate following simple curettage

K. Must be differentiated from giant cell tumor, aneurysmal bone cyst, and clear cell chondrosarcoma

L. Clinical correlation of age (< 20), site (strictly epiphyseal), and histology points to the correct diagnosis

M. May behave aggressively and invade soft tissue and pulmonary matastasis has been observed

VII. Unicameral Bone Cyst (UBC)

A. Often referred to as a "*solitary bone cyst*" or "*simple bone cyst*"

B. Represents a benign fibrous lesion characterized by an attenuated cortical wall that is lined by a thin fibrous membrane containing a clear yellow fluid

C. Two types of UBC's exist:
   1. Active type UBC
      a. Typically develops in patients under 10 years of age
      b. Represents an active type of lesion
      c. Lesion usually arises adjacent to the physeal growth plate
      d. Usually invades the entire metaphysis area
      e. Cortex is expanded
      f. May result in pathological fracture
      g. Recurrence is common (50%)
   2. Passive type UBC
      a. Typically develops in patients over 10 years of age
      b. More common type (90%)
      c. Cysts are usually latent

       d.   Less chance for recurrence (10%) with simple curettage and bone grafting

D. These lesions show predilection for the metaphysis and/or diaphysis of long tubular bones with 80% occurring in the proximal humerus and femur

E. In the foot, UBC *occurs almost exclusively in the calcaneus* **and is characteristically found under the middle facet with its apex towards the forefoot**

F. On a lateral radiograph, the lesion is located in the lateral aspect of the calcaneus

G. 90% occur in patients less than 20 years old

H. UBC's are usually asymptomatic until a pathological fracture occurs

I. Radiographic features include:
1. Radiolucent expansile lesions with well-defined margins (geographic pattern)
2. Length is always greater than width
3. No matrix mineralization is evident
4. No bony separations or loculations
5. May have central calcification of the lesion

J. Bone scans show a photon deficient area that corresponds to a geographic lesion

K. Any increased uptake will generally result from pathologic fracture

L. The *"fallen fragment sign"* **occurs late in disease process and is usually only present after a pathological fracture has occurred**
1. Represents a free fragment of cortical bone fallen by gravity in the fluid containing cyst

M. Traditional treatment has been simple curettage with or without bone grafting of the lesion
1. However, recurrence rates of up to 70% have been documented with simple curettage
2. Recurrence rates are higher in weightbearing areas such as the calcaneus

N. More recently UBC's have been treated with aspiration, flushing, and injection with methylprednisolone acetate steroid (95% heal with this aspiration technique)
1. Injecting 80-200 mg of methylprednisolone into the cavity

O. To avoid injecting a bone lesion other than a UBC, the following four criteria must be followed:
1. Typical radiographic findings of a UBC
2. Aspiration of clear yellow fluid
3. Arteriolar pressure between 15-28 mmHg
4. Complete filling of cyst with Renografin-76 injection

P. Pathologic fractures should be allowed to heal before an injection is performed

Q. UBC's should not be left untreated in the hope that they will regress

R. They will invariably become larger, making definitive treatment more difficult

VIII. Fibrous Dysplasia (FD)

A. Disorder which normal bone tissue is replaced by an abnormal proliferation of fibrous tissue

B. FD is usually monostotic (affecting one bone)

C. Men and women are equally affected

D. Extremely low incidence in foot (less than 2%)

E. There is no reaction by the normal bone to the lesion

F. The *"ground glass appearance"* (fibrous stroma containing bone spicules) **of the lesion is diagnostic and hallmark**

G. FD can result in marked deformities of bone (angular deformities and limb length discrepancies)

H. Uncommon before age 2 or after age 30

I. Occasionally FD is associated with **polyostotic** (many bones) involvement as well as melanotic pigmentation of the skin (café au lait spots) and disturbance of endocrine metabolism called "*Albright's Syndrome*"

J. **Unless excised and grafted, FD will progress rapidly and cause destruction of bone** (pathological fracture) and gross osseous disfigurement

IX. Aneurysmal Bone Cysts (ABC)

A. **Represents an uncommon expansile osteolytic lesion of bone consisting of a proliferation of vascular tissue that forms a large blood filled cystic lesion, however the exact etiology is unknown**

B. **One theory of the etiology of primary ABC's is that these lesions are secondary to increased venous pressure that leads to hemorrhage which causes osteolysis**

C. **ABC usually develops in the first two decades of life** (uncommon after 30) and has eccentric metaphyseal locations

D. **Incidence: only bone tumor with a female to male ratio of 3:1**

E. **Primary location is in the lower distal tibia metaphyseal area**

F. *Only osseous tumor in body that derives name from its radiographic appearance, rather than its histologic appearance*

G. **Radiographic features include:**
   1. Rapidly growing benign lesion with a thin shell of reactive periosteal bone
   2. The highly expansile lesion perched at the end of the bone has been described with the catch phrase "*finger in a balloon*"
   3. Classic "*soap-bubble*" appearance on plain radiograph secondary to internal septae and longitudinal striations
   4. Eccentric, *strictly metaphyseal* location with an interior radiolucency appearance

H. **MRI shows classic multiple "*fluid-fluid levels*" and the non-homogeneity of the lesion which is highly suggestive of the diagnosis but are not diagnostic**
   1. ABC appears on both T1 and T2 MRI with a low signal rim encircling the cystic lesion

I. **A three phase bone scan shows intense uptake in the margin of the lesion, with normal background or decreased uptake in its center**

J. **Depending on the location, the differential diagnosis includes an UBC, chondromyxoid fibroma, giant cell tumor, osteoblastoma and the highly malignant telangiectatic osteosarcoma**

K. **At biopsy the lesion consists of clotted and unclotted blood in a friable network of mesenchymal tissue**

L. **Treatment most commonly consists of intralesional curettage, application of high speed burr and bone grafting**
   1. May be complicated by profuse bleeding from the lesion
   2. Recurrence rates vary from 20% to 50% with simple curettage

M. **Other treatment options include percutaneous injection of a fibrosing agent, selective embolectomy of the nutrient artery and percutaneous injection of polymethylmethacrylate (PMMA)**

N. **All tissue should be submitted for histologic examination because ABCs may be a secondary feature of a more aggressive tumor**

O. **ABCs can be secondary to an underlying lesion such as non-ossifying fibroma, chondroblastoma, osteoblastoma, UBC's, chondromyxoid fibroma and fibrous dysplasia**

P. **Histological features include:**
   1. Lesion consists of blood-filled cavities surrounded by spindle-shaped fibroblastic cells

and multinucleated giant cells
   2. Fibrous septa have immature woven bone trabeculae and macrophages filled with
      hemosiderin, fibroblasts, capillaries and giant cells
Q. Recurrence is a possibility and conversion into a malignant lesion has been reported
R. Radiation may be needed in recurrent lesions but adds the additional risk of malignancy

X. Giant Cell Tumor (GCT)

A. This is a locally aggressive tumor of young adults (20 to 40 years of age) with a propensity
   for local recurrence and a low metastatic potential
B. The incidence in the foot is relatively uncommon
C. Radiographic features include:
   1. GCT's present as eccentric lytic lesions at the junction of the metaphysis and epiphysis of
      long bones
   2. Characteristic "*moth-eaten appearance*" on radiograph
   3. There is minimal normal bone reaction
   4. There is no matrix production
   5. Cortex is usually expanded and may appear destroyed on radiographs, but is usually
      intact at surgery
   6. There is no periosteal reaction in this lesion
**D. GCTs are not malignant de novo, but they demonstrate malignant potential after
   multiple local recurrences** (20% to 40% become malignant upon recurrence)
E. Each local recurrence increases the risk of malignant transformation
F. Treatment of GCT is through surgical removal
   1. Curettage is not recommended since recurrence rates of up to 80% have been
      documented
   2. En block excision (wide excision) is preferred
   3. Filling of the lesion with a suitable material, such as morcellized bone graft, bone graft
      substitute, or polymethylmethacrylate (PMMA) bone cement is recommended
   4. Amputation is reserved for a massive recurrence or malignant transformation
G. *Cryosurgery has been utilized more successfully than for any other type of bone tumor*
   1. Cryosurgery generally involves a thorough curettage of the lesion after which liquid
      nitrogen is poured directly into the cavity
   2. The liquid nitrogen ensures complete contact with the wall of the tumor so that any
      remaining tumor cells will be killed

XI. Non-Ossifying Fibroma (NOF)

A. Known as "*benign fibrous cortical defect*"
B. This is a benign fibrous tumor that presents at the metaphysis of long bones
**C. It presents during adolescence with a tendency to undergo spontaneous healing after
   skeletal maturity** (rare after puberty)
**D. Lesion has no clinical symptoms in children and is usually discovered on a plain
   radiograph that is taken for unrelated reasons**
E. Male to female ratio is 2:1
F. Radiographic features include:
   1. Well-defined lytic lesion
   2. Generally eccentrically located between the metaphysis and diaphysis of long bones
   3. Minimal periosteal reaction is seen

4. Lesion has a thin sclerotic border that is often scalloped
G. **Pathology fracture may occur and 90% occur in the lower extremity**
H. **Majority (75%) are found in tibia or fibula**
I. **The differential diagnosis includes: Brown tumor, Paget's disease, fibrous histiocytoma, desmoplastic fibroma, fibrous dysplasia, and osteosarcoma**

XII. **Chondromyxoid Fibroma (CMF)**
A. **This relatively rare tumor presents in children and young adults**
B. **75% of patients are younger than 30 and two-thirds are male**
C. *This unusual tumor has a striking predilection for the foot*
D. **Most tumors occur below the knee and 25% of the total involves the foot**
E. **The metatarsals, midfoot and hindfoot may be involved**
F. **Patients present with a slow growing mass and mild or moderate pain**
G. **Pathological fracture is rare (less than 5%)**
H. **Radiographic features include:**
1. Lesion is ovoid in shape with its long axis parallel to the bone
2. There is often a sclerotic margin and a lobulated contour
3. Ridges and grooves that appear in the margins secondary to scalloping falsely appear to be trabeculae
I. **CT helps define cortical integrity and confirms that there is no mineralization of the matrix, unlike other cartilage tumors**
J. **CMF has the same appearance on MRI as other cartilage tumors which is decreased signal on T1 weighted images and increased signal on T2 weighted images**
K. **MRI is helpful in pre-operative planning and staging**
L. **The radiologic differential diagnosis includes giant cell tumor, aneurysmal bone cyst, unicameral bone cyst, chondroblastoma and fibrous dysplasia**
M. **Treatment is by en bloc resection most commonly**
N. **The tumor may recur in the soft tissues from intra-operative seeding in simple curettage so surgeons should take care to avoid tumor spillage into the wound**
O. **Recurrences after curettage are common (40%)**
P. **Surgeons should thoroughly assess the soft tissue extension of the tumor to achieve complete local control**

XIII. **Eosinophilic Granuloma (EG)**
A. **This is a benign lesion which *arises from reticuloendothelial system* (RES) during the first decade of life (5-10 years)**
B. **Known as "*Langerhan's cell histiocytosis*", formerly known as "*histiocytosis X*"**
C. **EG is a destructive lesion that presents in a moth-eaten cortical pattern**
D. **It may undergo spontaneous healing**
E. **Not a true bone neoplasm** (non-neoplastic proliferation of histiocytes) and is often confused for benign bone tumor
F. **Most commonly in spine and is associated with vertebra plana**
G. **Classic "*punched-out*" borders appearing radiolucenies on radiograph**
H. **Often have pathological fracture associated with this neoplasm**
I. **The radiologic differential diagnosis includes Ewing's sarcoma, osteosarcoma, PVNS, metastases and hematogenous osteomyelitis**
J. **Associated with two systemic diseases:**

        1. Letterer-Siwe disease: fulminant systemic disease in children under 3 that is usually fatal

        2. Hand-Schuller-Christian disease: chronic disseminated form that occurs in older patients

           a.   Classic triad: diabetes insipidus, exopthalmos, and skull lesions

   K. **Treatment of EG depends on the form of the disease**

   L. **With localized disease, often a biopsy alone is enough to incite healing**

   M. **Other treatment modalities of EG include simple curettage, excisional resection, steroid injection, radiation and observation**

   N. **Chemotherapy is recommended for systemic disease**

XIV.   **Intraosseous Lipoma (IOL)**

   A. **Categorized as intraosseous, cortical, or parosteal lesions, according to their location in the bone**

   B. **Rare lesion, representing only 0.1% of all bone tumors**

   C. **Represents a non-aggressive lesion that is usually asymptomatic and found on the radiographic examination performed for other reasons**

   D. **Radiographic features include:**

      1. Lytic lesion with sharply defined sclerotic borders

      2. May have associated thinning of the cortex

      3. Frequent (80% cases) central ossification or calcification, which occasionally may have a radiolucent center

   E. **Magnetic resonance imaging shows, on T1- and T2-weighted images, that lesions have signals similar to those of subcutaneous fat**

   F. **Majority of cases are found in the calcaneus (80%)**

   G. **Incidence is slight male dominated**

   H. **Rare during the first decade of life**

XV. Pigmented VilloNodular Synovitis (PVNS)

   A. **Represents a rare tumor of the synovium and tendon sheath**

   B. **Two forms exist:**

      1. Localized type: usually affects one bone

      2. Diffuse type: often affects more than one bone

   C. **PVNS affects the knee most commonly (60%), but can also present in the ankle and midfoot**

   D. **Radiographs demonstrate "*juxta-cortical erosions*" of both sides of an affected joint**

   E. **The lesion has a pathognomonic MRI appearance**

      1. The T1-weighted images with a short TR/TE showed the lesion to have density similar to muscle, while on the T2-weighted images with a long TR/TE, the lesion is dark due to a signal void created by the ferromagnetic hemosiderin in the lesion

   F. **Synovial biopsy provides the definitive diagnosis**

      1. Upon joint aspiration, patients usually have a dark brown or serosanguineous fluid

   G. **PVNS is treated by surgical excision** (either marginal or in some cases radical) and complete synovectomy

   H. **Very high recurrence rates with incomplete resection**

XVI.   **Desmoplastic Fibroma (DF)**

   A. **Extremely rare tumor, especially in the foot and ankle regions**

    B. **Only 300 documented in the English literature**
    C. **Most common site is the mandible, followed by the femur and pelvis**
    D. **10% present with pathological fracture**
    E. **Radiographic diagnosis is extremely difficult**

XVII. **Epithelioid Hemangioendothelioma (EHE)**
    A. **Most commonly seen in second and third decades in the lower extremity**
    B. **Characteristic "*soap-bubble*" appearance on plain radiographs**
    C. **Often affects multiple bones**
    D. **Classified as benign aggressive lesion**
    E. **May transform into malignant lesion (20%)**
    F. **Extremely high recurrence rate with local excision (50%)**

XVIII. **Tumors That Affect More Than One Bone**
    A. **Epithelioid hemangioendothelioma**
    B. **PVNS**
    C. **Polyostotic fibrous dysplasia**
    D. **Enchondromatosis: Ollier's and Mafucci's**
    E. **Multiple hereditary osteochondromas**
    F. **Metastaic tumors: Angiosarcoma**
    G. **Pseudotumors: Gout, Gaucher's disease, hyperparathyroidism, Brown tumor**

MALIGNANT BONE TUMORS

I. **Introduction**
    A. **Primary bone tumors are usually malignant**
    B. **Ratio of malignant to benign is approximately three to one**
    C. **However, overall malignant bone tumors are a relatively infrequent lesion**
    D. **Almost all have a uniformly poor prognosis when compared to other sarcomas**
    E. **Has a tendency to arise in actively growing bone and as such, they strike mostly young people**
    F. **Their predilection for young people, often adolescents, stands in sharp contrast to the general pattern of malignant disease**
    G. **Malignant bone tumors have a tendency to arise in the metaphyseal region of long bones due to their especially active area of bone growth**

II. **History and Physical Examination**
    A. **History and physical examination should include standard questions regarding general health, weight loss, fevers, fatigue, night sweats, and relevant risk factors, such as, family history, smoking and dietary habits**
    B. **Physical examination should include palpation for lymphadenopathy and all masses**
    C. **Laboratory evaluation should include a CBC with differential, peripheral blood smear, ESR, serum chemistries** (such as BUN, calcium, phosphorus, albumin, and alkaline phosphatase) and serum immunoelectrophoresis (screens for myeloma)
    D. **Malignant bone tumors tend to manifest themselves first by producing pain**

III. Types of Malignant Bone Tumors

A. Osteosarcoma (OS)

1. Represents a high-grade malignant tumor, characterized by the production of tumor osteoid (immature bone) directly form the stroma
2. Most common malignant bone tumor with a predilection for long tubular bones, especially in the adolescent (75% between age of 15 and 25)
3. In patients over the age of forty, it is often associated with a pre-existing condition, most commonly Paget's disease
4. Most common sites are the bones of the knee joint (rare in foot <1%)
5. Serum alkaline phosphatase will be elevated, but it is not diagnostic since it is also elevated with other skeletal diseases
6. Pain is the most common complaint
7. A mass is often found
8. Systemic symptoms are rare
9. Growth of the tumor is very rapid
10. The blood stream is the major route of spread
11. The lungs are the most frequent site of metastasis
12. Death is most often due to this pulmonary metastasis
13. Radiographic findings include:
    a. Increased intramedullary radiodensity
    b. Area of radiolucency
    c. Pattern of permeative destruction
    d. Poorly defined borders
    e. Cortical lysis
    f. Periosteal elevation creating a Codman's triangle
    g. Extraosseous extension with soft tissue ossification
    h. 50% percent of OS will present with both sclerotic and lytic patterns, the remainder will be equally divided between strict lytic and strict sclerotic presentations
    i. The lytic type presents the most difficult diagnostic problems
    j. Classic *"sun-burst pattern"* of bone destruction
14. In the past, treatment consisted of amputation since metastasis to the lungs generally occurred within two years
15. More recently, chemotherapy and thoracotomy have increased the survival rate
16. When amputation is contemplated for OS, it is performed one joint level above the tumor containing bone
17. Limb sparing resection is becoming increasingly used to treat OS and consists of resection of the tumor, skeletal reconstruction through arthrodesis or prosthetic replacement, and soft tissue and muscle transfers
18. Overall cure rates now approach 50% to 60% when tumor resection is combined with chemotherapy
19. Osteosarcoma variants
    a. There are eleven variants of classic OS, but three are common:
        i. Parosteal OS
        ii. Periosteal OS
        iii. Small cell OS

B. Parosteal Osteosarcoma

1. Parosteal osteosarcoma arises from the cortex of the bone and occurs in older age groups
2. It is slow growing, slow metastasizing, and has a high rate of survival

3. It most commonly affects the distal posterior femur and proximal tibia
4. Radiographically, it presents as a large mass attached to the bone without involving the medullary canal
5. Treatment is by wide excision of the tumor and may require amputation

C. **Periosteal Osteosarcoma**
1. Periosteal osteosarcoma almost always arises superficially from the cortex of the tibial shaft
2. It presents as a small radiolucent lesion with some evidence of bone spiculation
3. Unlike parosteal OS that is radiodense, periosteal OS presents as a small scooped out lesion of the cortex
4. It is high grade malignant and requires amputation

D. **Small Cell Osteosarcoma**
1. Small (round) cell OS is rare and generally requires surgical ablation
2. It has the worst prognosis

E. **Chondrosarcoma (CS)**
1. This is a malignant tumor of bone consisting of anaplastic chondroblasts
2. It is the second most common primary malignant bone tumor (2% incidence in foot)
3. They occur in an older (after 35 years of age)
4. They grow much slower than osteosarcoma
5. Chondrosarcomas are often confused with a benign lesion such as a chondromyxoid fibroma
6. They afflict the bones of the trunk and the upper extremities most commonly
7. The majority arises de novo, but some chondrosarcomas arise from transformation of enchondromas
8. CS can become quite large without causing pain
9. An adult with a benign looking cartilage tumor on a radiograph that is associated with pain, most likely has a chondrosarcoma
10. Radiologically, two patterns may present
    a. Peripheral CS
       i. Presents as a well-defined lytic lesion with surrounding sclerosis with faint calcification
    b. Mesenchymal CS
       i. Presents as a lytic lesion with no sclerotic border
    c. In both, the key diagnostic sign is the so-called *"smoke ring calcification"* within the tumor
11. Treatment of CS is surgical removal
12. The fact that CS tends to be low-grade malignant makes it amendable to limb spearing procedures
13. Five-year survival rates of up to 90% have been recorded
14. Mesenchymal CS is more aggressive but occurs much less frequently
15. Peripheral CS tends to have higher survival rates when compared with central skeletal CS

F. **Malignant Fibrous Histiocytoma (MFH)**
1. This is a high-grade bone tumor without evidence of osteoid production
2. It involves the bones around the knee
3. It disseminates rapidly and may involve the lymphatic system
4. Pathological fractures are common
5. It presents as an osteolytic lesion, generally at the metaphysis of long bones, with a permeative pattern of destruction and minimal cortical reaction
6. There is no periosteal reaction and no evidence of matrix formation

7. It is commonly associated with Paget's disease and osteomyelitis
8. *Hardcastle's Syndrome* = diaphyseal medullary stenosis (DMS) + MFH
   a. Inheritance autosomal dominant
   b. Rare hereditary cancer syndrome with only four families identified worldwide
   c. Etiology unknown

G. Synovial Sarcoma (SS)

1. Are deep seated, well-circumscribed, multinodular, firm tenosynovial tumors that occur predominantly in the flexor aspect of the extremities close to joints
2. Although these tumors are of a synovial origin, they do not arise from joints
3. Associated with prolonged history of trauma (35-50%) or a pre-existing small mass lasting months to years
4. 15% to 20% involve the foot and ankle areas
5. Treatment is wide excision or amputation

H. Fibrosarcoma (FS)

1. FS is an uncommon, malignant spindle cell neoplasm
2. This is a fibrogenic tumor of bone that affects the long bones of middle age adults
3. Fibrosarcoma is found most commonly around the knee in the distal femur and proximal tibia followed by the pelvis
4. It rarely affects the foot (less than 35 are documented in the English literature)
5. The tumor produces a collagen matrix but does not produce osteoid or chondroid
6. It is a radiolucent lesion with minimal periosteal and cortical reaction
7. Destruction of cortical bone with irregular roughening and poorly defined margins is usually present
8. Extension into the soft tissue is common
9. Pathologic fracture occurs in approximately 30% of patients with fibrosarcoma
10. MRI helps define intraosseus spread and soft tissue extension
11. Bone scan demonstrates increased uptake
12. The differential diagnosis includes leiomyosarcoma, metastatic carcinoma, melanoma, malignant fibrous histiocytoma and multiple myeloma
13. Treatment is similar to those of other spindle cell sarcomas (radical surgical excision and adjuvant radiation therapy)
14. Prognosis is largely dependent on the tumor grade

I. Ewing's Sarcoma (ES)

1. Incidence: most patients male, 90% < 10 years old
   a. Ewing's sarcoma is a disease of childhood, although it does not present in children below the age of 5, mean age diagnosis in the foot is 17 years
2. Primary location: 80% tibia & femur
   a. It most frequently involves the flat bones of the axial skeleton
   b. If it presents in long bones, it involves the diaphyseal area
   c. ES has been documented to affect every bone in the foot
   d. 35% occur in the rearfoot, with 20% occurring in the calcaneus
3. Ewing's sarcoma is a "*round cell sarcoma*"
4. The most common round cell sarcomas are Non-Hodgkin's lymphoma and Ewing's sarcoma
5. Round cell sarcomas, unlike spindle cell sarcomas, are best treated with radiation and chemotherapy; and surgery is reserved only for special situations
6. Ewing's sarcoma will present with systemic signs, such as fever, anemia, and anorexia, as well as pain accompanied by significant diffuse swelling
7. The WBC count, ESR, and temperature are all usually elevated

8. Patients usually have symptoms for an average of 14 months prior to accurate diagnosis
9. Patients with rearfoot involvement have an average duration of symptoms of 22 months prior to diagnosis, whereas those in the forefoot have an average duration of symptoms of 7 months
10. ES is a highly destructive radiolucent lesion with no evidence of bone formation
11. There will be the following characteristic radiographic findings:
    a. *"Permeative pattern"* of bone destruction
    b. Multi-laminated periosteal elevation
    c. *"Onion-skinning"* of the periosteum
    d. Codman's triangle
    e. *"Hair-on-end"* appearance is common
12. When ES involves flat bones the above findings will be absent and in their place will appear a destructive lesion with a large soft tissue mass
13. The radiographic appearance of ES in the foot is highly variable
    a. Usually a small lytic lesion
    b. Permeative destruction of bone
    c. No matrix production
    d. No soft tissue calcification
14. A bone scan usually shows focal, intense uptake
15. CT and MRI are essential for surgical planning and demonstrate the soft tissue extent of the mass, as well as permeative bone destruction
16. Ewing's is highly lethal and rapidly metastasizes
17. The most common sites of metastasis are the lungs and other bones
18. ES may involve the lymphatic system and clinical examination of regional lymph nodes is necessary
19. A complete cancer staging work-up is required
20. Treatment usually consists of radiation therapy with adjunct chemotherapy
21. Because ES has extensive extra-osseous involvement, primary amputation is often required for lower extremity lesions
22. Use of radiation which is becoming an increasingly popular mode of treatment, however it increases the potential for development of secondary sarcomas within the irradiated fields
23. The five-year survival rate for ES is 70% in patients who are free of metastasis at the time of the diagnosis, otherwise the prognosis is extremely poor (0% to 10%)
24. When present in the forefoot a 70% five-year survival rate is seen and lesions in the rearfoot have less than 35% five-year survival rate
25. However, tumor size and delay before diagnosis also vary by site, and these factors are likely to have a greater impact on prognosis than the difference in site alone

O. **Round Cell Tumors**
1. Ewing's sarcoma
2. Metastatic neuroblastoma
3. Metastatic rhabdomyosarcoma
4. Non-Hodgkin's lymphoma/leukemia
5. Small cell osteosarcoma
6. Mesenchymal chondrosarcoma

METASTATIC CARCINOMA

I. **Introduction**

   A. **Metastatic carcinoma refers to skeletal metastasis of carcinomas from other tissues of the body**

   B. **The incidence of metastasis to the skeleton far outnumbers primary bone tumors (25:1)**

   C. **It is the most common bone tumor in patients over 40 years of age**

   D. **The hallmark of skeletal involvement is severe pain**

   E. **A patient with known cancer who develops skeletal pain is assumed to have bony metastasis until proven otherwise**

   F. **The most common sources of skeletal metastasis are cancers of the lungs, breast, prostate, and GI**

   G. **Whereas primary bone tumors usually arise in the metaphysis, metastatic cancers are found in the diaphysis of bones**

   H. **The most common sites of involvement are the spine, femur, and ribs**

   I. **Although metastatic carcinoma is the most common malignant tumor of bone in the elderly, it is seldom found distal to the knee**

   J. **Of the five carcinomas most likely to metastasize to bone (lung, breast, prostate, kidney, thyroid), bronchogenic carcinoma of the lung is most common to occur below the knee**

   K. **If another primary lesion is found in a metastatic location distal to the knee, the primary carcinoma often has already metastasized to the lung**

   L. **Treatment to prevent pathologic fracture or for palliation is indicated to maintain quality of life**

METASTASIS IN THE FOOT

I. **Statistics**

   A. **Metastasis to the foot is an extremely rare event**

   B. **About 1 in 10,000 primary malignancies metastasize to the foot**

   C. **In a recent series on the largest study in metastases to the foot, 13 of the primary tumors were from the LUNGS, KIDNEYS, or COLON**

   D. **Metastasis to the hand is twice as common as to the foot**

   E. **Supradiaphragmatic lesions have a tendency to metastasize to the hand, whereas subdiaphragmatic lesions metastasize to the foot**

   F. **Majority of metastasis are to the calcaneus (60%) and the metatarsals (20%)**

   G. **The highest incidence is men between 60 to 80 years of age**

OSSEOUS TUMOR BREAKDOWN BY LOCATION

I. **Goss and Walter classification by skeletal location**

   A. **The foot is broken down into 4 zones** *(see diagram)*

   B. **Represents the most common location for each osseous neoplasm when they occur in the foot**

C. Some osseous lesions only occur in one area, while others occur in more than one area
  1. **Zone I**: *phalanges*
     a. Bizarre parosteal osteochondromatosis proliferation (90%)
     b. Enchondroma (80%)
     c. Osteoid osteoma (30%)
     d. Chondromyxoid fibroma (30%)
  2. **Zone II**: *metatarsals*
     a. Osteochondroma (80%)
     b. Ewing's sarcoma (60%)
     c. Chrondromyxoid fibroma (60%)
     d. Giant cell tumor (40%)
     e. Chrondrosarcoma (30%)
     f. Osteosarcoma (30%)
  3. **Zone III**: *tarsal bones, except talus and calcaneus*
     a. Epithelioid hemangioendothelioma (80%)
     b. Plasmacytoma (70%)
     c. PNVS (50%)
     d. Osteosarcoma (20%)
  4. **Zone IV**: *talus and calcaneus*
     a. Fibrosarcoma (90%)
     b. Intraosseous lipoma (80%)
     c. UBC (70%)
     d. Osteoid osteoma (60%)
     e. Chrondrosarcoma (60%)
     f. Chondroblastoma (50%)
     g. Giant cell tumor (40%)
     h. Chondromyxoid fibroma (30%)
     i. Osteosarcoma (40%)
     j. Ewing's sarcoma (30%)

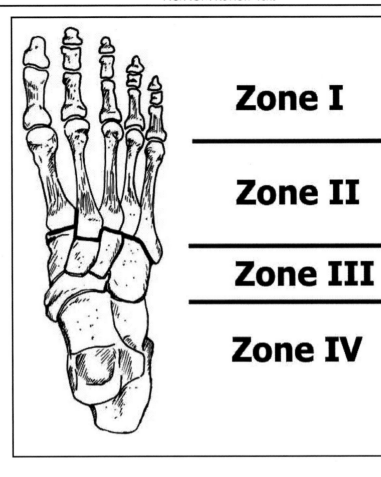

REFERENCES

Acharaya S, Pradhan NK, Rao PT: Giant cell tumour of bones of the foot. J Foot Surg 4(1):28-31, 1989.

Aisen AM, Martel W, Braunstein EM, McMillin KI, Phillips WA, Kling TF: MRI and CT evaluation of primary bone and soft-tissue tumors. Am J Roentgenol 146:749-756, 1986.

Appenzeller J, Weitzner S: Intraosseous lipoma of os calcis: case report and review of literature of intraosseous lipoma of extremities. Clin Orthop 101:171-175, 1974.

Aszodi K: Benign osteoblastoma: quantitative histological distinction from osteoid osteoma. Arch Orthop Unfallchir 88:359-368, 1977.

Bakotic B, Huvos AG: Tumors of the bones of the feet: The clinicopathologic features of 150 cases. J Foot Ankle Surg 40 (5):277-286, 2001.

Berlin S, Mirkin G, Tubridy S: Tumors of the heel. Clin Pod Med Surg 7:307–321, 1990.

Berrettoni BA, Carter JR: Mechanisms of cancer metastasis to bone. J. Bone Joint Surg 68A:308-312, 1986.

Beskin JL, Haddad RJ: Desmoplastic fibroma of the first metatarsal: A case report. Clin Orthop Rel Res 195:299-303, 1985.

Biscaglia R, Gasbarrini A, Bohling T, Bacchini P, Bertoni F, Pici P: Osteosarcoma of the bones of the foot: An easily misdiagnosed malignant tumor. Mayo Clin Proc 73:842– 847, 1998.

Burns TP, et al: Giant cell tumor of the metatarsal. Foot Ankle 8:223, 1988.

Carrasco CH, Murray JA: Giant cell tumors. Orthop Clin North Am 20(3):395-405, 1989.

Casadei R, Ferraro A, Ferruzzi A, Biagini R, Ruggieri P: Bone tumors of the foot: epidemiology and diagnosis. Chir Organi Mov 76:47-62, 1991.

Choll LB, Malawer MM: Analysis of surgical treatment of 33 foot and ankle tumors, Foot Ankle 15:175, 1994.

Choong PF, Qureshi AA, Sim FH, Unni KK: Osteosarcoma of the foot. A review of 52 patients at the Mayo Clinic. Acta Orthop Scand 70(4):361– 364, 1999.

Dahlin D, Salvador A: Chondrosarcomas of bones of the hand and feet: A study of 30 cases. Cancer 34:755, 1974.

Dahlin DC: Bone tumors, ed 4, Springfield, Ill, 1986, Charles C Thomas.

Dahlin DC: Bone Tumors: General Aspects and Data on 6,221 Cases, 3rd Ed. Springfield, IL, Thomas, 1978.

Dhillon MS, Singh DP, Mittal RL, Gill SS, Nagi ON: Primary malignant and potentially malignant tumours of the foot. Foot 2(1):19-26, 1992.

Enneking WF, Spanier SS, Goodman MA: A system for the surgical staging of musculoskeletal sarcoma. Clin Orthop 153:106– 120, 1980.

Enneking, WF (ed.): Musculoskeletal Tumor Surgery. New York, Churchill Livingstone, 1983.

Fink BR, Temple HT, Chiracosta F, Mizel MS, Murphey MD: Chondroblastoma of the foot. Foot Ankle Int 18:236-242, 1997.

Flandry E, Hughston JC: Current concepts review. Pigmented villonodular synovitis. J Bone Joint Surg 69A:942-949, 1987.

Frassica FJ, Waltrip RL, Sponseller PD, Ma LD, McCarthy EF: Clinicopathologic features of osteoid osteoma and osteoblastoma in children and adolescents. Orthop Clin North Am 27:559-574, 1996.

Friscia DA: Pigmented villonodular synovitis of the ankle: A case report and review of the literature. Foot Ankle Int 15:674-678, 1994.

Fuselier C, Binning T, Kushner D, et al: Solitary osteochondroma of the foot: An indepth study with case reports. J Foot Surg 23:3, 1984.

Gall RJ, Sim FH, Pritchard DJ: Metastatic tumors to the bones of the foot. Cancer 37:1492-1495, 1976.

Goss LR, Walter JH: Aneurysmal bone cyst of the distal tibia in a pediatric patient. JAPMA 87(3):136-40, 1997.

Greenfield GB: Radiology of bone disease. Philadelphia, J.B. Lippincott, 1990, pp. 649-701.

Greenspan A, Raiszadeh K, Riley GM, Matthews D: Intraosseous lipoma of the calcaneus. Foot Ankle Int 18:53-56, 1997.

Hattrup SJ, Amadio PC, Sim FH, Lombardi RM: Metastatic tumors of the foot and ankle. Foot Ankle 8:243-247, 1988.

Healey JH, Turnbull A, Miedema B, Lane JM: Acrometastases: a study of twenty-nine patients with osseous involvement of the hands and feet. J Bone Joint Surg 68-A:743–746, 1986.

Hudson TM: Fluid levels in aneurysmal bone cysts: a CT feature. Am J Roentgenol 141:1001-1004, 1984.

Jackson RP, Reckling FW, Mantz FA: Osteoid osteoma and osteoblastoma. Clin Orthop 128:303-313, 1977.

Johnson MR: Epidemiology of soft-tissue and bone tumors of the foot. Clin Pod Med Surg 10(4):581, 1993.

Kransdorf MJ, Sweet DE: Aneurysmal bone cyst: concept, controversy, clinical presentation, and imaging. Am J Roentgenol 164(3):573-580, 1995.

Kricum ME, Kricum R, Haskin ME: Chondroblastoma of the calcaneus: radiographic features with emphasis on location. Am J Radiol 128:613-616, 1977.

Leeson MC, Lippitt SB, Makley JT: Thermal aspects of the use of polymethyl methacrylate in large metaphyseal defects in bone. A clinical review and laboratory study. In New Developments for Limb Salvage in Musculoskeletal Tumors. Yamamuro, T. (ed.), Tokyo, Springer-Verlag, 1989, pp. 277-288.

Libson E, Bloom RA, Husband JE, Stoker DJ: Metastatic tumours of bones of the hand and foot: A comparative review and report of 43 additional cases. Skeletal Radiol 16:387-392, 1987.

Mankin HJ, Gebhardt MC: Advances in the management of bone tumors. Clin Orthop 200:73–83, 1985.

Marcove RC: A 17-year review of cryosurgery in the treatment of bone tumors. Clin Orthop 163:231-233, 1982.

Mechlin MB, Kricun ME, Stead J, Schwamm HA: Giant cell tumor of tarsal bones. Skeletal Radiol 11:266-270, 1984.

Meneses MF, Unni KK, Swee RG: Bizarre parosteal osteo-chondromatous proliferation of bone (Nora's lesion). Am J Surg Pathol 17(7):691– 697, 1993.

Miyayama H, Sakamoto K, Ide M, Ise K, Hirota K, Yasunaga T, Ishihara A: Aggressive osteoblastoma of the calcaneus. Cancer 71:346-353, 1993.

Mullins F, Beard CW, Eisenberg SH: Chondrosarcoma following synovial chondromatosis, Cancer 18:1180, 1965.

Murari TM, Callaghan JJ, Berrey BH, Sweet DE: Primary benign and malignant osseous neoplasms of the foot. Foot Ankle 10:68-80, 1989.

Ogose A, Unni KK, Swee RG, May GK, Rowland CM, Sim FH: Chondrosarcoma of the small bones of the hands and feet. Cancer 80:50–59, 1997.

O'Keefe RJ, O'Donnell RJ, Temple HT, Scully SP, Mankin HJ: Giant cell tumor of the foot. Foot Ankle Int 16:617-623, 1995.

Ozdemir MH, Yilmaz C, Yildiz Y, Saglik Y: Tumors of the foot and ankle: analysis of 196 cases. J Foot Ankle Surg 36(6):403-408, 1997.

Pandey S: Giant cell tumor of the talus. Int Surg 55:179-182, 1971.

Posteraro RH: Radiographic evaluation of pedal osseous tumors. Clin Pod Med Surg 10:633-653, 1993.

Poussa M, Holmstrom T: Intraosseous lipoma of the calcaneus: report of a case and a short review of the literature. Acta Orthop. Scand 47:570-574, 1976.

Salo J, Lewis J, Woodruff J: Malignant fibrous histiocytoma of the extremity. Cancer 58:1765, 1999.

Shereff MJ, Cullivan WT, Johnson KA: Osteoid osteoma of the foot. J Bone Joint Surg 65A:638-641, 1983.

Simon WH, Brooks ML, Mayer DP, Mitchell EI, Schmidt RG, Schwamm HA: Magnetic resonance imaging of calcaneal aneurysmal bone cyst. J Foot Surg 29:448-451, 1990.

Sundberg SB, Carlson WO, Johnson KA: Metastatic lesions of the foot and ankle. Foot Ankle 3:167-169, 1982.

West A, Polito MA: Aneurysmal bone cyst of the foot. J Am Pod Med Assoc 71:446-449, 1981.

Wilkins RM, Pritchard DJ, Burgert EO, Unni EE: Ewing's sarcoma of bone: experience with 140 patients. Cancer 58:2551-2555, 1986.

Williams RP, Pechero G: Management of soft-tissue and bone tumors of the foot. Clin Pod Med Surg 10(4):717-725, 1993.

Wu KK, Guise ER: Metastatic tumors of the foot. South Med J 71:807–808, 1978.

Wu KK: Ewing's sarcoma of the foot. J Foot Surg 28:166, 1989.

Wu KK: Fibrosarcoma of the foot. J Foot Surg 26:530, 1987.

Wu KK: Giant cell tumor of the foot. J Foot Surg 31:414-419, 1992.

Wu KK: Osteoblastoma of the foot. J Foot Surg 27:92-94, 1988.

Wu KK: Osteoid osteoma of the foot. J Foot Surg 30:190-194, 1991.

Yeager KK, Mitchell M, Sartoris DJ: Diagnostic imaging approach to bone tumors of the foot. J Foot Surg 30:197-208,1991.

Zindrick MR, Young MP, Daley RJ, Light TR: Metastatic tumors of the foot: case report and literature review. Clin Orthop 170:219-225, 1982.

CHAPTER 17
OSSEOUS TUMORS

1. Which of the following is **NOT** a tumor of unknown origin?

    A. Aneurysmal bone cyst
    B. Osteoid osteoma
    C. Giant cell tumor
    D. Ewing's sarcoma

2. Which of the following is **NOT** a primary radiographic sign of a malignant osseous tumor?

    A. Codman's triangle
    B. Buttress pattern of periosteal reaction
    C. Permeative lesion
    D. Onion skinning periosteal reaction

3. Which of the following is **NOT** in the Enneking classification of benign bone tumors?

    A. Active
    B. Latent
    C. Aggressive
    D. Non-reactive

4. Ollier's disease is associated with what osseous tumor?

    A. Osteochondroma
    B. Osteoblastoma
    C. Chondroblastoma
    D. Enchondroma

5. Which of the following neoplasms is located strictly in the epiphyseal location?

    A. Giant cell tumor
    B. Enchondroma
    C. Chondroblastoma
    D. Fibrous dysplasia

6. What is the most common osseous neoplasm in the body?

    A. Osteochondroma
    B. Osteoblastoma
    C. Chondroblastoma
    D. Enchondroma

7. Cryosurgery is most successful with what osseous tumor?

    A. Aneurysmal bone cyst
    B. Giant cell tumor
    C. Fibrous dysplasia
    D. Enchondroma

8.   Which benign bone tumor produces a **"bulls-eye"** configuration on a radiograph because of its radiolucent central nidus?

     A.   Osteochondroma
     B.   Enchondroma
     C.   Osteoblastoma
     D.   Osteoid osteoma

9.   What neoplasm is often confused with a benign bone tumor, but actually arises from the reticuloendothelial system and is know as **"Langerhan's cell histiocystosis"**?

     A.   Giant cell tumor
     B.   Eosinophilic granuloma
     C.   Malignant fibrosis histiocytoma
     D.   Chrondrosarcoma

10. **Albright's syndrome** is often associated with what benign bone tumor?

     A.   Osteochondroma
     B.   Giant cell tumor
     C.   Fibrous dysplasia
     D.   Eosinophilic granuloma

11. Which of the following are considered **"round cell tumors"**?

     A.   Ewing's sarcoma
     B.   Peripheral chondrosarcoma
     C.   Small cell osteosarcoma
     D.   Both A and C are correct

12. Which of the following carcinomas is most likely to metastasize to bones below the knee?

     A.   Breast
     B.   Lung
     C.   Prostate
     D.   Kidney

13. What high-grade bone tumor is most commonly associated with Paget's disease?

     A.   Chondrosarcoma
     B.   Ewing's Sarcoma
     C.   Osteosarcoma
     D.   Malignant Fibrous Histiocytoma

14. A giant cell tumor is classified as:

     A.   Benign latent
     B.   Benign aggressive
     C.   Benign active
     D.   Low-grade malignant

15.   Hand-Schuller-Christian disease is associated with what osseous neoplasm?

        A.   Unicameral bone cyst
        B.   Enchondroma
        C.   Eosinophilic granuloma
        D.   Parosteal osteosarcoma

The following are matching questions and are only used once.

16.	Fibrous dysplasia	A.	String sign
17.	Osteosarcoma	B.	Fallen fragment sign
18.	Enchondroma	C.	Ground glass appearance on radiograph
19.	Chondroblastoma	D.	Sunburst pattern
20.	Giant cell tumor	E.	Onion-skinning
21.	Ewing's sarcoma	F.	Fluid-filled levels on MRI
22.	Osteochondroma	G.	Popcorn appearance on radiograph
23.	Chondrosarcoma	H.	Smoke ring calcification
24.	Unicameral bone cyst	I.	Moth-eaten appearance on radiograph
25.	Aneurysmal bone cyst	J.	Stippled calcification on radiograph

DIABETES MELLITUS

By Jason T. Bruse, Todd C. Loftus and Gregg K. Young, based on a chapter originally written by Elizabeth Auger, Stephen Palmer, Dean Titemore and Gregg K. Young

PATHOGENSIS AND CLINICAL DIAGNOSIS

I. **Definition**

   A. **Diabetes Mellitus is a group of metabolic diseases characterized by hyperglycemia resulting from defects in insulin secretion, insulin action, or both.** The chronic hyperglycemia of diabetes is associated with long-term damage, dysfunction, and failure of various organs, especially the eyes, kidneys, nerves, heart, and blood vessels

   B. **Symptoms of diabetes include polyuria, polydipsia, weight loss, sometimes with polyphagia, and blurred vision.** Acute, life-threatening consequences of diabetes are hyperglycemia with ketoacidosis, or the non-ketotic hyperosmolar syndrome

II. **Classification of Diabetes Mellitus**

Note: Several classification systems have been employed in the past to describe diabetes mellitus. As a result of a better understanding of the disease process, the World Health Organization's Expert Committee on Diabetes has recommended a new classification system

   A. **Important changes in new and current classification scheme:**

      1. The terms insulin-dependent diabetes mellitus and non-insulin dependent diabetes mellitus and their acronyms IDDM and NIDDM have been eliminated. These terms erroneously classify patients by their treatment rather than etiology

      2. The terms Type 1 and Type 2 diabetes are retained with Arabic numerals rather than Roman numerals

   B. **Diabetes mellitus**

      1. Type 1 Diabetes mellitus:

         a. Characterized by Pancreatic Beta cell destruction usually leading to absolute insulin deficiency

2. Type 2 Diabetes mellitus:
   a. Characterized by insulin resistance with or without an insulin secretory defect. This category of patients is expected to be reclassified as more is learned about the various causes and treatments of the complexities of insulin resistance
3. Type 3 Diabetes: Other Specific Types
   a. Specific genetic defects in Beta cell function
   b. Specific genetic defects in insulin action
   c. Diseases of the exocrine pancreas (pancreatitis, trauma, neoplasia, etc.)
   d. Endocrinopathies (i.e., acromegaly, Cushing's syndrome, glucagonoma, etc.)
   e. Drug or chemical induced
   f. Infection induced (cytomegalovirus, congenital, rubella, etc.)
   g. Uncommon forms of immuno-mediated diabetes (i.e., anti-insulin receptor antibodies)
4. Gestational Diabetes Mellitus (GDM)
   a. Patients develop hyperglycemia during pregnancy. Glucose tolerance and control usually return to normal after pregnancy
   b. Patients have an increased risk of developing diabetes later in life

III. Pathogenesis of Type 1 and Type 2 Diabetes

A. Type 1 – Pancreatic Beta cell destruction

1. Stems from an autoimmune destruction of pancreatic Beta cells leading to reduced production or absence of insulin
2. Markers of the immune mediated destruction include islet cell antibodies (ICA), autoantibodies to insulin (IAA), autoantibodies to glutamic acid decarboxylase and autoantibodies to the tyrosine phosphatases IA-2 and IA-2B. Eighty to ninety percent of individuals with detected fasting hyperglycemia initially have one or more of these antibodies
3. Type 1 has strong HLA associations
4. Rate of Beta cell destruction is variable: faster in infants and children, slower in adults
5. Some patients are initially diagnosed when they present in diabetic ketoacidosis (DKA), while others have modest fasting hyperglycemia that can rapidly change to DKA in the presence of stress or infection, while still others have enough residual Beta cells and circulating insulin to prevent DKA for several years
6. Immune mediated diabetes commonly presents in childhood and adolescence, but can occur as late as the 8th or 9th decade of life
7. There are a minority of patients with Type 1 diabetes who have no autoimmune markers, and no HLA association. This idiopathic form of Type 1 diabetes usually occurs in patients of African or Asian decent, and appears to be inherited

B. Type 2

1. Seen predominantly in adults, but occasionally in juveniles
2. Characterized by insulin resistance and relative decrease (rather than absolute) decrease in insulin secretion
3. Likely has many different causes
4. Patients have circulating endogenous insulin, which is:
   a. Usually sufficient to prevent ketoacidosis
   b. Insufficient to prevent increased serum glucose due to insulin insensitivity
5. Most patients are obese;
   a. Obesity itself causes some degree of insulin resistance

6. Risk of developing Type 2 diabetes increases with age, weight gain, and inactivity
7. Patients often go undiagnosed for years because hyperglycemia develops slowly and patients do not recognize the classic symptoms of diabetes
8. No islet cell antibodies or other immune components are present
9. Occurs more frequently in women who had Gestational Diabetes previously
10. Occurs more frequently in patients with dyslipidemia and hypertension
11. Type 2 Diabetes has a strong genetic component, but the details are still poorly understood

IV. Clinical Diagnosis/Diagnostic Testing:

Because of past inconsistencies and controversy regarding the most appropriate test to diagnose diabetes, the diagnostic criteria for DM has recently been changed, and are summarized by the following table:

A. Criteria for the Diagnosis of Diabetes:

1. Symptoms plus casual plasma glucose levels ≥ 200 mg/dl. Casual is defined as any time of day without regard to time since last meal. The classic symptoms of diabetes include polydipsia, polyuria, and unexplained weight loss or
2. Fasting Plasma Glucose ≥ 126mg/dl. Fasting is defined as no calorie intake for at least eight hours or
3. Two-hour plasma glucose ≥ 200 mg/dl during an Oral Glucose Tolerance Test. The test should be performed using a glucose load containing the equivalent of 75 GM anhydrous glucose dissolved in water, as described by WHO
Notes: Any of the above criteria must be confirmed on a subsequent day to warrant the diagnosis of diabetes. Fasting plasma glucose is recommended in clinical settings because of ease of administration, convenience, lower cost, and acceptability to patients. Glycosylated hemoglobin is not recommended as a method for diagnosis of diabetes, but rather as a tool for monitoring treatments.

B. Type 1 Diabetes Mellitus

1. Most commonly seen in young adults: (under age 40)
   a. Can occur at any age
2. Strong family history of:
   a. Diabetes mellitus
   b. Thyroid disorders (i.e., Hashimoto's thyroiditis)
   c. Other autoimmune diseases
3. Ketosis prone
4. Screening: Because there are no accepted treatments to intervene with the natural progression of early Type 1 Diabetes, random testing or screening for genetic markers or autoantibodies in order to identify potential undiagnosed patients is not recommended at this time

C. Type 2 Diabetes Mellitus

1. Often asymptomatic at time of diagnosis
   a. Incidental finding on blood tests/urinalysis
2. Usually patient is over 40 years old; however, it is becoming more common in younger age groups
3. Often overweight/obese
4. May have family history of diabetes but not as consistent as in Type 1
5. Ketonuria & ketonemia are uncommon at time of diagnosis
6. Generally not ketosis prone

a. Can be seen in times of severe infections or surgical stress
7. Screening: Because it is suspected that up to eight million people currently have undiagnosed Diabetes Type 2, testing and screening is cost-effective in high-risk individuals. The criteria are as follows:

D. Criteria for testing for diabetes Type 2 in asymptomatic, undiagnosed individuals:
1. Testing should be considered in all individuals at age 45 years and above and, if normal, it should be repeated at three-year intervals
2. Testing should be considered at a younger age or be carried out more frequently in individuals who:
    a. Are overweight
    b. Have a first-degree relative with diabetes
    c. Are members of a high-risk ethnic population (African-American, Hispanic American, Native American, Asian American, and Pacific Islander)
    d. Have delivered a baby weighing > 9 lbs or been diagnosed with GDM
    e. Have hypertension
    f. Have an HDL cholesterol level ≤ 35 and/or a triglycerides level ≥ 250
    g. Have Impaired Glucose Tolerance (prior FBG of ≥ 110 mg/dl, but ≤ 126 mg/dl)

TREATMENT OF DIABETES MELLITUS

I. **Treatment Goals for Patients with Diabetes:**
   A. **The better the control, the lower the HbA1c, and the fewer the complications**
      1. HbA1c (test semi-annually) < 7.0%
      2. Blood Pressure < 130/80
      3. LDL Cholesterol (check every two years) < 100
      4. Foot Exam (check at least annually)
      5. Microalbumin/Creatinine Ratio (check annually) < 30
      6. Dilated Eye Exam (annually)
      7. Tight glucose control should be weighed against the risk of hypoglycemia

II. **Diet and Exercise**

Diet and exercise as sole treatment for diabetes is reserved for patients who have not experienced severe hyperglycemic symptoms, have had no significant weight loss, and have not been ketonuric. Additionally, proper diet and daily exercise may enable a patient who is taking insulin to decrease the insulin dosage

III. **Oral Medications**
   A. **Sulfonylureas** (Table 1)
      1. Act by stimulating endogenous secretion of insulin, although do not cause the biosynthesis of pro-insulin
      2. Second generation sulfonylureas restore the sensitivity of the Beta cell to glucose to a greater extent than the first generation drugs
      3. Vary in rapidity of onset of action (i.e., glipizide given 30 minutes before meals will have a greater effect on glucose levels from that meal than glyburide)

4. Duration of action varies between the sulfonylureas; this dictates dosage and timing of administration
5. Metabolism and excretion
   a. Highly bound to serum albumin, and therefore may compete for binding sites with other drugs
   b. Second generation sulfonylureas are less likely to have interaction with other drugs than are first generation agents because of their non-ionic nature
   c. Are metabolized by the liver and excreted by the kidney and in feces
6. Common drug interactions
   a. Hypoglycemia
      i. Aspirin and trimethoprim displace sulfonylureas from their binding sites
      ii. Alcohol, antihistamines, and anticoagulants are inhibitors of sulfonylurea metabolism
      iii. Probenecid and allopurinol inhibit urinary excretion of sulfonylureas
      iv. Beta-adrenergic blockers and sympatholytic drugs antagonize counter regulatory hormones
      v. Although uncommon, hypoglycemia from sulfonylureas tends to be severe and prolonged
   b. Hyperglycemia
      i. Barbiturates and rifampin will increase the metabolism of sulfonylureas
      ii. Thiazides and loop diuretics, beta-adrenergic blockers, and phenytoin will inhibit insulin secretion
      iii. Corticosteroids, growth hormone, estrogens, and catecholamines inhibit the action of insulin
7. Recommended for lean patients

Table 1: Sulfonylureas

Drug	Dose, mg	Doses/day	Duration of Action, hours	Metabolism/Excretion
FIRST GENERATION				
Tolbutamide	500 -3000	2-3	6-12	Liver
Tolazamide	100 -1000	1-2	12-14	Liver
Chlorpropamide	100 -500	1	60	Liver/Kidney
SECOND GENERATION				
Glyburide	1.25 - 20	1-2	to 24	Liver/Kidney
Glipizide	5 – 20	1-2	to 24	Liver/Kidney
Glimepiride	1 – 8	1-2	to 24	Liver/Kidney

B. **Biguanides - metformin**
   1. Thought to inhibit hepatic gluconeogenesis and may also enhance glucose utilization in muscle and adipose
   2. Does not cause hypoglycemia
   3. May cause weight loss but not weight gain, recommended for obese patients
   4. The most common side effect is gastrointestinal upset
   5. Can be used as mono therapy for patients who fail diet/exercise regimen, and is often added as adjunct
   6. Use must be monitored for lactic acidosis
   7. Dosage: 500 mg BID to 850 mg TID
C. **Thiazolidinediones – "glitazones"** (rosiglitazone, pioglitazone)
   1. These drugs are known as "insulin sensitizers", and have a mechanism of action

entirely different from the sulfonylureas, glucosidase inhibitors, or biguanides Thiazolidinediones are highly selective agonists for the peroxisome proliferator activated receptor (PPAR) that regulates the transcription of a number of insulin responsive genes

2. Unlike oral sulfonylureas, thiazolidinediones enhance tissue sensitivity to insulin, rather than stimulating insulin secretion. Both thiazolidinediones and sulfonylureas are ineffective in patients with insulin deficiency (Type 1 Diabetes)
3. Good option for patients who are intolerant to metformin
4. Edema can be significant side effect
5. Expensive
6. Contraindicated in heart failure
7. No resulting hypoglycemia
8. Dosages: rosiglitazone: 2–8 mg/day
                      pioglitazone: 15–5 mg/day

D. Glucosidase inhibitors

1. Glucosidase is an enzyme of the intestinal brush border that aids in the digestion and absorption of carbohydrates
2. Glucosidase blocks the digestion of starch, sucrose, and maltose, resulting in smaller increases of postprandial plasma glucose levels
3. Must be given before a main meal because the drug is a competitive inhibitor of glycosidase and must be present when the carbohydrates are present in the small intestine
4. Hypoglycemia does not occur when glucosidase inhibitors are the primary form of therapy
5. Most common side effect is gastrointestinal upset
6. Dose: 150-300 mg/day divided TID

E. Oral Medication Treatment Strategies/Principles

1. Tight control should never take precedence over the risk of hypoglycemia
2. Obese patient: begin with metformin. If not tolerated, then switch to a glitazone
3. Lean patient: begin with a sulfonylurea
4. Dosage should be maximized on a single oral agent before adding a second or a third agent
    a. Preferred combination: metformin with a sulfonylurea, metformin with a glitazone or a sulfonylurea with a glitazone
5. When combination of two oral agents fails, the next option is: three oral agents, a single oral agent + insulin, or basic insulin therapy protocol (see insulin section)
6. Patient should be seen and glucose levels checked at least every three weeks until stabilized. Average blood glucose should be under 140 mg/dl (both for fasting blood glucose and two-hour postprandial)

III. Insulin

Insulin is made from pork pancreas, or is made identical to human insulin through recombinant DNA technology. Insulin is available in short, medium, and long acting types that may be injected separately or mixed in the same syringe

NOTE: Again, tight glucose control should be weighed against the risk of hypoglycemia

A. Basic Insulin Therapy:

1. Calculate the predicted insulin need (PIN): obese – 1.1 u/kg, non-obese = 0.55 u/kg
2. Initially use 30-60 % of PIN in divided doses
    a. A.M.: 2/3 of total daily dose at breakfast, 2 parts NPH or lente, 1 part regular or humalog

b. P.M.: 1/3 of total daily dose at dinner, equal parts of NPH or lente and regular or humalog
3. The patient should report finger stick glucose levels daily for first five days at the following times: before breakfast, before lunch, before dinner, and at bedtime. When the BG falls outside of a stated parameter, adjust dosage per the following table:

Table 2: Insulin Types

Is A.M. FBG 90-140? If no, raise (high BG) or lower (low BG) P.M. NHP/Lente by 10-15%
Is before lunch BG 90-140? If no, raise or lower A.M. Regular/Humalog by 10-15%
Is before dinner BG 90-140%? If no, raise or lower A.M. NPH/Lente by 10-15%
Is bedtime BG 90-140? If no, raise or lower P.M. Regular/Humalog by 10-15%

4. If the patient experiences excessive hypoglycemia in the presence of uncontrolled hyperglycemia, he should be placed on intensive insulin therapy: an endocrine consult is needed. If the HbA1c cannot be lowered to less than 8, intensive insulin therapy is also recommended
5. Return visits should include a review of finger stick records and repeat HbA1c every three months

B. **Oral Agent plus insulin strategy:**
1. NPH, Lente, Ultralente, or Lantus is given in a single P.M. injection and used to control fasting A.M. BG
2. Oral agent is used to control daytime BG
3. It is almost always possible to control a.m. fasting blood glucose by increasing or decreasing the nighttime insulin injection
4. Once a.m. BG is controlled with insulin, daytime BG readings will often come under control with the oral agent
5. Dose oral agent + insulin starting dose of 0.1-0.2 u/kg of NPH, lente, ultralente, or lantus
    1. Initial adjustments of insulin dosage are made, increasing or decreasing by 10-20% until A.M. FBG is controlled
    2. Addition of one or two other oral agents may help daytime control (see oral strategies section)
    3. If average BG is not < 126 mg/dl, move to basic insulin therapy

C. **Intensive insulin therapy:**
1. Involves multiple factors and therefore patients should be referred to an endocrinologist or diabetes management team
2. The general treatment principles are as follows:
    a. Short acting insulin (humalog) is given before, at, or after meals and snacks
        i. Insulin dosage is calculated based upon carbohydrate counting of the meal/snack
    b. Long acting insulin (Ultralente or NPH) is used once or twice daily, generally in the evening to control overnight BG
3. Lantus:
    a. Administered once daily, usually at bedtime for Type 1 and Type 2 Diabetics who require long acting insulin for the control of hyperglycemia
    b. Cannot be diluted or mixed with other types of insulin
    c. Administer subcutaneously only—not IV
    d. Lantus is more expensive than other long-acting insulin

IV. Complications of Therapy:

A. Exercise induced hypoglycemia
1. May occur acutely and up to 24 hours post exercise (lag effect)
2. Counteract hypoglycemia with a carbohydrate snack (10g for exercise of short duration and up to 50g for exercise of high intensity and long duration), or decrease the insulin dose (5% decrease for low intensity exercise and up to a 30% decrease for exercise of high intensity and long duration)
3. Monitor BGL before and after exercise to better manage diabetes

B. Nocturnal hypoglycemia
1. Somogyi effect – an overnight hypoglycemic episode that occurs secondary to a high evening dose of intermediate or long acting insulin, resulting in a high AM fasting BG; the high fasting BG occurs because counter regulatory hormones are released in response to low BG and cause glycogenolysis and gluconeogenesis
   a. Check BG in the early morning hours (2-4 AM) to make diagnosis
   b. Treatment consists of decreasing the evening dose of insulin; the timing of insulin dose may need to be changed (i.e., pre-dinner intermediate acting insulin moved to bedtime)

C. Morning fasting hyperglycemia
1. Rule out Somogyi effect
2. Waning insulin – when the evening dose of insulin is not sufficient in duration of action to control BG in the early waking hours
3. Diagnosis consists of early morning blood glucose checks
4. Treatment includes longer acting insulin to be given or postponing the dosage to later at night

D. Dawn phenomenon – the secretion of growth hormone at night increases glucose production by the liver and a decreased sensitivity to the action of insulin
1. Usually occurs between 4:00 a.m. – 8:00 a.m
2. Diagnosis consists of early morning blood glucose checks
3. Treatment consists of giving intermediate acting insulin at bedtime

E. Medications
1. Nonselective beta-blockers may impair glucose recovery from hypoglycemia
2. Sulfonylurea therapy alone may induce hypoglycemia
3. Certain drugs that potentiate action of sulfonylureas:
   a. Alcohol, tricyclic antidepressant, antihistamines, phenylbutazone, chloramphenicol, probenecid, MAO inhibitors, clofibrate, warfarin, and other sulfonamides

F. Alcohol
1. Excessive alcohol intake in either insulin-dependent or non insulin-dependent diabetics will inhibit hepatic gluconeogenesis

G. Antibodies to insulin and the insulin receptor
1. Can result anytime insulin is the choice of treatment
2. Hypoglycemia may be caused by the release of bound insulin from the antibodies, action of the antibody-insulin complex on the insulin receptor, and/or prolongation of the circulating half-life of injected insulin

H. Extrinsic factors related to insulin resistance
1. Most common factor is obesity; there is a decreased responsiveness to insulin in all of the major target tissues (muscle, liver, and fat)
2. Other clinical states such as surgery, acute illness, infection, and ketoacidosis
3. Metabolic effects of glucocorticoids (i.e.. Cushing's disease, exogenous steroids)
4. Excessive levels of growth hormone

DIABETIC COMPLICATIONS

I. **Systemic vascular complications:**

   A. **Retinopathy**
       1. Non-proliferative diabetic retinopathy – Background Diabetic Retinopathy (BDR)
       2. Venous abnormalities, micro-aneurysms, retinal hemorrhage, edema, exudates
       3. Pre-proliferative retinopathy
       4. Proliferative retinopathy
       5. Neovascularization
       6. Glial proliferation
       7. Vitreoretinal traction

   B. **Treatment**
       1. Diabetic retinopathy is asymptomatic in its most treatable states. Blurred vision may reflect changes in the hydration of the lens or macular edema
       2. Floaters may indicate hemorrhage and flashing lights may indicate retinal detachment
       3. Good glycemic control and treating hypertension reduce the risk of retinopathy
       4. Diabetic retinopathy is best diagnosed by an Ophthalmologist
       5. Forty percent of Type 1 diabetics and 60% of Type 2 diabetics with proliferative retinopathy become blind within five years. Diabetics with proliferative retinopathy have a median survival time of 5.4 years
       5. Photo-coagulation
       6. Fluoroscein angiography

   C. **Coronary disease occurs more frequently in diabetics**
       1. Atherosclerosis
       2. Myocardial infarction
       3. Autonomic Neuropathy
       4. Cardiomyopathy
       5. Congestive heart failure

II. **Nephropathy**

   A. **Renal papillary necrosis**
       1. Infarction secondary to atherosclerosis
       2. Urinary retention

   B. **Cystopathy** (neuropathy of the bladder nerves)
       1. Difficulty initiating or maintaining a urinary stream
       2. Urinary retention
       3. Urinary tract infection
       4. Obstruction of urine flow

   C. **Glomerular pathology**
       1. Inter-capillary glomerulosclerosis
           a. Thickened glomerular basement membrane
           b. Hyaline cap
       2. Afferent and efferent arteriolosclerosis
       3. Microalbuminuria and proteinuria
           a. Microalbuminuria (30-300 mg/24h or greater than 20 mcg/min) – Often first lab evidence of Diabetic Renal Disease
           b. Proteinuria (greater than 300 mg/24h)

        c.   Renal insufficiency (Creatinine greater than 1.5 mg/dl)
     4. Nephrotic syndrome
     5. Azotemia
  D. Contrast media toxicity-patient can develop acute renal failure (acute tabular necrosis) can develop acute renal failure (acute tubular necrosis) after intravascular injection of radiographic contrast agents
  E. End state renal disease
     1. Dialysis
     2. Kidney transplantation

III. Treatment

  A. Team approach
  B. Protect against iatrogenic injury
     1. Limit contrast media
     2. Minimize nephrotoxic drugs, i.e., NSAIDs, amiloride, triamterene, spironolactone, and cyclosporin
     3. Avoid urethral instrumentation
  C. Control hypertension
     1. Diuretic
     2. ACE inhibitors
        a. Renal protective, consider for patients with microalbuminuria
     3. Vasodilators
     4. Calcium channel blockers
     5. Minoxidil
     6. Beta-blockers should be avoided if possible because of adverse effect on glucose control – block movement of K + into cells
  D. Monitor cardiac status:
     1. Renal salt retention simulates congestive failure
     2. Angina exacerbated by anemia
     3. Reduce digoxin dose in renal insufficiency
     4. Furosemide in large doses plus metolazone may be required for diuresis
  E. Rationalize diet:
     1. Reduce protein intake when microalbuminuria detected
     2. Restrict to 40g protein when creatinine clearance drops to 15 ml/min
     3. Adjust dietary salt according to ability to excrete (2-8 g/d)
     4. Encourage consistency in timing and size of meals
  F. Preserve bones:
     1. Reduce hyperphosphatemia in renal insufficiency by intra-gastric phosphorus binding (aluminum hydroxide or carbonate)
     2. Administer synthetic vitamin D3
     3. Rarely subtotal parathyroidectomy
  G. Anticipate reduced insulin requirement:
     1. Renal catabolism accounts for about 25% of insulin metabolism
  H. Cease all cigarette smoking!
     1. In defense of coronary arteries
     2. To prevent post-transplant pulmonary infections
  I. Tight glucose control:
     1. Lower risk of micro-vascular complications when the HbAlc is less than 7.5%

IV. Neuropathy

A. Diffuse neuropathy

1. Distal symmetric sensorimotor polyneuropathy
   a. Neuropathic: Foot ulceration
   b. Painful neuropathy – drugs first used to treat painful neuropathy include: Tricyclic antidepressants (amitriptyline – start at 25 mg qhs and increase to a maximum of 150 to 200 mg). Phenytoin, carbamazepine, gabapentin (initial dose 300 mg to a max of 2400 mg) and topical capsaicin. NSAIDs should be used carefully because of renal toxicity in patients with microalbuminuria. Narcotics have the potential for abuse and should be avoided
   c. Neuroarthropathy (Charcot arthropathy)
2. Autonomic neuropathy
   a. Abnormal papillary function
   b. Sudomotor dysfunction
   c. Distal anhidrosis
   d. Gustatory sweating
   e. Genitourinary autonomic neuropathy
   f. Bladder dysfunction
   g. Decreased sensation of bladder fullness
   h. Diminished frequency of urination
   i. Increased urinary tract infections
   j. Decreased bladder contraction
       i. Straining to urinate
       ii. Dribbling
       iii. Recurrent infections
   k. Sexual dysfunction
       i. Decreased vaginal lubrication
       ii. Decreased erectile function
   l. Gastrointestinal autonomic neuropathy
       i. Gastroparesis – treatment can include:
              Metoclopramide (10-30mg/ 1h ac and hs)
              Erythromycin (250mg/half hour ac)
              Domperidone (20-40mg/1h ac and hs)
              Cisapride (10-20mg/ac)
       ii. Gall bladder atony
       iii. Diabetic diarrhea – tetracycline can be used in one or two doses (200-500mg) Also, diphenoxylate with atropine can also be used
   m. Hypoglycemia unawareness (adrenal medullary neuropathy)
       i. Problematic in patients trying to achieve tight control
   n. Cardiovascular autonomic neuropathy
       i. Abnormal cardiovascular exercise performance
       ii. Postural hypotension
       iii. Cardiac denervation syndrome

B. Focal neuropathy

1. Mononeuropathy
2. Mononeuropathy multiplex
3. Plexopathy-unilateral injury to the femoral nerve plexus
4. Radiculopathy – generally resolve spontaneously over 6-24 months

5. Cranial neuropathy
    a. Often the elderly diabetic
    b. Affects the CNIII
    c. Patients will present with headache and lateral eye movement

THE DIABETIC FOOT

I. **Neuropathy**
    A. **Patients have a tendency of losing their sense of awareness with insensate parts and must be educated as to care for their feet**
    B. **Autonomic neuropathy results in dry skin** (sweat and sebaceous gland dysfunction)
        1. Petroleum based moisturizers tend to dry skin in individuals with normal sweat and sebaceous gland function. Water-based creams are probably better in these individuals
        2. Patients with sweat and sebaceous gland dysfunction should use petroleum based products following hydration of tissues (after bathing) to retain moisture
    C. **Ulcers and wounds of the foot** (See Infectious Disease chapter)
        1. Much has been learned in the salvage of tissue
        2. Greater efforts at preserving limbs and digits
        3. Diligent care of ulcers including debridement and encouragement of granulation tissues
        4. Hyperbaric oxygen therapy
        5. Increased arterial dilation/supply via Nitric Oxide pathway (L-arginine)
    D. **Peripheral vascular disease**
        1. Large and medium sized vessels
            a. Atherosclerosis occurs at the same rate as in the age-matched general population
        2. Small vessel disease
            a. Arteriolar disease
    E. **Signs and symptoms of vascular insufficiency**
        1. Intermittent claudication
        2. Cold feet
        3. Rest pain
        4. Pallor of the foot on elevation and delayed capillary filling
        5. Dependent rubor
        6. Atrophic skin changes
    F. **Specific Vascular problems**
        1. Blue Toe Syndrome
        2. Acute arterial occlusion

SKIN DISORDERS ASSOCIATED WITH DIABETES MELLITUS
(See chapter on Dermatology)

I. **Necrobiosis lipoidica diabeticorum:**
    A. **So named due to the degeneration of collagen in the dermis**
    B. **Accompanying atrophy of dermis with yellow plaques**
    C. **No well established treatment, but some success with pentoxifyline**

II. Granuloma annulare:

    A. Arciform plaques that form from the coalescence of red-brown papules

    B. Etiology unknown

    C. Treatment is empiric and includes topical steroids

III. Bullosis diabeticorum:

    A. Lesions arise from normal, non-inflamed skin

    B. Other than local care, no specific treatment recommended

IV. Acanthosis nigricans:

    A. Velvety dark-brown plaques seen on the neck, axilla and groin of diabetics

    B. Associated with insulin resistance syndromes, but often accompanies obese diabetics

    C. Alpha-hydroxy acids can improve the appearance

BIBLIOGRAPHY

The Expert Committee on the Diagnosis and Classification of Diabetes Mellitus; Diabetes Care, vol 25, Supplement 1, ppg S5-S17, January 2002.

Position Statement of the American Diabetes Association "Screening for Diabetes", Diabetes Care, vol 25, Supplement 1, ppg S21-S24, January 2002.

Hairejoshu D. Management of Diabetes Mellitus: Perspectives of Care Across the Life Span, 2nd Ed, Mosby Yr Bk, St. Louis, 1996.

Lebovitz, Harold E. Therapy for Diabetes Mellitus and Related Disorders, third edition. American Diabetes Assoc, Alexandria, 1998, ppg 290-470.

Wahlen, Jack, MD (committee chair). "Care Program Module", Intermountain Health Care Select Committee on Diabetes, 2001.

CHAPTER 18
DIABETES MELLITUS

1. The new classification system for Diabetes Mellitus recommends that health care providers do which of the following:

    A. Eliminate the names Type 1 and Type 2 Diabetes Mellitus
    B. Eliminate the terms IDDM, but retain NIDDM
    C. Eliminate both abbreviations: IDDM and NIDDM
    D. Add Type 3, 4, and 5 Diabetes Mellitus

2. The pathogenesis of Type 1 Diabetes Mellitus involves:

    A. Auto-immune destruction of pancreatic beta cells
    B. Auto-immune destruction of pancreatic alpha cells
    C. Auto-immune destruction of enzyes responsible for glycolysis
    D. Auto-immune destruction of all insulin receptors

3. The pathogenesis of adult-onset Diabetes Mellitus is best characterized by:

    A. A single genetic mutation on insulin receptors
    B. Multiple genetic and environmental factors that have yet to be well defined
    C. Beta cell antibodies
    D. Weak association with hypertension and obesity

4. The diagnosis of Diabetes Mellitus is **best** made by:

    A. A single casual glucose level above 126mg/dl
    B. Fasting plasma glucose levels above 126mg/dl on consecutive days
    C. HbAlc level above 7.0%
    D. Presence of <u>at least</u> two of the three classic symptoms: polydipsia, polyuria, or unexplained weight loss

5. Which of the following lab value/vital sign goals is **incorrect** when managing a patient with Diabetes?

    A. Blood Pressure < 130/80
    B. HbAlc < 8.0%
    C. LDL Cholesterol < 100
    D. Microalbumin/Creatinine Ratio < 30

6. Diabetic Nephropathy is characterized by:

    A. Low creatinine
    B. Low CFR
    C. Thickened glomerular basement membrane
    D. Absence of microalbuminuria

7.   During its most treatable stages, the symptoms of Diabetic Retinopathy are:

      A.   Blurred vision
      B.   Flashing lights
      C.   Often there are no symptoms during treatable stages
      D.   Two of the above
      E.   Three of the above

8.   Which of the following anti-hypertensives is "renal protective" for a patient with Diabetes?

      A.   Beta blockers
      B.   Calcium channel blockers
      C.   Ace inhibitors
      D.   Vasodilators (hydrazine)

9.   In treating painful Diabetic Neuropathy, NSAIDS are:

      A.   Used as a first line treatment
      B.   Used in conjunction with anti-depressants
      C.   Rarely used because of renal toxicity in patients with microalbuminuria
      D.   The most commonly used class of drugs for this condition

10.   Diabetics with peripheral vascular disease usually have:

      A.   Increased atherosclerosis in small vessels
      B.   Increased atherosclerosis in large vessels
      C.   Increased atherosclerosis in medium vessels
      D.   Increased atherosclerosis in all vessels

GENERAL PEDIATRICS

Ronald Valmassy

PEDIATRIC NEUROLOGY

I. Observation of child

    A. Evaluation of alertness

    B. Ability to suck/swallow

    C. Morphological features: Weight, length, head shape/circumference

    D. Symmetry and position of all limbs/digits

    E. Spinal/facial features

II. Evaluation of developmental landmarks

    A. At 3 months

        1. Baby produces vigorous movements

        2. Head bobs when baby is held upright

        3. Head held up when baby lies prone

        4. Baby is able to hold toy

        5. Baby smiles, follow an object

    B. At 6 months

        1. Baby is able to lift head up when lying supine

        2. Baby can roll from supine to prone

        3. Baby is able to support weight when in a standing position

        4. Baby can transfer a toy from hand to hand

    C. At 9-10 months

        1. Baby can pull self into an upright position

    D. At 12 months

        1. Toddler can stand unassisted

        2. Toddler can walk when led

    E. At 15 months

        1. Toddler can walk with a broad base of gait

    F. At 18 months

        1. Toddler can run with only occasional falls

G. **At 24 months**
1. Toddler can run without falling
2. Toddler can walk up and down stairs unassisted
3. Toddler can rise from a squatting position
4. Toddler can walk on heels to test ankle dorsiflexors
5. Toddler can walk on toes to test gastrocnemius
6. Balance may be assessed with toddler's feet together/cerebellar function may be assessed with toddler's eyes open
7. Joint position may be assessed with toddler's eyes closed while standing (Romberg's)

H. **At age 3 years**
1. Child can balance momentarily on one foot

I. **At age 4 years**
1. Child can run and jump

J. **At age 5 years**
1. Child can skip
2. Child can balance momentarily on one foot with eyes closed

III. **Formal examination of neurological status**

A. **Limb symmetry, muscle bulk, tone, strength, and reflexes should be compared on each side**

B. **Muscle strength should be tested in groups**
1. Ll, L2, L3 supply the hip flexors (iliopsoas)
2. L4, L5, S1 enervate the hip extensors (glutei)
3. L2, L3, L4 supply the knee extensors (quadriceps)
4. L5, S1, S2 enervate the knee flexors (hamstrings)
5. L4, L5 supply ankle dorsiflexion (tibialis anterior)
6. S1, S2 supply ankle plantar flexion (gastrocnemius)
7. L4 supply ankle inversion (posterior tibial)
8. L5, S1 supply ankle eversion (peroneals)

C. **Plantar response should be tested last**

D. **Dermatome evaluation based on**
1. Ll, L2, L3: Anterior thigh
2. L4: Anteromedial lower leg
3. L5: Anterolateral lower leg
4. Sl: Outer border of the foot and sole
5. S2: Back of the leg
6. S3, S4, S5: Over the buttocks

E. **Joint position sense:** Move fingers or toes with patient's eyes closed and ask direction of movement

F. **Vibration:** Tuning fork over bony prominence

G. **Cerebellar function:** Slurred speech (dysarthric), jerky eye movements (nystagmus), heel/shin test, and tandem gait

IV. **Assessment of abnormal neurological patterns**

A. **Upper motor neuron (UMN) damage:**
1. Weakness of extensor muscles in upper limbs and flexor group in lower limbs, with spasticity, hyperflexia, and extensor plantar response
2. Hip circumduction in gait (unilateral spasticity)

3. Scissored gait, plantar flexion, and inversion of feet (bilateral spasticity)

B. **Basal ganglion involvement:** Produces tremor, increased tone (rigidity), and slowed movement (hypokinesia)

C. **Cerebellar damage:** Evidenced by slurred speech, nystagmus, lack of coordination, wide-based antalgic gait

D. **Lower motor neuron disorders:** Produces wasting, fasciculation, hypotonia, weakness, areflexia, and flexor plantar responses

E. **Neuropathies:** Produces sensory and motor signs (e.g., loss of vibration, reduced reflexes, foot drop, steppage gait)

F. **Disorders of the neuromuscular junction:** Evidenced by fatiguable weakness without wasting, fasciculation, reflex changes, or sensory loss

G. **Primary muscle disorders** (e.g., polymyositis, Duchenne muscular dystrophy): Produces weakness with or without wasting in upper and lower limbs, normal reflexes, no sensory signs, and swaggering gait with rolling at the hips

V. **Diseases affecting the nervous system**

A. **Cerebral palsy**
   1. Defined as aberrant control or movement due to a central nervous system lesion, damage, or dysfunction; classified into three types:
      a. Spastic (quadriplegia, diplegia, hemiplegia)
      b. Ataxic
      c. Dyskinetic
   2. Most common cause: Intraventricular hemorrhage in preterm infants
   3. Treatment includes passive movement and braces. If surgery is to be utilized to improve ambulation, it should be employed after age 6

B. **Friedreich's ataxia**
   1. Most common form: Hereditary ataxia (autosomal recessive with a high spontaneous mutation rate)
   2. Classical presentation: Child with a clumsy ataxic gait
   3. Tendon reflexes absent in lower extremities. Vibration and position sense are lost
   4. Pes cavus and talipes equino varus are present in 75% of cases

C. **Spina bifida**
   1. Defined as a failure of closure of the spinal column leading to a defect in the vertebral column
   2. Varies in severity from asymptomatic spina bifida occulta to myelomeningocele
   3. Clinically is either flaccid paraparesis or paraplegia with loss of lumbosacral sensation and bladder atonicity

D. **Guillain-Barré syndrome**
   1. Defined as acute post infections and demyelinating motor neuropathy that predominantly involves the anterior spine root
   2. Fifty percent of patients relate a preceding upper respiratory tract infection or diarrheal sickness
   3. Some sensory symptoms but predominantly motor symptoms; onset of weakness occurs distally and asends
   4. Virological tests sometimes demonstrate increase in titer of Epstein-Barré virus
   5. Recovery of strength takes place over months, with a 10% mortality rate

E. **Charcot-Marie-Tooth disease**
   1. Autosomal dominant condition

    2. Type I: Presents in teens or 20s with slowly progressive foot drop secondary to peroneal wasting and peripheral nerve palpably enlarged; type III: Onset of muscle weakness occurs in adult life and peripheral nerve is not palpable

    3. Pes cavus and hammer toes noted: Lateral foot and ankle instability precedes frank weakness

    4. Distal weakness/wasting in the lower limbs, accompanied by tendon hyporeflexia and glove-stocking impaired sensation

    5. Progression is slow in both types

F. Myasthenia gravis

    1. Relapsing and remitting autoimmune disease in which autoantibodies are directed against the patient's own postsynaptic acetal choline receptors at the neuromuscular junction

    2. Neonatal, congenital, juvenile, and adult forms

        a. Neonatal: Appears transiently in 10%-20% of mothers with myasthenia gravis and results in spontaneous improvement

        b. Congenital: Rare; and not life threatening

        c. Juvenile: Similar to adult form, presents at approximately 8 years of age; females are affected 3-4 times more often than males; fatiguable muscle weakness noted; removal of thymus gland may produce improvement or long-term remission

G. Duchenne muscular dystrophy (DMD)

    1. A hereditary myopathy; an X-linked recessive dystrophy due to a mutation at position 21 on the short arm of the X chromosome, resulting in a defective gene (dystrophin); almost exclusively affects males; 1 in 25,000 live births

    2. Manifests itself prior to age 5, with a delay in walking, abnormal gait, frequent falling, and difficulty in climbing stairs

    3. Waddling gait, lordotic posture, abnormal run and hop, difficulty in rising from the floor due to weakness of pelvic girdle muscles (Gower's sign), and pseudohypertrophy of calves

    4. Associated low IQ, equino varus, scoliosis, and fixed flexion contractures

    5. Elevated serum creatine kinase levels and increased echogenecity on ultrasound of muscle

    6. Progressive loss of function, with eventual wheelchair bound usually by 12 years of age

    7. No effective treatment; however, extensive immobilization should be avoided and physical therapy encouraged

PEDIATRIC HISTORY

I. History of present illness

  A. Family history

    1. Include name; age; blood type; and RH of mother, father, brothers, and sisters

    2. Indicate whether anyone in the child's immediate family (parents, siblings, grandparents, uncles, and aunts) had any of the following: allergy, asthma, hay fever, eczema, sinus trouble, bronchitis, drug reactions, anemia, bleeding, diabetes, cancer, leukemia, tuberculosis, epilepsy, convulsive disease, emotional problems, and/or inherited disease

II. Past history

  A. Include birth history: Birthdate, due date, and weight and length at birth, APGAR score

Table 1. APGAR score

Sign		0 Points	1 Point	2 Points
A	Activity	Absent	Arms & legs flexed	Active movement
P	Pulse	Absent	<100 BPM	>100 BPM
G	Grimace	No response	Grimace	Sneeze, cough, pulls away
A	Appearance	Blue-gray, pale all over	Normal except extremities	Normal
R	Respiration	Absent	Slow, irregular	Good, crying

7-10 normal, 4-7 may require resuscitative measures, below 3 requires immediate resuscitation

    B. Determine whether mother had any of the following during pregnancy: anemia, bleeding, infections, surgery, weight gain over 20 pounds, edema, injuries, convulsions, high blood pressure, vomiting, and/or weight loss

    C. Include medications or vitamins taken by mother

    D. Include specifics of labor:
        1. Onset: Spontaneous or induced
        2. Length
        3. Type: Breach, vertex, or cesarean section
        4. Type of anesthesia
        5. Whether forceps were used

    E. Include whether baby required resuscitation, oxygen, or incubator

    F. Include any problems noted in nursery: jaundice, bleeding, breathing difficulties, rash, seizures, cyanosis, vomiting, or infection

III. Early developmental history

    A. Indicate the age at which the child performed the following tasks:
        1. Rolled over
        2. Sat without support
        3. Crawled
        4. Walked alone
        5. Talked in sentences
        6. Toilet trained

    B. Record immunizations
        1. DPT
        2. Oral polio
        3. Measles
        4. Mumps
        5. Rubella
        6. FHV
        7. Tuberculin testing

IV. Later development history and school history

    A. Include present grade

    B. Include school name

    C. Include estimated achievement: slow, average, high

    D. Include problems with speech, concentrating on a single project, distractibility, or hyperactivity

   E. **Record relevant behaviors:**
       1. Bed wetting
       2. Nail biting
       3. Constipation
       4. Nightmares
       5. Nervousness
       6. Speech problems
       7. Toilet problems
       8. Hyperactivity
       9. Ability to get along well with children, adults, and school structure
   F. **Record illnesses:**
       1. Measles
       2. Mumps
       3. Chickenpox
       4. Roseola
       5. Whooping cough
       6. Scarlet fever
       7. Pneumonia
       8. Bronchitis
       9. Croup
       10. Severe illnesses
       11. Injuries
       12. Hospitalizations/surgery

V. **General survey**
   A. **Central nervous system:** Frequent headaches, seizures, dizziness, head injury, or blackout spells
   B. **Ear, eye, nose, or throat problems**
   C. **Chest or lung problems**
   D. **Heart problems:** Murmur, palpations, or congenital heart defect
   E. **Infections:** Gastrointestinal, kidney, or bladder
   F. **Muscles and coordination problems:** with gait or walking, speech coordination, weak muscles, joint swelling, joint pain, fractures, or need for braces or special shoes
   G. **Skin problems:** chronic rashes or other skin problems
   H. **Allergies:** frequent colds, bronchitis, pneumonia, asthma, hay fever, sinus trouble, eczema, hives, or reactions to medications
   I. **Blood problems:** anemia or bleeding problems
   J. **Episodes of fever with no known cause**
   K. **Habits:** Diet, drug use, smoking, alcohol, sexual activity, exercise, sleep, medications, toxic exposures, social activities, friends, jobs, and hobbies

NORMAL AND ABNORMAL DEVELOPMENT OF THE PEDIATRIC PATIENT

I. **Musculoskeletal disorders**
   A. **Arthridities**
       1. Defined as inflammatory joint disease manifested by swelling, pain, stiffness, loss of

motion, and inflammation and warmth of the involved joint

2. Arthritis in childhood or diseases that mimic arthritis may be one of the following
    a. Rheumatic diseases of childhood
        i. Juvenile rheumatoid arthritis (JRA): Divided into polyarticular and posiarticular types
            (a) Polyarticular arthritis: Includes three subgroups:
                (i) Systemic onset of the disease: Spiking fever, rash, hepatospleenomegalgy, lymphadenopathy, polyserositis, myalgia, arthralgia, leucocytosis, and anemia; involves large and small joints, often symmetrical; average age at onset is 5 years, with equal sex distribution; serologic tests negative
                (ii) Median age of onset is age 3; more frequent in girls; 25% have positive ANA test
                (iii) Seropositive: Median age at onset is 12, with equal sex predilection, 75% with positive ANA test; subcutaneous rheumatoid nodules common
            (b) Posiarticular: Only a few joints involved and are generally large and asymmetrical
                (i) Type I: Median onset age 2, with equal sex predilection
                (ii) Type II: Median age at onset 10, with male predominance. Treatment: Goal is to establish relief of pain and to maintain joint motion: Salicylates (100 mg/kg/day to 3600 mg/day total), tolmetin, gold, physiotherapy, night splints, and joint replacement
    b. Infectious arthridities
        i. Joint infection or synovitis caused by bacteria without presence of organism
        ii. Often caused by penetrating wounds
        iii. Aspirative joint effusion contains WBCs greater than 50,000, predominantly PMN's organism on smear
        iv. Staph aureus most common cause in children younger than 4 year of age
        v. Children with sickle cell more prone to salmonella osteomyelitis
        vi. Treatment: Intravenous antibiotics for 2-4 weeks, with possible treatment via oral antibiotics
    c. Noninflammatory conditions
    d. Malignancies
        i. Musculoskeletal joint pain has known association with leukemia, neuro blastoma, Hodgkin's disease, histiocytosis, and rhabdomyosarcoma
        ii. Pain unrelieved by aspirin
        iii. Radiographs often normal at onset

II. **Osteomyelitis: A pyogenic infection, usually hematogenous in origin, which typically affects the metaphysis of long bones**

A. **Causative organisms**
    1. Staph aureus
    2. Haemophilus influenzae
    3. Streptococcus pyogenes
    4. Salmonella in patients with sickle cell anemia

B. **Characteristics**
    1. Epiphyseal plate of growing bone prevents spread to adjacent joint spaces
    2. Infected limb is painful

3. More commonly in males than in females

4. Increased incidence occurring in distal femur proximal to the distal radius, distal humerus, and calcaneus

5. Initial radiographs not usually diagnostic until several days after onset; bone scans are more appropriate to determine presence at earlier stage

6. White blood cell count typically elevated with a left shift. Elevation of the sedimentation rate demonstrates index of severity

7. Treatment includes aggressive antibiotic therapy, to include one, two, or more weeks of intravenous antibiotics followed by oral therapy until there is a clinical cure; lack of response to antibacterial therapy indicates possible necessity for surgical intervention

III. Slipped capital femoral epiphysis

A. Characteristics

1. Acute or chronic disruption of structural integrity of the epiphyseal cartilage plate of the proximal femur

2. Most common hip disorder in adolescents, although rare

3. Twenty-five percent bilateral involvement

4. Characterized by displacement of femoral head relative to the neck of the femur

5. Occurs most commonly during growth spurt in adolescence (because growth plate is more vertical in adolescence)

6. More common in boys

7. Obesity is an aggravating factor: More than 50% of patients demonstrate greater than 95th percentile in weight

8. Possible predilection toward underlying connective tissue disorders (i.e., Ehlers-Danlos disease or Marfan's syndrome)

B. Symptoms

1. Pain over anterior aspect of hip joint

2. Antalgic limp with affected leg externally rotated

C. Examination

1. Hip cannot be internally rotated

2. Tenderness overlying the anterior hip joint

3. AP and frog-leg lateral views confirmatory, films should be bilateral for comparison

4. Categories

   a. Slips classified as Grade I, II, and III

      i. Slips less than one third the diameter of the growth plate

      ii. Slips one third to one half the diameter of the growth plate

      iii. Slips greater than one half the diameter of the growth plate

5. Treatment

   a. Grade I and II require in situ pinning

   b. Grade III requires trochanteric osteotomy

IV. Legg-Calvé Perthes disease (Coxa plana)

A. Characteristics

1. Self-limiting disease process

2. Incidence one in 750 children

3. Fifteen percent bilateral

4. Etiology unknown, but factors interfering with blood supply is probable cause

5. Occurs in males 4-5 times more frequently than in females

6. Occurs between 4 and 5 years of age

B. Symptoms
1. Groin pain and limp
2. Obturator nerve involvement often precipitating knee pain

C. Examination
1. Range of motion decreased in abduction and external rotation
2. Atrophy of thigh muscles
3. Varied radiographs
4. Early radiographic changes demonstrate demineralization of the femoral head and neck and later fragmentation
5. Radiographic changes demonstrate a return of normal patterns, with the exception of the flattening of the femoral head

D. Classifications
1. Catterall's classifications
    a. Group I: Anterior head involvement without other changes and disease levels without sequelae
    b. Group II: Greater head involvement and intact lateral pillar in epiphyseal metaphyseal area; results are good
    c. Three quarters of the epiphysis is affected, with early collapse; Metaphyseal area and plate are involved; results often poor
    d. Entire epiphysis, involved, with severe collapse; results are generally poor

E. Treatment
1. Traction may be hazardous
2. Disease heals spontaneously within 2 years
3. Ambulation stabilized via a brace will maintain the femoral head within the acetabulum (abduction with internal rotation)

V. Dislocation of the hip (developmental dysplasia of the hip)

A. Terminology
1. Dislocation: Femoral head completely displaced from the acetabulum
2. Dislocatable hip: Femoral head normally in the acetabulum but can be forcibly displaced
3. Subluxation: Femoral head can be partially displaced from its normal position in the acetabulum
4. Dysplasia: Abnormal development of the acetabulum or femoral head

B. Characteristics
1. Incidence
    a. 1 in 1,000 live births for dislocation
    b. 10 in 1,000 live births for dislocatable/subluxable hip
    c. Occurs in females 4-6 times more frequently as in males
    d. Higher incidence in Italy, Israel, and Japan
    e. Sixty percent occurrence on the left extremity, 20% occurrence on the right extremity, 20% bilateral

C. Etiology
1. Heredity: Increased incidence with parental/sibling history
2. Environmental factors: Breach presentation associated with 20%-30% of congenital dislocation of the hip, first pregnancy, swaddling with legs in extension
3. Developmental: Flattened acetabulum
4. Hormonal: Increased relaxin from mother during labor

      5. Functional: Unstable hip with increased motion, which may lead to secondary flattening of acetabulum

D. Diagnosis
      1. History: As listed under Etiology above

E. Clinical signs
      1. Asymmetrical, inguinal, and gluteal folds (+ anchor sign)
      2. Restriction of abduction and external rotation with child in a supine position (< 60° is cause for suspicion)
      3. Galeazzi's sign (Allis' sign): With the child supine and the hips and knees flexed, short-leg side may be displaced; Galeazzi's sign is negative with bilateral dislocation (This test is also positive with a limb-length discrepancy)
      4. Barlow's maneuver: With the child supine and the hips and knees flexed, the leg is adducted and internally rotated, when gentle downward pressure is placed against the medial thigh, a dislocatable hip will slide out of the acetabulum under pressure (This test is not as widely utilized as in years past as a result of potential for precipitating injury)
      5. Ortolani's sign: With the infant supine, the hips and knees are flexed; the thigh is lifted anteriorly and then abducted and externally rotated; a palpable click indicates dislocation (Note - Galeazzi's sign and the adduction test remain the most reliable tests after the first 3-4 months of age)
      6. Telescoping: With the child on the back and the hip flexed to 90° or extended to 180°, the knee is held and a pistoning motion performed; an increased pistoning mobility noted at the hip is consistent with dislocated femur moving within the soft tissue
      7. Trendelenburg's sign: A positive hip drop on the unaffected side along with an abductor lurch noted in the ambulatory child

F. Radiographic evidence
      1. Four quadrants drawn over the affected hip, utilizing Hilgenreiner's horizontal line (Y line) and Ombredanne's (Perkins) vertical line: The ossifying head of the femur normally lies within the medial inferior quadrant
      2. Acetabular index on an AP projection: A line extending from the acetabular roof is drawn that crosses at the level of Hilgenreiner's line; the angle formed should be less than 30°; greater than 30° is suggestive of acetabular dysplasia with an increased likelihood of a dislocated hip
      3. Shenton's line: On an AP projection, a line is drawn along the medial border of the femur and femoral neck and then continued along the superior margin of the obturator foramen, with a broken line consistent with a dislocated hip
      4. Von Rosen's method: The Y line is drawn initially, with a second line drawn parallel to it through the upper margin of the symphysis pubis; if the limb is dislocated, the ossified femur will move up within the area between the lines and is consistent with a superior displacement of the hip
      5. Von Rosen's frog-leg view: An AP radiograph of the hips maintained in 45° of abduction with internal rotation is obtained; a line bisecting the femoral shaft should bisect the lateral corner of the acetabulum so that with a dislocated hip, the line bisects the ASIS

G. Other evidence
      1. Ultrasound: Technique involves short, focused transducers utilizing high-frequency high resolution with real-time equipment; this test demonstrates a sensitivity of approximately 95%, so all patients with a risk for dislocated hip should have ultrasound or minimally radiographic studies of the hips even with a normal clinical examination

H. Treatment
      1. Principle: To maintain the leg inflection along with external rotation and abduction

2. Early treatment includes use of the following:
   a. Pavlick harness
   b. Ilfeld's splint
   c. Von Rosen's splint
   d. Frejka splint
3. As a rule, treatment lasts twice the length of the child's age in months, from the time treatment was initiated; delayed onset of treatment will result in more aggressive treatment involving both traction and surgery.

BIBLIOGRAPHY

Apgar V. A proposal for a new method of evaluation of the newborn infant. Curr Res Nesth 32:360, 1953.

Avery MD, Taeusch HWJr. Schaffer's disease of the newborn, 5th ed. W.B. Saunders Co, Philadelphia, 1984.

Browne D. Congenital deformities of mechanical origin. Arch Dis Child 30:37, 1955.

Committee on Drugs: Section on anesthesiology guidelines for the elective use of conscious sedation, deep sedation and general anesthesia in pediatric patients. Pediatrics, 76:317, 1985.

Heinonen OP, Slone D, Shapiro S. Birth defects and drugs in pregnancy. Publishing Sciences Group, Littleton, MA, 1976.

Jackson LG. First-trimester diagnosis of fetal genetic disorders, Hosp Pract 20:39, 1985.

Jacob L. Pharmacologic properties of antibacterial agents and their clinical usage. J Am Podiatr Med Assoc 75:132, 1985.

Kaback MM, ed. Medical genetics. Pediatr Chn North Am 25:3, 1978.

Kaplan EB, et al. The usefulness of preoperative laboratory screening. JAMA 253:3576, 1985.

Korsch BM, Aley EF. Pediatric interviewing techniques. Curr Probl. 3:1, 1973.

Kunin CM. Antibiotic accountability (editorial). N Engl J Med 301:380, 1979.

Pagliaro L, Levin R, eds. Problems in pediatric drug therapy. Drug Intelligence Publication, Inc, Hamilton, IL, 1979.

Port M, et al. Prevalence of dermatologic problems of the lower extremity, Part H.J Am Podiatr Med Assoc, 70:445, 1980.

Rosenberg H. Malignant hyperthermia. Hosp Pract 20:139, 1985.

Salter RB, Harris WR. Injuries involving the epiphyseal plate. J Bone Joint Surg 45A:587, 1963.

Sgarlato TE. A compendium of podiatric biomechanics. College of Podiatric Medicine, San Francisco, 1971.

Shulman ST, et al. Bacterial endocarditis. AJDC 139:232, 1985.

Stickler GB. Polypharmacy and poisons in pediatrics: The epidemic of overprescribing and ways to control it. Adv Pediatr 27:29, 1980.

Tax HR. Podopediatrics. Williams & Wilkins Co, Baltimore, 1980.

Thomson P. Introduction to podopediatrics. W.B. Saunders Co, London, 1993.

Valmassy RL. Clinical biomechanics of the lower extremities. Mosby Year Book, St. Louis, 1995.

Wilson JG. Misinformation about risks of congenital anomalies. Prog Clin Biol Res 163:165, 1985.

Zier BG. Essentials of internal medicine in clinical podiatry. W.B. Saunders Co, Philadelphia, 1990.

CHAPTER 19
GENERAL PEDIATRICS

1.   At what age should children first be able to stand unassisted and walk when led?

      A.   3 months
      B.   6 months
      C.   9-10 months
      D.   12 months
      E.   15 months

2.   Which nerves are being tested during a muscle strength exam when one test ankle plantar flexion (gastrocnemious)?

      A.   L5, S1, S2
      B.   L4, L5
      C.   S1, S2
      D.   L4
      E.   L5, S1

3.   In a dermatome exam, what nerves are associated with the anterior thigh?

      A.   L1, L2, L3
      B.   L4
      C.   L5
      D.   S1
      E.   S2

4.   Which of the following is NOT associated with cerebellar function testing?

      A.   Tandem gait
      B.   Heel/shin test
      C.   Jerky eye movements (nystagmus)
      D.   Slurred speech (dysarthric)
      E.   Vibratory sensation

5.   Which gait pattern is found in patients with upper motor neuron damage?

      A.   Steppage gait
      B.   Wide-based antalgic gait
      C.   Scissored gait
      D.   Swaggering gait
      E.   Antalgic gait

6.   Which of the following diseases is classified into three types (spastic, ataxic, dyskinetic)?

      A.   Charcot-Marie-Tooth disease
      B.   Guillain-Barre syndrome
      C.   Spina bifida
      D.   Friedreich's ataxia
      E.   Cerebral palsy

7. The following are associated with infectious arthritis EXCEPT:

    A.   Children with sickle cell are more prone to salmonella Osteomyelitis
    B.   Treatment consists of IV antibiotics for at least 6 weeks
    C.   Joint aspirate contains WBCs greater than 50,000 and predominantly PMNs on smear
    D.   Staph aureus most common cause in children younger than 4 years of age
    E.   Often caused by penetrating wounds

8. Of the following, which is NOT generally a causative organism in Osteomyelitis in the pediatric patient?

    A.   Haemophilus influenzae
    B.   Bacteroides fragilis
    C.   Streptococcus pyogenes
    D.   Staph aureus
    E.   Salmonella

9. What percent of slipped capital femoral epiphysis is bilateral?

    A.   0%
    B.   10%
    C.   25%
    D.   50%
    E.   100%

10. Which of the following is true about dislocations of the hip (developmental dysplasia of the hip)?

    A.   Incidence of approximately 1 in 100,000 live births
    B.   Occurs more frequently in males than females
    C.   No increased incidence with parental/sibling history
    D.   Ortolani's sign is also known as Allis' sign
    E.   Trendelenburg's sign is positive with a hip drop on the unaffected side

COMMON PEDIATRIC DEFORMITIES

Ronald Valmassy

DIGITAL DEFORMITIES

I. Congenital curly toe

    A. Most commonly noted in third, fourth, and fifth toes usually bilateral symmetry

    B. Toe is typically underriding and in varus

    C. Flexible at birth, becoming more rigid with age; usually asymptomatic

    D. May spontaneously reduce, but some residual deformity persists if untreated

    E. Initial treatment with manipulation and tape splintage is sometimes beneficial primarily prior to weightbearing, but deformity often leads to surgery

    F. Flexor tenotomy or transfer beneficial in flexible deformity; osseous, surgery deferred until skeletal maturity

II. Digital elevatus

    A. Most common in second toe

        1. Toe is rectus but rests above common plane of other toes

        2. Toe does not purchase ground when child is weight bearing

    B. Commonly accompanied by underriding hallux

    C. Spontaneous reduction typical as standing and walking is achieved

    D. Resistant cases usually respond to splinting

        1. Tape toe in mild plantarflection at MPJ

        2. If child is weightbearing, dynamic splint may be used, as it holds toe against ground when forefoot loads

III. Overlapping fifth digit

    A. Triplane deformity, with dorsiflexion, adduction, and varus rotation of digit

    B. May respond at birth and early infancy to manipulation and tape splinting, but the

contracture typically is resistant to conservative therapy

  C. **Surgical correction generally involves a combination of skin plasty (dorsal and plantar at MPJ level), capsulotomy, and pin fixation**

    1. Prognosis good with surgical correction

 IV. **Juvenile bunion (hallux abductovalgus)**

  A. **Etiology:** Multifactorial and somewhat controversial

    1. Most likely a combination of genetics, intrauterine position, and pathomechanics

  B. **Two basic subtypes**

    1. Isolated hallux valgus resulting from epiphyseal dysplasia at base of proximal phalanx

    2. Hallux valgus as part of a biomechanically unstable foot type

      a. Hypermobile flat foot causing hyperpronation with secondary pathomechanical effects on foot

      b. Secondary to metatarsus adductus

        i. Increases intrinsic hallux abductus angle

        ii. Further exacerbated by shoes

      c. Secondary to equinus deformity

        i. Via pronatory impact on foot

      d. Secondary to skewfoot deformity

        i. Combination of hindfoot pronation and forefoot adductus

  C. **Treatment typically surgical**

    1. Defer until foot is skeletally (10 years or older) mature

    2. Osseous bunionectomy indicated

    3. Must also correct associated deformities or deforming forces (see above)

METATARSALS

 I. **Metatarsus adductus**

  A. **"True" metatarsus adductus is a single plane deformity (transverse) in which metatarsals are medially deviated on lesser tarsals**

  B. **Etiology: Unclear; evidence for both genetic and acquired factors**

  C. **Clinically presents as flexible, semirigid, or rigid**

    1. In flexible type, forefoot is manually reducible beyond rectus lateral border when abducted on the hindfoot

    2. Semirigid deformity allows some motion of forefoot in abduction, but typically a rectus lateral border is not attained or is attained with significant resistance

    3. Rigid deformity demonstrates minimal transverse plane motion available in abduction; cannot attain rectus lateral border

  D. **Deformity is idiopathic and should be distinguished from metatarsus varus, hallux adductus, or combination deformities** (e.g., skewfoot, talipes equinovarus [clubfoot])

  E. **Radiographic presentation**

    1. Prior to ossification of the navicular, metatarsus adductus is indistinguishable from forefoot adductus

    2. Bisection of second metatarsal relative to a line traversing the first and fifth metatarsal bases exceeds 25° (at birth), 20° (at 18 months), and 10° (in adulthood)

    3. Other important angles to evaluate:

        a. Kite's angle (normal or slightly increased in metatarsus adductus)

        b. Calcaneocuboid angle (abducted cuboid position indicative of transverse plane compensation at midfoot possible skewfoot deformity)

    4. Treatment based on degree of rigidity and age of patient

        a. Flexible deformity in newborn may respond well to manipulation and passive stretching by parents

        b. Commonly treated with manipulation and serial casting at weekly or biweekly intervals, which is followed by a "holding cast" once deformity is reduced

        c. Severe or unresponsive cases may require surgery (e.g., McCauley, H-H-S, metatarsal abductory osteotomies, lesser tarsal osteotomies, shortening procedures for lateral column)

        d. Orthotic, shoe, or bar therapy may be beneficial in flexible cases but is typically adjunctive after correction is obtained by other means

F. Congenital hip dysplasia: Due to frequency of metatarsus adductus occurring with an unstable hip, clinical and/or radiographic evaluation of hip congruency is recommended

HINDFOOT/ANKLE

I. Calcaneovalgus

A. Etiology: Intrauterine malposition

B. At birth, entire foot is dorsiflexed and everted relative to leg

C. Dorsum of foot is easily brought into apposition with anterior tibia

D. Foot demonstrates convex medial border and concave lateral border

E. Flexible deformity

F. Prognosis excellent

    1. Deformity usually spontaneously reduces with age and as child becomes weight bearing

    2. Occasionally serial casting required in more resistant cases

G. Important to distinguish clinically and radiographically from congenital vertical talus (congenital convex pes valgus) because of morbidity of the latter

II. Congenital vertical talus (congenital convex pes valgus)

A. Etiology: Multifactorial, including intrauterine malposition, genetic, and neuromuscular causes

    1. May present as an isolated deformity or as part of a variety of syndromes (e.g., congenital dislocated hip, arthrogryposis multiplex congenita, neurofibromatosis, autosomal trisomy)

B. Rigid deformity, with navicular dorsally dislocated and abducted on neck of talus and with corresponding severe plantarflexion of talus

C. Calcaneus rotated into equinus

D. Forefoot dorsiflexed and abducted on hindfoot

E. Associated contracture of triceps surae, dorsal ligaments, and extensor tendons

F. Radiographic presentation

    1. Key radiographic view is stress plantarflexion lateral

        a. If first metatarsal cannot be brought into alignment with talus, presumptive diagnosis is made

    2. Magnetic resonance imaging allows direct visualization of talonavicular dislocation

   G. Morbid deformity: Prognosis poor, with or without surgery
      1. Typically, partial reduction of deformity obtained with soft-tissue releases
      2. Follow-up triple or pantalar arthrodesis commonly performed when foot reaches skeletal maturity

III. Congenital clubfoot (talipes equinovarus): Two clinical types

   A. Intrinsic clubfoot
      1. Etiology
         a. Primary germ cell defect in which the head and neck of the talus are plantarflexed and adducted in relation to the body of the talus
      2. Clinical presentation
         a. Classic triad of forefoot adductus, hindfoot varus, and hindfoot equinus
         b. Fourth deformity of "horizontal breach" or medial malalignment syndrome present in ambulatory patients
         c. Rigid deformity
         d. Skin creases in medial arch and superior to calcaneus
         e. Contractures present in posterior and medial soft-tissue structures of foot
         f. Talar head prominent on lateral side of foot as a result of severe adduction of forefoot and inversion of hindfoot
         g. Navicular is medially subluxated on talus in more severe cases

   B. Extrinsic clubfoot
      1. Etiology
         a. Same gross deformity as intrinsic clubfoot with significant differences
         b. Deformity resulting from intrauterine malposition
         c. Flexible deformity
         d. No germ cell defect present
         e. Normal skin lines in arch and heel
         f. Prognosis excellent with manipulation and serial casting

   C. Radiographic presentation
      1. Kite's angle low to 0, reflecting stacking of tarsus
      2. Forefoot adductus angle markedly increased
      3. Stacking of metatarsal bases in AP (DP) view
      4. Talar bisection projects dorsal to cuboid on lateral view
      5. Parallelism of talar and calcaneal bisections on lateral view resulting from calcaneal position
      6. Calcaneus rotated into equinus relative to tibia (i.e., declinated)

   D. Associated anomalies
      1. Congenital dislocated hip
      2. Spina bifida
      3. Myelomeningocoele
      4. Streeter's dysplasia
      5. Larsen syndrome

   E. Treatment, nonsurgical
      1. Manipulation with serial casting often successful for a portion, or sometimes all, of the deformity
      2. Must reduce forefoot adductus and hindfoot varus before dorsiflexion will be satisfactory
      3. Premature attempts to dorsiflex ankle will result in subluxation of lateral column from stacking of tarsus

4. Ankle dorsiflexion (i.e., sagittal plane) correction the most difficult
   a. Often requires surgical reduction although other components have been manually reduced
5. Once reduction is obtained, maintenance in night splint, holding cast, and clubfoot prewalker shoe are necessary
6. Recurrence of at least a component of the deformity is common

F. Treatment, surgical
1. Most commonly posterior, medial, plantar, and lateral release performed, although surgeon may choose to address only isolated components of deformity as required
2. Turco, Carrol, and Cincinnati methods most commonly used

TORSIONAL/POSITIONAL ABNORMALITIES

I. Internal femoral torsion

A. Excessive internal transverse plane relationship between the femoral condyles and head and neck of femur
1. 30° angle at birth, decreasing to 8°-12° at adulthood
2. Normally there is gradual reduction of angle with age (1°-3°/year) or with growth spurts
3. Simultaneous reduction of external femoral position at hip from birth to adolescence results in frontal plane neutral position of patellae
4. Persistence of excessive angulation results in clinically adducted position of patella in neutral stance (i.e., "squinting patellae")

B. Clinical evaluation performed segmentally during stance and gait
1. During gait, check relationship of patellar position and angle of gait
   a. If patellae are rotating around saqittal plane but angle of gait is adducted, pathology is distal to femur
   b. If patellae are internally rotated while angle of gait is normal or abducted, at least a portion of the pathology is in femur
2. Check hip ROM flexed and extended
   a. At birth, ROM should be 100° or greater with 2-3:1 external to internal relationship
   b. Relationship should be 1:1 external to internal by 5-7 years of age
      i. If hip ROM and relative position change from flexed to extended position, problem is most likely positional
      ii. If hip ROM and relative position do not change from flexed to extended position, problem is most likely torsional
      iii. Torsional and positional components may exist together

C. Treatment includes modification of sitting and sleeping habits, use of bar or brace therapy in mild to moderate cases, and orthoses for compensatory pronation if child is ambulatory

II. Internal knee position

A. Also known as "pseudolack of malleolar torsion"

B. Soft-tissue deformity occurring at knee joint that usually reduces spontaneously

C. Present at birth and typically persists to approximately 3 years of age
1. Newborn or infant displays minimal transverse plane rotation with knee extended
2. With increased knee flexion, transverse plane rotation gradually increases, with preponderance of internal to external range

D. **Differentiated from internal tibial torsion with knee evaluated in extension**
   1. Relationship of transmalleolar axis to femoral condyles normal

III. Internal tibial torsion

A. **Tibial torsion evaluated clinically via transmalleolar position, which is indirect**
B. **Normal value of 0°-5° external at birth, increasing gradually to 18° to 23° external in adulthood**
C. **Evaluate patient with knee extended**
   1. Note angular relationship of transmalleolar axis relative to femoral condyles
   2. Angle will rarely be internal but will typically lag in relationship to patient's age
   3. Clinically, child will present intoed, often with complaint of tripping
D. **May be seen in association with internal femoral position**
E. **Treatment includes modification of sitting and sleeping habits, use of bar or brace therapy in mild to moderate cases, and orthoses for compensatory pronation if child is ambulatory**
   1. Aimed at producing stability in gait
   2. Restoration of neutral subtalar joint position will increase adducted angle of gait by eliminating compensatory mechanism, but stability in gait will be achieved

FRONTAL PLANE DEFORMITIES

I. Genu varum

A. **Persistent frontal plane angulation of knee beyond 15°-30° after age 4**
   1. Presence of physiologic genu varum normal until age 3-4 years
   2. May be increased in heavy children who are early walkers or who bypass a crawling phase
B. **In more severe cases, must rule out medial genicular epiphyseal dysplasia (Blount's disease) or rickets with radiographs**
C. **Consider orthoses in children with lateral instability or compensatory hyperpronation**
   1. Severe case may require stapling at proximal tibial epiphysis to improve alignment of leg to ground
D. **Condition may be confused with torsional/rotational disorder of leg as a result of spurious appearance of bowing secondary to calf musculature**
   1. Evaluate knee in full extension and "mask off" distal two thirds of leg to eliminate optical illusion created by calf musculature
   2. Knee joint should be rectus or in mild valgum, based on age of patient

II. Genu valgum

A. **Persistent frontal plane angulation of knee into adolescence or beyond**
   1. Physiologic genu valgum is typically present between ages 3 and 5 years and gradually reduces by 8 years
B. **May become clinically significant if it leads to compensatory hyperpronation of foot**
C. **Treated with orthoses for secondary pathomechanics referred to foot**
   1. Severe case may require stapling at proximal tibial epiphysis to improve alignment of leg to ground

BIBLIOGRAPHY

Bernard MA. Treatment of skewfoot by multiple lesser tarsal osteotomies and calcaneal osteotomy, J Foot Surg 10:504, 1990.

Bleck E. Metatarsus adductus: classification and relationship to outcome of treatment. J. Pediatr Orthop 3:2, 1983.

Campos de Paz A, DeSouza V, De Souza DC. Congenital convex pes valgus, Orthop Clin North Am 9:207, 1978.

DeValentine SJ, ed. Foot and Ankle Disorders in Children, Churchill Livingstone, N.Y., 1992.

Heyman C, Herndon C, Strong J. Mobilization of the tarsometatarsal and intermetatarsal joints for the correction of resistant adduction of the forepart of the foot in congenital clubfoot or congenital metatarsus varus, J Bone Joint Surg (Am) 44:299, 1958.

McGlamry, ED (ed), Comprehensive Textbook of Foot Surgery, Vol. 1, Williams and Wilkins, Baltimore, 1987.

McKay DW. New concept of and approach to clubfoot treatment. 11. Correction of the clubfoot, journal of pediatric orthopedics 3:10, 1983.

Rockwood C. Fractures in Children, J.B. Lippincott, Philadelphia, 1984.

Salter RS. Textbook of Disorders and In uries of the Musculoskeletal System, 2nd ed. Normal structure and function of musculoskeltal tissues, Williams and Wilkins, Baltimore, 1983.

Simons GW. A standardized method for the radiographic evaluation of clubfeet. Clinical Orthopedics 135:107, 1978.

Tachdjian MO. Pediatric Orthopedics, W.B. Saunders, Philadelphia, 1995.

Tachdjian MO. The Child's Foot, Saunders, Philadelphia, 1985

CHAPTER 20
COMMON PEDIATRIC DEFORMITIES

1.   Which of the following is NOT true about congenital curly toe?

        A.   Most commonly noted in 3rd, 4th, and 5th toes and in bilateral symmetry
        B.   Toe is typically under riding and in varus
        C.   Flexible at birth
        D.   Never treated surgically
        E.   Initial treatment can include manipulation and tape splintage

2.   Digital elevatus most commonly affects which toe?

        A.   1st toe
        B.   2nd toe
        C.   3rd toe
        D.   4th toe
        E.   5th toe

3.   Which of the following is NOT true about metatarsus adductus?

        A.   "True" metatarsus adductus is a single plane deformity (transverse)
        B.   Etiology is unclear but there is evidence for both genetic and acquired factors
        C.   Clinical presentation may be flexible, semi-rigid, or rigid
        D.   Kite's angle is significantly decreased
        E.   In patients with metatarsus adductus, evaluation of the hip should be performed due to the
                association of congenital hip dysplasia with metatarsus adductus

4.   The following are true about calcaneovalgus EXCEPT:

        A.   Etiology is intra-uterine malposition
        B.   Also known as vertical talus
        C.   Dorsum of foot is easily brought into apposition with the anterior tibia
        D.   Flexible deformity
        E.   Good prognosis

5.   Which of the following is true about congential clubfoot (talipes equinovarus)?

        A.   4 clinical subtypes
        B.   Must reduce forefoot adductus and hindfoot varus before dorsiflexion will be satisfactory
        C.   Classic triad of forefoot abductus, hindfoot varus, and hindfoot equinus
        D.   Contractures present in lateral and posterior soft tissue structures of the foot
        E.   Talar bisection projects plantar to cuboid on lateral view

6.   Which of the following is true about internal femoral torsion?

        A.   Evaluated by examining the relationship between the femoral condyles and head and neck of
                femur
        B.   Evaluation performed only during stance
        C.   Hip ROM examined only when flexed
        D.   Persistence of excessive angulation results in clinically abducted position of patella in neutral
                stance
        E.   Orthoses are never attempted for treatment

7.   The following are true about internal knee position EXCEPT:

      A.   Also known as "pseudo-lack of malleolar torsion"
      B.   Soft-tissue deformity at knee joint that usually reduces spontaneously
      C.   Present at birth
      D.   Persists to 3 years of age
      E.   Differentiated from internal tibial torsion with knee evaluated in flexion

8.   Which of the following values are normal values for tibial torsion?

      A.   0-5 external at birth
      B.   5-10 external at birth
      C.   10-15 external at birth
      D.   10-20 external in adulthood
      E.   20-40 external in adulthood

9.   Which of the following is NOT true about genuvarum?

      A.   Persistent frontal plane angulation of the knee beyond 15-30 after age 4
      B.   In severe cases must rule out epiphyseal dysplasia (Blount disease) and rickets
      C.   May require stapling at proximal tibial epiphysis to improve alignment
      D.   Genuvarum is never confused with torsional/rotational disorders of the leg
      E.   Knee joint should be rectus or in mild valgum, based on age of patient

10.   Physiologic genuvalgum is typically present in which age range?

      A.   1 to 3 years of age
      B.   3 to 5 years of age
      C.   5 to 10 years of age
      D.   10 to 15 years of age
      E.   15 to 20 years of age

Chapter 21

COMMUNITY MEDICINE, BIOSTATISTICS, EPIDEMIOLOGY, EVIDENCE BASED MEDICINE AND GERIATRICS

Jeffrey M. Robbins

(The author wishes to acknowledge the following students who were helpful in the preparation of the original chapter: Ruth Stelflug, Payman Ellison, and Veidra Ellison)

PUBLIC HEALTH AND COMMUNITY HEALTH

I. **Public health**
   A. **Definition**
      1. Physical, mental, and social well-being
      2. Art and science of preventing disease, prolonging life, promoting health and efficiency through organized community effort for sanitation; controlling communicable disease; maintaining hygiene; facilitating early diagnosis and preventive treatment; and maintaining health
   B. **Purpose**
      1. Prevent disease
      2. Promote health
      3. Measure and evaluate the population's health status

C. **Podiatric public health: The subset of public health that addresses the needs of the human foot** and seeks to prevent foot pathology; prolong optimum foot function; and promote foot health through primary, secondary, and tertiary preventive techniques, patient education, and research

II. Community health

A. Definition

1. Issues of public health, preventive medicine, and epidemiology as they relate to groups of people, rather than to individuals

   a. Epidemiology: The science of the study of health and disease in a population; looks for the distribution and determinants of health and disease in groups of people and asks four questions: Who, where, when, and how

   b. Biostatistics: The study of the methods and procedures for collecting, summarizing, and analyzing data about health and disease and for making scientific inferences from such data

III. Disease prevention and control

A. **Primary prevention: Efforts to prevent disease before it occurs**

B. **Secondary prevention: Screening for disease precursors in order to institute treatment before symptoms occur**

C. **Tertiary prevention: Efforts to arrest or retard the effects of a condition already established**

IV. Education

A. **Health education: Any combination of learning experiences designed to predispose, enable, and reinforce voluntary adaptations of individuals or collective behavior conducive to health; the defining characteristic of health education is the voluntary participation of individuals in determining their own health practices**

B. **Patient education: Process initiated by medical care personnel to strengthen the motivation and ability of patients to adhere to prescribed medical or self care regimens, including preparation for hospitalization, surgery, and rehabilitation**

C. **Self care education: Process designed to predispose, enable, and reinforce individuals or groups in diagnosing, managing, and monitoring their own health care needs; differs from health education because it seeks to educate the individual to make judgments and actions traditionally performed by health care personnel**

D. **School health education: Process initiated by personnel in preschool, school, or college to develop the motivation and skills required by students to cope with challenges to health and to build the foundation of knowledge required to comprehend the health learning schedule for their future**

VIII. Health promotion

A. **Health promotion**

B. **Health protection**

C. **Preventive health services**

PROVISION OF PUBLIC HEALTH SERVICES

I. **Preventive services groups**
   A. **Community services to populations as a whole wherein the people who benefit are usually not aware of their existence**
   B. **Personal services are provided to individuals**
   C. **Combined preventive services have both community and personal aspects**

II. **Public health services by state and local government; the majority of public health services in the United States are provided by the government**
   A. **State services:** Each state constitution defines the responsibilities of the state government for the protection of the health of its citizens, for which there is no consistency in how this is to be accomplished; as each state differs in how it manages the health concerns of its domain, generally speaking, most states are divided into divisions of bureaus and provide for certain services in common
      1. Communicable disease control
      2. Vital statistics
      3. Environmental sanitation
      4. Maternal and child health
      5. Public health laboratory service
      6. Public health nursing
      7. Health education
      8. Local health services
      9. Mental hygiene
      10. Industrial hygiene
      11. Administration
   B. **Local services:** Usually mandated by the state government
      1. Vital statistics
      2. Public health laboratory service
      3. Communicable disease control
      4. Environmental sanitation
      5. Maternal and child health
      6. Public health education

HOST-AGENT-ENVIRONMENTAL RELATIONSHIP

I. **Nineteenth century: Acute infectious communicable diseases were the most common cause of death**
   A. **Tuberculosis:** Large, inner-city populations aided in the transmission of the disease by close contact, increasing the likelihood of infection with aerosolized droplets
   B. **Pneumonia:** Community acquired through respiratory droplets or hospital acquired
   C. **Influenza:** Contracted by respiratory route, with ability to produce epidemics and pandemic, usually in the fall or winter
   D. **Smallpox:** Highly contagious virus eradicated through immunization and vaccinia virus in 1979; immune rates have, however, been declining

E. **Typhus**
1. Louse borne: Encouraged by crowded living conditions, famine, war, or any circumstances that predispose to heavy infestation with lice
2. Flea borne: Caused by being bitten by an infected flea; rare cases followed travel; recent cases linked to cat or opossum exposure and transmittal via the cat flea
3. Mite transmission: Depending on rodent population, which is related to waste disposal, overcrowding, and war

F. **Typhoid**
1. Contagious; immunization not always effective
2. Household contacts, travels to endemic areas, and epidemic outbreaks increase the risk of contraction
3. Adequate waste disposal and protection of food and water supplies from contamination are important public health measures to prevent contraction

II. **Today: Chronic degenerative diseases are the leading causes of death**

A. **Heart disease**
B. **Cancer**
C. **Stroke**
D. **Accidents**

III. **Top Ten List of Public Health Achievements**

A. **Vaccination**
B. **Motor vehicle safety**
C. **Safer Workplaces**
D. **Control of infectious diseases**
E. **Decline in deaths from CHD and stroke**
F. **Safer and healthier foods**
G. **Healthier mothers and babies**
H. **Family planning**
I. **Fluoridation of drinking water**
J. **Recognition of tobacco use as a health hazard**

IV. **Vaccine Preventable Disease**

A. **Smallpox**   **1798**
B. **Rabies**   **1885**
C. **Typhoid**   **1896**
D. **Cholera**   **1896**
E. **Plague**   **1897**
F. **Diphtheria**   **1923**
G. **Pertussis**   **1926**
H. **Tetanus**   **1927**
I. **TB**   **1927**
J. **Influenza**   **1945**
K. **Yellow Fever**   **1953**
L. **Polio**   **1955**
M. **Measles**   **1963**
N. **Mumps**   **1967**

O.	Rubella	1969
P.	Anthrax	1970
Q.	Meningitis	1975
R.	Pneumonia	1977
S.	Adenovirus	1980
T.	Hepatitis B	1981
U.	Type B Influen.	1985
V.	Japan enceph	1992
W.	Hepatitis A	1992
X.	Varicella	1995
Y.	Lyme Dis.	1998
Z.	Rotavirus	1998

V. **Host-agent-environment: The etiology of all disease includes host, agent, and environmental components**

   A. **Inherited disease:** Genetic and/or congenital; for example, the following systems developing in the fetus may be injured or affected by physical, chemical, or traumatic events to the mother during gestation: fourth week, limb buds; sixth week, palate and optic lens; eighth week, septal wall and hearing

   B. **Environmental effects**
      1. Overcrowding: Promotes disease infestation from lack of adequate waste disposal and sanitation and promotes increased concentration of transmission of disease
      2. Air, water, noise, and food pollution: Promote contamination of food and water, which can result in disease (e.g., typhoid fever)
      3. Social conditions: Can create stress as well as frank violence
      4. Radiation hazards
         a. X-rays and radiation therapy have caused significant morbidity when inappropriately applied
         b. Radon gas has been found in many private homes and has been implicated as a health hazard
         c. Nuclear materials from industry have been dumped within close proximity to housing complexes and have been implicated in several cases of cancer (e.g., Love Canal, Fernald)
      5. Drugs
         a. Over-the-counter medications are unrestricted and abused by many
         b. Prescription drugs, although regulated and controlled, continue to be a problem when indiscriminately prescribed or inappropriately used
         c. Illicit drugs (e.g., heroin, cocaine) continue to pour into the United States and are responsible for significant health problems in the users and for potential danger to victims of violent crime relating to the acquisition of drugs
         d. Poisons are a common cause of accidental death of children
            i. Irritant
            ii. Neurotoxins
            iii. Hemotoxins

   C. **Infectious process:** Increasingly resistant strains of bacteria are evolving and diseases that had been under control (e.g., tuberculosis) are re-emerging

   D. **Nutritional deficiency**
      1. Obesity

a. Contributes to many health problems, especially heart disease and stroke (from high blood pressure that results from the obesity); some forms of cancer; and adult-onset diabetes

b. Self-perpetuating
   i. Internal metabolic mechanisms readjust to maintain higher weight
   ii. Excess girth makes it difficult to move and leads to a sedentary life style

2. Bulimia
   a. Uncontrolled, recurrent episodes of binge eating; inappropriate compensatory behavior to avoid weight gain; excessive concern with body image
   b. Restricted caloric consumption between binges
   c. Maintains body weight at or above a minimally normal level
   d. Chronic, lasting for several years, or intermittent with remission alternated with relapse

3. Anorexia
   a. Greek for "lack of appetite", a misnomer because appetite loss is rare
   b. Overly preoccupied with food
   c. Very little is eaten because of a dread of gaining weight despite being seriously underweight
   d. Perceived body image damages self-esteem
   e. May not be food-restricting; may be binge and purge

4. Deficiency states
   a. Primarily due to inadequate food intake; secondarily as a result of illness
   b. Kwashiorkor: Protein deficiency in the presence of adequate calories
   c. Marasmus: Combined protein and calorie deficiency
   d. Alcoholism: Causing thiamin deficiency, vitamin B12 deficiency
   e. Additional: Blind-loop syndrome, surgical resections, Crohn disease, and pernicious anemia

5. Metabolic disturbances
   a. Primarily a result of diabetes: Significant lower-extremity morbidity and mortality

6. Allergic disturbances
   a. Food: Causing allergic gastroenteropathy, atopic dermatitis, asthma, anaphylaxis, urticaria, and angioedema
   b. Drugs: Causing urticaria and anaphylaxis

7. Aging and degenerative processes
   a. Characterized by the progressive construction of each organ system's homeostatic reserve
      i. No symptoms
      ii. No restrictions in activities of daily living
   b. Higher risk of disease, disability, and drug side effects

8. Accidental injuries
   a. Highest risk for males 16-35; resulting in serious injury and death from accidents and violence
   b. Guns in the home increase the likelihood of homicide by 2.7-fold and suicide by 5-fold

9. Cancer and neoplasms
   a. Cigarette smoking: Most significant preventable cause of cancer
   b. Skin cancer: Prevention consists of restricting exposure to ultraviolet light

ACQUIRED IMMUNODEFICIENCY SYNDROME

I. **Human T-lymphotrophic virus type III (HTLV III)**

II. **HIV**
   A. **Retrovirus transmitted through sexual activity, blood products, and perinatal exposure**
      1. Targets cells of the immune system
      2. Destroys the immune system at end stage
   B. **At-risk populations**
      1. IV drug users: Fastest growing population of AIDS victims
      2. Homosexuals: Largest current population of AIDS victims
   C. **Management**
      1. No cure, no vaccine
      2. Prevention is the best public health course
      3. Retarding progression
         a. AZT: First approved antiviral agent used to prolong survival
   D. **Epidemiology**
      1. Current prediction: Within 32 years or less, 100% of all HIV-positive individuals will have developed AIDS
      2. The World Health Organization estimates that 18 million adults and 1.5 million children have been infected with HIV, resulting in approximately 4.5 million AIDS cases worldwide
      3. The Centers for Disease Control (CDC) announced that AIDS is now the leading killer of all Americans age 25-44
      4. According to WHO estimates 37 million adults and 2.5 million children worldwide are living with HIV; the epidemic has left behind a cumulative total of 14 million AIDS orphans
   E. **CDC classification**
      1. Grade I: Acute infection
      2. Grade II: Asymptomatic infection
      3. Grade III: Persistent generalized lymphadenopathy
         a. Subgroup A: Constitutional disease: Weight loss, fevers, and night sweats
         b. Subgroup B: Neurologic disease: Central nervous system: Depression, changes in personality, difficulty in concentrating, and frank confusion
         c. Subgroup C: Secondary infections: Mouth lesions (candidal plaques, hairy leuko-plakia) and gingival and periodontal inflammation and ulceration
            i. Category C 1: Specific secondary infections: Disseminated Kaposi sarcoma
            ii. Category C2: Secondary infections, other: Herpes zoster, herpes simplex infec-tion, folliculitis, seborrheic dermatitis, onycholysis, retinal cotton-wool spots, and angular cheilitis
         d. Subgroup D: Secondary cancers: Kaposi sarcoma and lymphoma
         e. Subgroup E: Other conditions: Cytomegalovirus retinitis
   F. **Podiatric manifestations**
      1. Dermatology complications: Tinea pedia, onychomycosis, verruca, folliculitis, and psoriatic flares
      2. Vascular complications: Edema and thrombophlebitis
      3. Neurological complications

    a. Motor neuropathy: Proximal muscle weakness and varying degrees of muscle tenderness

        i. Muscle biopsy to distinguish HIV myopathy from drug-induced myopathy

    b. Sensory neuropathy: Tingling, numbness, and pain in the lower extremities

        i. Symptoms: Disproportionate to findings on gross examination

G. Prevention for health care workers

1. Workers at risk

    a. Category 1: Frequent direct contact with blood and body fluids: Phlebotomists, surgeons, laboratory technicians, and sanitation workers

    b. Category 2: Infrequent: X-ray technicians and EKG technicians

    c. Category 3: Seldom: receptionists

2. Universal infections control procedures

    a. Hand washing

    b. Barriers: Gloves, gowns, sleeves, aprons, masks, goggles, and face shields

    c. Needles and sharps: Disposed in puncture-proof container, needles not recapped, and blades removed with hemostat

    d. Fluid spills: Chemical germicides and hospital disinfectants

    e. Specimens: Sealed containers

    f. Instruments: Standard sterilization and disinfection procedures adequate: Cold sterile for noninvasive instruments and autoclave instruments that invade tissue or vascular system

3. Most likely exposures for podiatrists

    a. Needle sticks and cuts

    b. Splashed fluids to eye, mouth, or mucous membrane

    c. Cutaneous exposure through abraded skin

ROLE OF THE FEDERAL GOVERNMENT IN THE PROVISION OF PUBLIC HEALTH

I. **Agencies involved in health issues and their respective percentage of federal health care budget**

  A. **U.S. Department of Health and Human Services (DHHS):** 75% of health care budget

    1. Largest federal government department for budget and number of employees

    2. Replaced the U.S. Department of Health, Education, and Welfare in 1979; split into U.S. Department of Education and DHHS

    3. Major components

      a. Office of Human Development

      b. U.S. Public Health Service

        i. Alcohol, Drug Abuse, and Mental Health Administration: Defined by its name

        ii. Centers for Disease Control: Functions to prevent and control communicable disease, to direct foreign and interstate quarantine operations, and to improve the performance of clinical laboratories; serves as the national focus for developing and applying disease prevention and control, environmental health and health promotion, and health education activities designed to improve the health of the people of the United States

        iii. Food and Drug Administration: A monitoring agency which reviews products in order to protect the public against hazards of electronic and radiological products, ensuring the safety and efficacy of drugs, medical devices and biologicals, ensuring the purity of food, regulating the production of animal feeds and drugs, and ensuring the safety of cosmetics

iv. Health Resources and Services Administration: Operates several direct health care and support services; supports health sciences education, health planning, health facility construction, Community Health Centers program National Health Service Corps, and health maintenance organizations

   (a) Bureau of Health Professionals: Provides national leadership in coordinating, evaluating, and supporting the development and utilization of the nation's health personnel; provides grants for health professions; funds regional centers that provide education services and training; administers several loan programs supporting student training, and serves as a focus for technical assistance

   (b) Indian Health Service: Provides a comprehensive health services delivery system for American Indians and Alaska Natives with opportunity for maximum tribal involvement in developing and managing programs to meet health needs

   (c) Bureau of Resources and Development: Develops, coordinates, administers, directs, monitors, and supports federal policy and programs pertaining to health care facilities; national network associated with organ donations and transplants; and activities related to AIDS

   (d) Bureau of Primary Health Care: Serves to ensure the availability and delivery of health care services in health profession shortage areas, to medically underserved populations, and to those with special needs; provides project grants, and administers the National Health Service Corps Bureau, and National Health Services Corps Scholarship and Loan Repayment Programs

   (e) Maternal and Child Health Bureau: Addresses the full spectrum of primary, secondary, and tertiary care services and related activities conducted in the public and private sector that have an effect on maternal and child health

v. National Institutes of Health: Major national force in biomedical research

   (a) National Cancer Institute

   (b) National Heart, Lung, and Blood Institute

   (c) National Library of Medicine: Serves as the nation's principal source of medical information provided by medical library services and on-line bibliographic searching capabilities, such as MEDLINE, TOXLINE, and others

   (d) National Institute of Diabetes and Digestive and Kidney Disease

   (e) National Institute of Allergy and Infectious Diseases

   (f) National Institute of Child Health and Human Development

   (g) National Institute on Deafness and Other Communication Disorders

   (h) National Institute of Dental Research

   (i) National Institute of Environmental Health Sciences

   (j) National Institute of General Medical Sciences

   (k) National Institute of Neurological Disorders and Stroke

   (l) National Eye Institute

   (m) National Institute on Aging

   (n) National Institute of Alcohol Abuse and Alcoholism

   (o) National Institute of Arthritis and Musculoskeletal and Skin Diseases

   (p) National Institute on Drug Abuse

   (q) National Institute of Mental Health

   (r) Clinical Center: Designed to provide a setting in which scientists working in

the Clinic's laboratories can work in close proximity with clinicians caring for patients to collaborate on problems of mutual concern
- (s) Fogarty International Center: Promotes development of science internationally as it relates to health
- (t) National Center of Human Genome Research
- (u) National Center for Nursing Research
- (v) Division of Computer Research and Technology
- (w) National Center for Research Resources
- (x) Division of Research Grants

   vi. Office of the Assistant Secretary of Health
- (a) Founded in 1985
- (b) Offices of Disease Prevention and Health Promotion
- (c) Population affairs
- (d) Smoking and health
- (e) International health
- (f) Presidents Council on Physical Fitness and Sports
- (g) National Centers for Health Statistics
- (h) National Centers for Health Services Research

c. Center for Medicare and Medicaid (CMS) formerly known as Health Care Financing Administration (HCFA): Primary function is to run the government's two major treatment services: Medicare and Medicaid; oversees financing and management and direction and administration

   i. Social Security Act of 1937: Originally included two programs: Insurance for the elderly and unemployed and assistance for the blind, dependent children, and the aged

   ii. 1965 Amendments to the Social Security Act
- (a) Established Medicare in Title 18: Provides health care for the elderly, blind, and disabled
  - (i) Part A (involuntary)
    - Inpatient services ($520 deductible)
    - Extended care services
    - Home health services
    - Outpatient diagnostic services
  - (ii) Part B (voluntary)
    - Doctors' fees: $100 deductible; pays 80% of approved costs; additional 20% due from patient
- (b) Established Medicaid in Title 19: Provides medical care for indigent populations: Aid to the Aged; Aid to Families with Dependent Children; Aid to the Blind; Aid to the Disabled
  - (i) Funded by federal and state governments
  - (ii) Called Medicaid in 49 states; Medical in California
  - (iii) Arizona does not provide a Medicaid program for its residents
- (c) Did not include payment for podiatrists and did not cover podiatric care

   iii. 1967 Amendments to the Social Security Act
- (a) Added podiatrists to the list of physicians
- (b) Added podiatric care as a covered service
- (c) Excluded orthotics; treatment for subluxations; routine foot care for corns, calluses, nails, and other routine hygienic care

d. Social Security Administration

    B. Veterans Administration: 10% of health care budget

      1. Provides health services: Hospitals, nursing homes, domiciliary care, and outpatient medical and dental care to eligible veterans of military services in the Armed Forces

      2. Benefits

        a. Compensation and pension: Claims for disability compensation and pension, adaptive equipment, adaptive housing, survivors' claims for death compensation, dependency and indemnity compensation, death pension, and burial and lot allowance claims

        b. Education: Responsible for the Montgomery GI Bill, the Post Vietnam Era Veterans' Educational Assistance Program, the Survivors' and Dependents' Educational Assistance Program, school approvals, and compliance surveys

        c. Loan Guarantee: Establishes the eligibility of veterans for the program, passing on the ability of a veteran to repay a loan and the credit risk, and under certain circumstances, guaranteed refinancing loans

        d. Insurance: Life insurance operations for the benefit of service members, veterans, and their beneficiaries; includes complete maintenance of individual accounts, underwriting functions, life and death insurance claims awards, and any other insurance-related transactions

      1. Podiatric services: Established in 1976

    C. Department of Defense: 7% of health care budget

      1. Chief Medical Officer responsible for both treatment services and public health services for their installation

      2. Operates 170 hospitals of which 129 are in the U.S. Podiatric Services

      3. Positions currently available and filled: Army, 22 FTEs; Navy, 28 FTEs; Air Force, 27 FTEs

      4. Podiatrists are not given medical corps status: The Army and the Navy have medical service corps status, and the Air Force has biomedical science corps status; both medical services corps and biomedical services corps are non-physician corps, considered to be the administrative and allied health corps

    D. Other: 1.5% of health care budget

      1. Department of Agriculture: Responsible for human, animal, and plant health in the United States

        a. Food inspection

        b. Food Stamp program

        c. National School Lunch Program

      2. Department of Labor

        a. Environmental Protection Agency: Independent federal agency that controls air and water quality and pollution control, solid waste disposal control, pesticide regulation, radiation hazard control, noise reduction, and toxic substances

        b. Occupational Safety and Health Act (OSHA): General responsibility to protect employees against both safety and health hazards

        c. National Institute for Occupational Safety and Health (NIOSH): Research body that develops recommendations for occupational and safety standards to OSHA

EPIDEMIOLOGY AND BIOSTATISTICS

I. Biostatistics

    A. The application of statistical reasoning and methods to the solution of biological,

medical and public health problems

   B. **Scientific use of quantitative information to describe or draw inferences about natural phenomena**

II. Biostatistics process

   A. **Generate hypotheses – ask questions**

   B. **Design and conduct studies to generate evidence, make observations, collect data**

   C. **Describe the observations – descriptive statistics**

   D. **Assess the strength of the evidence for or against the hypothesis (evaluate the data) - statistical inference**

III. Organization of Data

   A. **Ordering Data**

   B. **Tallies**

   C. **Grouping Data**

   D. **Frequency distributions, percentiles**

   E. **Summarizing Data**

   F. **Measures of central tendency**

   G. **Displaying Data**

   H. **Tables and graphs**

IV. Summarizing Data

   A. **Measures of Central Tendency**

   B. **Mean** (average)

   C. **Median** (middle observation)

   D. **Mode** (most frequent)

   E. **Measures of dispersion or variability**

   F. **Range** (largest value – smallest value)

   G. **Variance** (average of squared difference of each observation from the sample mean)

   H. **Standard deviation**

V. Epidemiology

Study of variation in the occurrence of disease and the reasons for that variation. Entails making observations of occurrences of illness or injury and of those characteristics that distinguish affected from unaffected followed by inferences regarding the role those characteristics play in the disease or injury

VI. Clinical Epidemiology

   A. **The study of the variation in the outcome of illness and the reasons for that variation**

   B. **Observations: Fate of ill persons, who recovers, worsens, develops complications**

   C. **Inferences: Patient characteristics and his/her care that were responsible for the differences in outcome**

VII. Types of clinical studies

   A. **Randomized Controlled Trials - Gold Standard**

      1. Strengths of RCT
         a. Control over confounding factors (selection bias)
         b. Can estimate absolute incidence of bad outcomes
         c. Prospective as outcome most always occur after the study has been initiated
      2. Weakness of RCT
         a. If key outcome are rare number of patients needed can be difficult and costly
         b. Strict eligibility criteria or low participation can limit findings
         c. Non-compliance can interfere with testing true effect

B. Cohort Study
      1. Study groups or Cohorts are formed based on <u>exposure</u> status
      2. No random assignment only classification of exposure status
      3. Types of Cohort Studies
      4. Prospective – outcomes occurring after the initiation of the study
      5. Retrospective – outcomes have already occurred
      6. Strengths of Cohort Studies
         a. Exposure is known to proceed outcome
         b. Can directly measure the absolute incidence of adverse outcomes
         c. Easy to study multiple outcomes of a single exposure in the same study
      7. Weakness of Cohort Studies
         a. Inefficient for rate or long-delayed outcomes
         b. Prospective studies can be expensive if they require large samples or long follow-up periods

C. Case-Control Study
      1. Selection on the basis of outcome
      2. Relative numbers of subjects with and without outcome does not reflect true frequency (Many more without in population)
      3. When both cases and controls come from the same sample population the design is called nested case control
      4. Strengths of Case-Control Study
         a. Efficient for rare outcomes or long interval between exposure and outcome
         b. Permits multiple possible causes of an outcome using same comparison group
         c. Usually inexpensive and fast
         d. Can most often obtain a good estimate of the relative incidence of bad outcomes in exposed vs. non-exposed
      5. Weaknesses of Case-Control Study
         a. Can't directly estimate absolute incidence or prevalence of a bad outcome in exposed or non-exposed persons
         b. Selection of controls can be difficult
         c. Self-reported exposure data is subject to biased recall from subjects
      6. Cross-sectional Studies
         a. Assessing exposure and outcome status at a given point or period in time
         b. Can't always tell if exposure preceded outcome

D. Longitudinal Study
      1. Repeated assessment of outcome and/or exposure in same patients over long period of time

VIII. Rates

A. Prevalence rate

1. All cases of a given disease at a given time/estimated population X 1000
2. Example: In a population of 200 people, there are 25 people with tinea pedis on January 1, 2004; the prevalence rate for tinea pedis would be 25/200 X 1000 = 125/1000

B. Incidence
1. New cases of disease per unit time/estimated population X 1000
2. Example: In a population of 200 persons there are 12 people present with onychocryptosis in the month of January 2004 and 15 people present in the month of February 2004; the incidence rate for January would be 12/200 X 1000 = 60/1000, and the incidence rate for February would be 15/200 X 1000 = 75/1000

C. False positive: People without the disease positive to test/total nondiseased X 100

D. False negative: People without disease negative to test/total diseased X 100

E. Sensitivity: True positive: Number of positives with disease/total with disease present X 100

F. Specificity: True negative: Number of negatives without disease/number who are without disease X 100

G. Example: In a test population of 200 persons, 75 persons tested positive and 125 tested negative for fungus infection using the KOH test. DTM culture testing revealed that of the 75 testing positive, 50 actually had a fungus, and 25 did not. In addition, of the 125 testing negative, 15 actually had fungus, and 110 did not. The false positives in this scenario is calculated 25/125 X 100 = 18.5/100. The false negatives in this scenario is calculated 15/65 X 100 = 23/100. The sensitivity, or true positive, is calculated 50/65 X 100 = 77. The specificity, or true negative, is calculated 110/135 X 100 = 81

IX. Measures of central tendency: Used as summary measures to describe data

A. Mean: Numerical average: 16,18,20,22,24 has a mean of 20

B. Median: Middle-most value in a set of numbers of values: 16,18,20,22,24 has a median of 20

C. Mode: Most frequently occurring value or number: 16,19,21,21,22 has a mode of 21

IV. Measures of variability: Used as methods to measure scatter or dispersion

A. Range: Largest number or value minus the smallest number: 16,18,20,22,24 has a range of 8 (24-16+8)

B. Standard deviation: Most frequently used measure of variability; in a normal curve, 2 standard deviations = a central range in which 95.45% of the measurements lie and 3 standard deviations = a central range in which 99% of the measurements lie

V. Other

A. Statistical significance: Result that cannot be explained by chance

B. Null hypothesis: Negative reasoning that Treatment A is no different from Treatment B; if accepted in the study, then there is insufficient evidence to prove otherwise

C. Chi squared: Test of association; demonstrates whether there is an association between a factor or attribute and an outcome

EVIDENCE BASED MEDICINE
I. Strength of the Evidence

II. Quality of published evidence hierarchy:

A. Evidence from at least 1 properly randomized controlled trial

    B. **Evidence from well-designed controlled trials without randomization**

    C. **Evidence from well-designed cohort or case-control analytic studies, preferably from more than 1 center or research group**

    D. **Evidence from comparisons between times or places with or without the intervention. Dramatic results in uncontrolled experiments could also be included here**

    E. **Opinions of respected authorities, based on clinical experience, descriptive studies or reports of expert committees**

       (For more information http://www.ahrq.gov/clinic/evrptfiles.htm)

PSYCHOSOCIAL

I. **Abuse syndromes**

    A. **Child abuse:** Cause of 1300 deaths in 2001

      1. Signs and symptoms

         a. Subnormal growth: Weight, height, or both less than 5 percentile for age; decreased velocity for growth

         b. Head injuries: Bilateral black eyes, with history of single blow or fall; traumatic hair loss; and diffuse or severe central nervous system injury, with history of minor to moderate fall

         c. Skin injuries: Bruise or burn in shape of an object, bite marks, bruises of various colors and in various stages of healing, and injury to soft tissue areas normally protected (e.g., thigh, stomach, or upper arm)

         d. Injuries to genitourinary or gastrointestinal tract: Recurrent vomiting or diarrhea witnessed only by the parent, injury to genitals or rectum, and sexually transmitted disease

         e. Bone injuries: Rib fracture in the absence of major trauma, metaphyseal long-bone fracture in an infant, and multiple fractures in various stages of healing

      2. Reporting requirements: Since the 1960's, legislation in the United States and Canada has mandated that virtually any professional (a term that often includes teachers, psychologists, and social workers as well as physicians and nurses) must make a report to civil authorities if he or she suspects that a child has been abused or neglected by a caretaking adult, even if the professional has not seen the child face to face; most child abuse statutes specify that this reporting requirement supersedes all claims of professional-client privilege, and most statutes also prescribe penalties for failing to report abuse, while at the same time granting professionals immunity when they report suspicions in good faith

      3. Interventional strategies: Suspected child abuse or neglect reported to Child Protective Services agencies will intervene on behalf of the child; foster care, group therapy, individual psychotherapy, and family preservation programs (with services that include in-home help with child care, assistance with housing, food, transportation, and counseling)

    B. **Elder abuse:** Classified as physical, psychological, or financial/material abuse or neglect

      1. Signs and symptoms

         a. Excessive weight loss

         b. Progressive deterioration

         c. Pattern of physician and/or hospital "hopping"

         d. Unexplained delay of seeking treatment

e. Series of missed medical appointments
f. Previous unexplained injuries
g. Explanation of medical injuries inconsistent with medical findings
h. Previous reports of similar injuries
i. Fearful of family members
j. Reluctant to respond to questions
k. Conflicting accounts of incident
l. Family member overly concerned about medical costs
m. Family member attempting to prevent private interaction between the patient and the physician
n. Family member indifferent or angry toward patient and refuses to provide necessary assistance

2. Reporting requirements
   a. Mandatory reporting laws differ from state to state
   b. Office of Protective Services in every state
   c. Adult protective services programs in every state; listed in AMA "Diagnostic and Treatment Guidelines on Elder Abuse and Neglect"
   d. Ethical and, in most states, legal responsibility to act if abuse or neglect is documented

3. Intervention strategies
   a. Team approach preferred
      i. Social worker to provide counseling to help patient examine available options and choose the most suitable option for physical and emotional needs
      ii. Physicians to attain proper medical care
      iii. Rehabilitation facility
      iv. Counseling

II. Chemical dependency

A. **Illegal, prescription, over-the-counter, and "social" drugs:** Estimated that 74 million Americans have used at least one illicit substance in their lifetime. Illicit drug use results in approximately 20,000 deaths each year from overdose, homicide, suicide, motor vehicle injuries, diseases related to HIV, pneumonia, hepatitis, and endocarditis

   1. Substances of abuse: Alcohol, amphetamines (e.g., methamphetamine, "crystal," "speed"), cocaine/"crack", hallucinogens (e.g., lysergic acid diethylamide [LDS]), inhalants (e.g., glue, paint thinners), marijuana/hashish, opiates (e.g., heroin, morphine, codeine), phencyclidine (PCP), polysubstances (i.e., abuse of multiple substances at the same time), sedatives, hypnotics and anidolytics, tobacco, anabolic steroids, nitrous oxide, over-the-counter medications, and certain prescription medication

B. **Signs and symptoms:** Occult substances can be effectively identified by simple screening questions and careful attention to clinical indicators during history and physical examination

   1. History
      a. Personal history of previous substance abuse
      b. Family history of previous substance abuse
      c. History of infections common among drug abusers: Endocarditis, hepatitis B and C, tuberculosis, sexually transmitted diseases, and recurrent pneumonia
      d. Chaotic relationships, employment problems, and criminal incarceration
      e. Frequent emergency room visits
      f. CAGE: "Have you ever felt you should Cut down on your drinking or use? Have

people Annoyed you by criticizing your drinking or use? Have you ever felt Guilty about your drinking or use? Have you ever had a drink or use first thing in the morning to steady your nerves or to get rid of a hangover (Eye opener)?"

2. Physical exam: Nonspecific and often subtle
   a. Ocular findings
      i. Cocaine, amphetamines: Pupillary dilation and reduced pupillary response to light
      ii. Heroin, opiates: Pupillary constriction
   b. Needle marks/tracks; scars from prior skin abscesses; antecubital fossa tattoos; and attempts to hide needle tracks
   c. Perforation of the nasal septum (cocaine)
   d. Hypertension, tachycardia: Suggests withdrawal or intoxication

C. Interventional strategies
1. Referral to drug abuse treatment program

III. Psychosomatic disorders

A. The somatic patient (factitional):
Patient who presents with complaints and symptoms but has no organic or physiologic disease; often dismissed as hypochondriacs or may receive extensive costly tests and examinations; it has been estimated that as many as 50% of patients presenting to primary care physicians with medical complaints actually have psychosocial disorders

1. Psychosocial disorders
   a. Depression: Dffficulty sleeping, impaired concentration, poor appetite, and various pain states
   b. Anxiety: Dyspnea, palpitations, chest pain, choking, dizziness, and trembling
2. Somatoform disorders: Physical symptoms with no demonstrable physical findings
   a. Conversion disorder: Loss or alteration of physical functioning (e.g., paralysis, blindness, seizures)
   b. Hypochondriasis: Fear or belief of having a serious illness or disease
   c. Somatization disorder: Recurrent episodes of multiple somatic complaints
   d. Somatoform pain disorder: Preoccupation with pain in the absence of any physical signs
3. Adjustment disorder with physical symptoms: Stress-related physical symptoms without general impairment or emotional disturbance
4. Substance abuse: Causes multisystem symptoms related to the abused substance and not organic disease
5. Psychotic disorders: Patients with thought disorders may experience intractable physical symptoms that may be bizarre

B. Interventional strategies:
Referral to appropriate health care specialist for psychotherapy and possible pharmacologic therapy

IV. Counseling and management of patients with chronic, debilitating, and progressive disorders

A. General approach to patient counseling
1. Pain syndromes: The pain management clinic is a multidisciplinary health care team designed to evaluate and manage the patient with chronic pain and progressive debilitating conditions; early referral to a comprehensive multidisciplinary pain management clinic is essential for optimal patient functioning; the absence of a community pain clinic presents a much more difficult management challenge and

requires a coordinator to manage multiple referrals (e.g., internist, psychologist, psychiatrist, physiatrist, podiatrist, orthopedist, neurologist, physical therapist)

2. The dying patient: Hospital care programs for palliative and supportive services, including physical, physiological, social, and spiritual care for dying patients

B. Referral sources

1. Social services
2. Psychology/psychiatry
3. Informal supports (e.g., family, clergy)

GERIATRICS

I. Interdisciplinary geriatric assessment

A. Core team required to provide the geriatric patient with the necessary interdisciplinary approach for health care of the elderly patient

1. Geriatrician
   a. To assess the changes of normal aging as distinguished from disease effects
2. Nurse practitioner
   a. To assess the functional capacity of the patient by assessing the patient's ability to perform the basic activities of daily living (ADLs) that are needed for self-care
   b. The less incapacitated patient should be evaluated for instrumental activities of daily living (IADLs), which include shopping, money management, cooking, and so forth
   c. Assessment is necessary to determine the patient's level of independence
3. Social worker
   a. To assess the ability of the family, friends, and community agencies to provide supports that will allow the patient to remain at home
   b. Financial and family problems are often elucidated by the social worker

B. Assessment process

1. Evaluation: The core team performs a comprehensive evaluation
2. Prioritizing medical, nursing and social issues
3. Coordinating referrals and management
   a. Primary consultants include audiology, clinical psychology, dentistry, nutrition, occupational therapy, physical therapy, podiatry, speech pathology, and clergy
   b. Secondary consultants include neurology, ophthalmology, orthopedics, physiatry, surgery, and urology

II. Problems with cognition

A. Progressive dementia syndromes (Alzheimer's disease)

1. Signs and symptoms
   a. Early in the disease process, problems of memory, particularly recent or short-term memory, mild personality changes, and tendency to withdraw from social interactions
   b. Later in the disease, problems in abstract thinking or in intellectual functioning develop; further disturbances in behavior and appearance may be seen (e.g., agitation, irritability, quarrelsomeness, diminishing ability to dress appropriately); patient may appear to be confused or disoriented about the month or year, may begin to wander, may be unable to engage in conversation, may seem inattentive and erratic in mood, may appear uncooperative, and may lose bladder and bowel control

      c.   By the end of the disease, the patient will be incapable of caring for him- or herself

  2. Diagnosis

      a.   Clinical presentation with dementia, significant loss of intellectual abilities, insidious onset of symptoms, subtly progressive and irreversible course with documented deterioration over time, and exclusion of all other specific causes of dementia by history, physical examination, laboratory tests, psychometric, and other tests

      b.   There is no specific clinical test or finding that is unique to Alzheimer's disease

  3. Interventional strategies

      a.   Can involve support from the family, help of a homemaker or other aide in the home, employment of behavioral therapies, and/or use of medication

      b.   Sources can include family support groups (e.g., Alzheimer's Association), professional consultations of the patient and family with a mental health specialist, and a variety of community programs (e.g., day or respite care)

      c.   Every state has an agency on aging that provides information on services and programs (e.g., local Office on Aging, community mental health center, local medical society, local chapter of Alzheimer's Association)

B. Reversible dementia syndromes: Side effects of medication, substance abuse, metabolic disorders, circulatory disorders, neurological disorders, infections, trauma, toxins, and tumors

  1. Signs and symptoms: Forgetfulness in the absence of depression and inattentiveness, significant cognitive impairment, and changes in emotional behavior or personality

  2. Diagnosis: Based on history and on physical and mental status examinations, supplemented by careful review of the patient's medication list and alcohol intake, and by laboratory investigations to exclude other causes of cognitive impairment

  3. Interventional strategies

      a.   With acknowledgement of changes in the patient's behavior or cognitive function, medical treatment is necessary to search and correct the treatable factors influencing the onset of the dementia

      b.   Treatment should include discontinuation of nonessential medications, treatment for coexisting medical and psychiatric problems, and family assistance in dealing with the condition

III. Age-related physical changes

A. Normal age related physical changes

  1. In general, elderly patients experience an increase in body fat with decrease in total body water

  2. Eyes- and ears-related changes: Presbyopia, lens opacification, and decrease in high-frequency acuity

  3. Endocrine-related changes: Impaired glucose, decreased vitamin D absorption and activation, and decreased testosterone

  4. Respiratory-related changes: Decreased lung elasticity and increased chest wall stiffness

  5. Cardiovascular-related changes: Increased systolic blood pressure and decreased arterial compliance

  6. Gastrointestinal-related changes: Decreased gastric acidity, colonic mobility, anorectal function, and hepatic function

  7. Hematological and immune systems-related changes: Decreased T-cell function and increased autoantibodies

  8. Renal-related changes: Decreased glomerular filtration rate (GFR) and decreased urine concentration dilution

9. Genitourinary-related changes: Vaginal and urethral mucosal atrophy and prostate enlargement

10. Musculoskeletal-related changes: Decreased lean body mass and bone density

11. Nervous system-related changes: Brain atrophy, decreased stage 4 sleep, and decreased brain catechol and dopamingergic synthesis

B. Abnormal age-related physical changes

1. Caused by disease, not age

2. Include obesity, anorexia, blindness, deafness, diabetes mellitus, thyroid dysfunction, impotence, osteoporosis, osteomalacia, dyspnea, hypoxia, syncope, heart failure, heart block, cirrhosis, fecal impaction, fecal incontinence, anemia, autoimmune disease, symptomatic urinary tract infection (UTI), urinary incontinence, urinary retention, hip fracture, dementia, depression, Parkinson's disease, sleep apnea, and falls

BIBLIOGRAPHY

"Alcohol and Other Drug Abuse in Adolescents," American Family Physician, 50(8):1737-1739, 1994.

Burns S, Podiatric manifestations of AIDS, J Amer Pod Med Assoc 80:1, 1990.

Burton LE, Smith HH, Nichols SW, Public Health and Community Medicine. Williams and Wilkens, Philadelphia, 1980.

"Child abuse and neglect: review article." New England Journal of Medicine, 332(32):1425-1431, 1991.

DiMatteo, RM, "The psychology of health, illness and medical care: An individual perspective." Brooks/Cole Publishing Company, Pacific Grove, 1991.

Hefland, AD, Podiatric public health. In: Hefland AD, ed., Public Health and Podiatric Medicine. Williams & Wilkins, Baltimore, 1987.

"Identifying substance abuse in primary care." American Family Physician, 52(7):2029-2005, 1995.

Machello V, Faerella B, Shelley M, Progressive dementia: strategies to manage new problem behaviors. Geriatrics: Medicine for Midlife and Beyond. March:40-43, 1995.

Massachusetts Medical Society: First 500,000 AIDS cases - United States. MMWR 44:46, 1995.

Massachusetts Medical Society- Recommendations and reports, U.S. Public Health Service recommendations for human immunodeficiency virus: Counseling and voluntary testing for pregnant women. MMWR 44:RR-7, 1996.

National Institute of Health: National Institute of Mental Health pamphlet: Alzheimer's disease, 1994.

NBC Nightly News: "Child Abuse." December 5, 1995.

Patient care. "Eating Disorders: Keeping eating disorders at bay," 1995.

Peterson, M (series ed), Elder abuse and neglect: How to recognize warning signs and intervene. Geriatrics: Medicine for Midlife and Beyond. 50(4):47-51, 1995.

Rakel RE, Textbook of family medicine, 4th ed. WB Saunders Co, Philadelphia, 1990.

Robbins JM. Primary podiatric medicine. In: Robbins JM, ed. W.B. Saunders Co, Philadelphia, 1995.

Soloman D, National Institutes of Health consensus development conference statement: Geriatric assessment methods for clinical decision making. JAGS, 35:342-347, 1988.

Tierney Jr, Name LM, McPhee SJ, Papadakis MA, eds., Current medical diagnosis and treatment, 34th ed. Appleton and Lange, CT, 1995.

Tueth MJ, How to manage depression and psychosis in Alzheimer's disease. Geriatrics: Medicine for midlife and beyond. 50(l):43-49, 1995.

U.S. Government Manual, Office of Federal Register, National Archives and Records Administration, 1993-94, pp 306-325, 524-527.

JAMA Users' Guide to the Medical Literature, JAMA, November 3, 1993-Vol.270, No.17.

Class notes from the ERIC Summer Epidemiology Seminar, Seattle, June 2002.

CHAPTER 21
COMMUNITY MEDICINE, EPIDEMIOLOGY

1.   Public health is defined by which of the following?

    A.   Physical well-being
    B.   Mental well-being
    C.   Social well-being
    D.   Spiritual well-being
    E.   All of the above

2.   Primary prevention is defined as efforts to prevent disease before it occurs

    A.   True
    B.   False

3.   Secondary prevention is defined as screening for disease precursors in order to institute treatment before symptoms occur

    A.   True
    B.   False

4.   Tertiary prevention is defined as efforts to arrest or retard the effects of a condition already established

    A.   True
    B.   False

5.   Which disease was a more likely cause of death in the early 1900's?

    A.   Cancer
    B.   Heart Disease
    C.   Tuberculosis
    D.   Liver Disease
    E.   Diabetes

6.   What is the number one public health achievement of the 20th Century?

    A.   Vaccination
    B.   Motor vehicle safety
    C.   Safer Workplaces
    D.   Control of infectious diseases

7.   CDC classification of HIV disease which grade is characterized as asymptomatic infection?

    A.   Grade I
    B.   Grade II
    C.   Grade III
    D.   Grade III B
    E.   None of the above

8.   Which federal agency has the largest role in health care to the public and receives the most resources?

    A.   Department of Health and Human Services
    B.   Centers for Medicare and Medicaid Services
    C.   Veterans Health Administration
    D.   Department of Defense
    E.   Department of Agriculture

9.   Which type of study is considered the "gold standard" in the evidence based medicine model?

    A.   Cohort
    B.   Randomized Controlled Trial
    C.   Retrospective Study
    D.   Case Controlled Study
    E.   Prospective Study

10.   Which of the following is NOT considered a form of elder abuse?

    A.   Physical
    B.   Psychological
    C.   Financial/material abuse
    D.   Neglect
    E.   None of the above – all are considered forms of elder abuse

Common Foot Problems in the Older Patient Diagnostic and Therapeutic Considerations

Arthur E. Hefland, DPM

I. INTRODUCTION

A. Geriatric Foot Conditions
1. Common
2. May limit ambulation
3. Present as risk factors to elderly
   a. Disability
   b. Impairment
   c. Ambulatory dysfunction
   d. Gait imbalance
   e. Pain and discomfort
   f. May lead to amputations
4. Affects patient's ability to be functional and may generate psychological issues

II. PODIATRIC ASSESSMENT

A. Evaluation and examination
B. Recognize patient's concerns
C. Primary focus of care
1. Relieve pain
2. Restore patient to maximum level of function
3. Maintain function

    4.   Anticipate future changes

    5.   Provide assurance of patient's dignity

D. Demographic data

    1.   Living conditions

E. Chief complaints

    1.   In patient's own words

    2.   How does this affect their daily lives/activities

F. Systems review

G. Current medications

H. Past medical history

I. Review of conditions as listed in Medicare regulations

* Diabetes Mellitus

* Chronic Renal Disease

* Ventilator Dependence

* Arteriosclerosis

* Chronic Obstructive Pulmonary Disease

* Raynaud's Disease/Syndrome

* Ischemia

* Coronary Artery Disease

* Vitamin Deficiencies

* Burger's Disease

* Congestive Heart Failure

* Osteoarthritis

* Chronic Thrombophlebitis

* Hypertension

* Rheumatoid Arthritis

* Venous Stasis

* Edema

* Gout

* Peripheral Neuropathies

* Post-Trauma

* Obesity

* Malnutrition

* Leprosy

* Psoriasis

* Alcohol Abuse

* Neurosyphilis

* Urticaria

* Chemical/Substance Abuse

* Hereditary Disorders/Diseases

* Atopic Dermatitis

* Malabsorption

* Mental Illness

* Pruritus

* Pernicious Anemia

* Mental Retardation

* Hyperhidrosis

* Anemia

* Cerebral Vascular Accidents/Stroke

* Localized Neurodermatitis

* Hemophilia

* Transient Ischemic Attacks

* Hysterical Paralysis

* Cancer

* Thyroid Disease

* Psychogenic Tremors

* Drug Interactions

* Milroy's Disease

* Parkinson's Disease

* Toxic States

* Patients on Anticoagulants

* Functional Disability

* Multiple Sclerosis

* Hemiparesis or Quadriparesis

* Ambulatory Dysfunction

* Uremia

J. Past podiatric history and foot care history
  1. Self care
  2. List commercial foot procedures used

K. Past occupational, military and recreational history
  1. Foot related activities
  2. Footwear
  3. Exposure
  4. Geographic surfaces/flooring
  5. Degree of weightbearing

L. Social history
  1. Use of caffeine
  2. Tobacco
  3. Alcohol
  4. Recreational drugs
  5. Other sedatives/narcotics
  6. Above may be linked to patient's condition(s)

M. Patient subjective symptoms
  1. Dermatologic
      a. Suspicious hypopigmented or hyperpigmented lesions
      b. Painful or painless hyperkertoses
      c. Slow healing or nonhealing wounds or necrosis
      d. Skin color changes
          i. Redness
          ii. Ecchymosis
          iii. Cyanosis
      e. Chronic itching, scaly or dry feet
      f. Infections
          i. Paronychia
          ii. Tinea pedis
          iii. Onychomychosis
      g. Toenail pathology
  2. Vascular
      a. Change in skin temperature
      b. Pain in feet or legs with ambulation or at rest
          i. Intermittent claudication
  3. Musculoskeletal
      a. Gradual change in foot shape
          i. With or without symptoms
          ii. Change in shoe size
          iii. Weakness or instability with standing or ambulation
          iv. Joint changes and deformity
  4. Neurologic
      a. Sensory change
      b. Burning
      c. Tingling
      d. Clawing sensations
      e. Motor changes
      f. Weakness
      g. Foot drop

h. Autonomic, such as diminished sweating
5. Hyperkeratosis, onychial and dermayologic lesions
   a. Dryness of skin (xerosis)
   b. Chronic tinea pedis
   c. Keratotic lesions
   d. Subkeratotic hemorrhage (plantar and digital)
   e. Ulcerations (diabetic, pressure, vascular, carcinogenic)
   f. Diminished or absent hair growth
   g. Trophic nail changes (onychopathy)
        i. onychogryphosis (Ram's Horn nail)
        ii. onychauxis (hypertrophic and thickened nails)
        iii. onychomychosis (fungal nails)
        iv. onychophosis (callused nail grooves)
        v. onychocryptosis (ingrown toe nail)
   h. Onychia (inflammation)
   i. Paronychia (infection and inflammation)
   j. Subungual or subhyperkeratotic hemorrhage
   k. Cellulitis and or abscess
   l. Incurvated or involuted toenails
   m. Foot type
   n. Gait
   o. Postural deformities
   p. Palpation of pain
   q. Range of motion
   r. Angulation
   s. Frank deformities
   t. Arthropathy
6. Pedal vasculature

N. Medicare criteria for billing
1. Basic elements
   a. Class A
        i. Nontraumatic amputation of the foot or an integral skeletal portion thereof
   b. Class B
        i. Absent posterior tibial pulse
        ii. Absent dorsalis pedis pulse
        iii. Advanced trophic changes
        iv. Hair growth - decrease or absent
        v. Nail changes - thickening
        vi. Pigmentary changes - discoloration
        vii. Skin texture - thin and shiny
        viii. Skin color - rubor or cyanosis
   c. Class C
        i. Claudication
        ii. Temperature changes, e.g., cold feet
        iii. Paresthesias, e.g., abnormal spontaneous sensations in the feet
        iv. Burning
        v. Edema
2. Other criteria
   a. Vascular

    i. Absent popliteal or femoral pulses
   ii. Bruits
       iii. Dependent rubor and pallor with elevation
       iv. Prolonged capillary filling time (above 3 to 4 seconds)
        v. Arterial skin temperature
       vi. Blood pressure
       vii. Doppler, pulse volume recordings, oscillometric readings
  b. Radiographic studies
  c. Neurologic elements
      i. Gait review
     ii. Reflexes
        (a) Patellar
        (b) Achilles
        (c) And superficial plantar
     iii. Clonus
     iv. Vibratory sense
      v. Weakness
     vi. Sensory deficits
        (a) Proprioception
        (b) Pain and temperature
     vii. Hyperesthesia
     viii. Autonomic dysfunction
     ix. Manual muscle testing
  d. Drug history
      i. Antihypertensives
     ii. Antidiabetics
     iii. Cortisone
     iv. Sedatives
      v. Topicals
     vi. Antibiotics
     vii. Antiarthritics
     viii. Over the counter foot keratotic applications
  e. Functional imbalance
    * Pes Cavus
    * Spur Formation secondary to degenerative joint disease
    * Pes Valgo Planus
    * Enthesopathy (e.g., calcaneal spurs)
    * Plantar Imbalance
    * Bursitis
    * Prolapsed Metatarsal Heads
    * Fibrositis
    * Fasciitis
    * Neuritis
    * Myofasciitis
    * Neuroma
    * Tendonitis
    * Morton's Syndrome
    * Myositis
    * Soft Tissue Atrophy

* Hallux Abducto Valgus
* Digital and Phalangeal Deformities
* Hyperostosis
* Hallux Limitus/Rigidus
* Exostosis

f. Diabetes mellitus and pedal manifestaions
* Paresthesia
* Ischemia
* Sensory Impairment
* Trophic Changes
* Motor Weakness/Atrophy
* Neurotrophic Ulceration
* Reflex Loss
* Angiopathy
* Neurotrophic Osteoarthropathy
* Neuropathy
* Dermopathy
* Infection
* Onychopathy
* Necrosis and Gangrene
* Absent Pedal Pulses

g. Peripheral arterial insufficiency
* Muscle Fatigue (heavy legs)
* Atrophy of Soft Tissue
* Cramping
* Muscle Wasting
* Claudication
* Trophic Skin Changes
* Pain
* Dryness
* Coldness
* Hair Loss
* Pallor
* Absent Pedal Pulses
* Paresthesia
* Calcified Vessels
* Burning
* Edema

*   *Aforementioned objective dermatologic, vascular, neurologic, orthopedic, etc.*

LONG TERM CARE

"The Standards for Long Term Care" as developed by the Joint Commission on Accreditation of Healthcare Organizations includes foot health and care as a quality assurance issue. A similar component is currently being instituted for the current revision to the Medicare and Medicaid, "Conditions of Participation for Long Term Care". These documents suggest as a basic consideration, administrative projections to assure foot health and care for the patient per the following Guidelines:

LONG TERM CARE GUIDELINES

Foot care and/or podiatric services are organized and staffed in a manner designed to meet the foot health needs of patient/residents.

A podiatrist or another appropriately licensed practitioner with a podiatric practitioner as a consultant should provide the facility's foot health services.

A foot health program should be an integral part of the facility's total health care program.

Written policies and procedures should be developed to serve as a guide to the provision of podiatric/foot care services.

The consulting or supervising podiatrist participates in patient/resident care management as appropriate.

The quality and appropriateness of podiatric services are monitored as an integral part of the overall quality assurance program, consistent with other practitioner/professional services.

CONTINUING PROFESSIONAL EDUCATION

A program of professional, in-service and patient education should form a part of a total geriatric program. A projected outline for such an educational program includes:

    A. **Relationship of foot problems to the total Geriatric Patient**
        1. Needs
        2. Ambulation and Independence
        3. Risk Diseases
        4. Factors which modify foot care in society and health care
            a. Medicare and Medicaid
        5. Mental health considerations
        6. Long term care
        7. Rehabilitation
    B. **Primary Foot Care**
        1. Assessment and examination

2. Nail disorders
3. Skin disorders
4. Hyperkeratotic disorders
5. Foot orthopedic and biomechanical (pathomechanical) changes
6. Foot deformities associated with aging
7. Risk diseases
   a. Diabetes Mellitus
   b. Arthritis
   c. Gout
   d. Vascular insufficiency
8. Management
9. Interdisciplinary considerations

C. Foot Health Education
1. Professional and interdisciplinary
2. Patient

D. Care Delivery
1. Ambulatory care
2. Acute hospital considerations
3. Rehabilitation
4. Long term care
5. Home care
6. Mental health and retardation

E. Interdisciplinary Education
F. Footwear and Related Considerations

SUMMARY

The 1981 White House Conference on Aging, in its final Report, stated the following:

"Recommendation Number 148: Comprehensive foot care be provided for the elderly in a manner equal to care provided for other parts of the human body, to permit patients to remain ambulatory; Implementation: Remove current Medicare exclusions which preclude comprehensive foot care." The ability to ambulate requires appropriate and essential foot health.

If older persons are to maintain a high quality of life, it is crucial that they be kept ambulatory with minimal discomfort. It is vital that patients, spouses, family members or caregivers should inspect elderly patients' feet on a daily basis as a preventative measure. Good supportive, comfortable, and properly sized footwear should be worn.

Given the high prevalence of foot problems in the elderly, especially in those patients with chronic diseases and mental health problems, foot care needs are essential. Foot health care and its promotion on a national level should make all older Americans more aware of its importance. The ability to remain active and ambulatory is one way of assuring dignity and self esteem for the elderly.

TEMPLE UNIVERSITY SCHOOL OF PODIATRIC MEDICINE
Podogeriatric Assessment and Chronic Disease Protocol

THE FOOT
& ANKLE
INSTITUTE

Date of Service _____   MR # _____

Patient Name _____   Date of Birth _____ Social Security # _____

Address _____ City _____ State _____ Zip Code _____

Sex   M   F   Race   B   W   A   L   N/A   Weight_____ lbs   Height _____ in   Marital Status   M   S   W   D   Sep

Name of Primary Physician/Health Care Facility _____   Date of Last Visit _____

HISTORY OF PRESENT ILLNESS

___Swelling of Feet	___Infections	___Duration
___Painful Feet	___Cold Feet	___Context
___Hyperkeratosis	___Other	___Modifying Factors
___Onychial Changes	___Location	___Associated Signs & Symptoms
___Bunions	___Quality	
___Painful Toe Nails	___Severity	

PAST HISTORY

___Heart Disease	___Thyroid	___Hypercholesterol
___High Blood Pressure	___Allergy	___Gout
___Arthritis	___Diabetes Mellitis*	___History: Smoking: OH
___* Circulatory Disease	___IDDM ___NIDDM	___Family - Social

SYSTEM REVIEW

___Constitutional	___Hematologic	___Neurologic
___ENT	___Card / Vasc	___Endocrine
___Eyes	___Musculo-Skeletal	___GI
___Skin / Hair	___GYN	___Immunologic
___Respiratory	___Lymphatic	
___Psychiatric	___GU	

MEDICATIONS

DERMATOLOGIC

___* Hyperkeratosis	___Onychodystrophy	___Hematoma
___Onychauxis B-2-b	___* Cyanosis	___Rubor
___Infection	___Xerosis	___* Preulcerative
___* Ulceration	___Tinea Pedis	___Discolored
___Onychomycosis	___Verruca	

FOOT ORTHOPEDIC

___* Hallux Valgus	___* Pes Valgoplanus	___* Prominent Met Head
___* Anterior Imbalance	___* Pes Cavus	___* Charcot Joints
___* Digiti Flexus	___* Hallux Rigidus Limitus	___
___* Pes Planus	___* Morton's Syndrome Bursitis	Other

VASCULAR EVALUATION

___* Coldness C-2	___* Night Cramps	___* Amputation
___* Trophic Changes B-2-a	___* Edema C-3	___* AKA BKA FF T A-1
___* DP Absent B-3	___* Claudication C-1	___Atrophy B-2-d
___* PT Absent B-1	___Varicosities	

NEUROLOGIC EVALUATION

___* Achilles	___* Paresthesia C-4	___* Burning C-5
___* Vibratory	___Superficial Plantar	___Other
___* Sharp / Dull	___* Joint Position	

RISK CATEGORY - NEUROLOGIC

___- 0 = No Sensory Loss   ___* 2 = Sensory Loss & Foot Deformity
___* I = Sensory Loss   ___* 3 = Sensory Loss, Hx Ulceration & Deformity

RISK CATEGORY - VASCULAR

___ 0 - 0 No Change	___* I - 4 Ischemic Rest Pain
___* I - 1 Mild Claudication	___* II - 5 Minor Tissue Loss
___* I - 2 Moderate Claudication	___* III - 6 Major Tissue Loss
___* I - 3 Severe Claudication	

CLASS FINDINGS

___A1	Nontraumatic Amputation	___B2e Skin Color (rubor or redness)
___B1	Absent Posterior Tibial	___B3 Absent Dorsalis Pedis
___B2	Advanced Trophic Changes	___C1 Claudication
___B2a	Hair Growth (decrease or absent)	___C2 Temperature Changes (cold)
___B2b	Nail Changes (thickening)	___C3 Edema
___B2c	Pigmentary Changes (discoloration)	___C4 Paresthesia
___B2d	Skin Texture (thin, shiny)	___C5 Burning

Onychomycosis: Documentation of mycosis/dystrophy causing secondary infection and/or pain which result or would result in marked limitation of ambulation.

Discoloration	Onycholysis
Hypertrophy	Secondary Infection
Subungual Debris	Limitation of Ambulation and Pain

CLASSIFICATION OF MECHANICAL OR PRESSURE HYPERKERATOSIS

Grade	Description
0	No Lesion
1	No specific Tyloma Plaque, but diffuse or pinch Hyperkeratotic tissue present or in narrow bands.
2	Circumscribed, Punctate oval, or circular, well defined thickening of Kertinized Tissue
3	Heloma Milliare or Heloma Durum with no associated Tyloma
4	Well defined Tyloma Plaque with a definite Heloma within the Lesion
5	Extravasation, Maceration and early breakdown of structures under the Tyloma or Callus Layer
6	Complete breakdown of structure of Hyperkeratotic Tissue, Epidermis, extending to superficial Dermal involvement

PLANTAR KERATOMATA PATTERN

LT   1   2   3   4   5   RT   1   2   3   4   5

ULCER CLASSIFICATION

Grade - 0 - Absent Skin Lesions
Grade - 1 - Dense Callus but not Pre-Ulcer or Ulcer
Grade - 2 - Preulcerative Changes
Grade - 3 - Partial Thickness (Superficial Ulcer)
Grade - 4 - Full Thickness (deep) Ulcer but no involvement of Tendon, Bone, Ligament or Joint
Grade - 5 - Full Thickness (deep) Ulcer with involvement of Tendon, Bone, Ligament or Joint
Grade - 6 - Localized Infection (Abscess or Osteomyelitis)
Grade - 7 - Proximal spread of Infection (Ascending Cellulitis or Lymphadenopathy)
Grade - 8 - Gangrene of Forefoot only
Grade - 9 - Gangrene of Majority of Foot

ONYCHIAL GRADES AT RISK

Grade I Normal	Grade IV Hypertrophic
Grade II Mild Hypertrophy	Deformed
Grade III Hypertrophic	Onychogryphosis
Dystrophic	Dystrophic
Onychauxis	Mycotic
Mycotic	Infected
Infected	
Onychodysplasia	

FOOTWEAR SATISFACTORY   -   **HYGIENE SATISFACTORY**
     Yes   No   Yes   No

STOCKINGS: Nylon   Cotton   Wool   Other   None

ASSESSMENT

PLAN

___Podiatric Referral	___Medical Referral	___Vascular Studies	___Imaging
___Patient Education	___Special Footwear	___Clinical Lab	___Rx

1

SELECTED READINGS

Eng, WW., Geriatric Podiatry, Geriatric Curriculum Resource Guides for Health Professionals, Geriatric Education Center at Virginia Commonwealth University, 1986-1987.

Helfand, AE., Ed. Clinical Podogeriatrics, Williams and Wilkins, Baltimore, 1981.

Helfand, AE. & Bruno, Joseph, Ed., Rehabilitation of the Foot, Clinics in Podiatry, W. B. Saunders, August 1984, Philadelphia, 1984.

Helfand, AE., Public Health and Podiatric Medicine, Williams and Wilkins, Baltimore, 1987.

Helfand, AE., Assessment of the Foot Health Problems of the Elderly, Geriatric Services, Winning Strategies, Institute on Aging School of Medicine, Temple University, May 1989, Hershey, PA. Published, Temple University, 1990.

Helfand, AE., The Geriatric Patient and Considerations of Aging, Clinics in Podiatric Medicine and Surgery, Vol. Vol. 10, No. 1 & Vol. 10, No. 2, January and April 1993, W B Saunders Co., Philadelphia.

Helfand AE. Disorders and Diseases of the Foot In: Cobbs EL, Duthie ED, Murphy JB eds. Geriatric Review Syllabus: A Core curriculum in Geriatric Medicine, 5th ed. Maiden, MA, Blackwell Publishing for the American Geriatrics Society; pages 287-294, 2002.

Helfand AE, Assessing the Older Diabetic Foot, Pennsylvania Diabetes Academy, Pennsylvania Department of Health, Temple University, School of Podiatric Medicine, Harrisburg, 2001.

Neale, D and Adams, I, Common Foot Disorders, Second Edition, Churchill Livingstone, Edinburgh, 1985.

Reichel, William, Ed., Clinical Aspects of Aging, Third Edition, Williams and Wilkins, Baltimore, 1988.

Yale, Jeffrey A., Yale's Podiatric Medicine, Third Edition, Williams and Wilkins, Baltimore, 1987.

CHAPTER 22
GERIATRICS

1. Which one of the following disorders is not a qualifier for "foot care" with class findings under Medicare?

    A.   Parkinson's Disease
    B.   Diabetes Mellitus
    C.   Peripheral Arterial Insufficiency
    D.   Diabetes with Neuropathy

2. Of the following foot deformities, which one is considered as a degenerative arthritis?

    A.   Plantar Fasciitis
    B.   Pes Planus
    C.   Hallux Rigidus
    D.   Hallux Varus

3. Which one of the following is considered as an onychodystrophic change?

    A.   Onychomycosis
    B.   Onychorrhexis
    C.   Onychocryptosis
    D.   Paronychia

4. Which one of the following changes is usually associated with the older diabetic patient?

    A.   Reflex Loss
    B.   Onychomycosis
    C.   Hallux Valgus
    D.   Hallux Limitus

5. The primary initial measurement for diabetic neuropathy is the older patient today is:

    A.   Reflex Loss
    B.   Achilles Reflex Loss
    C.   Loss of Protective Sensation
    D.   Vibratory Loss

6. The number of pairs of "therapeutic shoes" that are covered by Medicare per year is:

    A.   1
    B.   2
    C.   3
    D.   4

INDEX

ANSWERS TO CHAPTER QUESTIONS

Chapter 1

1. B
2. A – Most vessel clips now are titanium so they can undergo an MRI at any time, however, the classic answer is 4-6 weeks if unsure.
3. C
4. D
5. C
6. B
7. C – Periosteal sarcoma is a soft tissue mass often with bony spicules and calcification; all others associated with bone lucency.
8. C
9. A
10. C

Chapter 2

1. A
2. E
3. C
4. D
5. B
6. D
7. B
8. E
9. D
10. A

Chapter 3

1. C
2. A
3. C
4. D
5. B
6. A
7. C
8. C
9. B
10. D

Chapter 5

1. B
2. C
3. A
4. B
5. C
6. A
7. B
8. A
9. C
10. C
11. B
12. A
13. D
14. B
15. C
16. A
17. D
18. B
19. A

20. C
21. D
22. A
23. D
24. D
25. D
26. B
27. B
28. B
29. B
30. A
31. D
32. C
33. C
34. B
35. D
36. C
37. C
38. D
39. B
40. A
41. C
42. A
43. A
44. B
45. D
46. C
47. A
48. C
49. D
50. B

Chapter 6

1. C
2. B
3. A
4. B
5. D
6. B
7. C
8. D
9. D
10. C
11. B
12. B
13. B
14. A

Chapter 7

1. A
2. D
3. D
4. D
5. C
6. D
7. B
8. C
9. A
10. B

Chapter 8

1. C
2. D
3. C
4. C
5. C
6. D
7. C
8. C
9. C
10. C

Chapter 9

1. B
2. D
3. B
4. D
5. C
6. A
7. E
8. E
9. E
10. D

Chapter 10

1. C
2. A
3. D
4. A
5. A
6. C
7. B
8. B
9. D
10. C

Chapter 11

1. D
2. B
3. A
4. A
5. C
6. C
7. D
8. A
9. C
10. B

Chapter 12

1. E
2. E
3. E
4. E
5. E
6. A
7. E
8. B
9. B
10. C

Chapter 13

1. A
2. A
3. C
4. B
5. B
6. B
7. D
8. B
9. A
10. A
11. C
12. C
13. A
14. D
15. C
16. E
17. E
18. A
19. D
20. D

Chapter 14

1. E
2. B
3. D
4. C
5. D
6. A
7. D
8. C
9. A
10. D

Chapter 15

1. D
2. D
3. B
4. A
5. B
6. E
7. B
8. A
9. E
10. C

Chapter 16

1. C
2. B
3. A
4. B
5. A
6. D
7. A
8. D
9. C
10. B
11. C
12. B
13. A
14. C
15. D

Chapter 17

1. B
2. B
3. D
4. D
5. C
6. A
7. B
8. D
9. B
10. C
11. D
12. B
13. D
14. B
15. C
15. C
17. D
18. G
19. J
20. I
21. E
22. A
23. H
24. B
25. F

Chapter 18

1. C
2. A
3. B
4. B
5. B
6. C
7. E
8. C
9. C
10. A

Chapter 19

1. D
2. C
3. A
4. E
5. C
6. E
7. B
8. B
9. C
10. E

Chapter 20

1. D
2. B
3. D
4. B
5. B
6. A
7. E
8. A
9. D
10. B

Chapter 21

1. E
2. A
3. A
4. A
5. C
6. A
7. B
8. A
9. B
10. E